ANXIETY DISORDERS IN ADULTS

Anxiety Disorders in Adults

A Clinical Guide

Second Edition

Vladan Starcevic, MD, PhD, FRANCP

Associate Professor, Discipline of Psychological Medicine
University of Sydney Faculty of Medicine
Head and Senior Staff
Specialist Psychiatrist
Academic Department of Psychological Medicine
Nepean Hospital, NSW
Australia

OXFORD
UNIVERSITY PRESS
2010

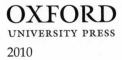

616.8522
5795a

OXFORD
UNIVERSITY PRESS

Oxford University Press, Inc., publishes works that further
Oxford University's objective of excellence
in research, scholarship, and education.

Oxford   New York
Auckland   Cape Town   Dar es Salaam   Hong Kong   Karachi
Kuala Lumpur   Madrid   Melbourne   Mexico City   Nairobi
New Delhi   Shanghai   Taipei   Toronto

With offices in
Argentina   Austria   Brazil   Chile   Czech Republic   France   Greece
Guatemala   Hungary   Italy   Japan   Poland   Portugal   Singapore
South Korea   Switzerland   Thailand   Turkey   Ukraine   Vietnam

Published by Oxford University Press, Inc.
198 Madison Avenue, New York, New York 10016

www.oup.com

Library of Congress Cataloging-in-Publication Data
Starcevic, Vladan.
   Anxiety disorders in adults : a clinical guide / by Vladan Starcevic. — 2nd ed.
      p.   ;   cm.
   Includes bibliographical references and index.
   ISBN 978-0-19-536925-0
   1. Anxiety.   2. Phobias.   I. Title.
   [DNLM: 1. Anxiety Disorders—psychology.
   2. Anxiety Disorders—therapy. WM 172 S795a 2010]
   RC531.S687 2010
   616.85′22—dc22

                                                                            2009008808

9 8 7 6 5 4 3 2 1

Printed in the United States of America
on acid-free paper

To KK, for patience and understanding

Acknowledgments

This book is a product of many years of clinical work, research, and collaboration with colleagues. Although it is difficult to single out among many people who have been influential, helpful, and supportive in my professional endeavors, I believe that I will do no injustice by mentioning Professor Eberhard H. Uhlenhuth and Professor Ljubomir Eric. Professor Uhlenhuth (Uhli) has been a dedicated mentor and a reliable friend; he has been consistently supportive, providing me with invaluable feedback and guidance when I needed it most. Professor Eric is "responsible" for sparking my interest in anxiety disorders and for showing me different roads that can be traveled to approach the subject of this book.

Preface to the Second Edition

More than four years have passed since the first publication of this book, arguably a lot of time in the life of a clinical guide containing much information that is subject to rapid change. Indeed, these four years have seen developments primarily in the realm of treatment of anxiety disorders and reconsideration of many conceptual issues in preparation for the next revision of the classification of mental disorders. This has suggested a need to update some information presented in the first edition of the book.

I was also prompted to consider another edition by the feedback I received from colleagues, other readers, and reviewers. I was encouraged by their endorsement of the book's practical and integrative approach. This has indicated to me that the book fulfills an unmet need and that making fundamental changes in its philosophy and general structure would be unnecessary. At the same time, I seriously took on board suggestions to give the book a more recognizable "personal touch" and enrich it with my "critical voice." With all this in mind, I set out to prepare the Second Edition.

The product of this endeavor is now in front of the reader. The main aims of the Second Edition have been to provide an update of the First Edition and broaden the scope of the book without a substantial increase in its size. With regard to the first aim, the reader will find main changes in the sections on treatment within each chapter. These sections have been thoroughly revised, especially discussion of the pharmacological and combined treatments. Sections on the epidemiology and etiology and pathogenesis have also been significantly updated to reflect new information and advances in these areas. Of course, there are also updates in other parts of the book, but they are not substantial.

Two sections have been added to each chapter on individual anxiety disorders to broaden the perspective. "Key Issues" now appear at the beginning of every chapter, with the purpose of providing a summary of the problems, "hot topics," and controversies associated with each anxiety disorder. "Outlook for the Future" appears at the end of six chapters, with a brief critical overview of further challenges and expectations for each anxiety disorder. "Key Issues" sets the stage for each anxiety disorder by pointing, especially to the more inquisitive readers, what to look for in the chapter, whereas "Outlook for the Future" provides a coda.

To further strengthen the emphasis on contention and controversy, I have provided a closer look at the main arguments and debates in the section "Diagnostic and Conceptual Issues" of each chapter. In addition to trying to find the right balance here, I had to keep this section relatively brief. This is to avoid being drawn into the details of various debates, as that would not be in accordance with the purpose of the book.

With the changes that I have outlined, I hope *Anxiety Disorders in Adults: A Clinical Guide* will remain a practical state-of-the-art reference work on the anxiety disorders. It builds on its key strengths and adds perspectives that will hopefully appeal not only to clinicians of different theoretical orientations and professional backgrounds, but also to a wider audience.

January 2009
Sydney, Australia   *V.S.*

Preface to the First Edition

Anxiety disorders are common in clinical practice. They often run a chronic course and have an adverse, though often overlooked, impact on the quality of life. Anxiety disorders often co-occur with other psychiatric conditions. This further complicates their course and treatment and leads to greater disability. Despite advances in their diagnosis and treatment, the recognition of anxiety disorders is still unsatisfactory, and many sufferers remain untreated. Others are not treated adequately, respond only partially to treatment, or are treatment resistant.

Although there has been much interest in the anxiety disorders as well as intense research activity over the last two decades, many issues remain unresolved, particularly in the area of etiology and pathogenesis. Also, the abundance of information and data on the treatment of anxiety disorders often produces conflicting effects, sometimes leaving therapists puzzled as to what treatment approach to use with a particular patient and in a given clinical situation.

This book was conceived mainly out of practical need to present the anxiety disorders as they occur and as they are treated in the "real world." That is, the main purpose of the book is to contribute in a practical way to both understanding and treatment of people with anxiety disorders. The book has been guided by clinical relevance of the problems that it addresses, regardless of whether these problems are of a conceptual and theoretical nature or pertain more to etiological and treatment issues. The book attempts to fill the gap between the textbook-like comprehensiveness and ultrapractical, reductionistic approach of some clinical and treatment guides.

The book is organized around the six main categories of anxiety disorders: panic disorder (with and without agoraphobia), generalized anxiety disorder, social anxiety disorder (social phobia), specific phobias, obsessive-compulsive disorder, and posttraumatic stress disorder. Each of these disorders is presented in a separate chapter, following a uniform style.

Thus, each chapter has sections on clinical features of the disorder, the relationship between that disorder and other conditions, assessment (which includes diagnostic issues, assessment instruments, and differential diagnosis), epidemiology, course and prognosis, etiology and pathogenesis, and treatment.

The emphasis of the book is on the phenomenology, etiology, and treatment of anxiety disorders, using a practical approach with frequent reference to clinical examples and scenarios. Thus, clinical features of each disorder are described in some detail, as the knowledge of these features is crucial for recognition and understanding of the underlying psychopathology. Each chapter also presents the most important models of etiology and pathogenesis, which serve as the basis for treatment of the corresponding disorders. Finally, main types of pharmacological and psychological treatment are described in a manner that clinicians will find useful, as the book contains practical tips, description of the relevant therapeutic procedures, and treatment guidelines for use in commonly encountered clinical situations.

The book does not "favor" any type of etiological explanation and treatment, but emphasizes models that have a heuristic and practical value and treatments whose usefulness has been demonstrated. The etiological models and treatments are presented critically, so that the reader can appreciate both their strengths and weaknesses. The book is a project that balances and integrates what is currently known about anxiety disorders and their treatment.

While the treatment approaches are presented mainly from an evidence-based (efficacy) perspective, the book also takes into account various treatment goals for patients, available resources, and applicability of the evidence-based treatments to real-life and complex clinical situations (effectiveness perspective). I acknowledge that I have been influenced by movements toward integration within psychological treatments and between pharmacotherapy and psychotherapy. Combined treatments are presented, however, with due consideration of the unresolved issues and caution about their unsatisfactory empirical status.

The book will be most useful to a professional audience, which includes psychiatrists, clinical psychologists, other mental health workers, primary care physicians, other medical specialists, and physicians-in-training. The book may also be of interest to students of medicine and psychology and to a general audience, particularly individuals interested in anxiety and those suffering from anxiety disorders.

Practicing clinicians will benefit from the multifaceted approach to conceptual issues and from practical treatment suggestions that will guide them in their clinical work. Indeed, the important aims of the book are to help clinicians make everyday clinical decisions about diagnosis and treatment and tailor their treatment approaches to the specific needs and characteristics of patients with various anxiety disorders. This is accomplished by describing not only what to do in treatment but also how to do it.

As the book is put to the test before its readers, I hope that it will help clarify some of the salient issues surrounding the anxiety disorders and help the readers feel better equipped to deal with the various challenges posed by anxiety disorders, without sacrificing appreciation of the complexity of these conditions.

Sydney, Australia   *V.S.*

Contents

ANXIETY DISORDERS IN ADULTS

1

Anxiety Disorders: Introduction

Anxiety disorders can be defined as conditions characterized by pathological anxiety that has not been caused by physical illness, is not associated
with substance use, and is not part of a psychotic illness. Therefore, the
concept of anxiety disorders is largely based on exclusion of several causes
of pathological anxiety—hardly a scientifically defensible position. Since
pathological anxiety has been postulated as the sine qua non of anxiety
disorders, it is important to first make a distinction between pathological
and "normal" anxiety. For the sake of clarifying this matter, the terms
anxiety and *fear* are used here interchangeably (as they both denote a
response to a perceived threat), although there is also a prominent view
that conceptual differences do exist between them (see also Table 2–21 and
Barlow's account of panic attacks in Chapter 2 for further discussion of
this issue).

There is broad agreement that pathological and normal anxiety can be
distinguished on the basis of the criteria listed in Table 1–1. These criteria
cut across all the components of anxiety: subjective, physiological
(somatic), cognitive, and behavioral. Although the criteria may seem
clear-cut, in practice it may be difficult to draw a precise boundary between
pathological and normal anxiety.

It is often assumed that normal anxiety has an adaptive role,
because it serves as a signal that there is some danger and that
measures need to be taken (e.g., a fight or flight response) to protect
oneself against that danger; both the danger perceived and the measures taken are considered appropriate (i.e., not exaggerated) in normal
anxiety. For example, a student who is anxious about failing the exam
correctly judges herself to be well below the sufficient level of knowledge and doubles the effort to catch up with her studies and minimize
the risk of failing. In contrast, pathological anxiety pertains to an
inaccurate or excessive appraisal of danger; protective measures taken
against this danger are way out of proportion to the real threat.

Table 1–1. Pathological Anxiety vs. Normal Anxiety

Criteria for Differentiation	Pathological Anxiety	Normal Anxiety
Intensity	Relatively high and/or out of proportion to the situation or circumstances	Relatively low and/or proportionate to the situation or circumstances
Duration	Generally longer lasting or recurrent	Generally shorter lasting
Preoccupation with anxiety	Yes	No
Quality of the experience	Distressing, overwhelming, incapacitating	Unpleasant, but not too distressing or not distressing for a long time
Effects on behavior and functioning	Causes long-standing changes in behavior, impairs functioning	Generally does not affect behavior more than temporarily, does not impair functioning

CONCEPTUALIZATION AND CLASSIFICATION

Anxiety disorders were introduced in 1980 as a distinct nosological group in the Third Edition of the *Diagnostic and Statistical Manual of Mental Disorders* (*DSM-III*; American Psychiatric Association, 1980). Before *DSM-III*, anxiety disorders were conceptualized as neuroses, and they encompassed four conditions: *(1)* anxiety neurosis, *(2)* phobic neurosis, *(3)* obsessive-compulsive neurosis, and *(4)* traumatic (or compensation) neurosis. In *DSM-III*, anxiety neurosis was divided into panic disorder and generalized anxiety disorder, whereas phobic disorder was split into agoraphobia, social phobia (social anxiety disorder), and simple (specific) phobia. Obsessive-compulsive neurosis became obsessive-compulsive disorder, and traumatic neurosis was largely transformed into a posttraumatic stress disorder. In the revision of *DSM-III*, *DSM-III-R* (American Psychiatric Association, 1987), agoraphobia was moved to the realm of panic disorder, in recognition of the close relationship between the two.

Anxiety disorders were retained as a distinct nosological group in the Fourth Edition, *DSM-IV* (American Psychiatric Association, 1994) and Text Revision of *DSM-IV*, *DSM-IV-TR* (American Psychiatric Association, 2000). The conceptualization and diagnostic criteria for all psychopathological entities within anxiety disorders underwent changes from *DSM-III* to *DSM-IV-TR*; the most important of these changes are presented in the chapters on individual disorders below. In *DSM-IV-TR*, the

Table 1–2. Disorders Included in the Group of Anxiety Disorders in *DSM-IV-TR*

Panic disorder without agoraphobia

Panic disorder with agoraphobia

Agoraphobia without history of panic disorder

Generalized anxiety disorder

Social anxiety disorder (social phobia)

Specific phobia

Obsessive-compulsive disorder

Acute stress disorder

Posttraumatic stress disorder

Anxiety disorder due to a general medical condition

Substance-induced anxiety disorder

Anxiety disorder not otherwise specified

group of anxiety disorders includes the following diagnostic entities (Table 1–2): panic disorder (with and without agoraphobia), agoraphobia without history of panic disorder, generalized anxiety disorder, social anxiety disorder (social phobia), specific phobia, obsessive-compulsive disorder, acute stress disorder, posttraumatic stress disorder, anxiety disorder due to a general medical condition, substance-induced anxiety disorder, and anxiety disorder not otherwise specified.

Of these conditions, anxiety disorder due to a general medical condition and substance-induced anxiety disorder do not "belong" in the group of anxiety disorders as they are defined more restrictively in this volume. Likewise, these two disorders have a dual status in *DSM-IV-TR*, because substance-induced anxiety disorder has also been classified among substance-related disorders, while anxiety disorder due to a general medical condition has also been classified among mental disorders due to general medical conditions. "Anxiety disorder not otherwise specified" is a residual diagnostic category, for use in those situations when a diagnosis of the specific anxiety disorder cannot be made.

In the latest version of the *International Classification of Diseases* (ICD-10; World Health Organization, 1992), anxiety disorders have not been granted a separate, independent status. Instead, they are a part of a large group of disorders labeled "neurotic, stress-related and somatoform disorders." Within such a group, anxiety disorders encountered in the *DSM* system are placed in four subgroups that resemble the pre-*DSM-III* classification (see Table 1–3). For most anxiety disorders, there are important differences between the way they are conceptualized and diagnosed in the *DSM* and *ICD* systems, and these differences are presented and discussed in the

Table 1–3. Classification of Anxiety Disorders in *ICD-10* [a]

Phobic Anxiety Disorders

Agoraphobia without panic disorder
Agoraphobia with panic disorder
Social phobias
Specific (isolated) phobias

Other Anxiety Disorders

Panic disorder (episodic paroxysmal anxiety)
Generalized anxiety disorder
Mixed anxiety and depressive disorder

Obsessive-Compulsive Disorder

Reaction to Severe Stress and Adjustment Disorders

Acute stress reaction
Posttraumatic stress disorder
Adjustment disorders

[a] "Other" and "unspecified" diagnostic categories are excluded from this table, as are the subtypes of obsessive-compulsive disorder and adjustment disorders.

chapters on individual disorders that follow. In addition, *ICD-10* has included with anxiety and related disorders conditions that are not present in the *DSM* system (e.g., mixed anxiety and depressive disorder) and conditions that are in the *DSM* system but classified elsewhere (e.g., adjustment disorders).

Conceptual, Diagnostic, and Classification Issues

Regardless of whether the *DSM* or *ICD* conceptualization and classification are adopted, the classification overhauls of anxiety disorders over the last several decades have resulted in splitting the four pre-*DSM-III* diagnostic entities into a large number of diagnostic categories. Moreover, the diagnostic categories within anxiety disorders have undergone further splitting, so that almost all the categories now have two or more subtypes. The upshot of this trend is a high likelihood for various anxiety disorders and their subtypes to co-occur. Therefore, high rates of co-occurrence among the anxiety disorders—or "comorbidity," as this phenomenon is often referred to—are not surprising. The rarity of pure cases of most anxiety disorders in clinical practice is a logical consequence of this situation. More often than not, however, the high rates of comorbidity do not reflect a genuine co-occurrence of independent disorders but rather are likely to represent an artifact of the splitting trends in classification and a consequence of a substantial overlap between the putatively separate disorders.

The creation of so many categories of anxiety disorders has seen challenges to their presumed distinctness and doubts about their validity. There have been calls to halt the proliferation of diagnostic categories and look more for what the individual anxiety disorders share than for the ways in which they differ. A longitudinal approach to the conceptualization of the anxiety disorders has been proposed (Starcevic, 2007, 2008), with the main underlying idea that most anxiety disorders (except for obsessive-compulsive disorder and posttraumatic stress disorder) are a consequence of a single diathesis, which only changes the way it expresses itself over time (Figure 1–1). Furthermore, the cross-sectional and temporal links between anxiety disorders, depression, somatoform disorders, and some personality disorders have been emphasized through the overarching concepts such as "general neurotic syndrome" (Tyrer, 1985; Tyrer et al., 1992). These attempts at "lumping" and integration have yet to be taken seriously by the architects of the major classification systems.

Anxiety disorders are grouped together on the basis of the assumption that pathological anxiety is their common, defining characteristic. But it is not clear that this is the case with all the disorders that are included in the *DSM-IV-TR* group of anxiety disorders, as emotions other than anxiety (fear) may be a predominant manifestation of some anxiety disorders. These include disgust, irritability, dysphoria, anger, shame, and guilt. Also, it has been argued, for example, that posttraumatic stress disorder is as much a disorder of memory, a dissociative disorder, or even a condition that should be placed in its "own" class of trauma-related disorders as it is an anxiety disorder (see Chapter 7). By contrast, some conditions that are not regarded as anxiety disorders in *DSM-IV-TR* (e.g., anxiety-related

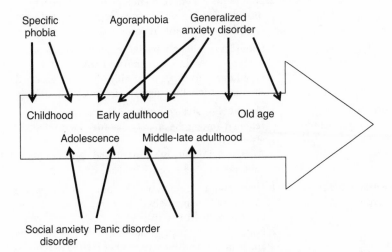

Figure 1–1. Longitudinal, "lumping" conceptualization of the anxiety disorders based on their usual sequence of occurrence (age of onset).

forms of hypochondriasis increasingly referred to as "health anxiety disorder" and personality disturbance such as avoidant personality disorder) have been considered for inclusion among the anxiety disorders. The conceptual and diagnostic dilemmas about specific anxiety disorders are summarized in Table 1–4 and discussed below with regard to individual disorders.

Table 1–4. Some of the Conceptual and Diagnostic Dilemmas About Specific Anxiety Disorders

Disorders	Dilemmas
Panic disorder	1. How useful is the conceptualization of the different types of panic attacks? 2. Should panic disorder have a diagnostic primacy over agoraphobia when both are present? Should agoraphobia be an entity in its own right or is it merely a subtype of panic disorder?
Generalized anxiety disorder	1. Is generalized anxiety disorder a diagnosis in search of its unique psychopathology? What combination of features of generalized anxiety disorder would ensure that it is better recognized in clinical practice? 2. Does generalized anxiety disorder really exist in the absence of depression or other anxiety disorders?
Social anxiety disorder	1. Where should the boundary be drawn between the "normal" social anxiety (shyness) and social anxiety disorder 2. Should the generalized subtype of social anxiety disorder be conceptualized as personality disturbance (avoidant personality disorder)?
Specific phobia	1. Should a specific phobia be split into its current subtypes, as separate diagnostic entities? 2. Should various types of specific phobia be grouped on the basis of whether they are driven by fear or disgust?
Obsessive-compulsive disorder	1. Should obsessive-compulsive disorder be retained among the anxiety disorders or be classified elsewhere? 2. Are there clinically meaningful and conceptually valid subtypes of obsessive-compulsive disorder?
Posttraumatic stress disorder	1. How should a trauma be conceptualized and is there a causal relationship between the trauma and posttraumatic stress disorder? 2. Is the syndrome of posttraumatic stress disorder unique, and how does it differ from other related psychiatric disorders?

ETIOLOGICAL MODELS

The etiological understanding of the anxiety disorders continues to be fragmented, as it is split into biological and psychological models. There is an increasing need, however, to combine the contributions of these models in an effort to arrive at a more comprehensive understanding of the etiology and pathogenesis of anxiety disorders.

Regardless of the preferred model, conceptualizing the predisposing, precipitating, and maintaining factors can afford better etiological understanding of the anxiety disorders. Also, this is where the main differences between various etiological models can be found: for example, biological models postulate that people are predisposed to develop anxiety disorders because of their genetic makeup, while psychological models find this predisposition in early childhood events, in certain personality features, or in the way that the symptoms are perceived and appraised. Whatever the nature of the predisposition, it is "dormant" until the precipitating factors—usually certain life events—activate this predisposition, bringing about a disorder. The factors that maintain anxiety disorders are particularly emphasized in behavioral and cognitive models, and these factors are targeted accordingly by the behavioral and cognitive therapies.

No biological mechanism has proved to be unique for any particular type of anxiety disorder, although some mechanisms may be relatively more specific for some anxiety disorders. In addition, various biological mechanisms may operate in the same anxiety disorder.

Several types of studies have examined the role of genetic factors in the etiology of anxiety disorders. They include family studies (studies of the first-degree relatives of probands with a particular anxiety disorder), twin studies, and genetic linkage studies. Family studies have been most commonly conducted, with findings of increased rates of specific anxiety disorders in first-degree relatives of probands with the same anxiety disorders being interpreted as a sign of possible genetic transmission. Such findings may also reflect influence of the shared environment on family members. Genetic studies generally suggest that there may be a genetic predisposition for some anxiety disorders in certain patients. It is not known, however, what this predisposition entails and what is inherited.

Studies of the neurotransmitter systems in anxiety disorders have largely been propelled by the efficacy of medications that act via the corresponding transmitters. Since several types of medications have been efficacious in several types of anxiety disorders, it is not surprising that many findings suggestive of specific neurotransmitter abnormalities are, in fact, nonspecific for any particular type of anxiety disorder. The only exception to this may be a relative specificity of the serotonin system abnormalities in obsessive-compulsive disorder. It is not clear whether some of the neurotransmitter abnormalities precede the onset of anxiety disorders, whether they are a consequence or a correlate of these disorders, or whether they are more associated with conditions that co-occur with particular anxiety disorders.

The psychological models of anxiety disorders that are most relevant for clinical practice include behavioral, cognitive, and psychodynamic approaches. Behavioral models are based on the learning theory. They provide an account of the acquisition of fear via conditioning and emphasize the crucial role of behaviors such as avoidance in maintaining anxiety disorders. The latter explains the focus on behavior modification in behavior therapy. Behavioral models are often criticized as simplistic, but behavior therapy has been the most successful psychological treatment across all the anxiety disorders, and its techniques should be given serious consideration for inclusion into any pragmatic treatment package.

Cognitive models of anxiety disorders emphasize the role of specific beliefs and appraisals of threat and of one's ability to cope. These models have become popular, perhaps because they attempt to give a fairly comprehensive account of anxiety disorders and seem credible in doing so. However, cognitive models have generally been less subjected to scientific scrutiny than the behavioral ones, and the treatment based on them has yet to demonstrate whether it is as effective as behavior therapy. The attractiveness of cognitive models—and cognitive therapy—also lies in their radical dismantling of the psychological mechanisms in anxiety disorders and in their proposition that therapeutic change should occur as a result of changes in the more fundamental patterns of thinking. At the same time, this ambitious proposition may be the reason that cognitive therapy seems less pragmatic and perhaps less applicable to *all* patients with anxiety disorders.

The psychodynamic models of anxiety disorders invoke several concepts that are now often considered controversial, if not untenable or outdated. These models are nonetheless reasonably well placed within the general psychodynamic theory. The main general aspect of psychodynamic models is the proposition that "neurotic" anxiety occurs as a result of intrapsychic conflicts between sexual or aggressive urges and defenses erected against these urges—and, more broadly, that such anxiety signals the existence of certain unconscious processes or phenomena. Therefore, the goals of psychodynamic treatment are an acquisition of insight into these unconscious conflicts and their resolution, which "releases" the person from anxiety. The efficacy of psychodynamic psychotherapy for anxiety disorders has barely been studied, but it is certainly not the type of treatment that should be or could be routinely offered to patients with these conditions.

TREATMENT

With current emphasis on evidence-based treatments in psychiatry, clinicians are in a better position to administer treatments that are likely to work. The reality of clinical practice, however, calls for treatment of patients who do not easily match patients on whom various evidence-based treatment guidelines and algorithms are based. The latter usually come from research or highly specialized settings in which randomized, controlled trials have been conducted, and they may have relatively "pure" and uncomplicated forms of psychopathology and are not necessarily representative of patients in the real world. Thus, we have a somewhat paradoxical situation: although there are many evidence-based treatment guidelines and algorithms for anxiety disorders, ordinary clinicians are often puzzled as to how to apply them to individual patients or do not apply them at all. Part of the reason that treatment guidelines and algorithms are difficult to implement is their frequent failure to take into account different treatment goals for different patients. That is, treatment guidelines and algorithms often assume that all patients have the same treatment goals. Because different treatment goals usually imply a need for different treatment approaches, it is reasonable to first agree on treatment goals and then consider various treatment options for achieving these goals.

Treatment goals for anxiety disorders should be openly discussed with patients and patients should be encouraged to formulate their own goals. Treatment goals may be expressed in many different ways. Typical patient statements, which reflect diverse expectations, are "controlling my anxiety," "getting rid of it," "not having to avoid things," or "wanting my normal life back." Some of these expectations may be rather unrealistic (e.g., "never again feeling anxious," "having full control over my life," "completely eliminating my anxiety") and when these are identified, it is important to point out to patients that such expectations cannot serve as the basis for formulating treatment goals. Actively engaging patients in formulating their treatment goals and in the treatment decision-making process is fundamental, because the responsibility for the course and outcome of treatment should be shared between patients and therapists. This is the foundation for *collaborative negotiation* between patients and therapists in the treatment process.

All treatment goals for anxiety disorders ultimately pertain to reducing the negative impact of anxiety. The disagreements, particularly among therapists, pertain mainly to how the negative impact of anxiety is to be reduced. Whereas some clinicians prefer to achieve this by suppressing the symptoms of anxiety with a medication, others use different strategies (Figure 1–2).

Different treatment goals are not mutually exclusive, especially at different stages of treatment. For example, a patient may initially request quick relief of anxiety and the associated physical symptoms, whereas later he or she may want to be free from the fear of anxiety and its symptoms. By the same token, treatment strategies used to achieve these goals are not inherently incompatible, hence a rationale for the sequential or simultaneous use of both pharmacotherapy and cognitive-behavioral therapy.

A. Where do various therapists and patients agree?

Reducing the negative impact of anxiety as the goal of treatment

B. Where is the disagreement about treatment goals?

How to go about reducing the negative impact of anxiety?

1. By suppressing/controlling the symptoms of anxiety

Pharmacotherapy

2. By controlling the symptoms of anxiety and/or eliminating behaviors that maintain anxiety disorders, such as avoidance

Behavior therapy

- Anxiety management techniques (e.g., relaxation, breathing retraining) to control the symptoms

- Exposure-based therapy to eliminate avoidance

3. By normalizing the assumptions, beliefs, and appraisals that contribute to the development of anxiety disorders or maintain them

Cognitive therapy

4. By uncovering and resolving the underlying intrapsychic conflicts and making the corresponding personality-level changes

Psychodynamic psychotherapy

Figure 1–2. Treatment goals for anxiety disorders and treatments used to achieve these goals.

Pharmacotherapy or Psychological Therapy? Or Both?

Ideological battles about the efficacy and usefulness of various treatments in anxiety disorders are still vehemently fought. The profession is no longer divided over the value of psychoanalysis and psychodynamic psychotherapy, as these forms of psychological therapy are not generally regarded as first-line treatment for anxiety disorders. The focus has now shifted to pharmacotherapy and cognitive-behavioral therapy, with their relative advantages and disadvantages often being bitterly debated. For example, an anonymous biological psychiatrist, cited in van Dyck and van Balkom (1997), had this to say about cognitive-behavioral therapy: "Exposure is not a real therapy, but the acquisition of a stoic attitude toward symptoms.... Cognitive therapy [is] a form of indoctrination" (p. 112). Tyrer (1999), in contrast, has made the following statement about the pharmacotherapy of anxiety disorders: "All new drug treatments of anxiety should be regarded as addictive until proved otherwise" (p. 117).

Such views not only fail to promote a dialogue between mental health professionals but also impede progress in our efforts to develop more effective treatments. Offering patients one type of treatment while denigrating the other does not take into consideration what particular patients need and therefore does not reflect a genuine intent to help; rather, such an attitude reflects the therapist's allegiance to a group within which beliefs about etiology and treatment are shared.

A well-balanced, nondogmatic approach to the choice of treatment of anxiety disorders involves matching treatment goals with treatment modalities (Figure 1–2). In addition, the clinician should take into consideration short-term and long-term treatment effects. Pharmacotherapy usually produces therapeutic effects faster than cognitive-behavioral therapy, it is easier to administer, and it is more widely available. But medications usually work in anxiety disorders only for as long as they are taken, and relapse rates following their discontinuation tend to be high. Cognitive-behavioral therapy generally takes longer to work; it is also more demanding and less available than pharmacotherapy. Its main advantage, however, is a greater likelihood of producing long-lasting treatment effects that tend to persist after the cessation of treatment, with relatively low relapse rates.

Since most patients with anxiety disorders usually want a relatively quick relief of their anxiety and distress, as well as long-term benefit of the therapy, ideal treatments should be able to produce both short-term and long-term therapeutic effects. In reality, such treatments rarely exist, and the two main treatment options may be offered initially on the basis of the patient's need, or lack thereof, to have anxiety or distress quickly alleviated (Figure 1–3). Thus, if the patient cannot tolerate anxiety or distress, the usual initial choice of treatment is pharmacotherapy; if the patient is able to tolerate anxiety or distress, cognitive-behavioral therapy may be offered from the beginning of treatment. Later in the course of treatment, these initial choices may be modified depending on the patient's response, but also on the basis of the patient's needs and preferences (Figure 1–3). The issues arising from combining pharmacotherapy and cognitive-behavioral therapy are addressed in more detail in Chapter 2.

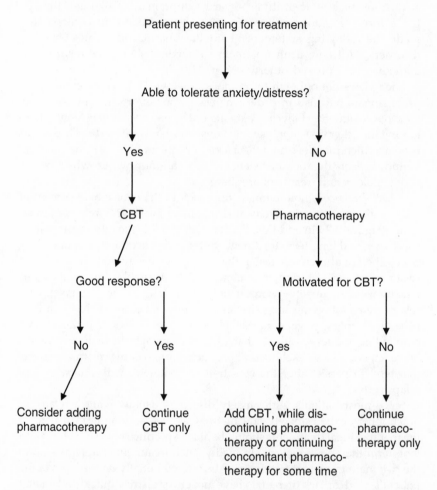

Figure 1–3. Initial and subsequent choice of treatment in anxiety disorders (simplified). CBT, cognitive-behavioral therapy.

Table 1–5. Factors that Affect Treatment Choice in Anxiety Disorders

Treatment-Related Factors

- Well-established efficacy (short-term efficacy: no advantage for pharmacotherapy or CBT, or may favor pharmacotherapy; long-term efficacy: generally favors CBT)
- Faster onset of therapeutic effects (favors pharmacotherapy)
- General ease of administration (favors pharmacotherapy)
- Wide availability (favors pharmacotherapy)
- Relatively low cost (may slightly favor pharmacotherapy; in the long run, this advantage may be lost to CBT)

Disorder-Related Factors

- Greater overall severity of the disorder (the more severe the disorder is, the more likely it is for pharmacotherapy to be used)
- Greater disability caused by the disorder (the more disabled patients are, the more likely it is for pharmacotherapy to be used)
- Presence of other disorders, especially depression (generally favors pharmacotherapy)

Patient-Related Factors

- Specific needs of patients, which determine treatment goals (pharmacotherapy or CBT may be preferred, depending on patient needs and treatment goals)
- Ability to tolerate symptoms, anxiety, and distress (the greater this ability is, the more likely it is for CBT to be used)
- Ability to withstand treatment-associated discomfort (e.g., side effects of medications or deliberate induction of anxiety in the course of CBT)
- Specific attitudes toward medications and psychological treatment (pharmacotherapy or CBT may be preferred, depending on the nature of these attitudes)
- Motivation, "psychological-mindedness," ambitiousness of treatment goals (the greater these are, the more likely it is for CBT to be used)

Clinician-Related Factors

- Clinician's preferences for or bias against pharmacotherapy or CBT
- Degree of familiarity with pharmacotherapy or CBT

CBT, cognitive-behavioral therapy.

In clinical practice, it is usually a combination of factors that is taken into account when treatment decisions are made; these factors and their impact are presented in Table 1–5.

2

Panic Disorder With and Without Agoraphobia

Panic disorder is characterized by two components: recurrent panic attacks and anticipatory anxiety. Panic attacks within panic disorder are not caused by physical illness or certain substances and they are unexpected, at least initially; later in the course of the disorder, many attacks may be precipitated by certain situations or are more likely to occur in them. Anticipatory anxiety is an intense fear of having another panic attack, which is present between panic attacks. Some patients with panic disorder go on to develop agoraphobia, usually defined as fear and/or avoidance of the situations from which escape might be difficult or embarrassing or in which help might not be available in case of a panic attack; in such cases, patients are diagnosed with panic disorder with agoraphobia. Those who do not develop agoraphobia receive a diagnosis of panic disorder without agoraphobia. Components of panic disorder are presented in Figure 2–1.

Patients with agoraphobia who have no history of panic disorder or whose agoraphobia is not related at least to panic attacks or symptoms of panic attacks are relatively rarely encountered in clinical practice. The diagnosis of agoraphobia without history of panic disorder has been a matter of some controversy, especially in view of the differences between American and European psychiatrists (and the *DSM* and *ICD* diagnostic and classification systems) in the conceptualization of the relationship between panic disorder and agoraphobia. The conceptualization adhered to here has for the most part been derived from the *DSM* system, as there is more empirical support for it.

KEY ISSUES

Although panic disorder (with and without agoraphobia) is a relatively well-defined psychopathological entity whose treatment is generally rewarding, there are important, unresolved issues. They are listed below and discussed throughout this chapter.

1. Are there different types of panic attacks based on the absence or presence of the context in which they appear (i.e., unexpected vs. situational attacks)? Should the "subtyping" of panic attacks be based on other criteria (e.g., symptom profile)?
2. Because panic attacks are not specific for panic disorder, should they continue to be the main feature of panic disorder? Can panic attacks occurring as part of panic disorder be reliably distinguished from panic attacks occurring as part of other disorders or in the absence of any psychopathology?
3. What is the relationship between panic attacks, panic disorder, and agoraphobia?
4. How can findings of an increased risk of suicidal ideation, suicide attempts, and suicide in people with panic disorder be explained?
5. What accounts for the link between panic disorder and increased cardiovascular morbidity and mortality? What are the clinical implications of this link?
6. In view of its association with increased suicide rates and cardiovascular morbidity and mortality, should panic disorder be regarded as a much more serious condition than it is usually assumed to be? And if so, should more efforts be made to target prevention of panic disorder and its early treatment?
7. Considering that several biological mechanisms have been implicated in the pathogenesis of panic attacks, are there panic attacks that are completely pathophysiologically distinct or is there a final common pathophysiological pathway leading to panic attacks?

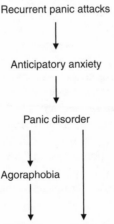

Figure 2–1. Components of panic disorder.

8. Is it realistic to expect that new drugs for use specifically in panic disorder will be developed? Or is it more likely that drugs that are broadly effective for depression and various anxiety disorders, including panic disorder, will continue to be used?

9. Does a dominant emphasis on easier access to and improved delivery of cognitive-behavioral therapy for panic disorder suggest that there is a general satisfaction with the effectiveness of cognitive-behavioral therapy?

10. How could pharmacotherapy and cognitive-behavioral therapy for panic disorder be combined in ways that would lead to better outcomes?

CLINICAL FEATURES

Panic Attacks

There is no universal description of a panic attack, because attacks differ in terms of their symptoms and how they are experienced. Panic attacks can nonetheless be defined as sudden episodes of severe anxiety that are characterized by physical symptoms and anticipation of dreadful consequences. The affected person typically believes that something horrific is about to happen and often has a tendency to escape right away, perhaps in an attempt to avert such a catastrophe. Panic attacks reach their peak very quickly—within 10 minutes according to *DSM-IV-TR*, but many patients report that attacks are most intense just a minute or two after the onset. There is greater variety in the duration of panic attacks, from several minutes to half an hour or an hour. After the attack, patients typically feel tired or exhausted. The frequency of panic attacks can vary greatly even in the same patient: from an occasional attack in months or years to more than 10–20 attacks a day.

Several features make panic attack a unique experience and not merely a more severe form of anxiety (Table 2–1). First, panic attacks occur abruptly and, at least initially, they are often described as "coming out of clear blue skies." Second, panic attacks reach the peak of their intensity very quickly. Third, panic attacks are characterized by prominent physical symptoms (e.g., heart racing or pounding, shortness of breath, dizziness), which often dominate the entire clinical presentation. Fourth, patients react to physical symptoms with a sense of an immediate catastrophe, as they believe that something terrible is going to happen to them because of their symptoms: they are going to die, lose control, or go mad. Fifth, there is a sense of urgency in the behavioral response to panic attacks; for example, patients have to escape immediately to a place perceived as safe. Sixth, panic attacks do not last very long—often 10–20 minutes—and only rarely is their duration longer than 1 hour; however, the duration of an attack may seem much longer to the sufferers.

The experience of a panic is usually puzzling and frightening, especially when it occurs for the first time. If there is nothing obvious in the person's

Table 2–1. Distinction Between Panic Attacks and Anxiety

Factor	Panic Attacks	Anxiety
Onset	Abrupt, sudden	More gradual
Reaching peak of the intensity of anxiety	Very quickly (maximum 10 minutes)	More slowly
Physical symptoms	Very prominent	Not necessarily prominent
Catastrophizing	Very typical and prominent, with a sense of immediacy	Lacking a sense of immediacy
Behavioral response	Immediate escape	Delayed escape, avoidance
Overall duration	Relatively short	Variable, but usually longer

life circumstances or current situation that might make it possible for him or her to understand the occurrence of a panic attack, as is often the case, the attack is experienced with even more bewilderment. The anxiety reaction precipitated by exposure to an objectively dangerous or life-threatening situation is usually not conceptualized as a panic attack, although it may have many characteristics of a panic attack.

It is intriguing to note not only what brings on panic attacks but also which mechanisms are involved in their cessation. Radomsky et al. (1998) have speculated that panic attacks cease because of physical exhaustion, which, in turn, is caused by autonomic hyperarousal. Some patients believe that they can terminate panic attacks by escaping from the situations in which attacks occur or by taking medications that act "very fast." But these are only examples of an illusion of having some control over the attacks. Patients may learn to abort panic attacks by slow breathing if hyperventilation is the main pathophysiological mechanism that triggers the attacks.

Types of Attacks

According to *DSM-IV-TR*, there are three types of panic attacks: unexpected, situationally predisposed, and situationally bound (Table 2–2).

Unexpected panic attacks occur "spontaneously," which means that the person does not associate their occurrence with any particular situation, object, or event. Of course, that does not mean that such attacks are never triggered by external influences; it is more likely that such influences are just not apparent to the person, and attacks are therefore experienced as occurring "for no reason." Unexpected attacks are typically seen in panic disorder without agoraphobia, especially during initial stages of the

Table 2–2. Types of Panic Attacks According to *DSM-IV-TR*

	Association With Particular Situations, Objects, or Events	Disorders in Which Type of Attacks Is Usually Seen
Unexpected	None	Panic disorder without agoraphobia
Situationally predisposed	Moderately strong (greater likelihood of the attacks occurring on exposure to certain situations, objects, or events)	Agoraphobia (panic disorder with agoraphobia) Less common in social anxiety disorder and specific phobias
Situationally bound	Very strong (attacks occur almost always and immediately on exposure to certain situations, objects, or events)	Social anxiety disorder and specific phobias May also be seen in agoraphobia (panic disorder with agoraphobia)

condition, before the patient has learned to expect panic attacks in certain situations.

Situationally predisposed panic attacks are more likely to occur in certain situations, but they do not occur every time the patient is in that situation; also, the attacks do not necessarily occur immediately upon exposure to that situation. For example, a patient may experience a panic attack after leaving home, but the occurrence of panic attacks cannot be reliably predicted by the patient being in that situation. Sometimes panic attacks do not occur at all, while at other times, they may occur hours after the patient has left home. This type of attack is characteristic of agoraphobia (and panic disorder with agoraphobia) but may also be seen among patients with social anxiety disorder and specific phobias.

Situationally bound panic attacks occur almost always and immediately upon exposure to a certain situation or object or while the patient is anticipating such an exposure. In other words, the exposure or anticipation of exposure almost invariably provokes a panic attack. For example, patients with a phobia of spiders have panic attacks upon seeing a spider or merely thinking that they are going to see a spider in certain situations. Situationally bound panic attacks are typical of social anxiety disorder and specific phobias but may also be seen in patients with agoraphobia.

Despite this three-way categorization, the usual distinction in clinical practice is that between unexpected and situational attacks. On phenomenological grounds, however, there is little if any, distinction. Some studies suggest that in comparison with other types of attacks, situationally bound panic attacks are characterized by fewer respiratory symptoms and less prominent fears of dying, losing control, or going crazy (e.g., Klein and Klein, 1989). The psychopathology and perhaps the pathogenesis of unexpected and situational panic attacks may differ significantly (Uhlenhuth et al., 2006); unlike situational attacks, unexpected attacks may be amenable to suppression by antidepressant medications (Uhlenhuth et al., 2000, 2002). Still, this categorization of panic attacks remains controversial (see Diagnostic and Conceptual Issues, below).

Physical Symptoms

Although the *DSM-IV-TR* diagnostic criteria stipulate that any combination of at least four symptoms is sufficient for the diagnosis of a panic attack, it appears that some physical symptoms are more frequent and more typical of panic attacks (Rapee et al., 1990a; Starcevic et al., 1993a; Cox et al., 1994b). Therefore, they could be termed "first-rank" panic symptoms (Table 2–3). These include heart racing (tachycardia) and pounding (palpitations), dizziness or lightheadedness, shortness of breath, choking sensations, chest discomfort or pain, sweating, and trembling. Of these first-rank symptoms, there are several (heart racing and pounding, dizziness or lightheadedness, shortness of breath, and choking sensations) that could be used for screening purposes. Patients in whom panic disorder is suspected should routinely be asked about these symptoms because at least one of them is likely to be present during a panic attack. Other physical symptoms are less common and less typical of a panic attack and could be considered "second-rank": hot and cold flushes, numbness or tingling sensations, and nausea or upset stomach.

There have been attempts to distinguish between respiratory and non-respiratory types of panic attacks on the basis of the presence or absence of

---

Table 2–3. Physical Symptoms During Panic Attacks

First-Rank Physical Symptoms, Also Useful for Screening Purposes

Heart racing (tachycardia) and pounding (palpitations)
Dizziness, lightheadedness, or fainting feeling
Shortness of breath
Choking sensations

Other First-Rank Physical Symptoms

Chest discomfort or pain
Sweating
Trembling

Second-Rank Physical Symptoms

Hot and cold flushes
Numbness or tingling sensations
Nausea or upset stomach

---

prominent respiratory symptoms (shortness of breath, choking sensations, hyperventilation) (Briggs et al., 1993; Biber and Alkin, 1999; Nardi et al., 2003, 2005; Abrams et al., 2006; Onur et al., 2007). Differences between these types of panic attacks have been reported in terms of the associated panic symptoms, degree of anxiety sensitivity, sensitivity to carbon dioxide, agoraphobic avoidance, family history of panic disorder, onset of illness, response to treatment, and other variables. Differences in treatment response were not consistent across the studies, as some authors reported that respiratory subtype responded better to imipramine (Briggs et al., 1993) whereas others found that the same subtype showed a faster response to clonazepam (Nardi et al., 2005). The practical utility of distinguishing between these types of panic attacks remains to be more firmly established.

Psychological Aspects

Although there are reports of nonfearful panic attacks, most patients describe panic attacks as being not only unpleasant but also frightening. Such an experience of panic is usually associated with an extremely negative, catastrophic appraisal of physical symptoms occurring during panic attacks. Broadly speaking, there are two types of catastrophes that panic patients anticipate (Table 2–4): one pertains to the physical consequences of an attack and the other to psychological and social consequences. As for physical consequences, patients are afraid that they might die suddenly (usually from a heart attack, stroke, or choking) or that they might collapse, lose consciousness, fall, and/or injure themselves.

The feared psychological and social consequences of panic attacks are reflected in frightening thoughts about losing control, going mad,

Table 2–4. Catastrophes Anticipated as a Consequence of Panic Attacks and Related Fears

Physical Consequences

Dying suddenly from

   Heart attack
   Stroke
   Choking

Collapsing, losing consciousness, falling, and/or injuring oneself

Psychological and Social Consequences

Losing control
Going mad
Appearing mentally ill
"Making a scene"
Embarrassing oneself

appearing mentally ill, "making a scene," and/or embarrassing oneself. Panic patients often feel that they do not know what they will be doing during the attack, that they might run aimlessly and "look crazy," that they might say something senseless, scream, or behave in an inappropriate or aggressive manner. Although these consequences of panic do not occur, this does not diminish patients' beliefs that "something dreadful" will happen. Patients often think that they were "lucky" in the past or that they did something to prevent the worst outcome but are certain that a catastrophe will occur next time.

Patients' ability to concentrate is often diminished during the attacks, and they may feel that they cannot plan or think rationally. This is true to a certain extent, as patients are typically immersed in the frightening experience and may have trouble focusing away from that experience and thinking clearly about other matters. However, their appraisal of their cognitive abilities is distorted in that they are much more able to act rationally than they think they are. In fact, the only "irrational act" to which patients may be prone during a panic attack is leaving suddenly or escaping; when they do that, it may seem somewhat unusual to others, but not "crazy," as patients often think.

Patients tend to feel that their panic experience sets them apart from others; they perceive panic as rather unique, unusual, and/or very difficult to describe. Patients often feel isolated because of panic and are surprised when they learn that other people also have panic attacks. Because panic is usually experienced in this manner, it is not unusual for patients to feel that no one can understand them. This may lead to a feeling that they are beyond the reach of any help. Recurrent panic attacks, accompanied by a feeling of helplessness and a strong sense of being unable to cope, may also undermine patients' hope and lead to demoralization.

Depersonalization and derealization experiences during panic attacks occur in various forms and are experienced with varying intensity. Patients typically state that they feel as if they were not real or as if their personality and identity had changed. In more extreme cases, patients report that they feel detached from their bodies, observing themselves as if they were at a certain distance. Panic patients usually respond to these experiences with fear that they signal a loss of control and onset of madness.

Behavioral Aspects

The most typical behavioral response to a panic attack is escape. Because they feel vitally threatened or fear that they might lose control, panic patients have an urge to "do something" to escape the danger. And because the danger is usually associated with the situation or a place in which the attack has occurred, patients feel compelled to flee to a place where they would feel safe. Depending on the nature of the underlying fear, that safety may be provided by one's home or the emergency room of a hospital.

Safety, comfort, and reassurance are usually sought from family members and friends or from health care professionals.

Many patients believe that during the attacks they lose the ability to act rationally and are often concerned that their performance will be impaired. This usually does not happen. If the panic attack occurs while patients are engaged in some activity—for example, driving—they react in different ways: some will continue with their activity (even as they feel apprehensive about panic and its symptoms) whereas others feel that they have to stop, at least for a brief period of time. Only a few feel so incapacitated that they are unable to continue driving for several hours. Contrary to their expectations, panic patients tend to behave rationally in situations of real danger and do not jeopardize themselves or others by their behavior (e.g., Starcevic et al., 2002).

Panic patients often believe that their attacks are visible to others and are therefore concerned that the panic might reveal their "weakness" or even mental illness. Other people are usually not aware that someone is experiencing a panic attack and may only guess that "something" is happening on those rare occasions when patients' behavior is unusual as a consequence of a panic attack (e.g., when they suddenly leave a social situation).

Variants of Panic Attacks

In addition to typical, full-blown panic attacks, there are several variants that either do not meet full diagnostic criteria for panic attacks or have special features. These variants include limited-symptom attacks, nonclinical attacks, nocturnal attacks, and nonfearful attacks (Table 2–5).

Limited-Symptom Attacks

Limited-symptom panic attacks are characterized by fewer symptoms—less than four according to *DSM-IV-TR*. They usually occur along with full-blown attacks. The demarcation on the basis of the number of symptoms, and not on the basis of their severity, is arbitrary. Patients who have panic

Table 2–5. Variants of Panic Attacks

Variant	Defining Characteristics
Limited-symptom attacks	Fewer symptoms during panic attacks (less than four according to *DSM-IV-TR*)
Nonclinical attacks	Panic attacks for which no help is sought
Nocturnal attacks	Panic attacks that occur during sleep
Nonfearful attacks	Fear is not experienced or reported during panic attacks

attacks with only two or three severe symptoms may be more disabled than those with full-blown attacks who have more than four symptoms of mild intensity. Except for the number of symptoms, limited-symptom panic attacks may in other respects be identical to full-blown attacks (Katerndahl, 1990). However, others have endorsed a view that limited-symptom attacks are generally less severe than the full-blown ones (e.g., Uhlenhuth et al., 2006). There is no difference in treatment approach to limited-symptom and full-blown panic attacks. During the treatment, the appearance of limited-symptom attacks and disappearance of full-blown attacks may indicate improvement. Some patients continue to occasionally experience limited-symptom panic attacks for a long time after their treatment has ceased.

Nonclinical Attacks

Nonclinical panic attacks have been observed in people who do not seek help for panic. These attacks are quite common in the population and are more frequently encountered among women. In comparison with full-blown panic attacks, nonclinical attacks are less severe and less frequent, they have fewer symptoms, and they are far less often accompanied by fears of dying, losing control, and/or going mad (Telch et al., 1989b; Cox et al., 1992). Nonclinical attacks appear in stressful situations, especially when the person's performance and behavior are under scrutiny from others—for example, when taking a test or being examined (Norton et al., 1986). It is not clear under what circumstances nonclinical attacks become attacks for which people seek help. It has been speculated that this occurs when persons become excessively concerned about the attacks and their potential consequences (Telch et al., 1989b).

Nocturnal Attacks

Nocturnal panic attacks usually occur along with panic attacks during the day, but some patients experience mainly nocturnal attacks. These attacks may characterize a more severe form of panic disorder (Labbate et al., 1994), but this view has been disputed (Craske et al., 2002). Typically, patients wake up in the midst of an attack, often with intense fear and severe symptoms, particularly shortness of breath and a choking feeling. Nocturnal attacks do not occur during the rapid eye movement (REM) phase of sleep and are not preceded by dreams or nightmares. Therefore, patients usually do not confuse nocturnal panic attacks with dreams and nightmares. The sleep is usually disturbed as a consequence of nocturnal attacks, and patients often have difficulty falling asleep after such attacks. Their memory for the details of nocturnal attacks is usually excellent. Patients with nocturnal panic attacks are less likely to develop agoraphobia and tend to respond to cognitive-behavioral therapy just as well as other panic patients (Craske et al., 2002).

Nonfearful Panic Attacks

These are a controversial type of panic attack (Kushner and Beitman, 1990) because they are not characterized by fear. They are also known as "somatic panic," "noncognitive panic," "alexithymic panic," and "masked anxiety." Since there is no reported fear, it may be difficult to recognize these episodes as panic attacks. Nonfearful panic attacks are characterized by a sudden surge of physical (usually cardiac) symptoms; they can be induced by lactate infusions, just like "regular" panic attacks (Russell et al., 1991). In view of the nature of their symptoms, particularly chest pain, patients with nonfearful panic attacks usually seek help from emergency department physicians and cardiologists. It is estimated that between 22% and 44% of all patients with panic disorder in cardiac settings may have a nonfearful subtype of the condition (Beitman et al., 1987, 1992; Fleet et al., 2000b; Bringager et al., 2004). Patients with nonfearful panic disorder are in many ways similar to those with panic disorder, except for a lower frequency of agoraphobia and co-occurring psychiatric disorders (Beitman et al., 1987; Fleet et al., 2000b; Bringager et al., 2004). They seem to be as impaired as those with panic disorder (Bringager et al., 2004). It is not clear how people with nonfearful panic attacks appraise their prominent physical symptoms and what their dominant emotional responses are. This variant of panic disorder does not appear to be amenable to cognitive therapy, and antipanic pharmacotherapy may be effective in its treatment (Russell et al., 1991; Bringager et al., 2004).

Anticipatory Anxiety

Anticipatory anxiety is as important as panic attacks for the conceptualization of panic disorder. There are several ways in which anticipatory anxiety can be defined (Table 2–6). Most broadly, anticipatory anxiety (sometimes also referred to as "fear of fear") can be defined as a persistent fear of having another panic attack (and/or fear of certain symptoms occurring during the attack). More specifically, this fear pertains to the anticipated consequences of panic attacks. These consequences may be of a physical, psychological, or

Table 2–6. Meanings of Anticipatory Anxiety

Persistent fear of:
  Having another panic attack
  Certain symptoms of panic attacks

Anticipated consequences of panic attacks:
  Physical consequences (death through a heart attack, stroke, choking, etc.)
  Psychological consequences (loss of control, becoming "crazy," etc.)
  Social consequences (embarrassment, shame, etc.)

social nature, with patients typically fearing that they might die, go crazy, or embarrass themselves as a result of panic attacks.

In *DSM-IV-TR*, anticipatory anxiety is deemed essential for the diagnosis of panic disorder and is conceptualized in the ways referred to above. If the patient does not have these typical features of anticipatory anxiety, *DSM-IV-TR* makes a provision that there should be a significant change in the patient's behavior, which is related to panic attacks and reflects anticipatory anxiety. For example, this change can pertain to avoidance of certain situations or undergoing numerous medical investigations.

It is an intriguing question as to why some individuals only experience occasional panic attacks whereas others are distressed by the anxious anticipation of the attacks. Persons who develop anticipatory anxiety (and thereby panic disorder) are likely to be predisposed to it; this predisposition may involve a belief that anxiety and its symptoms are dangerous (see Etiology and Pathogenesis, below).

Anticipatory anxiety may be more pronounced among patients with unexpected panic attacks because the occurrence of such attacks is unpredictable and cannot be prevented by avoidance. Anticipatory anxiety may be overshadowed by avoidance behavior in patients whose panic attacks are largely predictable, that is, bound to certain situations.

Agoraphobia

Among patients with panic disorder, agoraphobia is seen along the continuum of severity—from very mild cases that do not require treatment and in which phobic avoidance disappears with successful treatment of other components of panic disorder, to severe avoidance, when patients are homebound and treatment has to immediately address the agoraphobic component of illness.

As stated before, *agoraphobia* is defined as the fear and/or avoidance of various situations from which escape might be difficult or embarrassing or in which help might not be available in case of a panic attack. In accordance with this definition, there are two basic themes that link various situations that agoraphobic patients fear and avoid; these themes are related to different means of acquiring a sense of safety (Table 2–7).

The first theme pertains to the fear of being confined or trapped, and the corresponding concern that patients will not be able to escape *immediately* in case of a panic attack. The urge to escape is so strong because panic attacks are perceived as dangerous, and patients may believe that attacks will attenuate or disappear only if they know in advance that they can escape. Therefore, just being able to escape is for many agoraphobic patients of crucial importance and is also the main criterion that distinguishes between "safe" and "unsafe" situations. Indeed, not being able to escape may be the main reason that some agoraphobic patients are afraid of flying or traveling on trains or buses; patients typically state that they are more afraid when

Table 2–7. Underlying Themes in Agoraphobic Patients' Thinking and Means of Acquiring a Sense of Safety

Underlying Danger-Driven Beliefs	Means of Acquiring a Sense of Safety
It is dangerous to be in a confined place from which immediate escape might be difficult (in case of a panic attack)	Being able to escape immediately
It is dangerous if professional (medical) help is not immediately available (in case of a panic attack)	Being able to access medical help immediately

trains or buses make no stops, rendering their escape, in case of a panic attack, impossible.

The second theme is related to the patients' need to get *immediate* medical help in case of a panic attack. These patients believe that there will be dire consequences if help is not available right away. Therefore, they seek safety through physical proximity to individuals (e.g., doctors) and/or institutions (e.g., hospitals) that might help them. These patients often have to know the location of hospitals before they venture out, and especially if they travel to areas with which they are not familiar.

Three types of situations are generally feared and avoided by agoraphobic patients (Table 2–8). First, there are situations in which patients are alone and outside their own safety zone (e.g., traveling far away by themselves). The second type is represented by situations from which it would be physically difficult or impossible to escape (e.g., crowds and trains in motion). Finally, agoraphobic patients may be afraid of situations from which it would be awkward or embarrassing to escape in case of a panic attack (e.g., a social function that a patient would feel an urge to leave immediately).

The unique feature of agoraphobia is the multiple situations and/or places that are feared and avoided. Also, patients with agoraphobia may avoid more and more situations with the passage of time. The "profile" of the avoided situations may differ greatly from one patient to another and depends on the underlying themes described above. Local circumstances may determine whether patients with agoraphobia exhibit prominent avoidance of the specific situations or places, such as bridges, tunnels, or a subway, and whether they are disabled by such avoidance.

Some situations may be particularly difficult for agoraphobic patients and seem to be avoided at all cost. These are usually the situations in which patients had their first panic attack or in which anxiety symptoms and panic attacks were particularly severe or embarrassing. Among the symptoms that agoraphobic patients fear the most are lightheadedness, fainting feelings, and/or dizziness. Patients usually interpret these symptoms as a sign that they might faint, collapse, fall, and/or lose control, and they feel that the occurrence of these events in public would be particularly embarrassing.

Table 2–8. Types of Situations Feared and Avoided by Agoraphobic Patients

When Patients Are Alone and/or Outside Their Own Safety Zone

Leaving home alone
Traveling alone
Going far away alone
Driving alone
Staying at home alone

Where It Might Be Physically Difficult or Impossible to Escape (in case of a panic attack)

Crowded places
Trains, buses, and boats in motion
Airplanes during the flight
Controlled-access highways (e.g., freeways, turnpikes, motorways)
Underground railway (subway)
Elevators
Tunnels
Bridges

Where It Might Be Awkward or Embarrassing to Escape (in case of a panic attack)

Restaurants
Social functions
Hairdresser's chair or dentist's chair
Open public places (e.g., streets)
Theaters, cinemas
Shopping malls, department stores
Supermarkets
Standing in a line

The avoidance of agoraphobic situations may be subtle but still interfere with functioning. For example, patients may avoid traveling on buses or trains only during peak traffic hours and therefore come to work early or leave work late. The avoidance may, to a certain extent, be masked by the presence of a "phobic companion." That is, agoraphobic patients may not exhibit significant avoidance if persons whom they trust and who provide them with a sense of security accompany them. These are usually patients' partners or, less often, family members or friends. The functioning of such patients may be relatively good; for example, they may commute to work every day and hold a job for years if their partners regularly accompany them. The extent of phobic fear then becomes fully apparent when partners are no longer able or willing to accompany patients.

Onset of Panic Disorder

The first panic attack is usually well remembered by patients: it was so different from everything that they had experienced before that it usually remains vivid in their memory many years after its occurrence. However, the first panic attack often does not denote the onset of panic disorder and for this reason the precise onset of the disorder may be more difficult to ascertain.

Although many patients describe their first panic attack as quite sudden and unexpected and deny that there were any events preceding it, often there are prodromal symptoms leading up to the first panic attack and/or significant life events prior to the onset of panic disorder. Chronic worry and anxiety, generalized anxiety disorder, and hypochondriasis have been described as preceding panic disorder (Fava et al., 1988, 1992; Garvey et al., 1988). The first panic attack may occur in a variety of contexts and situations, such as interpersonal conflict, separation, traumatic experience, medical illness, physical exertion, excitement and agitation, sexual intercourse, and intoxication with or withdrawal from certain substances (e.g., alcohol, caffeine, amphetamine, cocaine, cannabis).

The circumstances of the first panic attack (particularly the location where it occurred and its intensity) may determine the person's initial response to the attack and whether the person will develop fear of further panic attacks and avoidance of the situations that remind him or her of the first attack (e.g., Lelliott et al., 1989; Amering et al., 1997). Thus, if the first panic attack was severe and occurred away from home—and particularly in situations from which a quick escape was impossible (e.g., being in a flying airplane) or in which urgent medical help was not available (e.g., while traveling far away from the nearest hospital)—there is an increased risk that the person will become afraid of another panic attack, that such an attack is anticipated outside the home, and that the person will ultimately develop agoraphobia, avoiding many situations away from home.

RELATIONSHIP BETWEEN PANIC DISORDER AND OTHER DISORDERS

Psychiatric conditions frequently co-occur with panic disorder, especially in clinical settings. Other anxiety disorders, mood disorders, hypochondriasis, and alcohol abuse are most common among these conditions. Various types of personality disturbance are also seen in patients with panic disorder.

The rates of another anxiety disorder co-occurring with panic disorder in clinical populations over a lifetime range between 35% and 93%; the most frequently co-occurring anxiety disorders include generalized anxiety disorder, specific phobias, and social anxiety disorder (de Ruiter et al., 1989; Sanderson et al., 1990; Starcevic et al., 1992b). Most of these co-occurring anxiety disorders usually precede the onset of panic disorder, and they can sometimes be considered to predispose to panic disorder.

The relationship between panic disorder and agoraphobia is of particular importance and it is discussed in some detail below. In addition, there are significant implications of the relationships between panic disorder on the one hand and generalized anxiety disorder, depression, hypochondriasis, and alcohol-related disorders on the other (Table 2–9). Finally, the

Table 2–9. Clinical Implications of the Relationship Between Panic Disorder and Other Disorders

Panic Disorder and Generalized Anxiety Disorder
- Generalized anxiety disorder often co-occurs with panic disorder, but it may be overshadowed by the more dramatic clinical picture of panic disorder and may therefore be unrecognized or missed
- Chronic worry and anxious apprehension in generalized anxiety disorder sometimes need to be distinguished from anticipatory anxiety in panic disorder
- Treatment implications are unclear; generalized anxiety disorder may need to be addressed at a later stage of treatment, after some relief has been obtained from panic disorder

Panic Disorder and Depression
- Many panic patients develop depression and should be closely monitored for any symptoms and signs of depression
- There are several pathways leading to depression; depression is not just a consequence of the panic-associated demoralization and the feelings of helplessness and hopelessness
- Both panic disorder and major depressive disorder tend to be more severe when they co-occur than when they appear alone; there is greater impairment in patients who suffer from both conditions; the presence of depression affects negatively the course and outcome of panic disorder, with further complications (e.g., suicide attempts) being more likely
- Vigorous treatment with antidepressants is needed, along with supportive measures and psychosocial interventions

Panic Disorder and Hypochondriasis
- There is a frequent overlap in clinical presentation between panic disorder and hypochondriasis; in most cases, features of hypochondriasis are secondary to panic disorder and abate with successful treatment of panic disorder
- Panic patients with prominent hypochondriacal features may "attract" some hostility and rejecting behavior, which are otherwise typical of the way patients with hypochondriasis are treated

Panic Disorder and Alcohol-Related Problems
- It is important to ascertain what role, if any, alcohol-related problems might have played in precipitating panic attacks (e.g., through withdrawals); diagnosis of panic disorder is not warranted if panic attacks occur only during alcohol withdrawals
- "Self-medicating" with alcohol may occur in panic patients, more often in men
- Benzodiazepines should be avoided (or used only with great caution) in patients with current or past alcohol-related problems

relationships between bipolar disorder and panic disorder and between panic disorder and personality disturbance are also reviewed.

Panic Disorder and Agoraphobia

Patients with panic disorder often resort to the avoidance of situations in which they expect to have panic attacks or some symptoms of the attacks. This is the path that leads to agoraphobia. Because agoraphobia is not solely and invariably a consequence of panic disorder, the relationship between panic disorder and agoraphobia has been a source of some controversy (see Diagnostic and Conceptual Issues, below).

In examining the relationship between panic disorder and agoraphobia from the perspective of panic disorder being a chronologically and conceptually primary condition, the main question is why some panic patients go on to develop agoraphobia whereas others do not. The research has identified several risk factors (Table 2–10) for developing agoraphobia among patients with panic disorder. The single most important risk factor is being female: women are three to four times more likely to develop agoraphobia than men, and there may be various cultural, psychological, and biological reasons for this (see Epidemiology, and Etiology and Pathogenesis, below).

Table 2–10. Risk Factors for Developing Agoraphobia Among Patients with Panic Disorder

Female gender

Cognitive factors

- Expectation that panic attacks will occur in certain situations (Craske et al., 1988; Rapee and Murrell, 1988; Adler et al., 1989; Telch et al., 1989a)
- Exaggerated expectation of negative social consequences of panic attacks (Telch et al., 1989a)
- Exaggerated expectation of negative consequences of panic attacks in certain specific situations (Franklin, 1987; Noyes et al., 1987a; Craske et al., 1988; Fleming and Faulk, 1989)
- Prominent fear of dying or "going crazy" during panic attacks
- Marked belief that one is not able to cope with panic attacks (Craske et al., 1988; Mavissakalian, 1988; Telch et al., 1989a; Clum and Knowles, 1991)

More prominent lightheadedness and dizziness during panic attacks (Noyes et al., 1987a; Telch et al., 1989a)

Occurrence of the first panic attack outside of the person's "safety zone" (e.g., far away from home, in a public place) (Lelliott et al., 1989; Amering et al., 1997)

Prominent dependency or dependent personality disorder (Kleiner and Marshall, 1987)

Embarrassment about having a panic attack (Amering et al., 1997)

Prominent social anxiety or social anxiety disorder (Rapee and Murrell, 1988)

In addition, various beliefs and expectations about panic attacks and panic symptoms may predispose panic patients to agoraphobia (Franklin, 1987; Noyes et al., 1987a; Craske et al., 1988; Mavissakalian, 1988; Rapee and Murrell, 1988; Adler et al., 1989; Fleming and Faulk, 1989; Telch et al., 1989a; Clum and Knowles, 1991). Agoraphobia was predicted by these cognitive factors better than it was by the severity and frequency of panic attacks (Clum and Knowles, 1991). More recent research, however, has questioned the role of cognitive factors in the development of agoraphobia among patients with panic disorder (Berle et al., 2008).

Panic Disorder and Generalized Anxiety Disorder

Generalized anxiety disorder co-occurs fairly frequently with panic disorder, in up to 68% of panic patients. Generalized anxiety disorder is usually diagnosed as a secondary condition, when panic disorder is the main reason for seeking help and treatment. However, generalized anxiety disorder often occurs before panic disorder, but because of the nature of generalized anxiety disorder (see Chapter 3), patients tend to seek help only after a condition such as panic disorder or depression has complicated its course. Generalized anxiety disorder and panic disorder may also occur at approximately the same time, or generalized anxiety disorder follows panic disorder. Criteria for distinguishing between panic disorder and generalized anxiety disorder are presented in Table 2–13 and clinical implications of the relationship between these two conditions are presented in Table 2–9. Clinical experience suggests that it may be more difficult to treat panic disorder co-occurring with generalized anxiety disorder.

Panic Disorder and Depression

Depression is often seen as a complication of panic disorder, especially in the context of agoraphobia (Thompson et al., 1989; Ball et al., 1994) and a long-standing and more severe panic disorder. In some cases, major depressive disorder and panic disorder develop at approximately the same time, while in the minority of patients, major depressive disorder precedes the onset of panic disorder. It is estimated that between 24% and 88% of patients with panic disorder have at least one major depressive episode in their lifetime (Breier et al., 1984; Lesser et al., 1988).

Such a common co-occurrence of panic disorder with depression has important implications (Table 2–9) in that panic patients need to be monitored for any symptoms and signs of depression and adequately treated if they develop depression. This is particularly significant in view of the findings that both major depressive disorder and panic disorder tend to be more severe when these two conditions co-occur (Breier et al., 1984; Andrade et al., 1994; Grunhaus et al., 1994). The impairment in patients who suffer from both panic disorder and depression is greater than that in those who suffer from either condition alone, and the presence of depression affects negatively the course and outcome of panic disorder (Scheibe and Albus, 1994). Finally, the risk of suicide attempts and suicide is increased when major depressive disorder co-occurs with panic disorder (e.g., Cox et al., 1994a; Warshaw et al., 2000).

Depression cannot be reliably prevented by antidepressant medication, and benzodiazepines may actually induce or worsen depression. Inasmuch as some cases of depression develop as a consequence of the panic-associated demoralization and the feelings of helplessness and hopelessness, vigorous treatment of panic disorder and the consequently improved functioning may help in the prevention of depressive episodes.

Panic Disorder and Hypochondriasis

Because of the overlap in clinical presentation between panic disorder and hypochondriasis (preoccupation with physical symptoms, persistent concerns about having a serious physical disease, seeking medical reassurance but apparently rejecting it at the same time, undergoing numerous medical investigations), it may be difficult to distinguish them (see Table 2–14 and Differential Diagnosis, below). From the cognitive perspective, the most conspicuous similarity between panic disorder and hypochondriasis is that both are based on catastrophic misinterpretation of innocuous bodily sensations and symptoms (Salkovskis and Clark, 1993).

The relationship between panic disorder and hypochondriasis is complex. Hypochondriasis can be a secondary feature of panic disorder, and many patients (45%–50%) with panic disorder exhibit significant hypochondriacal features (Starcevic et al., 1992a; Benedetti et al., 1997; Furer et al., 1997). These hypochondriacal features then diminish or disappear upon successful treatment of panic disorder. Less often, panic disorder and hypochondriasis coexist, with neither condition considered principal or chronologically primary; patients with this clinical presentation tend to have a more severe illness (Hiller et al., 2005). Hypochondriasis was also reported to precede panic attacks in some patients (Fava et al., 1990). To better understand the relationship between panic disorder and hypochondriasis, the crucial step is to ascertain whether hypochondriacal features (e.g., excessive bodily preoccupation, disease fear, disease suspicion) are better accounted for by panic disorder—that is, whether they occur primarily during panic attacks and/or as part of anticipatory anxiety.

Panic Disorder and Alcohol Abuse and Dependence

Alcohol abuse and alcohol dependence have been associated with panic disorder in 13%–43% of patients with panic disorder (Otto et al., 1992; Starcevic et al., 1992b, 1993b; Kessler et al., 1997a). Alcohol-related problems can precede the onset of panic attacks and can also play a role in the etiology of panic disorder by precipitating panic attacks during withdrawals from alcohol (see Table 2–9). Alcohol abuse and dependence can also develop in the course of panic disorder, as a result of patients' attempts to "self-medicate" and thus alleviate their symptoms and anxiety. This pattern happens less often than in patients with social anxiety disorder and posttraumatic stress disorder.

Bipolar Disorder and Panic Disorder

The relationship between bipolar disorder and panic disorder has increasingly been the focus of attention. This is likely a consequence of an increased scientific scrutiny of bipolar disorder in recent years, and findings about the relationship between bipolar disorder and panic disorder come mainly from studies of patients with primary bipolar disorder. Patients who present for treatment of panic disorder as their principal condition (e.g., in anxiety disorders clinics) show relatively low rates of the co-occurring bipolar disorder.

The lifetime prevalence of panic disorder among patients with bipolar disorder is approximately 20% (Chen and Dilsaver, 1995; McElroy et al., 2001). Higher rates of the co-occurring panic disorder have been reported in bipolar disorder patients with psychotic features and in patients with bipolar depression (Pini et al., 1997, 1999). It appears that the link between bipolar disorder and panic disorder has a stronger genetic component (Mackinnon et al., 1997). The presence of panic disorder and panic symptoms in patients with bipolar disorder has been associated with more severe depression, more suicidal tendencies, and delayed response to treatment (Frank et al., 2002). The co-occurrence of panic disorder and bipolar disorder may also have treatment implications in that some mood stabilizers, particularly valproate, may be effective in the treatment of panic disorder (Baetz and Bowen, 1998).

Panic Disorder and Personality Disturbance

The relationship between panic disorder and personality disturbance is important because of the implications it may have for the understanding of the psychopathology of panic disorder and for its treatment. Most personality disorders and personality traits that have been found in patients with panic disorder are nonspecifically associated with panic disorder. That is, the same or similar types of the personality-level psychopathology have been found in patients with other anxiety disorders and depression.

The proportion of panic patients with personality disorders varies, but is estimated at 40%–65% (Reich and Troughton, 1988; Brooks et al., 1989; Diaferia et al., 1993; Blashfield et al., 1994). This high prevalence of personality disturbance may be an overestimate due to a low threshold for diagnosing personality disorders. Predictably, most common among panic patients are *DSM* Cluster C ("anxious, fearful"; avoidant and dependent), followed by Cluster B ("emotional, dramatic"; histrionic) personality disorders (Diaferia et al., 1993); occasionally, Cluster A ("odd, eccentric") personality disorders are found among patients with panic disorder.

The relationship between panic disorder and personality disturbance can be understood in several ways (Starcevic, 1992). Certain personality disorders, particularly those from the *DSM* Cluster C, may predispose to panic disorder, but even when they appear to do so there is no evidence that this predisposition is specific for panic disorder. Therefore, it would be very difficult to estimate the likelihood of a person's developing panic disorder on the basis of that person having a particular type of personality disturbance. At least some changes in personality functioning, if not personality disorders, may be better conceptualized as a consequence of panic disorder, particularly when panic disorder has been severe, accompanied by agoraphobia, lasting for a long time, and/or with an early onset (e.g., in adolescence). For example, some patients with chronic, severe panic disorder with agoraphobia become extremely insecure and dependent, lose self-esteem, or exhibit extensive social withdrawal and isolation; this pattern may seem identical to that of dependent and/or avoidant personality disorders. Other patients become hypervigilant, extremely sensitive in interpersonal situations, mistrustful, and suspicious, traits that may resemble paranoid personality disorder.

The presence of certain personality traits and disorders usually implies a less favorable prognosis of panic disorder, with a greater likelihood of various problems occurring during treatment (e.g., Green and Curtis, 1988; Chambless et al., 1992; Hoffart and Martinsen, 1993). These problems include fluctuating motivation for treatment, secondary gain, poor compliance with pharmacotherapy and cognitive-behavioral therapy, and "sabotaging" one's own treatment. However, a successful treatment of panic disorder may sometimes lead to a significant decrease in certain personality traits (e.g., Mavissakalian and Hamann, 1987). Some studies do not support the notion that personality disorders are usually associated with poorer response to treatment of panic disorder (e.g., Dreessen et al., 1994).

ASSESSMENT

Diagnostic and Conceptual Issues

Diagnostic criteria for panic disorder in *DSM-IV-TR* are relatively straightforward. There needs to be a presence of recurrent, unexpected panic attacks and anticipatory anxiety for at least 1 month, and panic attacks must not be caused by a medical condition or a psychoactive substance. To qualify for the diagnosis of panic disorder, most panic attacks have to be unexpected, but some are situationally predisposed or situationally bound, especially in panic patients who also have agoraphobia. If most panic attacks are currently situationally predisposed or situationally bound, there has to be a history of unexpected attacks at the beginning of the disorder. Otherwise, the diagnosis of another anxiety disorder is more likely, as *DSM-IV-TR* stipulates that a diagnosis of panic disorder is warranted if its features cannot be better accounted for by social anxiety disorder, specific phobias, obsessive-compulsive disorder, posttraumatic stress disorder, and separation anxiety disorder. In other words, for the diagnosis of panic disorder to be made, panic attacks must not be a part of another psychiatric condition, but also, at least initial panic attacks have to be unexpected. As noted below, distinguishing between unexpected and situational panic attacks is not always easy.

The relationship between panic disorder and agoraphobia is also of diagnostic and conceptual importance (see below). In the *DSM* system, agoraphobia is conceived of as a complication of panic disorder or a condition secondary to panic disorder—hence the diagnosis of panic disorder with agoraphobia. In *ICD-10*, by contrast, the simultaneous presence of panic disorder and agoraphobia suggests that agoraphobia is a primary condition, and this combination is accordingly designated "agoraphobia with panic disorder." Moreover, *ICD-10* imposes a diagnostic hierarchy in that a diagnosis of panic disorder is precluded by the simultaneous presence of phobic disorders or major depressive disorder.

Panic attacks and anticipatory anxiety can be overshadowed by avoidance behavior in patients with severe agoraphobia. In such patients, even if panic attacks are "prevented" by avoidance, the fear of panic attacks does not vanish and can be found underneath extensive avoidance behavior.

The diagnosis of panic disorder first depends on the correct assessment of panic attacks. Many patients use terms *panic* and *panic attacks*, but their ideas of what constitutes panic may be very different from the description of panic presented here. It is worthwhile to emphasize that panic attacks should not be designated as such if they occur *only* on exposure to life-threatening situations. The most important features of panic attacks are their sudden, abrupt occurrence; very rapid culmination of their intensity; prominent physical symptoms; and catastrophic elaboration of these symptoms. If some components of this description are missing, it is likely that the patient is not experiencing panic.

It is usually not difficult to ascertain panic symptoms. However, some patients may focus on one or two dominant and/or the most distressing symptoms (e.g., heart racing and shortness of breath), whereas for comprehensive assessment, patients need to be specifically asked about the presence of other panic-associated symptoms. Sometimes anticipatory anxiety needs to be differentiated from worries that do not pertain to panic attacks. As presented in Clinical Features (above), anticipatory anxiety pertains strictly to panic attacks, even when it is conceptualized via changes in behavior, and its duration in *DSM-IV-TR* is at least 1 month.

There are two crucial steps in establishing the presence of agoraphobia: (1) ascertaining the type and number of situations that patients fear and/or avoid, and (2) asking patients about the reasons for avoidance. According to *DSM-IV-TR*, agoraphobia is present if panic patients fear and/or avoid at least two distinct agoraphobic situations, and avoidance (or phobic fear) has to be clearly related to panic attacks. The diagnosis of agoraphobia is warranted not only in the presence of avoidance behavior but also if patients endure agoraphobic situations with great distress and/or fear, or if they enter agoraphobic situations only when accompanied by the trusted other(s).

Types of Panic Attacks

As already noted, the distinction between unexpected and situational panic attacks entails assessment of whether they are associated with certain situations, objects, or events. There is increasing evidence that this assessment is often unreliable. For example, one epidemiological study has reported that many attacks initially believed to be unexpected subsequently turned out to be situational and that most panic attacks seem to be to some extent situational, even among people suffering from panic disorder without agoraphobia (Kessler et al., 2006). If unexpected panic attacks cannot be identified reliably, the concept of panic disorder without agoraphobia, based on this type of attack, is then undermined.

More broadly, the putative distinction between unexpected and situational panic attacks calls for reexamination of the idea that phenomena such as unexpected panic attacks occur in the absence of a psychological or social context. At the same time, the contextual, background factors that may determine whether a panic attack develops need to be identified.

Panic Disorder and Agoraphobia

Another conceptual issue that has received a large amount of attention is that of the relationship between panic attacks, panic disorder, and agoraphobia. In American psychiatry, as embodied in the *DSM* system, panic attack, especially spontaneous or unexpected panic attack, is regarded as a qualitatively different type of anxiety (Klein, 1981). When both panic attacks and agoraphobic avoidance are present, agoraphobia is seen as a consequence of panic attacks, whereas agoraphobia itself is defined through panic attacks or symptoms of panic attacks—as the fear of situations in which it would be embarrassing or difficult to escape in case of a panic attack or in which help might not be available, also in case of a panic attack. Therefore, in the *DSM* system agoraphobia is almost always regarded as part of panic disorder, with panic disorder being the main and primary diagnosis. Agoraphobia does exist as a separate nosological entity (under the name "agoraphobia without a history of panic disorder"), but it is rarely diagnosed and often considered spurious (e.g., Horwath et al., 1993).

In contrast, many European psychiatrists and the *ICD* system (as in *ICD-10*) postulate that there is a continuum of severity from normal fear through phobic fear to panic attacks. In other words, panic attacks are not seen as being qualitatively different from other types of anxiety (e.g., phobic or generalized anxiety), and they only denote greater severity of anxiety (Tyrer, 1984). Therefore, the presence of panic attacks in agoraphobic situations is viewed as an indicator of the severity of phobic anxiety. The main diagnosis in such situations is agoraphobia; hence the *ICD-10* diagnostic categories of agoraphobia with or without panic disorder.

There has been some support for both views, but the strength of evidence has generally favored the *DSM* position. Thus, most studies suggest that panic attacks precede agoraphobia in the vast majority of patients (e.g., Thyer and Himle, 1985; Uhde et al., 1985; Aronson and Logue, 1987; Franklin, 1987). Also, agoraphobic patients are usually not afraid of agoraphobic situations as such but are much more concerned about the physical symptoms of anxiety and their potential consequences (Buglass et al., 1977; Hallam and Hafner, 1978; Franklin, 1987). Moreover, unlike other phobias, where avoidance is likely to prevent phobic fear, avoidance in agoraphobia does not necessarily prevent panic attacks (Hallam, 1978). In many, if not most cases, agoraphobia can be viewed as an attempt to avoid certain physical symptoms (e.g., dizziness), sudden loss of control, or full-blown panic attacks, which patients believe are more likely to occur in certain places and situations.

Results of recent studies are likely to reignite a debate about the relationship between panic attacks, panic disorder, and agoraphobia as they suggest that in many cases agoraphobia is conceptually and diagnostically independent from panic attacks and panic disorder (Faravelli et al., 2008; Wittchen et al., 2008). Most of this evidence comes from epidemiological research. Studies in the community have consistently shown that incidence and prevalence rates of agoraphobia (with or without panic attacks and panic disorder) are higher than those of panic disorder (Somers et al., 2006); this is not in agreement with the *DSM* conceptualization of agoraphobia as usually being a consequence of panic attacks and panic disorder. In addition, prospective-longitudinal data regarding the progression, stability, and outcome of panic attacks, panic disorder, and agoraphobia also indicate that the links between them are much weaker than would be expected on the basis of the *DSM* conceptualization (Wittchen et al., 2008). All this points to a suggestion that several pathways may lead to agoraphobia; of these, some involve panic attacks and panic disorder, whereas others do not. In the latter case, agoraphobia may develop via separation anxiety disorder or some specific (situational) phobias. If so, perhaps the main distinction should be made between panic-driven and nonpanic-driven agoraphobia. The latter condition may be characterized by fears of being alone (or outside of one's own "comfort zone"), of being attacked on public transport, of getting lost during travel or in a crowd, of being involved in an accident, and so on (Wittchen et al., 1998).

Assessment Instruments

The recognition that panic disorder is a multifaceted condition has led to a construction of two instruments for separate assessments of different components and aspects of panic disorder (e.g., panic attacks, anticipatory anxiety, agoraphobic avoidance, health-related concerns, disability). These instruments are the Panic Disorder Severity Scale (Shear et al., 1997) and the Panic and Agoraphobia Scale (Bandelow, 1995, 1999). Both are designed for use by clinicians, but there are also patient, self-report versions. They enable clinicians to make a more thorough assessment of panic disorder and its components, and to monitor both global and specific changes in the course of treatment.

Several self-report instruments and assessment procedures can be used for the three main components of panic disorder (panic attacks, anticipatory anxiety, and agoraphobic avoidance) to complement clinician-based assessment.

Since retrospective recording of panic attacks is not reliable because of the possible memory bias, panic attacks are best monitored prospectively, in a diary format. A typical panic diary provides information on the frequency and severity of panic attacks, situations in which they occur, and other triggers that may precipitate the attacks. In addition to this "basic" panic diary, more detailed information may be obtained by asking patients to also record the symptoms, thoughts, and feelings that they experience during panic attacks, as well as the duration and type (unexpected or situational) of each attack.

There are two useful instruments for assessing various aspects of anticipatory anxiety. The first one is the Agoraphobic Cognitions Questionnaire (Chambless et al., 1984), which is used to assess the frequency of thoughts about negative (catastrophic) consequences of anxiety and panic. The other instrument is the Anxiety Sensitivity Index (Reiss et al., 1986), which measures the fear of symptoms of anxious arousal.

The Mobility Inventory (Chambless et al., 1985) is suitable for assessment of the degree of avoidance of typical agoraphobic situations. The distinct advantages of this instrument are its comprehensiveness and separate assessment of avoidance when patients are alone and when they are accompanied.

Differential Diagnosis

Differential diagnosis of panic disorder is important and complex for several reasons. First, because of the episodic occurrence of largely physical symptoms, diagnostic workup of panic disorder includes a consideration of several medical conditions. Second, panic attacks are often seen in the course of other psychiatric disorders and it is therefore important to ascertain whether panic attacks may be better conceptualized as part of another psychiatric condition. Finally, several disorders should be considered in the differential diagnosis of agoraphobia.

Medical Differential Diagnosis

In comparison with the general population and patients without panic disorder, patients with panic disorder are more likely to have certain medical conditions. Likewise, panic disorder is more likely to co-occur with a number of medical conditions. These include thyroid dysfunction (e.g., Lindemann et al., 1984), mitral valve prolapse (e.g., Margraf et al., 1988), asthma (e.g., Yellowlees et al., 1987; Shavitt et al., 1992), chronic obstructive pulmonary disease and other respiratory illnesses (e.g., Zandbergen et al., 1991), vestibular dysfunction (e.g., Jacob et al., 1996), irritable bowel syndrome (e.g., Walker et al., 1990; Lydiard et al., 1994), other gastrointestinal syndromes (e.g., Lydiard et al., 1994), and various allergies (e.g., Ramesh et al., 1991).

A large number of medical conditions can cause panic attacks (Table 2–11). Of these, the most clinically relevant are hyperthyroidism, cardiac arrhythmias, vestibular dysfunction, mitral valve prolapse, complex partial (temporal, psychomotor) epilepsy, and hypoglycemia. Not all panic patients need to go through extensive diagnostic testing for all these conditions, and organic workup in panic patients can be conceptualized as a sequential three-step process (Table 2–12). First, all patients should undergo routine physical examination and laboratory testing, including thyroid function tests. Second, if patients complain repeatedly of symptoms such as chest pain, abnormalities in the cardiac rhythm, dizziness, or depersonalization phenomena, relevant diagnostic investigations should be performed to check for the presence of the corresponding physical conditions. Finally, the full organic workup is warranted in all patients

Table 2–11. Medical Conditions That Can Cause Panic Attacks

More Clinically Relevant (in terms of higher frequency of association with panic attacks)

Hyperthyroidism (or less commonly, hypothyroidism)
Cardiac arrhythmias (e.g., paroxysmal atrial tachycardia)
Vestibular dysfunction
Mitral valve prolapse
Complex partial (temporal, psychomotor) epilepsy
Hypoglycemia

Less Clinically Relevant (in terms of lower frequency of association with panic attacks)

Hypoparathyroidism, hyperparathyroidism
Pheochromocytoma
Pulmonary embolus
Electrolyte disturbances
Cushing's syndrome
Menopause

Table 2–12. Sequential Three-Step Process in Organic Workup of Panic Patients

1. Diagnostic Investigations for All Panic Patients

- Routine physical examination
- Routine laboratory testing (complete blood count, electrolytes, calcium, glycemia)
- Thyroid function tests (levels of serum T_3, T_4, and TSH)

2. Additional Diagnostic Investigations for Panic Patients with Recurrent, Specific, and/or Severe Symptoms, such as Chest Pain, Abnormalities in Cardiac Rhythm, Dizziness, and Depersonalization Phenomena

- Electrocardiogram (ECG), cardiological examination (to check for cardiac arrhythmias)
- Echocardiogram (cardiac ultrasound), cardiological examination (to check for mitral valve prolapse)
- Vestibular function testing, neurological examination (to check for vestibular dysfunction)
- Electroencephalogram (EEG), neurological examination (to check for epilepsy)

3. Diagnostic Investigations for All Patients Whose Panic Attacks Occur for the First Time Later in Life (after age 45) or Whose Panic Attacks Have Atypical Features

- Full organic workup, with emphasis on those investigations that are relevant for each particular patient (and are based on the patient's symptom profile)

T_3, triiodothyronine; T_4, thyroxine; TSH, thyroid-stimulating hormone.

whose panic attacks occur for the first time later in life (after the age of 45) or in those cases where panic attacks have some atypical features. Examples of the latter include loss of consciousness or a "clouded" state of consciousness, urinary incontinence, severe headache, slurred speech, and amnesia.

The relationship between panic disorder and thyroid disease in general, and hyperthyroidism in particular, is complex. Hyperthyroidism can be considered a cause of panic attacks if in patients with both conditions, panic attacks subside following treatment with antithyroid therapy and normalization of thyroid function. In this situation, a diagnosis of panic disorder would be ruled out. In other cases, panic attacks do not abate after the thyroid disease has been treated successfully, and the thyroid condition (hyperthyroidism or hypothyroidism) may be thought of as playing a role in precipitating panic attacks but not accounting entirely for their appearance. Making a causal attribution might be so speculative that the question of whether panic attacks are better understood as a manifestation of thyroid dysfunction or as part of panic disorder is best left open and both conditions are treated regardless of the precise nature of their relationship.

Sudden tachycardia (up to 150 beats/minute) is commonly reported during panic attacks. Although such tachycardias are relatively benign, they can also occur as a consequence of life-threatening cardiac arrhythmias; therefore, the possibility of such an etiology should be further investigated.

Dizziness, lightheadedness, fainting feeling, loss of balance, and "walking on waves" are frequent symptoms during panic attacks; they may be more common among patients with agoraphobia. Depending on the severity of these symptoms and presence of any other symptoms suggestive of organic etiology (e.g., vertigo, nausea), vestibular dysfunction, inner ear disease, and neurological, cerebrovascular, and cardiovascular conditions may need to be investigated.

Panic disorder and mitral valve prolapse have several symptoms in common, including palpitations, chest pain, and manifestations of autonomic hyperarousal. The degree of association between panic disorder and mitral valve prolapse varies, but one meta-analysis has shown that mitral valve prolapse occurs twice more often among panic patients than among those without panic disorder (Katerndahl, 1993). Data on the prevalence of panic disorder among patients with mitral valve prolapse are less consistent, but it seems that panic disorder is not more frequent in patients with mitral valve prolapse than in the general population. There is a consensus that despite our lack of full understanding of the relationship between panic disorder and mitral valve prolapse, this link has no etiological importance and no implications for treatment.

Certain patients with panic disorder have various and for the most part nonspecific changes on electroencephalograms (EEG). Some of these patients have more prominent symptoms of depersonalization and/or derealization and may be irritable and aggressive during, just before, or immediately after panic attacks. Other symptoms unusual for panic (e.g., "déjà vu" phenomenon, marked hypersensitivity to light or sound) may also be present. Panic attacks in such cases may represent a manifestation of a seizure disorder or may occur with seizures that characterize temporal lobe (partial complex) epilepsy. In addition to an EEG, a detailed neurological examination and relevant investigations are warranted to establish the diagnosis.

Hypoglycemia is a relatively rare cause of panic attacks; in such cases, attacks occur only in states of hunger and disappear following the administration of intravenous glucose or intake of food.

Panic Disorder and Substance Use Disorders

Panic attacks can occur as a consequence of intoxication with cannabis and stimulant drugs (cocaine, amphetamine, caffeine) or in the context of alcohol, benzodiazepine, or opiate withdrawal. The diagnosis of panic disorder should not be made if there is close temporal proximity between the substance use and onset of panic attacks and if panic attacks disappear soon after substance use has been ceased. In other words, the diagnosis of panic disorder is justified if panic attacks persist for a long time after the intoxication or a withdrawal syndrome.

Psychiatric Differential Diagnosis

Psychiatric differential diagnosis of panic disorder may include quite a few disorders, but generalized anxiety disorder and hypochondriasis are of greatest conceptual and practical relevance. Generalized anxiety disorder can be distinguished from panic disorder on the basis of the criteria listed in Table 2–13. Still, the separation of the previous diagnostic entity of "anxiety neurosis" into panic disorder and generalized anxiety disorder remains somewhat controversial.

As already noted (see Relationship Between Panic Disorder and Other Disorders, above), panic disorder and hypochondriasis have much in common. However, there are ways of distinguishing between these conditions (Table 2–14). First, patients with panic disorder are troubled by physical symptoms that occur episodically, during panic attacks, whereas physical symptoms in hypochondriacal patients are more persistent. Physical symptoms in panic disorder are usually those of autonomic hyperactivity, whereas physical symptoms in hypochondriasis are more varied and often include aches and pains. The perceived threat in panic disorder is more immediate, with physical symptoms being appraised as suggesting a disease with quick, fatal outcome (e.g., myocardial infarct); the perceived threat in hypochondriasis is more remote, and physical symptoms are appraised as suggesting a disease with a somewhat slower progression, albeit with the same, fatal outcome (e.g., cancer) (Salkovskis and Clark, 1993). As a result of these differences in the appraisal of danger, panic patients are more likely to seek medical help promptly (when they have a

Table 2–13.　Distinguishing Between Panic Disorder and Generalized Anxiety Disorder

Criteria	Panic Disorder	Generalized Anxiety Disorder
Presence of panic attacks	Yes	No
Physical symptoms of anxiety	More pronounced, but occurring episodically (during panic attacks)	Less pronounced, but more persistent
Type of symptoms	Autonomic hyperactivity (arousal) symptoms more typical	Symptoms of tension (both somatic and psychological) more typical
Appraisal of symptoms	Typically catastrophic, with the catastrophe being anticipated quickly	Less often catastrophic, without the catastrophe being anticipated quickly
Onset	Usually abrupt	Gradual
Seeking help	Relatively quick	Usually delayed

Table 2–14. Distinguishing Between Panic Disorder and Hypochondriasis

Criteria	Panic Disorder	Hypochondriasis
Occurrence of physical symptoms	Mainly during panic attacks	More persistent
Nature of physical symptoms	Autonomic hyperactivity symptoms	Greater variety of symptoms
Nature of the perceived threat	More immediate (death from a rapidly developing disease)	More remote (death from a slowly progressing disease)
Seeking medical help	Prompt, urgent, but usually limited to panic attacks	Less urgent, but more persistent

panic attack) whereas patients with hypochondriasis seek such help with less urgency. Stated succinctly, panic patients are more likely to fear dying, whereas those with hypochondriasis are more likely to be afraid of death (Noyes, 1999).

With regard to other psychiatric disorders, the crucial step is ascertaining whether the panic attacks are better understood as being part of these disorders, and not a feature of panic disorder. To establish this, patients should be carefully examined for presence of other disorders (e.g., a psychotic illness or depression), and the nature of panic attacks needs to be clarified. Panic attacks may be exclusively situational, as in social anxiety disorder and specific phobias, or appear only in the specific contexts (e.g., trauma-related topics and stimuli in posttraumatic stress disorder and certain obsession-related situations in obsessive-compulsive disorder).

Differential Diagnosis of Agoraphobia

The most common issue in the differential diagnosis of agoraphobia (Table 2–15) is its distinction from specific phobias and social anxiety disorder. Patients with agoraphobia, specific phobias, and social anxiety disorder may fear and avoid the same or similar situations, but patients with agoraphobia are typically afraid of numerous and quite diverse situations (which are usually interconnected, however, by their common link to panic attacks). Reasons for fear and avoidance may be more useful in distinguishing between these phobic disorders than are the types of situations that are feared and avoided. Thus, fear and avoidance of agoraphobic situations are usually, though not always, related to panic attacks or symptoms of anxiety and panic (e.g., dizziness, urgent need to urinate). The types of specific phobias that may need to be distinguished from agoraphobia usually

Table 2–15. Differential Diagnosis of Agoraphobia

Other anxiety disorders
  Specific phobias, especially claustrophobia, fear of flying, driving phobia, and fear of heights
  Social anxiety disorder
  Obsessive-compulsive disorder
  Posttraumatic stress disorder
  Separation anxiety disorder
Depression
Psychotic disorder

include situational phobias (e.g., claustrophobia, fear of flying, driving phobia) and less often, phobia of heights. The relationship between these specific phobias and agoraphobia and the criteria for distinguishing between them are presented in more detail in Chapter 5. Likewise, the relationship between social anxiety disorder and agoraphobia and the criteria for making a distinction between them are further discussed in Chapter 4.

As for other anxiety disorders that are relevant in the differential diagnosis of agoraphobia, obsessive-compulsive disorder should be considered if fear of contamination appears to be the main reason for avoidance of going out. The avoidance in posttraumatic stress disorder may be widespread and resemble agoraphobia-associated avoidance, but all the situations avoided in posttraumatic stress disorder are directly or indirectly related to the trauma.

Separation anxiety disorder is typically seen in children, but it has also been described in adults. Patients with this condition are concerned about separating from attachment figures and being on their own; as a result, they avoid separation and loneliness, which may lead to an avoidance profile similar to the one seen in agoraphobia. However, patients with agoraphobia worry about catastrophes that may befall them, whereas patients with separation anxiety disorder are usually concerned that something terrible might happen to their attachment figures, which only strengthens their fears upon separating from these people.

Staying-at-home behavior is often seen in depression. Although it may resemble agoraphobic avoidance, such behavior is not driven by fear but is due to a pervasive loss of volition, interest, and energy. It is important to remember this distinction because many patients with agoraphobia become depressed, and the staying-at-home behavior may then be a consequence of depression rather than a manifestation of agoraphobia.

In relatively rare situations, a psychotic illness needs to be considered in the differential diagnosis of agoraphobia. This is the case with patients who avoid going out because of delusional beliefs that they are being followed, that someone might attempt to kill them, etc.

EPIDEMIOLOGY

The highlights of the epidemiology of panic disorder are presented in Table 2–16. Panic attacks are commonly seen in various psychiatric and medical conditions, and they also appear to be common in people who have no other health problems. Earlier estimates put the lifetime prevalence of panic attacks in the general population between 7.3% and 10% (Von Korff et al., 1985; Eaton et al., 1994). In the more recently conducted National Comorbidity Survey Replication, the lifetime prevalence of all panic attacks in adults in the United States was 28.3%, whereas the lifetime prevalence of isolated panic attacks (not occurring in the course of panic disorder or agoraphobia) was 22.7% (Kessler et al., 2006). According to these figures, most individuals who experience a panic attack at some point during their lives do not develop panic disorder or agoraphobia.

The three major epidemiological studies in the United States produced different prevalence findings for panic disorder. While the lifetime prevalence of panic disorder in the Epidemiologic Catchment Area study, based

Table 2–16. Epidemiological Data for Panic Disorder

- Lifetime prevalence of panic attacks in the United States: 7.3%–10% (*DSM-III/ DSM-III-R* criteria), 28.3% (*DSM-IV* criteria)
- Lifetime prevalence of panic disorder in the United States: 1.6% (*DSM-III* criteria, Epidemiologic Catchment Area Study), 3.5% (*DSM-III-R* criteria, National Comorbidity Survey), 4.8% (*DSM-IV* criteria, National Comorbidity Survey Replication; panic disorder without agoraphobia 3.7% + panic disorder with agoraphobia 1.1%)
- Lifetime prevalence in various countries, according to various diagnostic criteria: 0.13%–3.8% (for panic disorder), 0.73%–10.8% (for agoraphobia)
- Best-estimate lifetime prevalence rate across the world: 1.2% (for panic disorder), 3.1% (for agoraphobia)
- In the general population, panic disorder without agoraphobia is more common than panic disorder with agoraphobia, whereas in clinical settings, panic disorder with agoraphobia is more common than panic disorder without agoraphobia
- Women are more often represented than men (ratio of 2–2.5:1), particularly in clinical settings (ratio of 2.5–3:1); panic disorder with agoraphobia is 2.5 to 4 times more common in women
- More prevalent among separated, divorced, widowed, less educated, and urban dwellers
- Typical age of onset: third decade of life; mean age of onset: around age 25 years
- Bimodal distribution in the age of onset: the first peak in the age group 15–24, the second peak in the age group 45–54 years
- Characteristic help-seeking patterns: high prevalence in primary care, hospital emergency departments, and certain specialized medical settings (e.g., cardiology, gastroenterology, neurology, vestibular disorders clinics)

on the *DSM-III* criteria, was 1.6% (Regier et al., 1988; Eaton et al., 1991), the lifetime prevalence rate of panic disorder in the National Comorbidity Survey, based on the *DSM-III-R* criteria, was 3.5% (Eaton et al., 1994) and in the National Comorbidity Survey Replication, using *DSM-IV* criteria, it was 4.8% (Kessler et al., 2006). The latter figure is a sum of the lifetime prevalence rates for panic disorder without agoraphobia (3.7%) and panic disorder with agoraphobia (1.1%). With the use of the *DSM-III-R* and *DSM-IV* diagnostic criteria, there may have been a tendency to lower diagnostic thresholds for panic attacks, panic disorder, and agoraphobia, perhaps leading to an overestimation of their prevalence rates.

Not surprisingly, prevalence rates of panic disorder and agoraphobia are vastly different in different countries. The lifetime prevalence of panic disorder ranges from 0.13% in rural Taiwan (Hwu et al., 1989) to 3.8% in the Netherlands (Bijl et al., 1998), whereas the lifetime prevalence of agoraphobia ranges from 0.73% in Hong Kong (Chen et al., 1993) to 10.8% in Switzerland (Wacker et al., 1992). The main sources of variability in these prevalence rates are use of the different diagnostic criteria and different diagnostic instruments and social and cultural factors. Panic disorder and agoraphobia appear to be generally less common in Asian countries. The best-estimate lifetime prevalence rates across epidemiological studies published between 1980 and 2004 and conducted in various countries were 1.2% for panic disorder and 3.1% for agoraphobia (Somers et al., 2006).

As already noted, panic disorder without agoraphobia may be more than three times more prevalent than panic disorder with agoraphobia in the general population (Kessler et al., 2006). In contrast, panic disorder without agoraphobia is less often encountered in clinical samples than is panic disorder with agoraphobia, suggesting that individuals with panic disorder who seek help are more likely to have agoraphobia and that panic disorder with agoraphobia is a more severe variant of the condition.

The implications of epidemiological findings regarding the prevalence of agoraphobia have been controversial (see Diagnostic and Conceptual Issues, above). While agoraphobia without a history of panic disorder has been reported to occur so rarely that the usefulness of this diagnosis has been put into doubt (e.g., Goisman et al., 1995), the higher best estimate prevalence rates for agoraphobia than for panic disorder (Somers et al., 2006) suggest that agoraphobia may not be related solely to panic disorder.

Agoraphobia is less frequently encountered than specific phobias in the general population (e.g., Kessler et al., 1994; Magee et al., 1996), but this relationship is the reverse in clinical populations, with agoraphobia there being more prevalent than specific phobias. This indicates that agoraphobia tends to be more disabling than specific phobias.

Like most other anxiety disorders, panic disorder is more frequent among women; this has been a consistent finding in epidemiological studies conducted around the world. Across the studies, women in the general population appear to be 2–2.5 times more likely to have panic disorder than men (e.g., Regier et al., 1988; Eaton et al., 1991, 1994). In clinical populations, women with panic disorder outnumber men with the ratio of 2.5–3:1 (Katerndahl and Realini, 1993). Perhaps women are more likely to seek help for panic disorder because of the greater severity of panic disorder in women (especially when panic disorder is accompanied by agoraphobia) and women's greater propensity to seek help for health-related problems. Men with panic disorder, by contrast, may be more inclined to attempt to alleviate their distress through the use of alcohol, which may help explain a lower proportion of men in clinical samples of panic patients.

When panic disorder is associated with agoraphobia, the female-to-male ratio is 2.5–4:1, and 75%–80% of patients are women (Eaton et al., 1994; Yonkers et al., 1998). The preponderance of women among patients with agoraphobia is usually explained as a consequence of social and cultural factors; thus, agoraphobia has been portrayed as a "caricature of the traditional female roles," with society generally reinforcing dependence and avoidance as coping mechanisms in women (Clum and Knowles, 1991). Also, an expression of fear and avoidance behavior may be more socially acceptable in women (Fodor, 1974; Chambless and Mason, 1986).

Panic disorder is more common among the widowed, divorced, and separated than among married individuals (Lepine and Lellouch, 1994). People who live in an urban environment and have lower levels of education may also be more likely to have panic disorder (Eaton et al., 1994).

Although panic disorder can begin at any age, its onset is rare in children and the elderly. Most commonly, the onset of panic disorder is in a person's early to mid-20s, with the mean age of onset being around 25 years (Eaton et al., 1994). There also seems to be a bimodal distribution in the age of onset of panic disorder: the first peak was noted in the age group of 15–24 years, whereas the second peak was found in the age group of 45–54 years (Eaton et al., 1994). Thus, it is not at all rare to see the onset of panic disorder in mid-life, after the age of 40. Panic disorder with agoraphobia (and agoraphobia with or without panic attacks) may have an earlier onset than panic disorder without agoraphobia, but both usually begin in the third decade of life.

Patients with panic disorder have a characteristic pattern of help seeking. Because of their physical symptoms, they often seek help in hospital emergency departments and primary care settings; the current prevalence rate of panic disorder in the primary care setting in various countries was estimated to be around 1%, but varied from 0.2% to 3.5% (Ustun and Sartorius, 1995). About 13% of patients in primary care were found to have panic disorder in another study (Katon et al., 1986). The frequency with which panic disorder is found in certain specialized medical settings is often higher. Between 16% and 23% of outpatients in cardiac clinics may have panic disorder (Chignon et al., 1993; Barsky et al., 1996), and one study reported a lifetime prevalence of panic disorder of almost 22% among patients with noncardiac chest pain (angina-like pain in the absence of cardiac etiology) (White et al., 2008). Patients with panic disorder are also more likely to be seen in gastroenterology, neurology, and vestibular disorders clinics. Because of the somatic nature of their symptoms and the pattern of seeking help in medical settings, many cases of panic disorder are missed or misdiagnosed.

COURSE AND PROGNOSIS

The course of panic disorder is difficult to study for several reasons. Some of them are unique to panic disorder, whereas others are also applicable to long-standing conditions in general.

- First, it is difficult to find representative samples of persons with panic disorder who have not had any treatment. Studies of the course of panic disorder have almost invariably been conducted in patients who have received some treatment; hence, very little is known about the course of untreated panic disorder.
- Second, even after treatment has been completed, many panic patients occasionally or continuously receive additional pharmacological and/or psychological treatment, so that studying the course of panic disorder under absolutely "naturalistic" conditions (i.e., when patients receive no treatment at all) is difficult.
- Third, the course of treated panic disorder may depend on the type of treatment received, and numbers of patients who received different types of treatment should not be added to create larger samples.
- Fourth, there are no universally accepted definitions of improvement, response, remission, recovery, exacerbation, relapse, and recurrence of panic disorder. This means that criteria for characterizing the course of panic disorder are often arbitrary and differ from one study to another.
- Fifth, some patients exhibit significant improvement in one aspect of panic disorder (e.g., they may have only occasional panic attacks), while their improvement in other areas is much less impressive (e.g., they may still resort to some phobic avoidance). In such cases, it is difficult to characterize overall improvement.
- Finally, regardless of how long follow-up studies last, there are some patients whose status might change during further follow-up; it is unknown how many patients would experience such a change because of the need to impose a cross-sectional cutoff. Thus, patients who were panic-free and judged to be in remission at the end of a 5-year follow-up period might subsequently have a recurrence.

Keeping in mind these methodological problems, it is not surprising that results of follow-up studies of panic disorder are inconsistent. However, some conclusions about the course of panic disorder can still be made (Table 2–17).

Table 2–17. Long-Term Course of Treated Panic Disorder

Characterization of Course	Percentage Estimate
Recovery	30%–35%
Complete or almost complete remission	
No impairment in functioning	
No need for treatment	
Chronic, with Fluctuations	50%
Mild and/or occasional symptoms	
Minor and/or occasional interference with functioning	
Occasional, sometimes a prolonged need for treatment	
Chronic, without Fluctuations	15%–20%
Persistent and moderate to severe symptoms	
Complications of panic disorder more likely	
Continuous interference with functioning	
Continuous need for treatment	

First, panic disorder tends to be a chronic condition in the majority of patients. For example, after a 5-year follow-up of patients with panic disorder, only 12% had no symptoms at all and were not receiving any treatment (Faravelli et al., 1995). Similar findings were reported by two long-term follow-up studies, conducted 11 years (Swoboda et al., 2003) and 15 years (Andersch and Hetta, 2003) after pharmacological treatment of panic disorder. At 11-year follow-up, only one third of patients were considered to be in complete remission, although two thirds did not have a panic attack during the year preceding the follow-up. At 15-year follow-up, 18% of patients showed complete recovery (no panic attacks and no pharmacotherapy for 10 years prior to follow-up), whereas 13% were recovered but still taking medication. At 11-year and 15-year follow-up, the proportion of patients who met diagnostic criteria for panic disorder was 12.5% and 18%, respectively. At 15-year follow-up, 51% reported recurrent panic attacks. As for agoraphobia, significant avoidance was found in 46% of patients at 11-year follow-up and in 20% of patients at 15-year follow-up. These findings suggest that complete and permanent recovery in panic disorder—when all the relevant criteria for such a recovery are taken into account—does not occur often.

A second conclusion is that despite chronicity, the overall outcome of treated panic disorder is favorable. This means that most patients have relatively minor problems in one or more domains of panic disorder; these problems generally do not interfere with their functioning, interfere mildly to moderately, or interfere only at certain times. For example, in the 11-year and 15-year follow-up studies of panic disorder, the vast majority (78%–94%) of patients did not show impairment in functioning in the areas of work and family life (Andersch and Hetta, 2003; Swoboda et al., 2003).

Third, the precise proportion of panic patients with a fluctuating course is unknown, but rough estimates suggest that up to 50% exhibit this pattern over time (American Psychiatric Association, 2000). When panic disorder exhibits a fluctuating course, exacerbations can be precipitated by factors such as interpersonal conflicts, excessive consumption of caffeine, or hormonal changes during a premenstrual period. The frequency of panic attacks may decrease during pregnancy or the attacks may completely disappear during that time (e.g., Villeponteaux et al., 1992). In the postpartum period, however, panic attacks often return.

A fourth conclusion about the course of panic disorder is that in a minority of patients (15%–20% of all treated patients), various components of the disorder persist and patients usually remain impaired and require ongoing treatment. This group of patients is also most likely to develop complications, particularly depression and alcohol-related problems.

The course of agoraphobia may follow the course of panic disorder, so that with fewer and less severe panic attacks, agoraphobia also becomes less prominent, and vice versa. In other cases, there does not appear to be such a strong link between panic attacks and agoraphobic avoidance, and agoraphobia takes a course of its own. Thus, agoraphobia may persist in patients who have not had panic attacks for a long time.

Prognosis

Several follow-up studies have identified factors that are predictive of a more chronic course and a relatively poor prognosis of panic disorder (Table 2–18) (Noyes et al., 1993; Katschnig et al., 1995; O'Rourke et al., 1996; Andersch and Hetta, 2003). These factors include being single, earlier onset and longer duration of panic disorder before commencing treatment, greater severity of panic attacks and agoraphobia, presence of a personality disorder, co-occurrence of depression, and poor response to initial

Table 2–18. Factors Indicating a More Chronic Course and Relatively Poor Prognosis in Panic Disorder

Being single

Earlier onset of panic disorder

Longer duration of panic disorder before onset of treatment

Greater severity of panic attacks

Greater severity of agoraphobia

Presence of a personality disorder

Co-occurrence of depression

Poor response to initial treatment

treatment. Women seem to be more likely than men to have recurrences of panic disorder (Yonkers et al., 1998), but this effect may be mediated through women's greater propensity to develop agoraphobia, which is itself associated with a poorer prognosis.

Complications

Panic disorder may be complicated by depression and alcohol-related disorders. The links between these disorders are discussed in Relationship Between Panic Disorder and Other Disorders (above). Unlike patients with some of the other anxiety disorders, panic patients may be more aversive to other psychotropic substances, especially those that might have precipitated the first panic attack or exacerbated the course of the panic disorder (e.g., cannabis, cocaine).

Panic disorder has been associated with higher rates of suicide, suicide attempts, and suicidal ideation in comparison with the rates in the general population. Suicide was reported as a cause of death in 20% of patients with panic disorder (Coryell et al., 1982). Lifetime suicide attempt rates were 20% in an epidemiological study (Weissman et al., 1989; Johnson et al., 1990) and 42% in one clinical study (Lepine et al., 1993). Rates of suicidal ideation in panic disorder were 44% in an epidemiological sample (Weissman et al., 1989; Johnson et al., 1990) and 60% in a clinical sample (Lepine et al., 1993). These findings were intuitively surprising, as one would not expect more suicide and parasuicidal phenomena and behaviors among people who often have a very strong fear of death and dying.

Results of the subsequent research have suggested that the increased rates of suicidal ideation, suicide attempts, and suicide in panic patients may be attributed to the co-occurring conditions (e.g., depression, alcohol-related disorders, some personality disorders) known to be associated with a higher risk of suicide and parasuicidal phenomena and behaviors (e.g., Hornig and McNally, 1995; Warshaw et al., 2000; Vickers and McNally, 2004). There may be other mechanisms that increase this risk in panic patients. One population-based longitudinal study has confirmed a cross-sectional association of panic disorder or agoraphobia with suicidal ideation and suicide attempts, but it did not find a relationship between pre-existing panic disorder or agoraphobia and the subsequent suicidal ideation and suicide attempts (Sareen et al., 2005). Therefore, this link remains poorly understood and requires further research.

Another intriguing finding is a higher mortality rate among patients with panic disorder. Men with panic disorder seem to have a higher risk of cardiovascular and cerebrovascular diseases and die earlier from these diseases than men without panic disorder (Coryell et al., 1982, 1986; Weissman et al., 1990; Allgulander and Lavori, 1991; Kawachi et al., 1994). Postmenopausal women with panic attacks were also found to have a higher risk of cardiovascular morbidity and mortality (Smoller et al., 2007).

The clinical implications of the link between panic disorder and cardio-vascular disease are not entirely clear, except for making a stronger case for early and aggressive treatment of panic disorder as a way of decreasing the likelihood of this morbidity. It is not known whether this risk is a direct or indirect consequence of panic disorder. Panic disorder and panic attacks have been hypothesized to cause ventricular arrhythmias, coronary artery disease, myocardial infarction, and/or sudden cardiac death as a result of hyperventilation (Kawachi et al., 1994), sympathetic hyperactivity and "mental stress" (Katon, 1990; Fleet et al., 2000a), coronary vasospasm (Esler et al., 2004), myocardial perfusion defects (Fleet et al., 2005), or decreased vagal tone and the associated, decreased heart rate variability (Kawachi et al., 1995; Fleet et al., 2000a; Gorman and Sloan, 2000; Lavoie et al., 2004). It is possible that panic disorder confers an increased risk of heart disease because of its strong association with hypertension (White and Baker, 1986; Davies et al., 1999), high blood cholesterol levels (Bajwa et al., 1992), physical inactivity (as a consequence of the fear of the exercise-induced physical symptoms), and cigarette smoking (Pohl et al., 1992; Amering et al., 1999; Breslau and Klein, 1999). There may also be a link with cardiovascular disease via depression, which often accompanies panic disorder and has a well-established association with cardiovascular disease (Jiang et al., 2005).

Panic Disorder and Quality of Life

Panic disorder has an adverse effect on the quality of life (e.g., Markowitz et al., 1989; Candilis et al., 1999). The impairment in one or more domains of functioning as a result of panic disorder can be severe. Panic patients have often been found to have significant problems in marital and family func-tioning, general social and interpersonal functioning, and occupational and academic functioning. Because they often feel that no one understands them, panic patients may withdraw and find themselves socially isolated. Alternatively, they respond with anger and hostility toward partners, family members, and friends, creating marital, family, or interpersonal strife.

Many patients with panic disorder feel that they are unable to work or that their work performance is not satisfactory. Frequent absence from work may lead to loss of a job, and unemployment rates among panic patients are generally high (Leon et al., 1995). The consequences of unem-ployment include financial difficulties, and many panic patients receive financial assistance or disability payments (Klerman et al., 1991). Some patients find it difficult to attend school and feel that they have no choice but to drop out.

Panic disorder is associated with increased health care utilization. Panic patients seek treatment in hospital emergency departments and various medical and psychiatric settings and use primary care and specialized medical services far more often than patients with other psychiatric disorders and patients without psychiatric illness (Markowitz et al., 1989; Klerman et al., 1991; Leon et al., 1995; Katon, 1996; see also Epidemiology, above). Panic patients' frequent presentations to medical facilities and relatively poor recognition of panic disorder in such settings (e.g., Fifer et al., 1994; Fleet et al., 1996) result in substantial costs, mainly because of the expensive and often unnecessary medical procedures (e.g., Salvador-Carulla et al., 1995; Katon, 1996).

ETIOLOGY AND PATHOGENESIS

Etiological factors unique to panic disorder have not been elucidated. It is often assumed that panic disorder is a consequence of various interactions between etiological factors. People who develop panic attacks and panic disorder seem to carry a certain predisposition, but it is not clear whether the presence of some predisposing factors is necessary for *all* panic attacks and *all* cases of panic disorder. The predisposition is usually conceptualized in terms of genetic and/or psychological vulnerability. Panic attacks may then occur through various pathophysiological (e.g., hyperventilation) and/or cognitive and other psychological (e.g., catastrophic appraisal of physical sensations) mechanisms. However, reasons for triggering these mechanisms (and not others) remain elusive. The main models that account for etiology and pathogenesis of panic disorder are presented below.

BIOLOGICAL MODELS

Table 2–19 summarizes the hypothesized pathophysiological mechanisms that may be relatively specific for panic attacks and panic disorder.

Genetic Factors

In family studies, the lifetime prevalence rate of panic disorder among first-degree relatives of probands with panic disorder has been 10%–17.3%, which compares to the lifetime prevalence rate of panic disorder among control subjects of 0.8%–3.5% (Crowe et al., 1983; Noyes et al., 1986; Mendlewicz et al., 1993; Weissman, 1993; Fyer et al., 1995). Compared to first-degree relatives of persons without panic disorder, first-degree relatives of persons with panic disorder may be 17.7 times more at risk of developing panic disorder (Weissman, 1993). This risk is partly related to the age of onset of panic disorder: the earlier the age of onset (prior to the age of 20), the more likely it is for first-degree relatives to also have panic disorder (Goldstein et al., 1997). Thus, early-onset panic disorder may have a stronger familial or genetic component than panic disorder with a later onset in life. A higher prevalence of panic disorder in certain families and

Table 2–19. Hypothesized Pathophysiological Mechanisms That May Be Relatively Specific for Panic Attacks and Panic Disorder

- An abnormally sensitive anxiety-regulating mechanism (originating in the amygdala) lowers the threshold for tolerating sensory information, so that ordinary sensory information activates autonomic responses (through brain-stem nuclei) and the accompanying catastrophic cognitions (through the cortex), leading to a panic attack
- Panic attacks can be artificially induced by increasing the respiration rate (hyperventilation), inhaling carbon dioxide, or disrupting the acid-base balance
- Acute hyperventilation leads to a panic attack via hypocapnia and alkalosis
- A panic attack may result from hypersensitivity to carbon dioxide of the brain-stem chemoreceptors, so that they react excessively to an even minor increase in concentration of carbon dioxide
- A panic attack is a consequence of the premature and inappropriate activation of the alarm mechanism, which aims to prevent choking and ensure survival. This alarm mechanism involves hyperventilation and attempts to lower the concentration of carbon dioxide in an individual who is hypersensitive to carbon dioxide and therefore has a lower threshold for activating the alarm mechanism (theory of the false suffocation alarm)
- A panic attack is a consequence of the increased central noradrenergic activity (hypersensitivity of the presynaptic α-2 receptors, increased firing rate of the locus coeruleus)
- Failure of the GABA system to inhibit the locus coeruleus leads to a panic attack

among first-degree relatives of persons with panic disorder, however, does not constitute evidence that panic disorder is a genetically based condition.

There may also be a genetic link between panic disorder, major depression, alcoholism, social anxiety disorder, and bipolar affective disorder. In comparison with first-degree relatives of persons without panic disorder, first-degree relatives of persons with panic disorder had higher rates of social anxiety disorder and major depression (Goldstein et al., 1994; Maier et al., 1995), whereas alcoholism was almost four times more common among male relatives (Crowe et al., 1983). Panic disorder was also more common among relatives of persons with major depression than among relatives of individuals without major depression. The occurrence of panic disorder in people with bipolar affective disorder may be determined by genetic factors (Mackinnon et al., 1997).

Studies of panic disorder among twins have produced conflicting results. While some studies found a higher concordance rate for panic disorder among monozygotic twins than among dizygotic twins (Torgersen, 1983; Skre et al., 1993; Tsuang et al., 2004), there was no such difference in at least one twin study (Andrews et al., 1990). In addition, the concordance rate for panic disorder in monozygotic twins was 31%

(Torgersen, 1983; Tsuang et al., 2004), suggesting that nongenetic factors play an important role in the development of the condition. The risk of inheriting panic disorder, calculated in a female twin study, was estimated at 30%–40% (Kendler et al., 1993); this estimate is considerably lower than the corresponding figures for schizophrenia and bipolar affective disorder.

The mode of inheriting panic disorder is not known, but a single-gene transmission appears unlikely (e.g., Maron et al., 2005). It is also not known what exactly is inherited that constitutes a predisposition to develop panic disorder. A general vulnerability to develop anxiety may be more likely to be inherited than panic disorder itself (Krystal et al., 1996).

Induction of Panic Attacks

The purpose of panic induction studies has been to shed more light on the mechanisms involved in the occurrence of panic attacks. Various substances have been administered to induce panic attacks. Some of them, such as carbon dioxide, sodium lactate, and sodium bicarbonate, change the acid-base balance and affect levels of carbon dioxide and respiration rate, leading to panic. This mechanism involves hypersensitivity to carbon dioxide and/or hyperventilation (both described below). Other substances (e.g., yohimbin, fenfluramine, m-chlorophenylpiperazine, flumazenil, and cholecystokinin) induce panic attacks by acting on the noradrenaline, serotonin, or gamma-aminobutyric acid (GABA) neurotransmitter systems.

The most important finding of panic induction studies is that panic attacks are much more likely to be induced in individuals with panic disorder than in those without panic disorder. For example, panic attacks were induced by sodium lactate infusions in 67% of individuals with panic disorder, 7%–22% of those with other psychiatric disorders, and 13% of people without any psychiatric disorder (Liebowitz et al., 1985; Cowley and Arana, 1990). This finding has been a subject to two different interpretations. First, the occurrence of panic attacks may be a direct consequence of the pathophysiological changes produced by "panicogenic" substances; second, cognitive factors (e.g., fear of physical symptoms, catastrophic appraisal of physical symptoms) account for the occurrence of panic attacks, as physical symptoms are induced in almost all individuals, whereas only some go on to develop a panic attack. The main problem with panic induction studies has been the uncertainty about the extent to which their findings might be generalized to naturally occurring panic attacks.

Role of Hyperventilation

Acute hyperventilation (rapid, shallow breathing) causes many symptoms of panic. However, hyperventilation is not always sufficient, nor is it necessary for panic attack to occur, as many panic attacks are neither preceded by nor associated with hyperventilation.

The pathophysiological changes in acute hyperventilation occur as a result of the deficit of carbon dioxide: carbon dioxide lost through over-breathing is not compensated for by its production through metabolism. The consequently decreased blood level of carbon dioxide (hypocapnia) and alkalosis lead to symptoms typical of panic attacks. Hypocapnia causes cerebral vasoconstriction and decreased delivery of oxygen to the brain tissue, which is clinically manifested through lightheadedness, dizziness, fainting feeling, blurred vision, and even depersonalization, derealization, disorientation, confusion, and agitation. Alkalosis leads to hypocalcemia, and this in turn causes numbness or tingling sensations. The clinical consequences of further pathophysiological changes are tachycardia, palpitations, chest pain or tightness in the chest, and shortness of breath.

In chronic hyperventilation, all the pathophysiological changes are compensated for, except for hypocapnia. Therefore, persons who habitually hyperventilate may develop symptoms of acute hyperventilation with minimal increase in their breathing rate. Patients with panic disorder, however, were not found to be more likely to exhibit chronic hyperventilation than people without panic disorder (Brown et al., 2003).

Other Respiratory Dysfunction in Panic Disorder

Inhalation of 5%–35% carbon dioxide is much more likely to induce panic attacks in patients with panic disorder than in persons who have never experienced panic attacks (Gorman et al., 1984). The pathophysiological mechanism involves respiratory acidosis, hypercapnia, and hypercalcemia, which cause dyspnea, choking feeling, and panic. This state may trigger hyperventilation to compensate for the respiratory and metabolic changes, but hyperventilation only leads to further symptoms of panic (Gorman et al., 1988). These findings have led to a hypothesis that panic attacks are a consequence of the hypersensitivity to carbon dioxide of the brain-stem chemoreceptors (Gorman and Papp, 1990; Papp et al., 1993). Because of this hypersensitivity, chemoreceptors react excessively to an even minor increase in the concentration of carbon dioxide, causing dyspnea and choking feeling followed by hyperventilation, all of which lead to panic.

According to the "false suffocation alarm" theory (Klein, 1993), panic attack is a consequence of the premature and inappropriate activation of the alarm mechanism, which aims to prevent choking and ensure survival. This alarm mechanism involves hyperventilation—and an attempt to lower the concentration of carbon dioxide in an individual who is hypersensitive to carbon dioxide and therefore has a lower threshold for activating the alarm. The reaction is triggered especially in those situations that signal a possibility of lack of oxygen and the consequent suffocation (e.g., being in a small, enclosed space). Several clinical findings have been listed in support of this theory. For example, dyspnea is a frequent symptom during panic attacks but it is not a manifestation of "normal" anxiety, and panic disorder is the most common anxiety disorder among people with respiratory diseases. The false suffocation alarm theory has undergone some testing of its main tenets, with mixed results.

Neuroanatomy and Pathophysiological Mechanisms

Neuroanatomical Model of Panic Disorder

The first version of this theory (Gorman et al., 1989) has proposed that panic attacks originate in brain-stem structures, specifically locus coeruleus and raphe nuclei. The limbic system was believed to play the main role in the development of anticipatory anxiety, whereas the prefrontal cortex was thought to be involved in panic-related avoidance.

In its revised version (Gorman et al., 2000), the model has suggested that individuals who go on to develop panic disorder inherit and/or develop early in life an abnormally sensitive mechanism that regulates anxiety. The brain structure crucial for the functioning of this mechanism is believed to be the central nucleus of the amygdala, which is well connected with the prefrontal cortex, hippocampus, thalamus, hypothalamus, periaqueductal gray matter, locus coeruleus, and other parts of the brain stem. The overly sensitive anxiety-regulating mechanism lowers the threshold for tolerating sensory information, so that ordinary sensory information activates autonomic responses (through brain-stem nuclei) and the accompanying catastrophic cognitions (through the cortex). Medications that reduce intensity and/or frequency of panic attacks do so by decreasing the activity of the amygdala; cognitive-behavioral therapy and other efficacious psychotherapies, by contrast, affect higher brain structures connected with the amygdala, especially the hippocampus and prefrontal cortex.

Neuroimaging Studies

Numerous neuroimaging studies have been conducted in people with panic disorder. They involved structural and functional imaging, magnetic resonance imaging, and positron emission tomography, and imaging both using and not using anxiety- and panic-provocation paradigms. The results have not been very consistent and pointed to many areas of brain that could be implicated in panic disorder. These include the amygdala, hippocampus, raphe, insula, anterior cingulate cortex, orbitofrontal cortex, parietooccipital cortex, temporal lobes, and others (e.g., Vythilingam et al., 2000; Bystritsky et al., 2001; Hasler et al., 2008; Nash et al., 2008; Uchida et al., 2008). It has been suggested that panic disorder may be characterized by an impairment of frontal-limbic coordination in the modulation of anxiety responses (Hasler et al., 2008).

Neurotransmitter Systems

There is no neurotransmitter abnormality that is specific for panic disorder. It appears that the noradrenaline (norepinephrine), serotonin, and GABA systems are involved, in proportions and combinations that vary from one person to another.

Noradrenaline Early studies of the pathophysiology of panic disorder focused on the role of the locus coeruleus, which is located in the pons and contains at least one half of all noradrenergic neurons in the central nervous system. The locus coeruleus appears to play a key role in coordinating the functioning of the sympathetic nervous system, as it is well connected with the hippocampus, amygdala, limbic system, and cerebral cortex (particularly the frontal lobe). Through the descending pathways that originate in the locus coeruleus, it also affects peripheral sympathetic activity.

Two lines of evidence suggest that there may be an increased central noradrenergic activity in panic disorder. One is the finding from animal studies that stimulation of the locus coeruleus leads to anxiety reactions that are very similar to panic attacks in humans (Redmond, 1979). The other is that several medications effective in panic disorder (e.g., tricyclic anti-depressants and benzodiazepines) decrease the firing rate of the locus coeruleus. However, the locus coeruleus may have a broader role and appears to play a part in general arousal responses and responses to novel stimuli (Aston-Jones et al., 1984). Also, not all medications that decrease the firing rate of the locus coeruleus (e.g., propranolol, morphine) show efficacy in the treatment of panic disorder.

In patients with panic disorder, panic attacks can be induced by yohimbin, an α-2 central adrenergic antagonist that increases the activity of the locus coeruleus and noradrenergic function (Charney et al., 1984). Likewise, symptoms of panic and anxiety can be alleviated by clonidine, an α-2 central adrenergic agonist that inhibits the locus coeruleus. This has led to a hypothesis that panic disorder may be characterized by hypersensitivity of presynaptic α-2 receptors (Charney and Heninger, 1986) and the consequently increased noradrenergic stimulation. Such presynaptic hypersensitivity may be counteracted by imipramine, which would help explain the efficacy of imipramine in the treatment of panic disorder.

Serotonin The administration of fenfluramine (which enhances the release of serotonin) and *m*-chlorophenylpiperazine (which is an agonist at some serotonin receptors and antagonist at other serotonin receptors) to patients with panic disorder tends to induce anxiety and panic attacks. Numerous studies suggest a role of the serotonin system in the pathogenesis of panic disorder, but the exact mechanisms through which this occurs are not well understood. It has been hypothesized that the serotonin 1_A receptor dysfunction may be relatively specific for panic disorder (Lesch et al., 1992), but this has not been corroborated. In view of these uncertainties, it is not surprising that the mechanisms accounting for the efficacy of the selective serotonin reuptake inhibitors in panic disorder remain unclear.

Gamma-aminobutyric acid   The GABA system has been implicated in the anxiety disorders in general. Administration of antagonists at the benzo-diazepine-GABA$_A$ receptors (e.g., flumazenil) induces panic attacks in patients with panic disorder (Nutt et al., 1990), whereas administration of agonists (e.g., benzodiazepines) alleviates anxiety and panic. It is largely on the basis of these findings that alterations at the level of the benzodiaze-pine-GABA$_A$ receptors have been hypothesized in panic disorder.

Since GABA normally inhibits functioning of the locus coeruleus, thereby decreasing anxiety and preventing panic attacks, it has been hypothesized that the GABA system fails to inhibit the locus coeruleus. This may occur as a consequence of various primary mechanisms. For example, individuals with panic disorder may have fewer benzodiazepine-GABA$_A$ receptors, a possi-bility suggested by the finding of decreased benzodiazepine receptor binding in imaging studies (Malizia et al., 1998; Bremner et al., 2000a). Another possibility is that levels of GABA are decreased in patients with panic disorder (Goddard et al., 2001b). The sensitivity of benzodiazepine-GABA$_A$ receptors may be decreased in panic disorder (Roy-Byrne et al., 1990) or, more generally, their functioning is altered (Nutt et al., 1990; Hasler et al., 2008). Finally, there may be a deficiency in endogenous anxio-lytic substances or an excess of endogenous, anxiogenic/panicogenic sub-stances, which act via benzodiazepine-GABA$_A$ receptors.

PSYCHOLOGICAL MODELS

Cognitive Approaches

All cognitive theories of panic disorder (Table 2–20) share a view that the main feature of panic disorder, as well as other anxiety disorders, is the exaggerated perception of threat. It is the *nature* of this threat that distin-guishes panic disorder from other anxiety disorders. While the perceived threat in conditions like phobias is mainly external, the perceived threat in panic disorder is of an internal nature. That is, the threat in panic disorder is perceived to originate within one's body, which accounts for panic patients' hypervigilance about and fear of physical sensations and symptoms and their proneness to misinterpret certain physical events.

Catastrophic Misinterpretation of Benign Physical Sensations and Symptoms

The most influential cognitive model of panic disorder was postulated by Clark (1986, 1988). Its main idea is that panic attack is a consequence of catastrophic misinterpretation of benign physical sensations and

Table 2–20. Cognitive Aspects of Panic Disorder

Common to All Anxiety Disorders

Exaggerated perception of threat

Relatively Specific for Panic Disorder

The threat is perceived to originate within one's body

Hypervigilance about physical sensations and symptoms and bodily functions

Greater likelihood of misinterpreting physical sensations and symptoms as a sign of impending catastrophe

Beliefs about dangerousness of anxiety and its (physical) symptoms, leading to fear of anxiety and its (physical) symptoms

Greater need for control over physical sensations and symptoms and bodily functions

---

symptoms. In other words, physical sensations and symptoms do not lead to a panic attack unless they have been misinterpreted in a catastrophic fashion, that is, unless they have been appraised as dangerous and portending a disastrous outcome (death or a life-threatening medical condition, or, less often, loss of control or loss of sanity).

Physical symptoms, such as those of autonomic hyperactivity, initially occur as a physiological component of anxiety and are subsequently subjected to misinterpretation. For example, palpitations are typically misinterpreted as meaning that the person is having a heart attack and is about to die; this misinterpretation then intensifies anxiety and leads to further arousal and more physical symptoms. These symptoms are in turn further misinterpreted in a catastrophic manner, which creates a vicious cycle and a panic attack. Sensations and symptoms most likely to be misinterpreted are usually those that occur suddenly, that have not been experienced before, or for which the person does not have a ready explanation.

The proneness to misinterpret physical sensations and symptoms catastrophically may be a consequence of interacting with the parents who are preoccupied with health, symptoms, and bodily functions; as such, this proneness may be present long before the very first panic attack. It may also be reinforced by the attention and care that the person received after the first panic attack. If the tendency to make catastrophic misinterpretations persists after the first panic attack, the person will be likely to become apprehensive about future panic attacks, and thus develop panic disorder.

According to Clark's theory, panic disorder is maintained by one or both of the following mechanisms:

1. Persistent hypervigilance about physical sensations and symptoms lowers the threshold at which they are experienced. As a result, there are more "opportunities" to misinterpret sensations and symptoms catastrophically.

2. Avoidance of all physical activities (e.g., physical recreation, exercise, sport) that could induce feared physical sensations and symptoms prevents the person from finding out that these sensations and symptoms are not dangerous.

The catastrophic-misinterpretation model of panic disorder has received substantial support, although it has not been able to give a convincing account of all instances of panic attacks (e.g., nocturnal panic attacks). Also, panic attacks are not always preceded by catastrophic misinterpretation of physical sensations and symptoms (Rachman et al., 1988; Wolpe and Rowan, 1988), so that such an appraisal is not always necessary for panic attacks to develop. In accordance with the model, however, a panic attack can be prevented if symptoms induced by hyperventilation or other panic induction procedure are not appraised catastrophically. This has been used in treatment, as part of the cognitive therapy of panic disorder.

Beliefs About the Dangerousness of Anxiety

This model of panic disorder, sometimes referred to as the "expectancy model," was derived from the concept of anxiety sensitivity (Reiss and McNally, 1985; Reiss, 1991). This concept denotes a fear of anxiety-related sensations and symptoms, based on beliefs that anxiety and its symptoms have dangerous consequences, with these consequences being physical (e.g., a serious disease, death), psychological (e.g., loss of sanity), or social (e.g., humiliation). Anxiety sensitivity is akin to a stable personality dimension and represents a specific risk factor for developing panic disorder (McNally and Lorenz, 1987; Reiss, 1991). That is, strong beliefs that anxiety symptoms are dangerous are present before the first panic attack and predict the occurrence of panic disorder. High levels of anxiety sensitivity may be genetically determined (Stein MB et al., 1999a), but may also result from parental reinforcement of the child's sick role (Watt et al., 1998) or parental threatening, hostile, and rejecting behaviors (Scher and Stein, 2003).

Two issues have dominated research on the role of anxiety sensitivity in panic disorder. The first is the issue of anxiety sensitivity as a specific risk or vulnerability factor for panic disorder. The findings have been mixed. Some studies have supported the notion that high levels of anxiety sensitivity predict the occurrence of panic disorder (e.g., Maller and Reiss, 1992; Schmidt et al., 1997, 1999). Other studies have reported that high levels of anxiety sensitivity predict only panic symptoms and panic attacks, but not panic disorder (Plehn and Peterson, 2002; Struzik et al., 2004), or that they denote vulnerability for the development of hypochondriasis (Watt and Stewart, 2000).

The other issue is the nature of the link between anxiety sensitivity and panic disorder. Although levels of anxiety sensitivity tend to be higher among people with panic disorder than among those with other disorders, anxiety sensitivity was not found to have an exclusive relationship with panic disorder. High levels of anxiety sensitivity also characterize some of the other anxiety disorders (Taylor et al., 1992; Orsillo et al., 1994; Cox et al., 2001) and major depression (Otto et al., 1995; Taylor et al., 1996). It appears that only one component of anxiety sensitivity—concerns about physical consequences of anxiety—might be specifically associated with panic disorder (Zinbarg et al., 1997). This is in accordance with panic patients' hypervigilance about physical symptoms.

The concept of anxiety sensitivity has been of great interest and value in the study of the psychopathology of panic disorder. The account of panic disorder based on anxiety sensitivity can be combined with the catastrophic-misinterpretation theory in that people with high levels of anxiety sensitivity are more likely to misinterpret certain physical symptoms of anxiety as dangerous, because their underlying beliefs about and fears of these symptoms predispose them to do so. In other words, heightened anxiety sensitivity may reflect a catastrophic thinking style associated with panic disorder, other anxiety disorders, and hypochondriasis (Cox et al., 2001).

Panic Attacks as False Alarms

Barlow (1988) has proposed a model of panic disorder that includes components from biological, basic emotion, learning (behavioral), and cognitive theories. His theory first makes a distinction between fear and anxiety (Table 2–21). Fear is one of the "basic emotions" with a distinct physiological pattern (autonomic hyperarousal), which represents an acute, short-lasting response to the perceived, immediate threat ("true alarm"). Anxiety is a longer lasting "state of mood," which lacks a distinct physiological pattern and is more cognitive in nature, being characterized by

Table 2–21. **Distinctions Between Fear and Anxiety and Between Panic Attacks and Anticipatory Anxiety** [a]

Characteristics	Fear and Panic Attacks	Anxiety and Anticipatory Anxiety
Appraisal of threat	Clear and immediate	Somewhat vague and more distant (in the future)
Physiological response	Autonomic hyperarousal	Less clear, often absent
Behavioral response	"Fight or flight"	No clear and immediate behavioral response
Onset, course, and duration	Abrupt onset, acute, short lasting	Gradual onset, chronic, long lasting

[a] Distinctions according to Barlow (1988).

apprehension about harm and danger in the future. Within this framework, panic attack is conceptualized as fear but, more precisely, as a "false alarm," because real danger is not present. Except for the presence or absence of real danger, there is no difference between panic attacks and fear in terms of biological (autonomic hyperarousal), cognitive (appraisal of threat as immediate), and behavioral ("fight-or-flight") responses.

Barlow (1988) has suggested that there has to be both a biological and psychological vulnerability for the first panic attack to develop. Biological vulnerability refers to a susceptibility to be easily aroused, especially in response to stress; psychological vulnerability, which results from adverse childhood events and interactions with parents, pertains to the lack of security and a strong sense that one has little or no control over one's life. The theory accounts for two further developments after the initial panic attack. The first is the occurrence of the specific type of anxiety or anxious apprehension about having another panic attack. Panic is then usually perceived as even more unpleasant, uncontrollable, and dangerous, which contributes to the maintenance of panic disorder.

In the second development, following the first panic attack, a link is established between the experience of the false alarm on one hand and physical symptoms and the accompanying "negative" cognitions on the other—a process called "interoceptive conditioning." As a result, the occurrence of physical symptoms or certain associated thoughts may trigger panic attacks; these conditioned panic attacks are referred to as "learned alarms."

Through the false-alarm model of panic disorder, an important attempt has been made to integrate knowledge about panic and anxiety from different perspectives. Certain components of the model are somewhat controversial—for example, the distinction between panic (fear) and anxiety—but overall, the model has been widely accepted and used as a foundation for a specific and effective type of cognitive-behavioral therapy, panic control treatment.

Other Cognitive Factors

Another phenomenon that may be important in the development of panic disorder is a loss of the sense of control, often described by patients as the hallmark of their experience of a panic attack. If this is the case, can a restoration of this sense of control, even if it is an illusion, prevent panic attacks? This has been tested in a study in which panic attacks were induced by carbon dioxide inhalations (Sanderson et al., 1989). Subjects who were led to believe that they had some control over the situation by changing the concentration of carbon dioxide during inhalations, and thereby decreasing the likelihood of having panic attacks, had significantly fewer panic attacks than those who did not have this illusion of control. This study shows that, at least in some individuals, loss of the sense of control is associated with panic attacks. But this loss may precede panic attacks, just as it may be a consequence of panic disorder.

Expectations of panic attacks in general, and expectations of the attacks in certain situations in particular, have been associated with the occurrence of agoraphobia (see Table 2–10). The more a person expects a panic attack to occur, the more likely it is for panic to actually occur (Margraf et al., 1986). This is so because the vigilance and arousal accompanying such expectations make it easier for physical symptoms to appear; a catastrophic appraisal of such symptoms then leads to a panic attack.

Psychodynamic Approaches

Modern psychodynamic accounts of panic disorder (Table 2–22) all share a view that panic attacks are not spontaneous (unexpected); rather, panic attacks are usually preceded by events that have a unique, unconscious meaning for the person. This meaning then triggers a panic attack by automatically activating relevant neurophysiological mechanisms.

What are the unconscious meanings and mechanisms that could trigger a panic attack? According to the integrative model (Shear et al., 1993), panic attacks are triggered by the frightening thoughts and fantasies related to the fear of separation and abandonment by the mighty parental figures and others. This particular fear is a consequence of the interaction between the innately anxious, inhibited child and the overcontrolling, critical parents and the consequent conflict between dependence and independence. Other manifestations of this unresolved conflict are the following, alternating or simultaneously present, phenomena: excessive reliance on others, fear of interpersonal intimacy, and failure to attain a satisfying measure of independence. As a result of these dynamics, panic patients often harbor negative, angry, and hostile feelings toward their parents and other persons important in their lives, but at the same time they are extremely afraid of

Table 2–22. Psychodynamic Themes in Panic Disorder

- Panic attacks are triggered by events that have a unique, unconscious meaning for the person
- Fears of separation and abandonment
- Unresolved conflict between dependence and independence
    Excessive reliance on others
    Fear of interpersonal intimacy
    Failure to attain a satisfying measure of independence
- Ambivalent attitudes toward significant others
- Finding a bearable "interpersonal distance," so that significant others are neither too close (controlling) nor too far (impossible to rely on)

---

such feelings and use various defense mechanisms to avoid them. The main problem that panic patients face is to find a bearable "interpersonal distance" so that significant, mighty others are neither too close nor too far.

While the mainstream psychodynamic approach to panic disorder emphasizes underlying intrapsychic conflicts, self-psychology proposes a "deficit model." According to this approach, panic disorder is conceptualized as a result of a structural defect, with consequent deficiencies in the control of anxiety (Kohut, 1971, 1977). This defect is attributed to the parents' inability to empathize with the child, so that the child cannot feel secure. A fragile and incohesive self then develops and, as such, it is prone to fragmentation, which is the essence of the experience of panic (Diamond, 1985, 1987).

Psychological Accounts of Agoraphobia

The straightforward explanation of agoraphobia is that it is a consequence of recurrent panic attacks and anticipatory anxiety. As a result of conditioning, patients learn to fear those places and situations where they have had unpleasant, frightening panic attacks and symptoms (and where they now expect to have another attack). The avoidance of such places and situations reinforces agoraphobia, because avoidance decreases the possibility of having panic attacks, panic symptoms, and, more generally, anxiety and discomfort. The avoided situations are believed to be dangerous because of their link with panic attacks and panic symptoms: these are situations from which patients might have difficulty escaping in case of a panic attack or in which they might feel embarrassed and there would be no one to help in case of a panic attack. The avoidance behavior prevents disconfirmation of beliefs about such situations and about panic attacks and symptoms.

In other accounts of agoraphobia, panic attacks are not postulated as being so crucial in the development of agoraphobia. Instead, the avoidance behavior might have meanings and purposes other than just reducing the possibility of having a panic attack. The psychodynamic model of agoraphobia is a prime example of such an approach.

The classical psychoanalytic explanation (Fenichel, 1945; Miller, 1953) is that agoraphobia serves the purpose of "protecting" women from unconscious, forbidden sexual drives that suggest promiscuous tendencies. By developing agoraphobia and ultimately by becoming homebound, such women no longer have an "opportunity" to be unfaithful to their partners, who are often depicted as controlling and jealous. In this scenario, agoraphobia may also serve the purpose of "saving the marriage" (or saving the relationship, in a wider sense), and this is the secondary gain from having agoraphobia. Partners of agoraphobic patients may also "benefit" from agoraphobia, as it allows them to have better control over the agoraphobia sufferers. This is consistent with the observations (e.g., Hafner, 1977) that husbands of agoraphobic patients are often reluctant to change the agoraphobic status quo, that they may sabotage the treatment of patients, and that they actually get worse (become more jealous or develop sexual dysfunction) as patients get better.

The hypothesis that agoraphobia has the "marriage-saving" function has not been confirmed: studies generally show that marital functioning improves, rather than deteriorates, in the course of behavioral treatment of agoraphobia, and that treatment does not affect patients' partners in a negative way (Lange and van Dyck, 1992; Emmelkamp and Gerlsma, 1994). Moreover, studies could not confirm that marriages of most patients with agoraphobia differed significantly from the marriages of persons without agoraphobia (Buglass et al., 1977; Arrindell and Emmelkamp, 1986; McLeod, 1994). There is a subset of patients with agoraphobia, however, who are in a dysfunctional marital relationship such as that outlined above, and that is very prominent and precedes the onset of agoraphobia. This may play some role in the development of agoraphobia. One review has concluded that the issue of the role of marital dysfunction in the development of panic disorder with agoraphobia remains open (Marcaurelle et al., 2003).

Patients with agoraphobia who have significant marital problems often exhibit a paralyzing ambivalence about what to do. They want to leave their partners or seek a divorce, but are equally afraid of doing so; weighing the reasons for and against separation may be all-encompassing and exhausting. Such ambivalence may reflect an underlying conflict between autonomy and attachment (or independence and dependence), which was presumed to be an important factor in agoraphobia (Frances and Dunn, 1975).

More broadly, agoraphobia is portrayed as a prototype of dependent behavior. Patients with agoraphobia, however, do not necessarily feel "comfortable" about such dependence and may be quite resentful and hostile toward the person(s) on whom they have become dependent.

There has been some speculation about childhood "precursors" of agoraphobia. Agoraphobic patients may come from families in which mothers had a dominant and controlling position, and in which independent behavior and open expression of feelings and needs were discouraged or even punished (Goldstein and Chambless, 1978). Children growing up in such families adopt a style of avoidance in dealing with problems and leave it to others to take responsibility and "do things" for them, because they do not feel capable of acting responsibly and functioning on their own. Although there may be a link between these features in childhood and behaviors typical of agoraphobia in adulthood, the specificity of this link is questionable.

FACTORS AT THE BIOLOGICAL/PSYCHOLOGICAL INTERFACE

Childhood Separation Anxiety and School Phobia or Refusal

Separation anxiety in infants and young children has been conceptualized as a biologically determined, automatic response to separation from the mother or the mothering figure (Klein, 1981). This response is seen as the child's effective protest and serves the purpose of "assuring" that the mother will return as quickly as possible. Ultimately, separation anxiety is important for survival of the individual and the humankind. A panic attack occurs because of the inborn lowered threshold at which separation anxiety is activated. In other words, hypersensitivity to separation is at the root of a panic attack, as the attack may occur even when separation is merely being thought about or anticipated.

The findings that separation anxiety is more prominent among girls (Zitrin and Ross, 1988; Silove et al., 1993) and that it has a genetic basis only in females (Silove et al., 1995) have also been interpreted in terms of the theory of evolution. That is, strong separation anxiety in women (but not in men) was seen as adaptive and helping the survival of the species, because it "forced" women to stay with their children and thereby protect the children and care for them (Silove et al., 1995). If this is the case, then agoraphobia could be understood as a result of the conflict between these traditional, survival-driven feminine roles and expectations by contemporary Western society that women take on various social roles, be independent, and compete with men. This account of agoraphobia might also help explain why men are so underrepresented among individuals with agoraphobia.

Separation anxiety plays a pivotal role in Bowlby's (1973) attachment theory. According to this theory, separation anxiety is the prototype of any and every anxiety; it can be neutralized only through a secure attachment to the mother (or the mothering figure). If the mother fails to provide security to the child, an "insecure attachment" develops, while the separation anxiety persists. Therefore, agoraphobia will ensue in a child, who as a result of insecure attachment, feels that reliance on parents (and thus on others in general) is not possible but at the same time is afraid of separating from them.

Studies have shown that patients with panic disorder are more likely to have a history of childhood separation anxiety and school phobia (e.g., Gittelman and Klein, 1984). Also, patients with agoraphobia more often experienced prolonged separation from their mothers in childhood and were more likely to report separation or divorce of their parents and parents' deaths during childhood (Faravelli et al., 1985).

Other research has not found that there is a specific link between childhood separation anxiety and separation experiences on one hand and panic disorder or agoraphobia on the other. That is, childhood separation anxiety and separation experiences have been found just as frequently in patients with generalized anxiety disorder, social anxiety disorder, specific phobias, obsessive-compulsive disorder, depression, and eating disorders. Therefore, childhood separation anxiety may be one of the nonspecific risk factors for developing not only panic disorder and agoraphobia but also a range of other psychiatric conditions in adulthood.

Behavioral Inhibition in Childhood

Childhood behavioral inhibition is another etiological explanatory construct often used by theorists, clinicians, and researchers of various orientations. It refers to the inborn dimension of temperament, characterized by caution, inhibition, withdrawal, and physiological hyperarousal on exposure to novel stimuli and situations. When this behavior is prominent and persistent, it prevents exploration of the surrounding world, use of cognitive potentials, and self-assertion. Childhood behavioral inhibition was found to be a nonspecific risk factor for several anxiety disorders, including panic disorder, agoraphobia, and social anxiety disorder (Rosenbaum et al., 1988). The link between behavioral inhibition and social anxiety disorder is stronger and somewhat more specific, and the corresponding theory is presented in greater detail in Chapter 4.

Role of Other Developmental Factors and External Influences

Patients with panic disorder are more likely to report the occurrence of various unpleasant and/or traumatic events during their childhood, including physical and sexual abuse. They also tend to report difficulties in relationships with family members and a "family climate" characterized by strife (Raskin et al., 1982). Patients with panic disorder are more likely to perceive their parents as being overprotective, controlling, too critical and too strict, lacking in warmth and care, and/or being less interested in their children (Arrindell et al., 1983; Leon and Leon, 1990; Faravelli et al., 1991; Silove et al., 1991).

There are two fundamental problems with research of this kind. One is the retrospective methodological approach, which can be biased. The other is a lack of specificity of the research findings: traumatic experiences in childhood, unfavorable family constellation, and negative perception of parents have been found in adult patients with very different conditions.

Life Events Research

In the year preceding the onset of panic disorder, more negative life events were found among patients with panic disorder than among control group subjects. Among these life events, particularly common were separation or divorce and serious illness or death (especially sudden death) of a close family member or friend. The underlying meaning and significance of these events may be in their leading to abandonment or portending danger, in addition to such events often being experienced as loss of control (Roy-Byrne et al., 1986; Faravelli and Pallanti, 1989).

The onset of panic disorder is preceded not only by clearly unpleasant or painful events but also by such events as getting married or having a child. This suggests that some people who develop panic disorder may be particularly sensitive to any changes in their lives (Lteif and Mavissakalian,

1995). These findings have led to a hypothesis that the nature of life events preceding panic disorder is not as important as their negative interpretation (Rapee et al., 1990b); in turn, such an interpretation may be determined by various contextual factors (e.g., current health problems, perceived lack of support), personality-related factors (e.g., neuroticism), and/or childhood factors (e.g., loss of parents during childhood).

Perhaps life events that suddenly demonstrate the extent of a person's vulnerability and lack of control activate biological alarm mechanisms. Once set in motion, these mechanisms continue to operate and thus maintain panic attacks, long after the occurrence of the unpleasant or traumatic precipitating event.

TREATMENT

In view of the chronic course of panic disorder in most cases, short-term treatment is usually not sufficient. Even when significant improvement occurs after several weeks or months of treatment with medications or cognitive-behavioral therapy (CBT), as it does in 70%–80% of patients, some treatment measures need to remain in place because of the possibility of relapse and complications.

When patients with panic disorder first present for treatment, they are typically distressed by panic attacks and frightened of their consequences. They are likely to urgently seek some plausible explanation for their symptoms, reassurance that the feared catastrophe will not happen, and quick relief from at least some of their symptoms. All this can be achieved through relatively simple measures, such as psychoeducation and provision of support, in addition to administration of medication, if appropriate. The subsequent course of therapeutic action is a matter of negotiation between patients and their therapists, and ideally this occurs after patients have been well informed about available treatment options. In this process, it is important to identify patients' expectations from treatment and explore any discrepancies between these expectations and treatment realities.

Regardless of the treatment modality used, short-term (3–6 months) goals of treatment of panic disorder generally include a significant decrease in the frequency and intensity of panic attacks, and decrease in the intensity of anticipatory anxiety and panic-related avoidance. Although maintenance of the previously achieved treatment gains and further symptomatic improvement are important treatment goals in the long term (more than 3–6 months) treatment of panic disorder, the focus of treatment shifts largely to improving quality of life, minimizing impairment and likelihood of relapses and complications, and decreasing vulnerability to panic disorder (Starcevic, 1998). Long-term treatment of panic disorder takes different forms, such as maintenance pharmacotherapy, weekly sessions of psychotherapy, occasional "booster" sessions of CBT, or any combination of these treatment modalities.

PHARMACOLOGICAL TREATMENT

Indications for Pharmacotherapy and Goals of Pharmacological Treatment

Medications are usually used in the treatment of panic disorder when the condition is of moderate to severe intensity, when patients are in such distress that a quick relief is needed, and/or when panic disorder co-occurs with another psychiatric disorder, especially depression.

To the extent that panic disorder is characterized by the preponderance of unexpected panic attacks *at the time of commencing treatment*, antidepressant therapy may be useful, because antidepressants have been found to have a specific, suppressing effect on unexpected panic attacks, without significant effects on other components of panic disorder (Uhlenhuth et al., 2000, 2002). In other words, antidepressants alone may be sufficient in the treatment of panic disorder without agoraphobia, whereas treatment of panic disorder with agoraphobia may require more than an antidepressant.

The main short-term goals of pharmacotherapy of panic disorder are a decrease in the intensity and frequency of panic attacks and decrease in general symptoms of anxiety. Pharmacotherapy may also aim to suppress panic attacks. As already noted, pharmacotherapy is less effective in alleviating anticipatory anxiety and panic-related avoidance, but when this does occur, it is usually a consequence of the primary effect on (unexpected) panic attacks. The main long-term goals of pharmacotherapy are prevention of complications of panic disorder and improvement in quality of life.

Choice of Medication

Three groups of medications (selective serotonin reuptake inhibitors [SSRIs], tricyclic antidepressants [TCAs], and high-potency benzodiazepines [alprazolam, clonazepam]) and venlafaxine are approximately equally efficacious in the treatment of panic disorder. Of the SSRIs, the evidence of efficacy exists for paroxetine (Oehrberg et al., 1995; Lecrubier et al., 1997; Ballenger et al., 1998), sertraline (Londborg et al., 1998; Pohl et al., 1998; Pollack et al., 1998), fluvoxamine (den Boer et al., 1987; Black et al., 1993; Hoehn-Saric et al., 1993b), citalopram (Wade et al., 1997), fluoxetine (Michelson et al., 1998), and escitalopram (Stahl et al., 2003). As there are certain clinically meaningful differences between individual SSRIs, the choice of an SSRI for treatment of panic disorder (and other anxiety disorders) is based on the efficacy data, side effect profiles, likelihood of clinically significant interactions with other drugs, and likelihood of discontinuation symptoms following cessation of pharmacotherapy (see Long-term Pharmacological Treatment, below).

Venlafaxine (in its extended-release [XR] formulation), which is a serotonin and noradrenaline reuptake inhibitor, has also demonstrated efficacy in panic disorder (Ferguson et al., 2007; Pollack et al., 2007).

Of the TCAs, imipramine (Cross-National Collaborative Panic Study, 1992) and clomipramine (Cassano et al., 1988; Johnston et al., 1988; Fahy et al., 1992; Modigh et al., 1992; Gentil et al., 1993) were found to be efficacious in panic disorder. When clomipramine was compared with imipramine (Cassano et al., 1988; Modigh et al., 1992; Gentil et al., 1993), it was found to be somewhat more efficacious, with an earlier onset of efficacy.

Although various benzodiazepines have been used in the treatment of panic disorder, the convincing evidence of their efficacy exists for alprazolam (Ballenger et al., 1988; Cross-National Collaborative Panic Study, 1992) and clonazepam (Tesar et al., 1991).

It is important to note that the placebo response rates in pharmacological studies of panic disorder are often quite high, up to 51% in some studies (Pohl et al., 1998). Apart from raising concerns about the methodology and interpretation of results of various drug trials, this finding suggests that nonspecific treatment factors (such as expectations from the treatment that patients may have and the therapeutic relationship with the physician) may play an important role in the treatment of panic disorder.

Because there are no differences in efficacy between SSRIs, venlafaxine XR, TCAs, and benzodiazepines, the choice of medication depends on the factors listed in Table 2–23. The relative importance of each of these factors in every patient with panic disorder then determines which medication is used.

Although SSRIs, venlafaxine XR, and TCAs are considered first-, second-, and third-line choices of treatment, respectively (Table 2–24), they can

Table 2–23. Factors to Be Taken Into Consideration When Choosing a Medication for Treatment of Panic Disorder

Factors	SSRIs	Venlafaxine XR	TCAs	BDZs
Side-effect profile and general tolerability	++	+/++	0	+++
Presence of co-occurring mental disorders, especially depression (and history of depression)	+++	+++	+++	0
History of alcohol or other substance abuse or dependence	+++	+++	+++	0
Speed of therapeutic (antipanic) response	0	0	0	+++
Safety in overdose	+++	+/++	0	+++

SSRIs, selective serotonin reuptake inhibitors; Venlafaxine XR, venlafaxine extended-release; TCAs, tricyclic antidepressants; BDZs, benzodiazepines
+++ Clear advantage
++ Some or relative advantage
+ Minimal advantage
0 No advantage

Table 2–24. Choice of Medication in Treatment of Panic Disorder

Rank	Medication
First-line	a. SSRIs (especially sertraline, paroxetine, and escitalopram) b. SSRI + high-potency BDZ (alprazolam, clonazepam)
Second-line	a. Venlafaxine XR b. Venlafaxine XR + high-potency BDZ (alprazolam, clonazepam)
Third-line	a. TCAs (clomipramine, imipramine) b. TCA + high-potency BDZ (alprazolam, clonazepam)
Fourth-line	High-potency BDZs (alprazolam, clonazepam) only

SSRI, selective serotonin reuptake inhibitor; Venlafaxine XR, venlafaxine extended-release; TCA, tricyclic antidepressant; BDZ, benzodiazepine.

initially be administered together with a benzodiazepine, or treatment can be commenced with a benzodiazepine only. This decision is likely to depend on the combination of factors listed in Table 2–23.

One study suggests that making decisions about pharmacotherapy of panic disorder is fairly complex, without these decisions necessarily being based on current treatment guidelines (Bruce et al., 2003). This study indicates that benzodiazepines continue to be the most commonly used form of pharmacotherapy for panic disorder in the United States and that a majority of patients taking SSRIs also use benzodiazepines at the same time. The two most likely reasons for the apparent preference of benzodiazepines over SSRIs are their rapid onset of action and better tolerability (Bruce et al., 2003). An earlier study has already indicated that in comparison with patients treated with imipramine, panic patients treated with alprazolam were less likely to drop out of treatment and more likely to experience substantial relief from panic attacks (Schweizer et al., 1993).

Selective Serotonin Reuptake Inhibitors, Venlafaxine Extended-Release, and Tricyclic Antidepressants in Treatment of Panic Disorder

There are several reasons for the current status of SSRIs as the first-line pharmacological treatment for panic disorder (see Table 2–23). Their side effects are generally better tolerated than the side effects of TCAs, and they are safer in overdose than TCAs (an important consideration for many patients with panic disorder who develop depression and become suicidal). They are also not associated with dependence to the extent that benzodiazepines are, and SSRIs are often efficacious in pharmacological treatment of many disorders that tend to co-occur with panic disorder (e.g., generalized anxiety disorder, social anxiety disorder, depression). Perhaps the greatest disadvantage of the SSRIs is the fact that their full antipanic efficacy appears only after they have been administered continuously for 4–6 weeks. This delayed efficacy may be even more pronounced with TCAs, where antipanic effect often appears after 8–12 weeks of treatment.

Comparisons between clomipramine and SSRIs did not show significant differences in efficacy, but SSRIs tended to be better tolerated (den Boer et al., 1987; Lecrubier and Judge, 1997; Lecrubier et al., 1997; Wade et al., 1997). One meta-analysis has confirmed that there are no differences in efficacy between TCAs and SSRIs, but the number of dropouts was significantly higher among panic patients treated with TCAs (Bakker et al., 2002b). However, another review of the comparative efficacy and tolerability of SSRIs and TCAs found no differences (Otto et al., 2001), adding to the growing impression that good tolerability of SSRIs in panic disorder might have been somewhat overestimated.

Indeed, side effects of SSRIs can be troublesome, accounting for their premature discontinuation in a substantial proportion of panic patients (e.g., Cowley et al., 1997). Because the occurrence of side effects is unpredictable, patients should be well informed about them before commencing treatment. Most common are nausea, vomiting, diarrhea, other gastrointestinal disturbances, agitation, headache, dizziness, and insomnia. If the side effects are severe, some patients describe them as "worst ever experience." To prevent insomnia, SSRIs should generally be administered in the morning. A hypnotic medication can be taken on an as-needed (prn) basis if patients have already developed insomnia. Side effects may be particularly prominent at the beginning of treatment and usually abate with continued pharmacotherapy.

Although venlafaxine XR appears to perform just as well as paroxetine in the treatment of panic disorder, it is often considered a second-line pharmacotherapy option for panic disorder (e.g., National Institute for Clinical Excellence, 2004). The main reason for this is a less favorable side-effect profile of venlafaxine XR in higher doses (>225 mg/day), with increased blood pressure and possible cardiotoxicity. Also, there have been reports of lethal outcomes of overdoses with venlafaxine XR. Its side effects at lower doses (75–150 mg/days) are similar to the side effects of SSRIs. Less common side effects that may emerge in the course of treatment with venlafaxine XR include dry mouth, constipation, dizziness, sedation, and sweating.

The occurrence of side effects of TCAs is more predictable than that of SSRIs; for example, most patients taking a TCA will have dry mouth. The main issue is whether patients can tolerate the side effects of TCAs (which most commonly include anticholinergic symptoms, such as dry mouth, blurred vision, constipation, and urinary hesitancy, plus sedation, weight gain, postural hypotension, tachycardia, sexual dysfunction, and lowering of the seizure threshold). Some of these side effects are dose-dependent (e.g., sedation) and may disappear with a reduction in dose, whereas others occur regardless of dosage. In view of their side-effect profile and specific organ toxicity, TCAs are contraindicated in patients with cardiac arrhythmias, enlarged prostate, glaucoma, and epilepsy.

If SSRIs, venlafaxine XR, or TCAs are commenced at their usual antidepressant dosage, agitation, restlessness, and increased anxiety ("jitteriness syndrome") are particularly common. This phenomenon seems to be relatively specific for panic disorder. Therefore, it is important to start an SSRI or venlafaxine XR at one quarter to one half of its initial antidepressant dose. In practice, this means that sertraline should be commenced at 12.5–25 mg/day, paroxetine at 5–10 mg/day, escitalopram at 2.5–5 mg/day, and venlafaxine XR at 37.5 mg/day. When using a TCA, the starting dose should be 10 mg/day of imipramine or clomipramine. The initial doses should be increased as quickly as possible, depending on side effects. For an SSRI, venlafaxine XR, or a TCA to reach therapeutic dosage, several weeks may need to elapse; the rate of increasing the dose should be tailored to each individual patient. This phase of treatment is often critical, as patients do not yet experience the benefits of pharmacotherapy while possibly having prominent side effects. It is not surprising, then, that dropout rates are highest during this period.

The other commonly used strategy to counteract initial agitation and increase in anxiety with SSRIs, venlafaxine XR, or TCAs is to coadminister alprazolam or clonazepam. This combination is also useful for quick alleviation of distress and panic symptoms and for producing an earlier response, as confirmed by the results of studies in which clonazepam was coadministered with sertraline (Goddard et al., 2001a) and paroxetine (Pollack et al., 2003). The combined treatment with an SSRI, venlafaxine XR, or a TCA and alprazolam or clonazepam should last for 6–12 weeks—a period during which the dosage of an SSRI, venlafaxine XR, or a TCA is gradually increased to a therapeutic range, while a benzodiazepine is subsequently discontinued. Alternatively, combined antidepressant-benzodiazepine treatment can be continued for prolonged periods of time, depending on the circumstances of individual patients.

The usual medication doses for panic disorder are shown in Table 2–25. A target dose among SSRIs has been established only for paroxetine: 40 mg/day (Ballenger et al., 1998). However, if the patient responds fully to a daily dose of 20 or 30 mg of paroxetine, there is no need to further increase the dose. Sertraline was found to be efficacious in all three doses (50 mg/day, 100 mg/day, 200 mg/day) that were used (Londborg et al., 1998). Citalopram and fluoxetine may be more efficacious in doses of 20–30 mg/day and 20 mg/day, respectively, than in lower doses (Wade et al., 1997; Lepola et al., 1998; Michelson et al., 1998). If there is no satisfactory response to a dose of fluoxetine of 20 mg/day, patients may benefit from a higher dose (Michelson et al., 2001).

The doses of venlafaxine XR that have been efficacious in treating panic disorder range from 75 mg/day to 225 mg/day (Ferguson et al., 2007; Pollack et al., 2007). This indicates that noradrenergic properties of venlafaxine XR, associated with higher doses, may not be necessary for efficacy in panic disorder.

Table 2–25. Medication Dosages Efficacious in Treatment of Panic Disorder

Medication	Dose Range
Selective serotonin reuptake inhibitors	
Sertraline	50–200 mg/day
Paroxetine	20–60 mg/day
Escitalopram	10–20 mg/day
Citalopram	20–60 mg/day
Fluvoxamine	100–300 mg/day
Fluoxetine	20–40 mg/day
Venlafaxine XR	75–225 mg/day
Tricyclic antidepressants	
Clomipramine	75–250 mg/day
Imipramine	100–250 mg/day
Benzodiazepines	
Alprazolam	1.5–6 mg/day
Clonazepam	1–4 mg/day

A higher dose of imipramine (e.g., 200 mg/day) was associated with greater likelihood of response and more treatment gains (Mavissakalian and Perel, 1989, 1995). Therefore, the dose of imipramine should be pushed relatively quickly to at least 100–150 mg/day, unless patients experience intolerable side effects.

Benzodiazepines in Treatment of Panic Disorder

Some patients are so troubled by their symptoms and the overall experience of panic that they urgently seek alleviation of anxiety and panic. Because of the quick onset of anxiolytic and antipanic action, benzodiazepines are particularly advantageous in short-term treatment of such patients, as patients experience significant relief, with a complete disappearance of panic attacks within days or 1 to 2 weeks. In addition, benzodiazepines are generally well tolerated, and, if taken alone, are safe in overdose. The main disadvantages of benzodiazepines include therapeutic drug dependence and lack of efficacy for co-occurring depression and some of the other anxiety disorders (e.g., obsessive-compulsive disorder).

The most important and most common side effect of benzodiazepines is sedation, which patients typically experience through drowsiness and/or difficulty keeping their attention focused. If sedation is accompanied by problems with motor coordination, skills needed for driving or other complex activities may be impaired. Sedation and the accompanying impairment in motor coordination are made worse by the use of alcohol, and patients should be warned of the potential consequences of sedation and should be advised not to use alcohol along with benzodiazepines. Sedation is dose-dependent and tolerance to sedation develops quickly, so that higher doses of benzodiazepines are required to produce the same initial degree of sedation. In clinical practice, this means that sedation usually occurs at the very beginning of treatment or immediately after a dose of a benzodiazepine has been increased; there is usually no need to decrease the dose because of sedation. However, if sedation does persist, the dose may be decreased.

Another relatively common side effect of benzodiazepines is certain memory impairment, usually in the form of clinically nonsignificant anterograde amnesia. Some patients exhibit "paradoxical reactions" to benzodiazepines, which refers to irritability and disinhibited or aggressive behavior, instead of the expected effects of anxiolysis and sense of calm.

Alprazolam and clonazepam are the most commonly used benzodiazepines in the treatment of panic disorder. The initial dose of alprazolam is usually 1 mg/day, while the initial dose of clonazepam is 0.5 mg/day. The dose is then gradually increased, according to response and side effects (e.g., sedation). Clonazepam may have an advantage over alprazolam in that it has a longer duration of action and is therefore less likely to be associated with discontinuation problems. In addition, because of the same property, it is easier to administer clonazepam—usually twice a day—whereas the total daily dosage of alprazolam needs to be divided into three to four doses. For clonazepam it appears that doses of 1 mg/day and above are more efficacious than a dose of 0.5 mg/day; the dose of 1–2 mg/day is also well tolerated (Rosenbaum et al., 1997).

The optimal length of treatment of panic disorder with benzodiazepines is not known. There is general agreement that because of dependence issues (see below), benzodiazepines should be used for as brief a time as possible; this usually translates to 6–12 weeks of treatment. It appears, however, that quite a few patients require long-term treatment with benzodiazepines, which may extend over several months or even years.

Long-Term Pharmacological Treatment

Because panic disorder tends to have a chronic course, pharmacological treatment should be continued for at least 6–12 months after the patient has attained remission and the panic attacks have either disappeared completely or their frequency and severity have decreased significantly. In practice, patients often take medications for longer periods of time. After 1 year, a physician needs to review whether pharmacotherapy is to continue. In doing so, the physician should bear in mind that there is a high risk of relapse upon cessation of medication, unless the patient has learned strategies for coping with panic symptoms and anxiety. A decision to stop medication should be made jointly by the physician and patient after the patient has been well informed of the risks involved in medication cessation. It is also important that the patient feels ready for discontinuing pharmacological treatment.

Relapse seems to occur even in the course of adequate long-term pharmacotherapy, with as many as 46% of patients reporting a relapse after they had achieved remission (Simon et al., 2002). Relapse figures upon discontinuation of medication vary, with about 37% of panic patients relapsing within 6 months after cessation of antidepressants (Mavissakalian and Perel, 2002), and 67% relapsing over the course of 3 years (Toni et al., 2000). An even greater number of panic patients may relapse after the cessation of benzodiazepines (Noyes et al., 1991).

What can be done to minimize the risk of relapse after discontinuing pharmacotherapy? Several strategies have been proposed. The first is an administration of antipanic medication for longer periods of time (e.g., for 18 months rather than 6 months); as far as imipramine is concerned, this approach has not been supported convincingly (Mavissakalian and Perel, 1992, 2002). The other strategy is to add psychological interventions, most notably CBT, to the ongoing pharmacotherapy (see Combined Treatments, below). Clinicians may also try to detect a relapse early on, and then reinstitute treatment; risk factors for recurrence of panic disorder following discontinuation of antidepressants have been identified—for example, high level of anxiety sensitivity (Mavissakalian and Guo, 2004).

Except for paroxetine in some cases, most patients either do not gain weight or gain weight only minimally in the course of long-term treatment with SSRIs. The most troublesome long-term side effects of SSRIs and venlafaxine XR are various problems with sexual functioning. The SSRI- and venlafaxine-associated sexual dysfunction usually takes the form of ejaculatory disturbances (delayed or absent ejaculation) in men and anorgasmia in women. Less commonly, patients taking SSRIs or venlafaxine XR have erectile problems and decreased sexual desire. Of all the SSRIs, paroxetine may be most likely to be associated with sexual dysfunction.

In the long-term pharmacological treatment of panic disorder, medications do not seem to exhibit a decrease in efficacy (Uhlenhuth et al., 1988; Lecrubier and Judge, 1997; Lepola et al., 1998; Michelson et al., 1999). Therefore, the dose of medication during long-term treatment does not need to be increased, and it is likely to be the same as the one that initially produced remission of panic disorder.

Discontinuation or withdrawal symptoms occur in many patients who stop taking SSRIs or venlafaxine XR abruptly. These symptoms include restlessness, headache, dizziness, sweating, nausea, exhaustion, muscle pain, and flu-like symptoms, but various other symptoms may appear as well. Discontinuation symptoms are more likely to be seen after cessation of paroxetine than after cessation of other SSRIs—for example, sertraline (Bandelow et al., 2004). These problems usually do not occur with fluoxetine, because of its longer half-life. It is good clinical practice to decrease the dose of SSRIs and venlafaxine XR gradually, before their complete cessation. Depending on the dosage and type of SSRI used, this process usually takes between 1 to 2 weeks and 2 to 3 months; with venlafaxine XR, the taper should be longer rather than shorter.

Specific Issues in the Course of Long-Term Treatment With Benzodiazepines

The main issue during long-term treatment with benzodiazepines is therapeutic dependence on these medications, often labeled "addiction." Although therapeutic drug dependence and dependence on alcohol and certain illicit drugs ("addiction") are both characterized by the occurrence of withdrawal symptoms upon abrupt cessation of the drug, there are important differences between the two. Unlike addiction, therapeutic dependence on benzodiazepines is *not* associated with tolerance (increasing the dosage to produce the same initial anxiolytic effect or the initial dose producing a decreased effect). This was demonstrated by studies in which patients usually showed no tendency to escalate the dosage nor to develop tolerance to the anxiolytic effects of benzodiazepines over long-term treatment (Nagy et al., 1989; Pollack et al., 1993; Schweizer et al., 1993; Worthington et al., 1998). Moreover, patients using benzodiazepines over long periods of time do not crave the medication and show no adverse health and/or social consequences (e.g., an all-encompassing preoccupation with benzodiazepines).

There is no evidence that panic patients are more likely to abuse benzodiazepines in the absence of current or past alcohol or other substance use disorder (e.g., Salzman et al., 1993; Andersch and Hetta, 2003). Therefore, it is erroneous to assume automatically that benzodiazepines are "addictive" and on that basis deprive panic patients of these drugs' potential benefits. However, benzodiazepines should generally not be prescribed to panic patients with current or past substance use problems. Caution is also warranted when administering benzodiazepines to patients who have a family history of a substance use disorder and personality features (e.g., dependent) that might make it more difficult for them to stop taking benzodiazepines.

Benzodiazepine withdrawal symptoms are more likely to occur if the patient has been taking a benzodiazepine with a shorter half-life (e.g., alprazolam), if its dose has been higher (e.g., more than 2 mg of alprazolam per day), and if a benzodiazepine has been taken continuously over a longer period of time (generally more than 1–2 months). Benzodiazepine withdrawal syndrome is an unpleasant experience, which is rarely life-threatening. It may resemble a recurrence of anxiety disorder, and symptoms such as increased anxiety, tension, restlessness, agitation, insomnia, and panic attacks are quite common, especially a short time after a benzodiazepine has been ceased. If they occur, severe withdrawal symptoms usually appear later: tachycardia, hypertension, profuse sweating, nausea, vomiting, tremor, muscle pain, unstable gait, transient hallucinations, and, rarely, grand mal seizures. The prevention of a severe withdrawal syndrome entails its early recognition on the basis of the relatively specific symptoms (hypersensitivity to light, sound, smell or taste, various perceptual disturbances, distorted body image, tinnitus, tingling sensations, depersonalization, derealization) and early treatment.

After a sudden cessation of benzodiazepines, the withdrawal syndrome is not the only potential consequence. Patients may experience a "rebound," which is the worsening of initial symptoms of an anxiety disorder. The symptoms of rebound often overlap with those of benzodiazepine withdrawal syndrome; it is important to attempt to distinguish between the two because their course and treatment implications are different. While the withdrawal syndrome is transient (duration no longer than 10–20 days) and calls for general supportive measures, rebound essentially means a recurrence of the original disorder, for which a long-term treatment strategy is necessary.

The best way to prevent the benzodiazepine withdrawal syndrome is to taper benzodiazepines very gradually and carefully before their discontinuation. In addition, CBT can be helpful in the process of tapering benzodiazepines (Otto et al., 1993; Spiegel et al., 1994). As the dosage is being decreased, it is crucial to address patients' fears of the withdrawal symptoms, as these fears often determine the outcome of the taper. Although the rate of taper depends primarily on the duration of treatment with a benzodiazepine and its dosage, the rate should be adjusted according to the characteristics of the individual patient. The rate of taper should always be negotiated with the patient, without any pressure or hurry and in a flexible manner. It is more important that patients do not experience withdrawal symptoms (which can occur even with a relatively slow taper) and feel comfortable as they go through a tapering process than it is to complete this process within a set, predetermined period. Thus, there are large variations in the duration of taper, and it is not unusual for this to last 6 months or longer. In principle, a decrease in the total daily dosage by 0.25–0.5 mg of alprazolam per week or 0.125–0.25 mg of clonazepam per week is adequate to minimize the risk of withdrawal symptoms.

Pharmacotherapy of Treatment-Resistant Panic Disorder

Treatment resistance in panic disorder is not well defined and rests more on clinical judgment than on research-derived criteria. For practical purposes, a patient with panic disorder can be considered resistant to pharmacological treatment if he or she has not responded to an adequate trial (6–8 weeks of treatment in a therapeutic dose) of two SSRIs, venlafaxine XR, one of the TCAs (imipramine or clomipramine), a high-potency benzodiazepine, and a combination of one of these antidepressants with a benzodiazepine. Some patients may reach the stage of treatment resistance not only through a lack of efficacy of the first-, second-, third-, and fourth-line pharmacological agents, but also if they are unable to tolerate some of these drugs or if some medications cannot be prescribed to them. It is estimated that 20%–30% of panic patients do not respond to pharmacotherapy. Apart from using CBT or other psychological treatments, there are several pharmacotherapy options for these patients (Table 2–26).

A number of other antidepressants have shown promise in the treatment of panic disorder. The efficacy for phenelzine (45–90 mg/day), a classical and irreversible monoamine oxidase inhibitor (MAOI), was found only in one controlled study (Sheehan et al., 1980). This finding has not been replicated, and because phenelzine is associated with numerous side effects and potentially dangerous interactions with many other drugs, and requires a tyramine-free diet, it is considered a pharmacotherapy option for treatment-resistant panic disorder. The efficacy of other antidepressants—reboxetine (Versiani et al., 2002), moclobemide (Loerch et al., 1999; Uhlenhuth et al., 2002), mirtazapine (Carpenter et al., 1999), and milnacipran (Blaya et al., 2007)—was either inconsistent across the studies or was shown only in small, pilot, or open-label studies. Therefore, these drugs can be used if there has been no response at all to the first-, second-, third-, and fourth-line medications.

Anticonvulsants are another class of medications that could be used in treatment-resistant panic disorder, but evidence of their efficacy comes

Table 2–26. Pharmacological Options for Treatment-Resistant Panic Disorder

Lack of Response to First-, Second-, Third-, or Fourth-Line Pharmacotherapy

Monotherapy with another antidepressant
  Phenelzine
  Reboxetine
  Moclobemide
  Mirtazapine
  Milnacipran
Monotherapy with an anticonvulsant
  Gabapentin
  Valproate
  Levetiracetam
  Tiagabine
  Vigabatrin
Monotherapy with olanzapine

Partial Response to First-Line Pharmacotherapy

Augmentation strategies
  SSRI + olanzapine
  SSRI + pindolol
  SSRI + TCA

SSRI, selective serotonin reuptake inhibitor; TCA, tricyclic antidepressant mainly from small or uncontrolled studies of valproate, levetiracetam, vigabatrin, and tiagabine. One controlled trial of gabapentin did not find it to be superior to placebo, and significant improvement occurred only in gabapentin-treated patients with moderate to severe panic disorder (Pande et al., 2000). The use of anticonvulsants in panic disorder is of interest on theoretical grounds, because of a certain, still poorly understood relationship between panic attacks and various seizure disorders.

Second-generation antipsychotic drugs may represent another option for patients with pharmacotherapy-resistant panic disorder. It has been suggested that monotherapy with olanzapine might be useful for these patients (Hollifield et al., 2005).

If there has been a partial response to treatment with a first-line (SSRI) medication, augmentation strategies can be considered (Table 2–26). Olanzapine, a second-generation antipsychotic, has been used as augmentation therapy in a fixed dose of 5 mg/day (Sepede et al., 2006). A combination of an SSRI with pindolol has received some empirical support (Hirschmann et al., 2000). Treatment with an SSRI can also be augmented with imipramine or clomipramine, but this option is reserved for the most resistant cases because plasma levels of imipramine or clomipramine may increase dramatically and patients need to be closely monitored for any signs of TCA toxicity.

PSYCHOLOGICAL TREATMENT

Cognitive Therapy

Cognitive therapy of panic disorder is based on the cognitive theory of panic disorder and, more specifically, on the assumption that panic attacks are a consequence of catastrophic appraisals (misinterpretation) of benign physical sensations and symptoms. Hence, the immediate goal of cognitive therapy of panic disorder is to normalize appraisals of physical sensations and symptoms. Furthermore, cognitive therapy is undertaken with the goal of decreasing or eliminating the fear of anxiety symptoms and panic attacks. In order to achieve this, cognitive therapy has to "dismantle" the underlying ideas or beliefs about the dangerousness of anxiety and panic. The emphasis in cognitive therapy is *not* on the control and total disappearance of anxiety, panic, and its symptoms; rather, the goal is for panic patients to be able to appraise anxiety and panic in a nonthreatening manner and thereby cope with them more effectively. Cognitive therapy of panic disorder proceeds through several steps (Table 2–27) that are described below.

Identification of Specific Panic- and Anxiety-Relevant Catastrophic Cognitions

The first step is to identify catastrophic cognitions that patients have about specific anxiety symptoms and panic. This is done by directly asking patients

Table 2–27. Process of Cognitive Therapy of Panic Disorder

1. Identification of catastrophic cognitions (appraisals, beliefs) about specific anxiety symptoms and panic
2. Challenging the identified catastrophic cognitions

    Looking for evidence that catastrophic cognitions are (in)correct
    Proposing alternative, normalizing appraisals of the relevant physical sensations and symptoms
    Weighing "pros" and "cons" of catastrophic cognitions

3. Using behavioral experiments to provide more convincing evidence that the alternative appraisals are correct
4. Replacing catastrophic cognitions with normalizing, rational appraisals

what they think would happen as a result of the symptoms. The appraisals of symptoms may be easy to access, as in the case of patients who state that they believe they are going to lose control when they feel dizzy. In other cases, it is more difficult to grasp the underlying appraisal, and patients need to be led from one question to another to access it. Thus, patients who feel dizzy may appraise dizziness as leading to fainting and falling, and thereby either humiliating themselves or sustaining a serious injury.

Challenging Identified Catastrophic Cognitions

The next step in cognitive therapy is to challenge the previously identified catastrophic cognitions. This step involves several procedures.

Looking for Evidence that Specific Catastrophic Cognitions Are (In)correct This procedure consists of asking patients questions such as "How do you know that you will lose control when you feel dizzy?" or "What makes you think that you will injure yourself when you are dizzy?" The reasons patients come up with suggest to them that their appraisals are not well founded.

Proposing Alternative, Normalizing Explanations The next procedure is offering alternative explanations for the relevant physical sensations and symptoms, and discussing them with patients. Implementation of this technique is crucial, as it introduces a normalizing interpretation of the symptom(s) and of the overall panic experience, and asks patients to consider this instead of clinging to their catastrophic appraisal. The successful use of this technique depends on patients' understanding (previously achieved through psychoeducation) of the basic physiological processes involved in the anxiety response. For example, it can be suggested to patients that dizziness often results from the pathophysiological chain of events that occur during hyperventilation; in turn, hyperventilation and panic are explained as having no serious consequences, regardless of how unpleasant they may be.

Weighing "Pros" and "Cons" of Catastrophic Cognitions   After patients have been presented with alternative explanation(s) for their symptoms, their task is to weigh pros and cons of their particular appraisals. For example, patients who think that they will faint and collapse when they feel dizzy may try to support this appraisal of dizziness by asserting that because of their usually low blood pressure, they will faint and collapse. This line or reasoning should be contrasted with information, provided by the therapist, that blood pressure usually rises during panic attacks, which makes it rather unlikely for patients to faint and collapse, despite feeling dizzy. The weighing of pros and cons may take some time, as patients often need to rehearse this part of the process of challenging their catastrophic appraisals. Ultimately, they should be able to replace these appraisals with normalizing, rational interpretations.

Behavioral Experiments   It may not be sufficient for patients to go through the process of challenging their cognitions, and they may seek more convincing evidence that the alternative explanation is correct. In such cases, using behavioral experiments (Clark and Beck, 1988) may be particularly useful. This technique consists of the deliberate induction of one or more symptoms of anxiety that patients are particularly afraid of; after patients have induced this symptom, they try to modify their catastrophic appraisal of it on the basis of the alternative explanations presented to them. For example, for patients who are afraid of dizziness and have a catastrophic appraisal that they will faint and collapse because of dizziness, the behavioral experiment consists of asking them to hyperventilate for a few minutes. Hyperventilation produces dizziness among other symptoms, and patients find out that while dizziness is unpleasant, it does not lead to fainting and collapsing. For many patients, this direct demonstration that the feared symptom (e.g., dizziness) does not lead to a catastrophe (e.g., fainting, collapsing) is quite convincing and makes them more likely to abandon their catastrophic appraisals.

Replacing Catastrophic Cognitions with Normalizing, Rational Interpretations

Replacement of catastrophic cognitions with normalizing appraisals of sensations, symptoms, and panic occurs throughout the treatment, and not as any particular stage of cognitive therapy. It can be conceived of as both the mechanism of cognitive change and one of the treatment goals.

Other Aspects of Cognitive Therapy

Another aspect of cognitive therapy is focusing on dysfunctional expectations of panic attacks. Because many panic patients believe that expectations of attacks lead to the actual occurrence of attacks, it is important for them to realize that this association is not inevitable and that expecting a panic attack does not necessarily make it happen. Moreover, instead of focusing on the expectation of panic attacks, patients are encouraged to learn strategies for coping with anxiety and panic. Once they have learned to cope with them more effectively, it will be less relevant whether panic attacks are expected or not expected, and indeed, whether panic attacks occur or do not occur.

In the course of cognitive therapy, general anxiety-related cognitive distortions are addressed, so that panic patients become better equipped to recognize them and change these dysfunctional patterns of thinking (e.g., the "all-or-nothing," dichotomized, rigid style of thinking, underestimation of one's own abilities, exaggerated perception of threat). Through Socratic dialogue and challenging of entrenched assumptions, interpretations, and beliefs, it is demonstrated to patients that this cognitive style only contributes to the maintenance of anxiety in general and panic disorder in particular.

The use of cognitive therapy techniques is not simple and requires at least some degree of patients' psychological-mindedness. It may be difficult for some patients to accept the idea that the goal of treatment is not necessarily elimination of symptoms but learning how to cope with symptoms and anxiety. Other patients may have difficulty accepting alternative, rational explanations for their symptoms and panic attacks, as if having adopted a stance that "reason and logic cannot cure." This may be due to the general lack of common sense and logic in the "neurotic paradox:" regardless of how many times patients have experienced certain symptoms and panic attacks without a catastrophe occurring, they may believe that the catastrophe is still looming and that it has not occurred yet because they were "lucky" or because they escaped in time. Some of these beliefs need to be addressed for the treatment to proceed successfully.

The role played by "safety behaviors" (e.g., avoidance) and "safety devices" (e.g., medications that are carried around at all times) in maintaining panic disorder is considered important in cognitive therapy. The purpose of safety behaviors is to prevent the feared catastrophe; most commonly, this is avoidance, even if subtle, of various situations or activities (e.g., exercising) in which patients might experience the feared sensations and symptoms. If patients cling to their safety behaviors or safety devices, they may reinforce an erroneous belief that owing to their use, they have been able to prevent a catastrophe. This issue needs to be discussed with patients in some detail, and they should be encouraged to identify and abandon their own safety behaviors and safety devices.

Probably the most difficult component of the cognitive therapy package is participation in behavioral experiments. Many panic patients are understandably concerned about the technique in which the feared symptoms are being deliberately induced. Therefore, the rationale for conducting behavioral experiments and the corresponding procedures need to be carefully explained to patients.

Efficacy of Cognitive Therapy and Its Limitations

Cognitive therapy is an efficacious treatment modality for panic disorder, with 90% of patients in one study being panic-free upon completion of treatment, and 70% remaining panic-free at 1-year follow-up (Clark DM et al., 1994). Cognitive therapy was found to result in decrease in catastrophic misinterpretations of bodily sensations and symptoms during panic attacks; this outcome correlated with decreased severity and frequency of panic attacks (Bakker et al., 2002a). Studies of the efficacy of cognitive therapy in panic disorder should rely more on specific and relevant outcome measures, such as appraisals of panic symptoms and their consequences, because these reflect the goals of cognitive therapy more adequately than general outcome measures such as the severity and frequency of panic attacks.

Because of the demanding nature and somewhat radical goals of treatment, cognitive therapy in its unmodified form may be suitable for some panic patients only. Modifications often include use of symptom control or symptom alleviation techniques. "Pure" cognitive therapy has been considered useful in the treatment of panic attacks, but less so in the treatment of agoraphobia, whereas behavior therapy (exposure) has been deemed more efficacious for agoraphobia than for panic attacks (van den Hout et al., 1994). The logical implication is that cognitive and behavioral techniques should be combined in the presence of both panic attacks and agoraphobia.

Panic Control Treatment

Panic control treatment (Barlow, 1988; Barlow et al., 1989) is a commonly used form of CBT, with greater emphasis on behavioral components of treatment. It is based largely on the model of panic attacks as false alarms and the concepts of interoceptive conditioning and learned alarms. In contrast to the goals of treatment in cognitive therapy, the main goal of panic control treatment is a better control of symptoms of anxiety and panic.

The key technique of panic control treatment is interoceptive exposure, which is similar to behavioral experiments used in cognitive therapy. However, the rationale for using these techniques and the way in which they are administered are different. In interoceptive exposure (Table 2–28), the emphasis is on exposure to the deliberately induced symptoms, along with techniques for controlling symptoms (e.g., relaxation and controlled, slow breathing) and reattribution of symptoms to innocuous causes (i.e., normalization of patients' interpretations). The aim of interoceptive exposure is to enable patients to have a greater sense of control over their symptoms, anxiety, and panic. Alleviation of anxiety occurs through habituation to the symptoms and eventual extinction of the conditioned anxiety response.

Table 2–28. Components of Interoceptive Exposure

1. Exposure to deliberately induced symptoms
2. Use of symptom control techniques (e.g., relaxation, controlled, slow breathing)
3. Reattribution of symptoms to innocuous causes (normalizing patients' appraisals) following the challenging of catastrophic symptom appraisals

In behavioral experiments, the emphasis is on demonstrating to patients that deliberately induced, feared symptoms do not lead to the expected catastrophes. Also, symptom control techniques are not used in "pure" cognitive therapy; they are actually regarded by some cognitive therapists as a safety device. Cognitive therapists would argue that there is no need for patients to control symptoms because they are learning through cognitive therapy that they have no reason to fear symptoms.

Various symptoms can be induced, depending on what particular patients find most distressing. Exposure to these symptoms is gradual and in accordance with the hierarchical principles embedded in general exposure-based therapies (see Exposure-based Therapy for Agoraphobia, below). Interoceptive exposure may be contraindicated in patients with asthma, other respiratory diseases, or heart disease because the symptoms (e.g., shortness of breath, chest pain, accelerated heart rate) induced during interoceptive exposure would be indistinguishable from symptoms of the primary medical condition. In addition, there is a possibility of interoceptive exposure exacerbating respiratory or cardiac disease.

After several sessions of interoceptive exposure, in which symptoms are induced through an "artificial" procedure (usually hyperventilation), patients should expose themselves to the naturally occurring physical symptoms. That means that patients should resume physical activities that they have been avoiding for fear of provoking these symptoms. The panic control treatment is conducted over 12–15 sessions, with a frequency of one session per week. There are various modifications to this regimen, and the treatment has also been used in a group format.

Panic control treatment has been found to be efficacious in panic disorder. Between 79% and 87% of patients were symptom-free at the end of this treatment (Barlow et al., 1989; Klosko et al., 1990), whereas 83% were panic-free at 6-month follow-up (Telch et al., 1993) and more than 80% were panic-free at 2-year follow-up (Craske et al., 1991).

Panic Symptom Control Techniques

The most common techniques used for alleviation of symptoms of anxiety and panic are controlled, slow breathing (breathing retraining) and relaxation.

Controlled, Slow Breathing (Breathing Retraining)

The use of controlled, slow breathing can avert hyperventilation or restore normal breathing pattern in patients who are already hyperventilating. Insofar as the panic symptoms are caused by hyperventilation, restoration of the normal breathing pattern can alleviate or even eliminate these symptoms.

Controlled, slow breathing relies on three components: primary use of the diaphragm (instead of the chest) for breathing, normal-sized breaths (rather than deep breaths), and pacing the breathing rhythm so that the respiratory rate decreases to approximately 10 cycles/minute. The latter means that the patient needs to learn to breathe in cycles that consist of 3 seconds of inhaling and 3 seconds of exhaling. The technique of controlled, slow breathing is relatively easy to learn. It has to be practiced on a daily basis, however, before patients feel confident to use it after the occurrence of initial panic symptoms and in various situations, including those in which they expect to have a panic attack.

Relaxation

Various relaxation techniques have been used in the treatment of anxiety states, most notably generalized anxiety disorder (see Chapter 3). A modified progressive muscle relaxation technique, called "applied relaxation" (Öst, 1987a, 1988), has been used for panic disorder. Its goal is to quickly produce a relaxed state, which will neutralize autonomic arousal and provide patients with some sense of control. As with controlled, slow breathing, applied relaxation should be practiced regularly and used after the occurrence of initial manifestations of autonomic arousal and upon exposure to situations in which anxiety symptoms are anticipated.

Exposure-Based Therapy for Agoraphobia

The behavioral technique of exposure is the key component of the treatment of agoraphobia. Even if the formal exposure-based therapy is not used, at least some basic principles of exposure should be incorporated into every treatment approach to agoraphobia.

Gradual exposure in vivo is by far the most common type of exposure therapy for agoraphobia (Table 2–29). Its use entails a construction of phobic hierarchies on the basis of a behavioral analysis, with initial exposure to situations that elicit the least amount of anxiety (and that are least avoided). Patients need to remain in agoraphobic situations during exposure until the level of anxiety has started to subside; they should also make every effort not to escape from the situations. They should work simultaneously on two to three agoraphobic situations at any stage of the treatment.

Table 2–29. Aspects of Gradual Exposure in Vivo for Agoraphobia

- Gradual exposure to the hierarchically constructed agoraphobic situations
- Self-directed exposure is the cornerstone of treatment
- Therapist-assisted exposure at the beginning of treatment for some patients with very severe forms of agoraphobia (e.g., those who are homebound)
- Partner-assisted exposure at certain stages of treatment
- Exposure to two to three agoraphobic situations at any stage of the treatment
- Regular, continuous exposure (several hours every day) is preferable
- Shorter duration of exposure and "exposure-free" days should be avoided

The exposure is to be conducted by patients (self-directed exposure) after they have been adequately informed through psychoeducation about the purpose of treatment and its technical aspects. The main roles of the therapist are to plan exposure together with patients and to review the progress that they are making. Patients should be encouraged to take responsibility for conducting the treatment, as that enhances their sense of ownership of the treatment results.

The therapist should not accompany patients during exposure, except in the initial stages of therapy of some patients with very severe agoraphobia (i.e., those who are homebound and are extremely disabled by agoraphobia). The patients' partners, family members, or friends may accompany them occasionally, during exposure to particularly difficult situations.

Patients should conduct exposure every day for at least 1 hour. It is preferable that exposure exercises last several hours and that patients not skip a day or two in the course of treatment. To facilitate monitoring and review of treatment, it is very important that patients keep a good record of their exposure exercises, which includes the following: *(1)* type of situation to which they expose themselves; *(2)* degree of fear or discomfort experienced in these situations, rated on a scale, usually from 0 to 10; *(3)* symptoms that occur during the exposure; and *(4)* duration of each exposure session. The exposure to a particular situation is completed after the level of the recorded fear or discomfort has been reduced to manageable or negligible levels, and physical symptoms experienced in this situation have ceased to be disabling.

Patients can use various techniques to reduce their anxiety during exposure: relaxation, controlled, slow breathing, paradoxical interventions (e.g., imagining the "worst possible scenario" during exposure), and cognitive therapy techniques. The use of medications during exposure-based treatment is controversial; this issue is discussed in Combined Treatments (below).

The typical length of treatment of agoraphobia with exposure in vivo is between 8 and 12 weeks. The usual frequency of therapist sessions is once to twice a week, with self-directed exposure proceeding between these sessions. There have been trends to reduce both the number of therapist sessions and the overall duration of treatment to make exposure-based therapy more cost-effective.

It may be difficult for some patients to initiate or complete exposure in vivo, and refusal or dropout rates may be as high as 40%. Some of the problems that occur before and during exposure that affect the compliance with treatment and its outcome include fluctuating levels of motivation and therapist trust, a too quick progression through the hierarchy of phobic situations (with consequently unmanageable, high levels of anxiety induced by exposure), failure to remain in the situation long enough for habituation to take place, discontinuous exposure, and excessive use of companions, safety devices (e.g., medications), or safety behaviors (e.g., taking a seat only at the end of a row in a movie theater, which would allow easy escape in case of panic) during treatment. It is very important for patients to understand how these issues impede treatment progress and work collaboratively with the therapist to overcome them.

Exposure in vivo has been clearly efficacious in the treatment of agoraphobia. Numerous studies have shown that between 60% and 75% of patients are symptom-free or exhibit only minimal avoidance at the end of treatment (McPherson et al., 1980; Munby and Johnston, 1980; Jansson and Öst, 1982; Burns et al., 1986; Jacobson et al., 1988; Trull et al., 1988; Fava et al., 1995). Moreover, this improvement tends to be maintained over prolonged periods of time (Munby and Johnston, 1980; Burns et al., 1986; Jansson et al., 1986; Margraf et al., 1993; Marks et al., 1993; Fava et al., 1995); in one study, 67% of patients who remitted after exposure-based therapy remained in remission at 7-year follow-up (Fava et al., 1995).

Some minor avoidance may persist after exposure-based therapy has been completed; although patients are usually not distressed by such avoidance, they may resort to full-scale agoraphobic avoidance, usually in the context of a stressor. If the fear of certain symptoms (e.g., dizziness) persists and drives patients to continue with avoidance, despite gains previously made during exposure, this fear needs to be specifically addressed (e.g., through cognitive therapy techniques or interoceptive exposure).

The variants of exposure-based therapy for agoraphobia include a combination of exposure in vivo and imaginal exposure (for those situations where in vivo exposure is not practical) and massed or ungraded exposure ("flooding") for those patients who are able to tolerate high levels of anxiety upon immediate exposure to the most anxiety-eliciting situations. Good results have been reported for self-help-based and computer-assisted (Internet- or virtual reality-delivered) exposure therapy, with very little or no therapist involvement. However, in the more complex and severe cases of agoraphobia, more therapist involvement and time are needed.

Several mechanisms of change and improvement in the course of exposure therapy have been postulated. These include habituation (decrease in anxiety upon repeated exposure to phobic stimuli), extinction (decrease in anxiety because it is not reinforced by further phobic avoidance), improved perception of self-efficacy, and gradual loss of catastrophic appraisals and beliefs related to phobic situations. It has also been suggested that exposure therapy represents a form of cognitive intervention that specifically decreases the expectancy of harm (Hofmann, 2008). This view implies that a strict dichotomy between cognitive and behavioral therapies might be artificial and that it should perhaps be abandoned.

Supportive Psychotherapy

There appear to be few aspects of supportive psychotherapy that are relatively specific for panic disorder. This treatment seems to be used often, but because of its nonspecific nature, it is usually considered an auxiliary rather than a main modality for bringing about relevant therapeutic changes.

In view of the general characteristics of panic patients and issues that they often present with, supportive psychotherapy aims to foster their sense of security, overcome mistrust, and facilitate reliance on others. This is also done with a further aim of building strong therapeutic alliance and securing patients' active participations in other, more specific treatment modalities. Panic patients who are struggling with ambivalence and indecisiveness often ask for advice or reassurance and sometimes attempt to engage the therapist in making decisions for them. The therapist may have to walk a very fine line between providing patients with reasonable support, encouragement, and reassurance, and discouraging their excessive dependence. The therapist's task is to promote the notion that patients can cope on their own and help patients enhance their coping skills.

Marital or Couple Therapy

Marital or couple therapy may be indicated when pathological interactions between patients and their partners seem to play a pivotal role. This may be more likely in patients with agoraphobia; as already noted, a dysfunctional relationship between the partners may contribute to the persistence of agoraphobia, and in such cases, marital or couple therapy may be both appropriate and useful. However, marital or couple therapy is not a substitute for other, more specific psychological treatment approaches, such as cognitive, behavioral, and cognitive-behavioral therapies.

Marital or couple therapy is usually not the initial treatment for panic disorder. Many patients do improve in their functioning with partners after they have undergone a course of the more specific psychological therapy. A decision to use marital or couple therapy is likely to be based on the persistence of significant problems in the marital or partner relationship after treatments such as exposure in vivo have been used to reduce panic-related avoidance. Less often, CBT may not be effective because the agoraphobic patients' partners sabotage treatment or the interference of pathological partner relationships with CBT is too strong.

Patients' partners need to be highly motivated for marital or couple therapy to be useful. This may or may not entail partners' realization that they share some responsibility with patients for the development and maintenance of the disorder. Marital or couple therapy can itself be based on behavioral and cognitive principles or other theoretical models. Perhaps the most important component of this treatment is fostering of open communication between the partners. This involves direct expression of feelings and needs as well as expectations that partners may have of each other but have not been able to articulate before. Their understanding of these issues and willingness to deal constructively with areas of conflict are crucial for overall improvement in their relationship and, consequently, for improvement in some of the clinical manifestations of panic disorder and agoraphobia.

Psychodynamic Psychotherapy and Psychoanalysis

Psychodynamic therapy and psychoanalysis are used if general indications for these forms of psychotherapy are present. These include the patient's ability to make meaningful connections between various experiences, phenomena, symptoms, and external events, along with the willingness to understand these connections and relationships in relevant context ("introspectiveness"), ability to withstand unpleasant emotions and frustrations, delay gratification, resist impulsive urges and form reasonably mature interpersonal relationships, motivation for change and psychological growth, and willingness to invest time and energy into a treatment process.

In the course of the psychodynamic psychotherapy of panic disorder, the relatively specific issues that are worked through are fears of separation and abandonment, fear of one's own anger and aggressive feelings, and conflictual and ambivalent feelings about attachment and dependency (with the alternating, varying degrees of interpersonal mistrust and idealizing tendencies). The treatment aims are understanding of the psychological significance of panic and agoraphobia and gaining insight into the origin of the underlying unconscious conflicts. In other words, dynamic (developmental) understanding of these conflicts and of their relevance in the here-and-now situation is sought, along with their resolution through therapeutic use of the transference.

Of all the anxiety disorders, panic disorder seems to have received the most attention from psychodynamically oriented psychotherapists. A specific form of treatment, termed "panic-focused psychodynamic psychotherapy," has been developed (Milrod et al., 1997). It differs from traditional psychodynamic or psychoanalytic psychotherapy in that it is manualized, more structured, proceeds through well-defined phases, and is limited to 24 twice-weekly sessions. In addition to goals common to other psychodynamic psychotherapies, goals of panic-focused psychodynamic psychotherapy are specific for panic disorder and pertain to alleviation or disappearance of the main components of panic disorder. In contrast to CBT, this treatment does not use exposure techniques and homework assignments.

Promising results of an open, pilot study of panic-focused psychodynamic psychotherapy led to a randomized controlled trial in which this treatment was found to be more efficacious than applied relaxation training (Milrod et al., 2007a). It has been suggested that panic-focused psychodynamic psychotherapy might appeal to and help treat patients with panic disorder who do not find CBT suitable. In another report, panic patients with any *DSM* Cluster C (obsessive-compulsive, avoidant, dependent) personality disorder demonstrated greater improvement with panic-focused psychodynamic psychotherapy than did panic patients without Cluster C personality disorders (Milrod et al., 2007b). Therefore, patients with panic disorder more likely to benefit from psychodynamic psychotherapy might be those with a co-occurring, "anxious" type of personality disturbance.

Psychodynamic psychotherapy has also been used in conjunction with pharmacotherapy, whether simultaneously or following a sufficient decrease in symptoms by means of pharmacotherapy. One randomized controlled study has shown that the treatment of panic disorder with manualized, brief (12 weekly sessions) dynamic psychotherapy and clomipramine was associated with a significantly lower relapse rate than was treatment with clomipramine alone (Wiborg and Dahl, 1996). This finding suggests that psychodynamic psychotherapy may decrease panic patients' vulnerability to relapse.

Interpersonal Psychotherapy

Interpersonal psychotherapy is a potentially promising psychological treatment for panic disorder. It has shown efficacy for depression and is widely used to treat that condition. Interpersonal psychotherapy is time-limited, structured, manualized, and focuses on the interpersonal context in which panic disorder occurs. Like CBT, interpersonal psychotherapy emphasizes psychoeducation and requires the therapist to be more active, while exploring and addressing various interpersonal issues (e.g., separation, loss, fear of abandonment and dependency) that are often associated with panic disorder.

COMBINED TREATMENTS

The rationale for combining effective pharmacological and psychological treatments for panic disorder is that they might act in a complementary fashion and thereby lead to better outcomes. The issue of combined treatments is important for clinical practice, albeit one that has divided the profession. The reader should bear in mind that many of the problems identified in the context of panic disorder also apply to other anxiety disorders.

Whenever two treatment procedures are combined, the fundamental question is about the benefit of such a combination. In other words, does a combination of pharmacotherapy and CBT (as psychological treatment for which there is greatest evidence of efficacy) in panic disorder achieve better results than either treatment alone? If it does, there is justification for its use; if it does not, pharmacotherapy alone or CBT alone may be sufficient. It is this issue that has generated the most controversy.

Many CBT therapists regard a combination of CBT and pharmacotherapy as unnecessary because they argue that it is less effective than CBT alone or at best equally effective as CBT alone. Psychiatrists who rely more on pharmacotherapy than on CBT seem less opposed to combined treatment and more willing to admit that combination treatment works better than pharmacotherapy alone. After all, there is compelling evidence that when compared to pharmacotherapy alone, combined therapy is associated with a lower likelihood of relapse after cessation of treatment, regardless of whether CBT (Biondi and Picardi, 2003) or brief psychodynamic psychotherapy (Wiborg and Dahl, 1996) is used.

Establishing efficacy of combined treatment in panic disorder has been difficult because of the many methodological problems. It is not surprising that research findings in this area have often been contradictory or difficult to reconcile with clinical practice. Furthermore, merely identifying instances in which medications have been combined with psychological treatment has sometimes been difficult: in some studies of psychological treatment of panic disorder, concomitant use of medications is not reported at all, it is reported only in a cursory fashion, or if reported, it is often assumed that medication does not affect the outcome if its dose during psychological treatment does not change, with potential benefits of medication being downplayed. For example, one study that reported good results of exposure therapy in the treatment of panic disorder with agoraphobia made only cursory mention that patients were permitted to use benzodiazepines and that one fourth of the patients were taking these drugs at the conclusion of the study (Fava et al., 1995). Thus, the first obstacle to investigating the efficacy of combined treatment may be recording what treatments patients actually receive.

Discrepancies and Controversies

A small body of earlier research has found that medications such as imipramine might have a beneficial effect on exposure therapy for agoraphobia (Zitrin et al., 1980; Telch et al., 1985; Mavissakalian and Michelson, 1986b). It has been suggested that imipramine improves motivation and thereby makes it more likely for patients to engage in CBT for agoraphobia, especially self-directed exposure between sessions (Telch et al., 1985). One meta-analysis of the treatment of panic disorder found combination treatment (pharmacotherapy plus CBT) to be more efficacious than either pharmacotherapy or CBT alone (van Balkom et al., 1997).

Only a few studies suggest that a combination of CBT and pharmacotherapy confers no benefit over and above CBT alone (or some components of CBT, such as exposure therapy) in short-term treatment of panic disorder (Marks et al., 1983; Wardle et al., 1994). Research findings generally support a notion that combined treatment tends to produce better results than monotherapy with either CBT (de Beurs et al., 1995; Oehrberg et al., 1995; Barlow et al., 2000; Mitte, 2005; van Apeldoom et al., 2008) or medication (Barlow et al., 2000; Craske et al., 2005; Roy-Byrne et al., 2005) during a short-term (acute) treatment of panic disorder and/or before discontinuation of medication. One systematic review of randomized controlled trials in panic disorder comparing CBT (or various components of CBT) alone, antidepressant treatment alone, and a combination of CBT and antidepressants reported the same result in the acute treatment of panic disorder (Furukawa et al., 2006).

However, this advantage of combined treatment seems to diminish or even disappear over long-term treatment and/or after the cessation of pharmacotherapy and CBT, especially when compared to CBT alone (Mavissakalian and Michelson, 1986a; Marks et al., 1993; Otto et al., 1996; Barlow et al., 2000; Mitte, 2005). The aforementioned systematic review reported that after the acute treatment, the combined therapy was still superior to antidepressants alone, but was as effective as CBT alone, leading to a suggestion that either a combination of CBT and an antidepressant, or CBT alone, should be considered first-line treatment for panic disorder (Furukawa et al., 2006). From the cost-effectiveness perspective, it has been argued that CBT is preferable to combined treatment for panic disorder (McHugh et al., 2007). Another systematic review of randomized controlled trials in panic disorder with agoraphobia comparing exposure therapy alone, treatment with a benzodiazepine alone, and a combination of exposure therapy and benzodiazepines reported similar results, with combination therapy showing some tendency to be inferior to exposure alone after the acute phase of treatment (Watanabe et al., 2007). However, these results were based only on two methodologically rigorous studies.

Because panic disorder tends to have a chronic course and long-term treatment effects carry more weight, these research findings generally do not favor combined treatment. In contrast, combined treatment has been popular in clinical practice. The combining of pharmacotherapy and CBT (or components of CBT) is apparently preferred by patients (Craske, 1996), perceived by patients as the most effective form of treatment (Ballenger and Lydiard, 1997), and endorsed by international experts (Uhlenhuth et al., 1999) and treatment guidelines for panic disorder (e.g., American Psychiatric Association, 1998). One study conducted in a naturalistic setting, which investigated relationships between CBT and the use of various drugs for panic disorder, found that SSRIs, but not benzodiazepines, were associated with poorer outcomes (Arch and Craske, 2007). Use of benzodiazepines in this study actually decreased in the course of CBT, which runs contrary to the often-emphasized difficulties in discontinuing benzodiazepines. Finally, it has been suggested that pharmacotherapy does not have an adverse effect on the long-term outcome of CBT (Oei et al., 1997).

Possible Explanations for Discrepancies

How can these conflicting research findings be explained and clinical practice reconciled with research? As noted before, there are numerous methodological issues when studying the efficacy of any two treatments administered together, especially when these treatments are so different in nature and their proponents often ideologically intolerant of one another. These issues should always be taken into account when evaluating research results. Overall, however, it appears that combined treatments for panic disorder may be more likely to offer a short-term than a long-term advantage. A potential long-term disadvantage of combining pharmacotherapy with CBT may be accounted for by several mechanisms listed below. They all represent a variation on the theme, "no pain, no gain." In other words, if treatment progress primarily entails better coping with anxiety and panic, this can be achieved only if patients confront anxiety-provoking situations and panic symptoms without the facilitating effects of the concomitantly administered medication.

1. By decreasing anxiety, medications may promote passivity and reduce motivation for participation in CBT. Therefore, patients may not fully benefit from CBT, which becomes apparent only during and after long-term treatment.

2. During the concomitant administration of pharmacotherapy and CBT, there is no precise way of knowing what proportion of improvement is due to medication and what proportion is a result of CBT. If panic patients attribute progress to medication more than to learning new skills through CBT and personal mastery, they may run a risk of recurrence once the medication has been ceased (e.g., Marks et al., 1993; Basoglu et al., 1994). The recurrence may be a consequence of patients' difficulty in developing a sense of ownership of their treatment gains.

3. Medications may interfere with the acquisition of new skills through CBT because of the "state-dependent" learning of these skills. That is, the skills learned while patients are taking a medication cannot be effectively used in various situations outside treatment or when patients no longer take the medication. There has been mixed support, however, for the existence of state-dependent learning, and more broadly, for the interference of medications with learning that occurs during CBT (e.g., Jensen and Poulsen, 1982; Lister, 1985; Wardle et al., 1994; Morissette et al., 2008).

4. Medications may serve as safety devices when taken in the course of CBT; as such, medications perpetuate the erroneous notion that physical symptoms of anxiety and panic are dangerous and should be best dealt with by suppression. When the medication is ceased, patients may feel unprotected and fully exposed to the perceived danger of their symptoms, anxiety, and panic.

These potential mechanisms of interference do not necessarily imply that medications and CBT should not be combined in panic disorder. Instead, clinicians should be aware of them, discuss them openly with their patients, and attempt to minimize their impact. A complete understanding of how medications interact with CBT is lacking, but clinicians need to be pragmatic and combine these treatments whenever they believe that doing so might work better than monotherapy. If future studies pay more attention to the issues of when and how to combine treatments to maximize, not minimize, the benefits of such a combination, perhaps the discrepancy between research and clinical practice will diminish.

When Should Combined Treatment Be Used?

As noted above, a lack of clarity about when to use combined treatment has contributed to the ongoing controversy and confusion about its value. It appears that a combination of pharmacotherapy and CBT might be useful in the following situations and for the following purposes (Table 2–30):

1. When panic disorder is more severe, including a more severe agoraphobia (Spiegel and Bruce, 1997; American Psychiatric Association, 1998; Starcevic et al., 2004).
2. In the presence of other psychiatric conditions and/or psychiatric complications of panic disorder (e.g., depression) (Starcevic et al., 2004).
3. When it is difficult to conduct CBT because of the high level of anxiety and/or frequent or severe panic attacks (Spiegel and Bruce, 1997).
4. When there has been an insufficient response to either pharmacotherapy or CBT alone (American Psychiatric Association, 1998).
5. When the aim is to decrease the likelihood of relapse, particularly after the cessation of pharmacotherapy (Biondi and Picardi, 2003).

How to Combine Pharmacotherapy and Cognitive-Behavioral Therapy?

Sequencing

In terms of the sequence, there are basically three ways in which pharmacotherapy and CBT can be combined (Table 2–31).

Table 2–30. Possible Indications for Combining Pharmacotherapy and Cognitive-Behavioral Therapy in Panic Disorder

- Greater severity of panic disorder, including a more severe agoraphobia
- Co-occurrence of psychiatric conditions or presence of psychiatric complications of panic disorder (e.g., depression)
- Difficulty in conducting cognitive-behavioral therapy because of the high level of anxiety and/or frequent or severe panic attacks
- Insufficient (partial) response to either pharmacotherapy or CBT alone
- Decreasing the likelihood of relapse, particularly after the cessation of pharmacotherapy

Table 2–31. Sequencing of Treatments in Combined Treatment of Panic Disorder

Initially Administered Treatment	Subsequently Administered Treatment	Rationale for Combining Treatments
Pharmacotherapy	CBT	• Partial response to pharmacotherapy • Severe and persistent agoraphobia • Improving patient's coping with anxiety • Increasing the likelihood that treatment gains will last longer (relapse prevention)
CBT	Pharmacotherapy	• Partial response to CBT • High levels of anxiety or greater severity of panic disorder, which makes it difficult for patients to engage in CBT • Presence of psychiatric conditions (e.g., depression) or complications of panic disorder that may respond to pharmacotherapy
Pharmacotherapy and CBT commenced at approximately the same time		Maximizing the benefits of combined treatment from the very beginning of treatment

CBT, cognitive-behavioral therapy.

First, CBT may be added to the initially used pharmacotherapy. This seems to be the most common way of combining treatments in clinical practice: many patients are first treated with a medication, and by the time they present to a facility in which CBT is offered, they are likely to be using pharmacotherapy (e.g., Wardle, 1990). Indeed, when the clinician encounters a panic patient in specialized settings such as anxiety disorders clinics, the patient is likely to have been taking, and may still be taking, a medication; more often than not, this medication is a benzodiazepine. In this situation, CBT may be added if there has been only a partial response to pharmacotherapy, if the patient has severe and persistent agoraphobia, and/or with the goals of improving patient's coping with anxiety or increasing the likelihood that treatment gains will last longer.

Second, pharmacotherapy may be added to the initially used CBT. This may occur when patients are too distressed to participate in CBT because of the severity of anxiety and/or panic disorder, but it is somewhat controversial (from the perspective of some CBT therapists) whether a medication should be used to decrease levels of anxiety in this situation. Other reasons for adding pharmacotherapy to CBT include a partial response to CBT alone and presence of psychiatric conditions (e.g., depression) or complications of panic disorder that may respond to pharmacotherapy.

Finally, both CBT and pharmacotherapy may be commenced at approximately the same time. This does not seem to occur very often, as most clinicians prefer one treatment approach initially, and then add the other treatment modality if the initial one does not produce a desired effect or if they want to augment the response to the initially administered treatment. Most research of combined treatment has entailed administration of both treatments from the very beginning, thereby creating a somewhat artificial situation. The outcome of combined treatment studies would perhaps be different if they were to reflect the sequence in which individual treatments are administered under more natural circumstances.

Psychoeducation and Clinician Attitude

Regardless of the sequence in which CBT and pharmacotherapy are administered, it is crucial not to combine them "mechanically" (e.g., Biondi and Picardi, 2003) but in a manner that makes clinical sense. It is particularly important that patients understand the rationale for using combined treatment because they might have been receiving conflicting messages about the value of different treatments and different underlying models of psychopathology. While patients need to know what the global treatment plan is at the beginning of treatment and agree to it, they should also be prepared for treatment changes that may need to be introduced (including addition of another treatment modality), depending on their progress. Moreover, the clinician should not favor one type of treatment and suggest indirectly that he or she does not value the other treatment as much. In other words, the combined treatment is less likely to work if the clinician lacks a positive attitude toward all of its components.

Antidepressants or Benzodiazepines for Combined Treatment?

It is not known which type of medication might be better to combine with CBT for panic disorder, as antidepressants and benzodiazepines have not been directly and systematically compared in this regard. However, benzodiazepines tend to be regarded more negatively and are usually considered to interfere more with CBT. This is because of the (unsubstantiated) assumptions that patients have a greater tendency to attribute treatment gains to benzodiazepines and use these medications as safety devices, and that state-dependent learning is more readily associated with benzodiazepines.

Although some studies did not find a combination of benzodiazepines and situational exposure useful (e.g., Echeburua et al., 1993; Marks et al., 1993; Wardle et al., 1994; Otto et al., 1996), other studies indicated that the benefit of such a combination might depend on the sequence of administering these treatments (Spiegel and Bruce, 1997) and on whether benzodiazepines are administered regularly or on an as-needed (prn) basis (Westra et al., 2002). In particular, as-needed use of benzodiazepines in conjunction with CBT was associated with a negative outcome of CBT, whereas regular use of benzodiazepines did not interfere significantly with CBT (Westra et al., 2002).

OUTLOOK FOR THE FUTURE

A decision to designate recurrent panic attacks as a separate disorder has been controversial ever since panic disorder was introduced into psychiatric nosology. The survival of panic disorder as a diagnostic entity first depends on demonstrating that unexpected panic attacks are not a product of fiction. If unexpected panic attacks cannot be reliably distinguished from situational attacks on the basis of the criteria other than lack of context in which they appear, the raison d'etre for panic disorder may cease to exist. For panic disorder to be a viable concept, it would then need to be redefined, perhaps by proposing a set of different defining features. Once panic disorder is reconceptualized, its detection and recognition will hopefully improve, especially at the levels of primary and emergency care.

Future research needs to elucidate whether there are pathophysiologically distinct panic attacks. This could make possible a more accurate classification of panic attacks and better understanding of the role that they play in panic disorder, agoraphobia, and other conditions. Clarifying the links between panic disorder and agoraphobia would put an end to an increasingly fruitless debate about the primacy of panic disorder or agoraphobia when both are present.

Considering its complex relationship with various medical problems, panic disorder is perhaps the most "physical" of all the anxiety disorders. An important aspect of this status of panic disorder is its link with cardio-vascular morbidity. More prospective research is needed to understand to what extent and under what circumstances panic disorder constitutes a risk factor for heart disease. If it turns out that panic disorder (or some "type" of it) is indeed akin to a life-threatening condition, it will certainly require a different treatment approach, perhaps pharmacotherapy that would target its components more specifically. In that case, too, there would hardly be any role for psychological treatments that essentially provide reassurance that panic attacks and panic disorder cannot (ultimately) lead to a somatic catastrophe.

Because of the potentially serious complications of panic disorder, there is no room for complacency about the relatively good results of current pharmacological and psychological treatments. More effort is needed to prevent occurrence of panic disorder in predisposed individuals, deliver treatment early, improve access to it, and minimize dropout. As a result, CBT for panic disorder may be modified accordingly (e.g., through Internet-based delivery and various self-help approaches) and on the basis of greater appreciation of how its ingredients work to bring about a meaningful therapeutic change. Identifying who is more likely to benefit from which type of treatment is another task. The main challenge to the pharmacotherapy of panic disorder comes from a high risk of recurrence following the cessation of treatment, and future research needs to illumi-nate ways of minimizing this risk. Yet another task is to investigate how pharmacotherapy and CBT could be combined to improve the outcome.

3

Generalized Anxiety Disorder

The main characteristics of generalized anxiety disorder (GAD) are chronic pathological worry, other manifestations of nonphobic anxiety, and various symptoms of tension. Physical symptoms of anxiety are usually less prominent in GAD than in panic disorder, but they can still be an important component of clinical presentation. Behaviors that are often seen in other anxiety disorders, such as overt avoidance, are conspicuously absent. Unlike all other anxiety disorders, it is more likely for GAD in clinical setting to co-occur with a primary condition for which help has been sought—usually depression or other anxiety disorder—than to be the main reason for seeking professional help. Generalized anxiety disorder is one of the more controversial members of the family of anxiety disorders: it seems that almost every aspect of GAD has provoked debates that do not show signs of abating.

KEY ISSUES

Paradox, disagreement, debate, and controversy are the words most commonly associated with GAD. It is small wonder then that the list of "hot topics" related to GAD could be very long indeed. Listed below is a selection of issues thought to represent adequately a more comprehensive list.

1. What are the characteristic features of GAD that would help in its conceptualization? Pathological worry, other cognitive aspects of anxiety, manifestations of tension, and/or (some) symptoms of autonomic arousal? What combination of these features would ensure that GAD is diagnosed adequately and recognized in clinical practice?
2. What is the relationship between pathological worry and GAD?
3. How can different views on what constitutes the essence of GAD be reconciled? Is GAD a single entity or are there two or more "types" of GAD with distinct clinical characteristics?

4. How is GAD related to depressive disorders, other anxiety disorders, and personality disturbance? Where are its boundaries? In view of its close relationship with depression, should GAD be classified along with depression and perhaps renamed accordingly?

5. Can GAD exist on its own, without depression or other anxiety disorders? What could be features specific enough for GAD that would allow it to establish itself as an independent and valid psychopathological and diagnostic entity?

6. What are the pathophysiological correlates of pathological worry and other aspects of chronic anxiety in GAD?

7. What are the underlying mechanisms and purpose of pathological worry in GAD? What is the meaning of chronic anxiety?

8. How distinct is pharmacological treatment of GAD from that of depression? Are "broad-spectrum" antianxiety and antidepressant effects of medications sufficient to treat GAD?

9. What should be targeted by psychological treatments for GAD? Has the overemphasis on pathological worry turned psychological treatment of GAD into a "worry management program?" What are the alternatives in psychological treatment approaches to GAD?

CLINICAL FEATURES

Generalized anxiety disorder has been called the "basic" anxiety disorder (Barlow, 1988). This implies that many of its features characterize all anxiety disorders, and it is not surprising that singling out clinical features that might be specific for GAD has been difficult. Bearing this in mind, GAD encompasses in various proportions the following "clusters" of clinical features: (1) pathological worry and other cognitive aspects of chronic anxiety, (2) symptoms of tension and consequences of tension and anxiety, and (3) various physical symptoms, most of which reflect autonomic hyperactivity.

Pathological Worry and Other Cognitive Aspects of Chronic Anxiety

In *DSM-IV-TR*, GAD has been defined as a condition in which pathological worry is the most conspicuous feature. Also following *DSM-IV-TR*, pathological worry is conceptualized as being excessive, out of proportion to the actual problem (if such a problem exists), uncontrollable, pervasive, present almost constantly, and relating to several topics or domains (Table 3–1). In addition, pathological worry often pertains to events and circumstances in the remote future, and this may be one feature that is relatively specific for GAD (Dugas et al., 1998a).

Table 3–1. Characteristics of Pathological Worry

1. Excessive in intensity and/or out of proportion to the actual problem (if such a problem exists)
2. Almost constant (present more often than not; most of the day, nearly every day)
3. Pervasive
4. Uncontrollable; although it is self-initiated, it has an intrusive quality (e.g., the person states that he or she is unable to stop worrying)
5. Relates to several topics or domains (e.g., the person worries about health, finances, and work at the same time)
6. Associated with negative affect
7. Tends to prevent the person from shifting focus, inhibits problem solving, and interferes with decision-making process

Characteristics of Pathological Worry More Likely to Be Seen in Generalized Anxiety Disorder

1. Escalating pattern of "what if . . ." style of questioning
2. Worry usually pertains to remote future circumstances, with negative perception of the future
3. Presence of negative beliefs about worry
4. Poor tolerance of ambiguity and especially, poor tolerance of uncertainty

Patients with GAD worry about matters that may seem minor or unrealistic, but they also worry about health of loved ones, marital relationship, performance at work or in school, and so on. Worry often pertains to something in the future, and GAD patients perceive the future negatively and with much apprehension, as they might get sick, lose a job, or have no money, their children might have an accident, etc. Patients tend to overestimate the probability that events they worry about will happen. The worry themes are not unusual or odd in themselves, as many people without GAD do worry about similar things. Therefore, for the conceptualization of pathological worry, it is more important *how* people worry rather than *what* they worry about. The process of worrying is characterized by repetitive, prolonged, and fruitless thought activity, which is associated with negative affect and tends to inhibit problem solving.

Patients with GAD usually worry about more issues or matters than "normal" worriers. Also, the worry in GAD is almost constant, and it seems to patients that they have been troubled by worries for a very long time ("I have always been a worrier" is a typical statement made by GAD patients). Patients often realize that they worry excessively but feel that they cannot do anything to stop worrying. There is also a component of intrusiveness in the experience of pathological worry. As a result, worries are often described as "unwanted," but patients are preoccupied with worrying to the extent that they find it difficult to distract themselves, focus on something else, and fully experience or enjoy their lives.

Pathological worry is often accompanied by certain beliefs about worry. It has been demonstrated that "positive" beliefs (e.g., believing that it is beneficial to worry) characterize many if not all worriers, whereas "negative" beliefs (e.g., believing that worrying is dangerous and has some catastrophic consequences) are more typical of worriers who also suffer from GAD (Wells, 1995, 1997; Ruscio and Borkovec, 2004).

The thought processes of patients with GAD are often characterized by the escalating pattern of "what if..." style of questioning, whereby one imagined catastrophe leads to another. For example, a patient with health-related worries expressed the corresponding concerns in the following sequence: "What if they find that I have cancer? What if I have to undergo surgery? Will I be allergic to the anesthetic? What if my children have to watch me dying? How will they manage financially after my death?"

Many GAD patients have trouble tolerating any ambiguity and uncertainty (Ladouceur et al., 1997). They tend to interpret ambiguous situations as implying some hidden danger, which further "justifies" their worrying. The sense of uncertainty undermines their confidence and makes them more vigilant. Uncertainty also implies more risks than patients can tolerate, and because the decision-making process involves taking some risk, they have trouble making decisions. Intolerance of uncertainty is more specifically related to pathological worry than is intolerance of ambiguity (Buhr and Dugas, 2006).

Sometimes patients with GAD have difficulty identifying what they worry about or are vague about it. They may have nonspecific concerns about some existential and philosophical issues (such as the meaning and purpose of life and death) or state that they are anxious "about everything." They may also experience what has been referred to as "free-floating anxiety"—a pervasive anxious feeling, without a clear focus of anxiety.

The relationship between worry and anxiety is not well understood. Many view worry as an aspect of anxiety, especially as its cognitive component (O'Neill, 1985). According to another view, worry is different from anxiety, on grounds that worry can occur in the absence of fear (Levy and Guttman, 1976), that worry and anxiety correlate poorly in patients with GAD (Meyer et al., 1990), and that in comparison with anxiety, worry is more strongly associated with depression, confusion, lack of emotional control, and lack of control over problem solving (Zebb and Beck, 1998). If worry and anxiety are indeed, different phenomena, they should be assessed separately (see Assessment, below). Regardless of the precise nature of their relationship, there seems to be much overlap between these concepts.

Instead of pathological worry, other cognitive aspects of chronic anxiety have been presumed to characterize GAD (see Diagnostic and Conceptual Issues, below). These have been referred to as "apprehensive expectation," "apprehension," "anxious expectation," and so on, but they have not been described as well as pathological worry and probably have much in common with the concept of pathological worry.

Symptoms of Tension and Consequences of Tension and Anxiety

Patients with GAD are troubled by tension that can be experienced in many different ways (Table 3–2). Thus, patients often state that they are constantly nervous, keyed up, on edge, unable to relax, restless, "cranky," "ready to explode," unable to tolerate anything, and the like. As a result of the ongoing, excessive perception of threat, GAD patients tend to be hypervigilant: they are constantly on alert, expect something bad to happen, and get startled easily by ordinary, innocuous, and suddenly occurring stimuli, such as a knock on the door or the telephone ringing.

A very common physical aspect of tension is muscle tightness or stiffness (or muscle tension), which often leads to pain. As a result, GAD patients often complain of a stiff neck, back pain, or shoulder pain. Tension headache is another typical feature of GAD, with the headache usually being located in the back or frontal regions or described as "aching all over." Muscle tension was found to have a "unique relation" to pathological worry and was therefore assumed to be relatively specific for GAD (Joormann and Stöber, 1999). Patients may also complain of muscle spasms, tic-like movements, jerks, and fine tremor. These symptoms may be particularly prominent in eyelids and other facial muscles. Another manifestation of tension is difficulty in

---

Table 3–2. Manifestations of Tension in Generalized Anxiety Disorder

Psychological and Behavioral Aspects of Tension
- Nervousness
- Feeling keyed up, on edge, unable to relax
- Inner restlessness
- Irritability: feeling "cranky" or "ready to explode," getting easily annoyed or angry, having decreased tolerance for frustration
- Hypervigilance: feeling constantly on alert, expecting something bad to happen, getting startled easily
- Agitation

Physical (Somatic) Aspects of Tension
- Muscle tightness or stiffness (muscle tension): stiff neck, back pain, shoulder pain, tension headache
- Muscle spasms
- Tic-like movements, jerks
- Fine tremor
- Difficulty in swallowing ("psychogenic dysphagia")—fear of choking on food

Consequences of Tension and Anxiety
- Difficulty concentrating
- Sleep disturbance: trouble falling asleep, "broken sleep," unrefreshing sleep
- Fatigue, exhaustion, getting tired easily

---

swallowing, sometimes referred to as "psychogenic dysphagia"; this may lead to the fear of choking on food.

The consequences of tension and anxiety include difficulty in concentrating and inability to quickly shift the focus of attention from one subject to another, feeling tired or becoming tired too easily, and disturbed sleep. Patients usually have trouble falling asleep, but many have "broken sleep" or wake up feeling that their sleep has not been refreshing.

Other Physical Symptoms

Generalized anxiety disorder is also characterized by various other physical symptoms, which sometimes dominate the clinical presentation. Although the emphasis in the current *DSM* conceptualization of GAD is on pathological worry and tension, some patients with GAD present mainly with physical symptoms. In such cases, patients are more likely to seek help in primary care or other medical settings. Physical symptoms are not specific for GAD, as they often appear in other anxiety disorders, particularly panic disorder. Unlike panic disorder, in which physical symptoms are usually severe but appear episodically during panic attacks, physical symptoms in GAD are usually less intense but more chronic.

Many of the common physical symptoms in GAD reflect autonomic hyperarousal: tachycardia, palpitations, sweating, dry mouth, and trembling or shaking. Patients with GAD relatively frequently complain of gastrointestinal symptoms, such as nausea, upset stomach, and diarrhea. Other symptoms that may be seen among GAD patients include dizziness, lightheadedness, hot and cold flushes, numbness, and tingling sensations. Breathing difficulties, chest tightness, and chest pain are sometimes severe and lead patients to seek help in cardiology clinics, not unlike panic patients (Logue et al., 1993).

Physical symptoms may be the main vehicle through which GAD patients express distress, whereas expression of distress is often determined by personal and cultural factors. Thus, GAD patients in Asian countries are more likely to present with physical symptoms than GAD patients in the United States (e.g., Hoge et al., 2006). Unexplained physical symptoms attributed to the process of somatization are not rare among patients with GAD.

RELATIONSHIP BETWEEN GENERALIZED ANXIETY DISORDER AND OTHER DISORDERS

The relationship between GAD and other disorders is unique in that GAD almost "needs" other disorders to be present in order for it to be noticed. That is, GAD is usually diagnosed as a condition co-occurring with another disorder and less often as the only disorder for which help is being sought.

This has led to some doubt that GAD is an independent diagnostic entity and to a suggestion that GAD is no more than a precursor or a complication of other psychiatric disorders. For example, when GAD is a chronologically primary condition, it may represent a risk factor or predisposition for the development of some conditions with which it commonly co-occurs; this temporal relationship often exists between GAD and depression (major depressive disorder or dysthymic disorder). In contrast, when GAD develops after panic disorder, it may be regarded as a complication or a consequence of panic disorder.

Most patients with GAD have other psychiatric disorders; as many as 89% of GAD patients in the primary care setting have been diagnosed with at least one additional psychiatric condition (Olfson et al., 1997). In contrast to other anxiety disorders in which the rates of co-occurrence of other disorders are often much higher in clinical than in general populations, GAD has similar rates of co-occurrence in both populations. Psychiatric conditions that most frequently co-occur with GAD are major depressive disorder (up to 46% of patients currently and up to 64% over lifetime), social anxiety disorder (59% over lifetime), specific phobias (55% over life-time), dysthymic disorder (39.5% over lifetime), and panic disorder (27% over lifetime) (Brawman-Mintzer et al., 1993; Wittchen et al., 1994; Brawman-Mintzer and Lydiard, 1996; Wittchen and Jacobi, 2005). The most important relationship is the one between GAD and depressive disorders. Generalized anxiety disorder also has strong links with panic disorder (see Chapter 2) and with some of the other anxiety disorders (see Generalized Anxiety Disorder and Social Anxiety Disorder, and Differential Diagnosis, below).

Generalized anxiety disorder also has some association (in up to 15% of patients) with alcohol abuse and dependence (Brawman-Mintzer and Lydiard, 1996). Alcohol-related problems, however, are less prominent in patients with "pure" GAD than in those with some other anxiety disorders, especially social anxiety disorder and posttraumatic stress disorder. Generalized anxiety disorder may occur in people who have been abusing alcohol, for example, following alcohol withdrawal. Some symptoms of withdrawal from alcohol or other substances may be difficult to distinguish from autonomic hyperactivity and tension symptoms seen in patients with GAD. Alcoholism may also appear some time after the onset of GAD, as part of the patients' self-medicating strategy for coping with anxiety; how-ever, this is less common than with patients suffering from social anxiety disorder.

Personality disturbance may be present in a substantial number of GAD patients, with dependent and avoidant personality disorders being most common (Mavissakalian et al., 1993; Grant et al., 2005a). The relationship between GAD and personality disorders is discussed in more detail in Differential Diagnosis and Etiology and Pathogenesis, below.

Generalized Anxiety Disorder and Depression

It has been suggested that GAD is more closely related to depressive disorders than to the other anxiety disorders (Brown et al., 1998). This is somewhat paradoxical for a condition once considered to be the "basic" anxiety disorder. Studies of the structure of psychopathology have consistently reported that GAD, along with major depressive disorder and dysthymic disorder, belongs to a group characterized by "anxious-misery" and subsequently called "distress disorders" or "dysphoric disorders" (Krueger, 1999; Vollebergh et al., 2001; Slade and Watson, 2006). These studies did not group GAD together with "fear disorders" (panic disorder, agoraphobia, social anxiety disorder, and specific phobias).

Twin studies have found that GAD and major depressive disorder share a single genetic diathesis and are genetically indistinguishable (Roy et al., 1995; Kendler, 1996), prompting a suggestion that as far as genetic risk factors are concerned, GAD and major depressive disorder represent one disorder (Kendler et al., 2007). Other studies have reported that GAD and major depressive disorder have common vulnerability traits and other personality-level risk factors, such as high levels of neuroticism and negative affect/emotionality (e.g., Watson et al., 2005). Primary GAD has been found to be a significant predictor of the subsequent depression (Bruce et al., 2001) and to have the strongest power to do so of all the anxiety disorders (Hettema et al., 2003; Wittchen et al., 2003). This close relationship between GAD and depressive disorders has led to GAD being considered the main challenger of the dichotomy between anxiety and depression (Starcevic, 2008).

On clinical grounds, the relationship between GAD and depression is important for several reasons (Table 3–3). Perhaps most fundamentally, both are characterized by a predominantly dysphoric mood or negative affect (Clark and Watson, 1991). Their clinical presentation often overlaps,

Table 3–3. Clinical Implications of the Relationship Between Generalized Anxiety Disorder and Depression

Aspects of the Relationship Between GAD and Depression	Clinical Implications
Overlap between symptoms of GAD and depression	Difficulties in distinguishing between GAD and depression
Depression is the most frequent complication of GAD and the most common reason for GAD patients to seek help	When GAD patients present for help and treatment, there is a high likelihood that they have a co-occurring depression
High likelihood that a substantial proportion of GAD patients will develop depression	Treatment of GAD may prevent the development of depression

and the differentiation between GAD and depression may sometimes be very difficult. In fact, some of the GAD symptoms and the corresponding diagnostic criteria are also seen in depression. This pertains to sleep disturbance, concentration difficulties, and fatigue or exhaustion. Even pathological worry, considered a key feature of GAD in the *DSM* system, was found to characterize major depressive disorder to the same extent (Starcevic, 1995). Pathological worry in GAD and ruminations in depression may be indistinguishable, although theoretically, the former is more future-oriented, whereas the latter are more past-oriented, and also, their themes are supposed to be different: patients with GAD are concerned about multiple threats, whereas depressed patients tend to ruminate somewhat monothematically about losses, mistakes, wrongdoings, and/or guilt (Craske et al., 1989; Segerstrom et al., 2000; Watkins et al., 2005). Poor tolerance of uncertainty may also characterize both GAD and depression (Miranda et al., 2008).

The symptoms that can most reliably distinguish depression from chronic anxiety and GAD are loss of interest and anhedonia (Clark DA et al., 1994; Mineka et al., 1998). Symptoms that are most likely to suggest anxiety disorder as the main condition are those of autonomic hyperactivity and arousal (Clark and Watson, 1991); however, these symptoms may be more typical of panic disorder than of GAD.

Depression is the most frequent complication of GAD and the most likely reason for GAD patients to seek help. Therefore, by the time GAD patients see a physician or other therapist, the presence of co-occurring depression should always be kept in mind. A high probability for GAD patients to develop depression has important practical implications, because it may be possible for depression to be prevented by an early treatment of GAD.

Although it is more typical for depression to appear some time after the onset of GAD, different temporal patterns have been reported. For example, in one longitudinal study, GAD preceded major depressive disorder in 42% of the cases, but in 32% major depressive disorder was a chronologically primary condition and preceded GAD, and in 26% there was a concurrent onset of GAD and major depressive disorder (Moffitt et al., 2007a). These and other research findings indicate that GAD and major depressive disorder may be distinct, although closely related, and that they are unlikely to be different forms of the same disorder. Thus, a shortened rapid eye movement (REM) latency has been found in major depressive disorder, but not in GAD (Papadimitriou et al., 1988), and the two conditions had relatively few common childhood risk factors (Moffitt et al., 2007b). There is a need to clarify and better understand the relationship between GAD and depressive disorders, and this relationship is therefore a subject of much ongoing research.

Generalized Anxiety Disorder and Social Anxiety Disorder

Generalized anxiety disorder and social anxiety disorder often co-occur in clinical practice, with rates of social anxiety disorder in primary GAD ranging between 23% and 59% (Sanderson et al., 1990; Brawman-Mintzer et al., 1993). Generalized anxiety disorder and social anxiety disorder have some features in common, including early and gradual onset. Both disorders may have a similar origin, but the perceived threat in GAD spreads to various issues and areas, whereas the perceived threat in social anxiety disorder remains in the realm of social and interpersonal interactions and situations. Thus, GAD is a wider psychopathological concept, which may encompass some features of social anxiety disorder. It is not surprising, then, that even in the absence of a diagnosis of social anxiety disorder, concerns about performance and negative evaluation may be in the focus of worries of GAD patients. Generalized anxiety disorder and the generalized type of social anxiety disorder also have in common the pervasiveness of clinical features and their frequent construal as a form of personality disturbance rather than a mental state (*DSM* Axis I) disorder.

ASSESSMENT

Diagnostic and Conceptual Issues

There are several issues surrounding the diagnostic conceptualization of GAD and contributing to the uncertainty about the conceptual status of GAD. They include differences between various diagnostic criteria, non-specific nature of most features of GAD, and high rates of co-occurrence of GAD with other disorders.

Different Diagnostic Criteria

Diagnostic criteria for GAD have been changing too frequently within the *DSM* system. Generalized anxiety disorder has gone from a residual diagnostic category in *DSM-III* (to be used only if diagnostic criteria for other anxiety disorders and depression have not been met) to a condition characterized by both physical and psychological symptoms in *DSM-III-R* and then to a disorder whose key feature is pathological worry in *DSM-IV* and *DSM-IV-TR*. The lack of continuity in the conceptualization of GAD is a significant problem because it is uncertain whether different "versions" of *DSM*-defined GAD refer to the same condition. This conceptual instability is one of the main reasons for the finding that of all anxiety disorders, GAD had the lowest diagnostic reliability (Brown et al., 2001).

In addition, there are important differences between the *DSM-IV-TR* and *ICD-10* concepts of GAD and between the corresponding diagnostic criteria (Table 3–4). While GAD is basically viewed as a worry disorder or worry-tension disorder in the *DSM* system, it is largely regarded as an autonomic arousal disorder in the *ICD* system. As a result, although the *DSM*- and *ICD*-defined GAD overlap, they are not identical disorders.

Table 3–4. Differences in Conceptualization of Generalized Anxiety Disorder in DSM-IV-TR and ICD-10

Criteria	DSM-IV-TR	ICD-10
Nosological status	Independent diagnostic category	Residual diagnostic category; cannot be diagnosed if criteria for diagnosing other anxiety disorders, depression, or hypochondriasis have been met
Pathological worry	Must be present for diagnosis to be made	Not necessary for diagnosis
Symptoms of autonomic hyperactivity and other physical symptoms	Not necessary for diagnosis	Must be present for diagnosis to be made
Duration of symptoms	At least 6 months	Several months

These contrasts in the way GAD is viewed have further consequences and implications and make GAD a great "dichotomizer" because it has polarized mental health professionals and researchers on several levels and in several domains (Table 3–5).

Nonspecific Symptoms

The next set of issues relates to the fact that most features of GAD are not specific enough for this condition. Much research in this area has focused on the specificity of pathological worry for GAD. Many individuals with chronic and severe worry were not found to meet diagnostic criteria for GAD (Ruscio, 2002), suggesting that chronic and severe worry may not be sufficient for the diagnosis of GAD. Although some research has reported

Table 3–5. Generalized Anxiety Disorder as a "Dichotomizer"

- DSM-IV-TR vs. ICD-10
- Cognitive aspects of anxiety vs. somatic aspects of anxiety (reinforcer of the mind-body dichotomy)
- Cognition (worry) vs. emotion (anxiety)
- Clinical psychologists (emphasizing worry in GAD) vs. psychiatrists (emphasizing anxiety, especially somatic anxiety, in GAD)
- Measurement of worry vs. measurement of anxiety in the assessment and treatment studies of GAD

higher levels of pathological worry in GAD than in other anxiety disorders (Hoyer et al., 2001; Chelminski and Zimmerman, 2003; Fresco et al., 2003) and depression (Becker et al., 2003; Chelminski and Zimmerman, 2003; Gladstone et al., 2005), in other studies levels of pathological worry have been as high in GAD as in some other anxiety disorders (Mohlman et al., 2004; Gladstone et al., 2005; Starcevic et al., 2007) and depression (Starcevic, 1995). A specific association of pathological worry and GAD has been deemed uncertain (Becker et al., 2003), and a significant and strong relationship was found to exist between pathological worry, GAD, and social anxiety disorder, thus failing to support a notion that pathological worry is exclusively related to GAD (Starcevic et al., 2007). Several researchers have raised doubt about the validity of diagnosing GAD via pathological worry in view of the questionable specificity of pathological worry for GAD (Bienvenue et al., 1998; Rickels and Rynn, 2001; Ruscio et al., 2005).

Many symptoms of tension and consequences of tension and anxiety (e.g., difficulties with concentration, sleep disturbance, fatigue) are also nonspecific for GAD and are encountered among people with other anxiety disorders and depression. As noted before, physical symptoms of anxiety are the least characteristic of GAD and are also found in panic disorder and a range of other conditions.

Because of the insufficient symptom specificity, one of the main challenges for the future conceptualization of GAD is to develop a set of diagnostic criteria that would be more specific for this condition.

While pathological worry is not a perfect concept, it is less vague than the alternatives of "anxious expectation," "anxious apprehension," "apprehensive expectation," and "free-floating anxiety." Pathological worry may become more useful as a diagnostic criterion for GAD if its features that are more likely to be associated with GAD are included. These refer to various negative beliefs that people with GAD often have about worrying, strong focus of worrying on the future (along with the negative perception of future), poor tolerance of uncertainty, and the associated, escalating pattern of "what if . . ." style of questioning (see Table 3–1).

There seems to be a consensus about inclusion of the symptoms of tension and at least some consequences of tension and anxiety in any conceptualization of GAD. However, the minimum number of these symptoms may need to be increased to strengthen the specificity of the diagnosis (e.g., Brown TA et al., 1995; Starcevic and Bogojevic, 1999).

Certain autonomic arousal symptoms may be more common among patients with GAD: nausea or abdominal distress, sweating, dry mouth, palpitations or tachycardia, and trembling or shaking (Hoehn-Saric and McLeod, 1985; Marten et al., 1993; Brawman-Mintzer et al., 1994; Starcevic et al., 1994a; Abel and Borkovec, 1995; Starcevic and Bogojevic, 1999). It has been proposed that at least one of these symptoms should be required for the diagnosis of GAD (Starcevic and Bogojevic, 1999). This could also improve the specificity of the diagnosis and go some way toward reducing the dichotomy between GAD as a worry disorder (or worry-tension disorder) and GAD as an autonomic arousal disorder.

High Rates of Co-occurrence

As already noted, GAD co-occurs so frequently with other psychiatric disorders that it is rarely seen in relative isolation from them, prompting some to call it a "comorbid disease" (Nutt et al., 2006). As a result, GAD is more likely to be a secondary condition than a disorder for which patients seek help, and many clinicians do not regard it as particularly useful for clinical practice. This has led to a view that GAD represents no more than a prodrome, residual, or severity marker of another disorder, especially major depressive disorder.

Epidemiological data suggest that in the community, the rates of co-occurrence of other disorders with GAD are not significantly higher than the corresponding rates for other anxiety and other *DSM* Axis I disorders (Wittchen et al., 1994; Kessler et al., 2001; Grant et al., 2005a). High rates of co-occurrence in clinical samples of GAD patients might be due to a help-seeking bias, with a greater likelihood for people with GAD presenting in clinical settings to have more than one diagnosis solely because they seek treatment. However, these considerations do not seem to have changed clinicians' perception of GAD as a disorder with dubious clinical validity.

Controversies surrounding high rates of co-occurrence of GAD with other disorders underlie the ultimate issue in GAD—that of its conceptual status. There continues to be some doubt about GAD as an independent diagnostic category, mainly because of the many characteristics it shares with depression and other anxiety disorders (e.g., Watson et al., 2005; Kendler et al., 2007). In contrast, it has been argued that GAD is an independent psychopathological entity with regard to major depressive disorder, on the basis of the distinct neurobiological (neuroanatomical, neurotransmitter, neuroendocrinological, and polysomnographic) underpinnings, risk factors, and impairment profiles (e.g., Grant et al., 2005a; Moffitt et al., 2007b; Kessler et al., 2008). The latter proposition also rejects a view that GAD and major depression are only different manifestations of a single underlying syndrome (Grant et al., 2005a; Kessler et al., 2008). Other aspects of the relationship between GAD and depression are addressed in the Relationship Between Generalized Anxiety Disorder and Other Disorders (above).

Assessment Instruments

The most commonly used instrument for assessment of the degree of pathological worry (not necessarily related to GAD) is the Penn State Worry Questionnaire (Meyer et al., 1990). This is a brief, easy-to-administer, self-report measure, which is also useful for monitoring changes in the degree of pathological worry during treatment.

The Hamilton Anxiety Rating Scale (Hamilton, 1959) is one of the most frequently used instruments for measuring the degree of general anxiety, which cuts across various anxiety disorders. This clinician-administered instrument has served as a gold standard in pharmacotherapy trials of GAD. The scale assesses both the psychological and somatic symptoms of anxiety, but it does not specifically address worry; symptoms of autonomic arousal considered less important for GAD in *DSM-IV-TR* are emphasized. The Hamilton Anxiety Rating Scale can be useful for treatment monitoring purposes if administered along with the Penn State Worry Questionnaire.

As an alternative to the Hamilton Anxiety Rating Scale, a self-report Beck Anxiety Inventory (Beck et al., 1988) can be used because its administration is simpler. The Beck Anxiety Inventory emphasizes somatic symptoms of anxiety, which are not specific for GAD.

In an attempt to develop a brief, yet comprehensive measure of the severity of GAD, Sheehan and co-workers have proposed the Worry-Anxiety-Tension Scale (Sheehan et al., 2000). This self-report instrument generates a total score for the severity of GAD and separate scores for the severity of its main components by measuring separately the degree of pathological worry, general anxiety, and tension. Another instrument that measures the severity of GAD, the Generalized Anxiety Disorder Severity Scale (Shear et al., 2006), has been constructed using similar principles as the Worry-Anxiety-Tension Scale, except that it is a clinician-administered measure. It yields a total score of the severity of GAD and separate scores on six subscales: frequency of worries, distress due to worrying, frequency of associated symptoms (including tension), severity and distress due to associated symptoms, impairment/interference in work functioning, and impairment/interference in social functioning.

Differential Diagnosis

Generalized anxiety disorder needs to be distinguished from normal worries and various medical and psychiatric conditions, as well as substance-induced disorders (Table 3–6).

Generalized anxiety disorder may resemble "normal" anxiety. Criteria for distinguishing between normal worries and GAD have been spelled out in Clinical Features (above) and in Table 3–1. In addition, normal worries are not accompanied by the degree of tension, multiple manifestations of tension, and/or physical symptoms of anxiety seen in GAD, and there is no interference with functioning and no impairment in people with normal worries and normal anxiety.

Table 3–6. Differential Diagnosis of Generalized Anxiety Disorder

1. Normal worries or normal anxiety
2. Medical conditions (e.g., hyperthyroidism)
3. Substance use disorders

   Intoxication with psychostimulants (e.g., amphetamine)
   Caffeinism
   Alcohol withdrawal syndrome
   Benzodiazepine withdrawal syndrome

4. Psychiatric disorders

   Mood disorders (major depressive disorder, dysthymic disorder)
   Mixed anxiety and depressive disorder
   Panic disorder
   Obsessive-compulsive disorder
   Hypochondriasis
   Specific phobias
   Posttraumatic stress disorder
   Adjustment disorders
   Personality disorders (avoidant, dependent)

Medical Differential Diagnosis

Symptoms of GAD may appear in the course of hyperthyroidism and, less often, as part of asthma, chronic lung disease, various heart conditions, hypertension, diabetes mellitus, and certain neurological, metabolic, and other endocrinological diseases. A diagnosis of GAD is not warranted if it seems that GAD-like features are secondary to any medical condition, particularly if successful treatment of the medical condition brings about a disappearance of the symptoms of GAD. If the features of GAD persist despite improvement in medical condition, it is not likely that these features are attributable to the medical condition and a diagnosis of GAD is probably justified. Generalized anxiety disorder is relatively frequently seen in patients with irritable bowel syndrome, but the etiological significance of this association, if any, is not well understood.

Medical workup of patients with GAD should include routine laboratory analyses with thyroid function tests. Depending on the age of the patient, symptoms, and specific circumstances, the workup may also include a cardiological examination with electrocardiogram. A thorough medical workup is particularly important in elderly patients with features of GAD because of the increased probability of an association with various medical conditions.

Substance Use Disorders and Generalized Anxiety Disorder

Generalized anxiety disorder may need to be differentiated from intoxication with stimulant substances, such as amphetamine. In clinical practice, the most common stimulant-related disorder is intoxication with caffeine, and all patients with GAD-like clinical presentation should routinely be asked about their consumption of coffee and caffeinated beverages. It is important to distinguish between GAD and caffeine intoxication, as the two may share some clinical features (e.g., upset stomach and other gastrointestinal problems, tachycardia or other heart rhythm disturbances). Caffeine intoxication is more likely to be accompanied by symptoms such as frequent urination.

Sometimes GAD may also need to be distinguished from alcohol or benzodiazepine withdrawal syndromes.

Psychiatric Differential Diagnosis

In the psychiatric differential diagnosis, the first task is to distinguish GAD from a depressive disorder (both major depressive disorder and dysthymia) because of the significant overlap between their typical symptoms. The relationship between GAD and depression and criteria for distinguishing between the two are presented in Relationship Between Generalized Anxiety Disorder and Other Disorders (above).

Mixed anxiety and depressive disorder exists in *ICD-10* but not in the *DSM* system (except as a provisional diagnosis that requires further study). It can be used if neither the diagnosis of a specific anxiety disorder, including GAD, nor the diagnosis of a depressive disorder can be made. In other words, mixed anxiety and depressive disorder has been construed as a residual diagnosis for patients with diagnostically "subthreshold" manifestations of GAD and depression. This is a controversial proposition because it is not logical for an apparently common condition such as mixed anxiety and depressive disorder to be treated as a residual diagnostic category. Second, it may be more meaningful for mixed anxiety and depressive disorder to encompass full-blown anxiety and depressive disorders (for example, when GAD and major depressive disorder co-occur) rather than for these co-occurring anxiety and depressive disorders to be listed separately. A clinically relevant combination of the symptoms of anxiety and depression has been referred to as "cothymia" (Tyrer, 2001).

With regard to other anxiety disorders, the concept of worry has a place analogous to that of panic attacks. That is, just as panic attacks occur in various disorders and do not characterize only panic disorder, pathological worry is not confined only to GAD and is found in other psychiatric conditions, and other anxiety disorders in particular (e.g., Starcevic et al., 2007). For this reason, it is erroneous to equate pathological worry with GAD. Pathological worry in GAD may to some extent be differentiated from pathological worry in other anxiety disorders on the basis of the criteria listed in Table 3–1, its focus and pervasiveness. The focus of worry in other anxiety disorders is more circumscribed: patients with panic disorder are excessively concerned about future panic attacks and their consequences, whereas those with social anxiety disorder worry about being judged too harshly by others. Not only do patients with GAD worry about matters and issues from different domains but they may also worry about worrying—a phenomenon referred to as "meta-worry"

(Wells, 1994). In clinical practice, however, it may be difficult to be certain whether pathological worry is attributable to GAD or to another anxiety disorder or depression.

Criteria for differentiating between GAD and panic disorder are listed in Table 2-13.

Obsessive-compulsive disorder sometimes needs to be considered in the differential diagnosis of GAD because of the similarities between obsessions and pathological worry that characterize these conditions: both of these phenomena are experienced as uncontrollable and repetitive. In addition, obsessions involving doubting and centered on the need to check may seem similar to pathological worry and are often both related to a poor tolerance of uncertainty (Tolin et al., 2003). There may also be an overlap between worries and obsessions, so that worries with ego-dystonic features and obsessions with some basis in reality are difficult to categorize as worries and obsessions, respectively (Langlois et al., 2000). In most cases, however, GAD and pathological worry can be differentiated from obsessive-compulsive disorder and obsessions (see Table 3–7 and Chapter 6).

Patients with GAD who worry excessively about health and disease usually do not suspect that they already have a serious physical disease, as in hypochondriasis. Likewise, GAD patients do not exhibit typical hypochondriacal behaviors, such as seeking reassurance and subjecting themselves to numerous medical investigations.

Patients with GAD differ from patients with some types of specific phobias, particularly phobia of choking and disease phobia, in terms of having a broader anxiety. Also, their fears lack a phobic quality and these patients typically do not exhibit avoidance behavior.

Table 3–7. Distinguishing Between Generalized Anxiety Disorder and Obsessive-Compulsive Disorder

Criteria	Pathological Worry in GAD	Obsessions in OCD
Quality of the experience	Ego-syntonic, not alien, "crazy," or inappropriate	Ego-dystonic, alien, "crazy," or inappropriate
Content	Real-life problems (health, work, school, relationships, finances)	Referring to something abhorrent or shameful (e.g., contamination, aggressive or sexual urges) and/or implying one's personal involvement or responsibility
Relation to images	Usually not present	Often very strong
Need to neutralize	Usually not present	Usually very strong

OCD, obsessive-compulsive disorder.

Generalized anxiety disorder differs from posttraumatic stress disorder and adjustment disorders in that it is not necessarily preceded by and is not etiologically associated with a trauma or a stressful event.

Because of its chronic course and early onset in many of its sufferers, GAD may resemble some personality disorders, especially avoidant and dependent personality disorders. While personality disorders from the *DSM* Cluster C are often characterized by long-standing manifestations of anxiety, the pattern of pathological worry, various symptoms of tension, and other somatic symptoms is usually absent. Unlike GAD, avoidant and dependent personality disorders are characterized by marked patterns of social avoidance and excessive dependency, respectively.

EPIDEMIOLOGY

Highlights of the epidemiology of GAD are shown in Table 3–8. In the U.S. National Comorbidity Survey, the lifetime prevalence rate of GAD was

Table 3-8. Epidemiological Data for Generalized Anxiety Disorder

- Lifetime prevalence in the United States: 5.1% (*DSM-III-R* criteria, National Comorbidity Survey), 8.9% (*ICD-10* criteria, National Comorbidity Survey), 5.7% (*DSM-IV* criteria, National Comorbidity Survey Replication), 4.1% (*DSM-IV* criteria, National Epidemiologic Survey on Alcohol and Related Conditions)

- Lifetime prevalence in various countries, according to various diagnostic criteria: 1.9%–31.1%

- Best-estimate lifetime prevalence rate across the world: 6.2%

- Rarely occurs alone: about two thirds have at least one additional current disorder (most commonly depression, social anxiety disorder, and panic disorder); more than 90% have at least one additional disorder co-occurring with GAD during their lifetime (with depression and panic disorder being most common)

- Often diagnosed as a condition co-occurring with another disorder (e.g., depression) for which help was originally sought

- Occurs about twice more often among women than among men

- More common among separated, divorced, widowed, unemployed, homemakers, urban dwellers, and people with lower income

- Relatively high prevalence in all age groups

- Typical age of onset: between late teens and late 20s; onset occurs in childhood and early adolescence in a sizable proportion, but may also start later in a significant number of sufferers

- Characteristic help-seeking patterns: majority of persons with GAD do not seek help at all; there is often a period of many years between onset and the time of seeking help; help is usually sought in primary care for a condition that complicates the course of GAD (e.g., depression)

- One of the most common psychiatric disorders in primary care

5.1% based on the *DSM-III-R* criteria and 8.9% according to the *ICD-10* criteria (Wittchen et al., 1994). In the more recent National Comorbidity Survey Replication, which used the *DSM-IV* criteria, the lifetime prevalence of GAD in the United States was 5.7% (Kessler et al., 2005). Another study, the National Epidemiologic Survey on Alcohol and Related Conditions, which also used the *DSM-IV* criteria, reported a lower lifetime prevalence rate of GAD in the United States, at 4.1% (Grant et al., 2005a).

Lifetime prevalence rates of GAD in the world vary significantly and range from 1.9% in Switzerland (Wacker et al., 1992) to 31.1% in New Zealand (Oakley-Browne et al., 1989). The most important sources of this variability are different diagnostic criteria and different diagnostic instruments used in various epidemiological surveys. It is also possible that cultural and social factors affect prevalence rates of GAD. A tendency has been noted for lifetime prevalence rates of GAD to be lower in Europe than in other places in the world (Somers et al., 2006). The best-estimate lifetime prevalence rate for GAD across epidemiological studies published between 1980 and 2004 and conducted in various countries was 6.2% (Somers et al., 2006). This confirms that GAD is a common condition and one of the most frequently occurring anxiety disorders.

The lifetime prevalence of GAD without any co-occurring conditions was found to be much lower—only 0.5% (Wittchen et al., 1994). This finding suggests that GAD rarely occurs alone, not only in the clinical population but also in epidemiological samples. In the community, 66.3% of people with GAD had at least one additional current disorder, most commonly major depression, social anxiety disorder, and panic disorder; the lifetime rate of psychiatric disorders co-occurring with GAD was 90.4%, with major depression and panic disorder being the most common co-occurring disorders (Wittchen et al., 1994).

Generalized anxiety disorder occurs about twice more often among women than among men (Blazer et al., 1991; Wittchen et al., 1994; Grant et al., 2005a) and is encountered more often among separated, divorced, widowed, and unemployed persons and homemakers (Wittchen et al., 1994; Grant et al., 2005a). It may be more frequent among people with lower income (Grant et al., 2005a) and in urban populations.

Generalized anxiety disorder has been reported to be common both among the elderly (Uhlenhuth et al., 1983; Kessler et al., 2005) and in children and adolescents (Bowen et al., 1990; McGee et al., 1990). Data for children include overanxious disorder, which is considered to be a precursor of GAD in that age group. In terms of its prevalence across different ages, from childhood to old age, GAD is different from panic disorder and more akin to social anxiety disorder and specific phobias.

It may be difficult to precisely determine the onset of GAD because it usually develops gradually and many patients say that they have "always" worried and have "always" been anxious, nervous, or tense. Still, it has been estimated that the onset of GAD occurs most commonly between the late teens and late 20s (Barlow et al., 1986; Burke et al., 1991; Kendler et al., 1992a; Rogers et al., 1999), although in a sizable number, first manifestations of GAD appear in childhood and early adolescence. One study has reported a later average age of onset of GAD at 32.7 years (Grant et al., 2005a). In contrast to the gradual and insidious onset of GAD in adolescence and in the third decade of life, its onset later in life may be more acute and is often associated with a stressful event (Hoehn-Saric et al., 1993a).

In North America, only about 40% of people with GAD seek treatment (Kessler et al., 1997b) and one third seeks help in the year of onset of GAD (Olfson et al., 1998). People with GAD who seek help later delay doing so for many years. This lengthy delay before help and treatment are sought is similar to the corresponding delay in social anxiety disorder and specific phobias. Even when GAD sufferers seek help, this is often for a condition that complicates the course of GAD, such as depression. Generalized anxiety disorder may be overshadowed by psychiatric disorders that receive primary therapeutic attention and the presence of GAD may then be overlooked.

Although people with GAD usually have an early onset of this illness, their delay in seeking professional help means that they often present for treatment in their 30s or even later in life. By contrast, panic disorder usually has an onset at a later age than GAD, but persons with panic disorder do not wait very long before seeking help. Therefore, patients with panic disorder are often younger than those with GAD in clinical settings.

About one half of persons with GAD seek help from primary care physicians (Wittchen et al., 1994). Generalized anxiety disorder is one of the most common psychiatric disorders seen in primary care, with the prevalence of 7.9% being second only to that of depression (Goldberg and Lecrubier, 1995). Generalized anxiety disorder may be the most frequent anxiety disorder in primary medical care (Wittchen et al., 2002). People with GAD also tend to see various medical specialists, most commonly gastroenterologists (Kennedy and Schwab, 1997), but they seem to attend specialized medical clinics generally less often than persons with panic disorder.

COURSE AND PROGNOSIS

Generalized anxiety disorder is a chronic condition. While its clinical features tend to persist, the course of GAD is often characterized by the waxing and waning of its symptoms and by symptoms becoming more severe at times of stress. There have been reports that in a substantial proportion of sufferers, a course of GAD can be better described as recurrent, with symptom-free periods between exacerbations (e.g., Angst et al., 2009).

It is difficult to conduct follow-up studies of "pure" GAD because it so often co-occurs with other disorders. Still, a 5-year follow-up study of treated GAD patients revealed that only 18% were in remission, while more than 50% continued to have symptoms, with impairment in various areas of functioning (Woodman et al., 1999). Most other studies paint a similar picture of the course of GAD. Thus, Noyes et al. (1987b) have found that only one fourth of GAD patients have "remissions," defined as 3-month periods without any symptoms. In another study, one half of patients continued to have symptoms of GAD 16 months after the completion of treatment (Mancuso et al., 1993). Yonkers et al. (2000) have reported that over a 5-year follow-up, less than 50% of people with GAD experienced a full or partial remission. In contrast, some research suggests that people with GAD may show a greater tendency to improve over long periods of time (e.g., Angst et al., 2009). Another study, conducted over a 40-year period, has also reported improvement in more than 80% of GAD patients and a tendency for GAD to be replaced by somatization and somatoform disorders after the age of 50 (Rubio and López-Ibor, 2007).

As already noted, GAD is often complicated by depression and less often by panic disorder and alcohol-related problems. The longitudinal stability of the diagnosis of GAD seems to be rather poor: in one follow-up study, only 3% of patients with GAD retained this diagnosis after 12 years, 28% were diagnosed with dysthymic disorder or major depressive episode, and 11% received diagnoses of other anxiety disorders (Tyrer et al., 2004). If depression develops, patients' overall condition tends to be more severe, their functioning more impaired, treatment more difficult, and prognosis worse (Bruce et al., 2001; Hunt et al., 2002; Wittchen, 2004). The occurrence of depression in the course of GAD also increases the suicide risk.

Factors suggesting poor prognosis of GAD include early onset; long duration before it is treated; female gender; presence of depression, personality disorders, and other psychiatric conditions; and disturbed marital or other relationships (Mancuso et al., 1993; Yonkers et al., 2000; Bruce et al., 2001; Tyrer et al., 2004; Rubio and López-Ibor, 2007).

Generalized anxiety disorder is associated with substantial impairment in occupational and social functioning and adverse effects on quality of life. In particular, GAD has been associated with decreased work productivity (Greenberg et al., 1999; Kessler et al., 1999a; Wittchen et al., 2000a), unemployment, and/or likelihood of receiving welfare or disability financial packages (Massion et al., 1993). While the degree of impairment is higher when GAD is accompanied by depression, GAD has been associated with considerable impairment even in its pure form (Wittchen et al., 2000a; Kessler et al., 2001; Grant et al., 2005a). People with GAD tend to perceive themselves as being in poor health and are more likely to use health care services (e.g., Kessler et al., 1999a; Maier et al., 2000; Wittchen et al., 2002). Some research suggests that GAD may be associated with an increased risk of coronary heart disease, even in the absence of major depressive disorder (Barger and Sydeman, 2005).

ETIOLOGY AND PATHOGENESIS

There are generally two broad ways of conceptualizing the etiology and pathogenesis of GAD. Like other anxiety disorders, GAD may be conceived of as a condition that develops on the background of a specific and non-specific predisposition, following certain precipitating events; within this framework, factors that maintain GAD can also be identified. Relatively specific for GAD among all the anxiety disorders except for generalized social anxiety disorder is the fact that GAD has also been conceptualized as being akin to a personality disorder. When GAD is viewed as primarily a personality-level disturbance, a different etiological model—one in which a distinction between the predisposing and precipitating factors is largely irrelevant—would need to be elaborated.

In this section, contributions from the major theoretical perspectives to the current understanding of etiology and pathogenesis of GAD will be reviewed. A hypothesis that GAD is primarily a personality disorder will also be presented.

BIOLOGICAL MODELS

Genetic Factors

There is some indication that GAD may have a genetic component. This is suggested by the finding that GAD occurs several times more frequently among first-degree relatives of individuals with GAD (19.5%) than among first-degree relatives of normal controls (3.5%) (Noyes et al., 1987b). The heritability of GAD among female twins was estimated at 30% (Kendler et al., 1992a). However, other findings do not support the notion that GAD is a genetically based disorder (e.g., Torgersen, 1983), and it is possible that higher rates of GAD in some families reflect hereditary factors less than the influence of the shared environment.

Other studies have examined the genetic relationship between GAD and depression. One proposal is that genes involved in GAD and major depressive disorder might be linked, so that GAD might be inherited only if a gene for depression is also inherited (Skre et al., 1993). A genetic link between GAD and depression has been postulated in women, with genetic predisposition for GAD and depression presumed to be the same. According to this model, the development of GAD or depression then depends on environmental and developmental factors and life events (Kendler et al., 1992b; Kendler, 1996). As already noted, twin studies suggest that GAD and major depressive disorder have the same genetic diathesis (Roy et al., 1995).

Neuroanatomy and Pathophysiological Mechanisms

Neuroimaging Studies Neuroimaging studies of GAD have produced somewhat conflicting findings. One early positron emission tomography investigation has suggested that the large areas of the brain—the occipital, temporal, and frontal lobes, as well as the cerebellum and basal ganglia, but not the amygdala—might be implicated in the pathogenesis of GAD (Wu et al., 1991). Other brain imaging studies suggest that GAD might be characterized by dysfunction of the amygdala (DeBellis et al., 2000; Monk et al., 2008) or that GAD might be associated with reduced response to fearful facial expressions in the amygdala (McClure et al., 2007; Blair et al., 2008a). Neuroimaging studies of adolescents with GAD indicate a dysfunction of the ventrolateral and ventromedial prefrontal cortex (Monk et al., 2006, 2008).

One study has suggested that GAD could be distinguished from generalized social anxiety disorder on the basis of the activation of different brain areas in response to emotional facial expressions and patterns of response: while patients with generalized social anxiety disorder showed an increased response to fearful expressions in several brain regions, including the amygdala, patients with GAD showed increased response to angry expressions in lateral frontal cortex, especially a lateral region of the middle frontal gyrus (Blair et al., 2008a). Moreover, symptom severity in GAD correlated with the lateral frontal cortex response to angry expressions, whereas symptom severity in generalized social anxiety disorder correlated with the amygdala response to fearful expressions (Blair et al., 2008a).

Although not definitive, these findings converge to suggest that a more specific neural correlate of GAD might be a dysfunction of the frontal cortex. The role of the amygdala in the pathogenesis of GAD remains to be clarified.

Neurotransmitter Systems

Several neurotransmitter systems have been implicated in the etiology and pathogenesis of GAD: noradrenaline, serotonin, gamma-aminobutyric acid (GABA), and cholecystokinin. Studies of some of these systems have been undertaken in conjunction with findings of the efficacy of medications that act via the corresponding transmitters. Thus, the efficacy of buspirone (and later, the efficacy of selective serotonin reuptake inhibitors) in the treatment of GAD largely inspired investigations of the pathogenetic role of serotonin; similarly, the efficacy of benzodiazepines was instrumental in promoting studies of the GABA system. A finding that there are abnormalities in the noradrenaline system in GAD provided some explanation for the efficacy in GAD of medications such as imipramine.

The results of these studies have not been consistent and did not point to any neurotransmitter system as being more important for GAD than others. It cannot be presumed that some neurotransmitter abnormalities are specific for GAD and it is not clear whether they precede the onset of GAD or whether they are a correlate or a consequence of GAD. Some of the neurotransmitter abnormalities involved in GAD are presented in Table 3–9.

Table 3–9. Potential Neurotransmitter Abnormalities in Generalized
          Anxiety Disorder

Neurotransmitter Systems	Potential Abnormalities
Noradrenaline	Hyperactivity (e.g., Sevy et al., 1989; Kelly and Cooper, 1998)
Serotonin	– Hyperactivity or underactivity (role of serotonin neurotransmitter abnormalities unclear, with potential abnormalities in GAD speculated on the basis of corresponding abnormalities in other anxiety disorders) – Administration of m-chlorophenylpiperazine (a nonspecific 5-HT$_1$ and 5-HT$_2$ agonist) to GAD patients increased anxiety (Germine et al., 1992)
GABA	– Altered (decreased) function of GABA$_A$ receptors in the left temporal pole (Tiihonen et al., 1997) – Excessive release of noradrenaline, serotonin, and/or cholecystokinin via GABA

GABA, gamma-aminobutyric acid.

Other Neurobiological Aspects

Research suggests that GAD may be characterized by changes in the functioning of the hypothalamic-pituitary-adrenal axis, which plays a major role in response to stress. Some studies have reported chronically increased cortisol levels in GAD, indicating an exaggerated response to stress (e.g., Tiller et al., 1988).

There is also a possibility of an autonomic nervous system dysfunction in GAD. A general autonomic inflexibility in GAD is suggested by the findings of a weakened response to stress, prolonged recovery from stress (e.g., slower return to baseline of skin conductance after stress), and slower habituation to novel stimuli and stress (Hoehn-Saric et al., 1989; Brawman-Mintzer and Lydiard, 1997). Patients with GAD may also have a lowered vagal (parasympathetic) tone (Thayer et al., 1996).

Panic induction studies have shown that panic attacks can be induced in a much smaller percentage of patients with GAD compared to those with panic disorder (e.g., Cowley et al., 1988; Verburg et al., 1995; Perna et al., 1999). This finding supports a notion that GAD differs significantly from panic disorder.

PSYCHOLOGICAL MODELS

Cognitive Approaches

The reconceptualization of GAD as a condition primarily character-ized by cognitive activity, worrying, was largely a result of the growing number of cognitive models of GAD. This reconceptualization has in turn led to the formulation of additional cognitive accounts of pathological worry and GAD, sometimes treating pathological worry as if it were a proxy for GAD. These models better account for the ways in which pathological worry and GAD are maintained than for their causes. Nevertheless, the models are valuable for their contribution to a better understanding of the processes involved in pathological worry and GAD. Table 3–10 lists the main aspects of cognitive models in GAD.

The cognitive abnormalities in GAD have several consequences: patients often have great difficulty in distinguishing between threatening and non-threatening situations and cues; they feel less capable of detecting threat and of understanding where the danger is coming from; and they nonetheless feel very strongly that there is much danger out there and that they should do something about it (e.g., protect themselves). As a result, patients are puzzled about the nature of their worry (what it is that they "really" worry about and/or why), which only increases their apprehensiveness and a sense of dread.

Psychodynamic Approaches

No psychodynamic model has been specifically developed for GAD, and a psychodynamic approach to GAD is based on psychoanalytic theories of anxiety in general. Psychodynamic formulations of anxiety (Freud, 1926/1959; Karasu, 1994) are still relevant for clinical practice in that they can help clinicians better understand the underlying issues and the nature and meaning of anxiety in their patients. Modern psychodynamic approaches make a distinction between two types of anxiety ("automatic" and "signal") that may be present in GAD. Their origins are then traced to specific developmental issues (Table 3–11). Although it is difficult to separate them precisely along diagnostic lines, it appears that automatic anxiety is more characteristic of panic disorder, whereas signal anxiety is more typically encountered in GAD.

Role of Developmental and Childhood Factors

Patients with GAD tend to report various traumatic experiences in childhood, such as separation from parents, death of parents, and physical and sexual abuse. While this link does not appear to be specific for GAD (e.g., Raskin et al., 1982), other studies suggest that there may be a relatively specific relationship between GAD and these traumatic childhood experiences (e.g., Hubbard et al., 1995; Windle et al., 1995). Patients with GAD often view their parents as overprotective, controlling, and rejecting, and their families of origin as dysfunctional (e.g., Rapee, 1997), but this is very similar to how many panic patients perceive their parents and primary

Table 3–10. Cognitive Models of Worry and Generalized Anxiety Disorder

Model	Main Components of Model
Worry as cognitive avoidance	Worry is predominantly a thought activity, in contrast to mental imagery-related activity (Borkovec and Inz,1990)
	Emotions expressed through a thought activity (worry), in contrast to emotions expressed through imagery-related activity, are not associated with sympathetic nervous system hyperactivity (Vrana et al., 1986)
	Since worry inhibits autonomic arousal, it serves the purpose of avoiding somatic symptoms that accompany strong emotional states ("cognitive avoidance"); worry is maintained by the avoidance of both unpleasant emotions and the accompanying autonomic arousal (Borkovec et al., 1991, 1998)
Beliefs about benefits of worry	Worry is maintained by beliefs that it is necessary to worry to avoid danger, prevent harm, prepare oneself for a bad outcome, and/or promote better coping (Rapee, 1991; Freeston et al., 1994)
	These beliefs are maintained by nonoccurrence of the events that one worries about (Borkovec et al., 1998; Dugas et al., 1998b)
Intolerance of uncertainty as the central cognitive feature of GAD	Intolerance of uncertainty perpetuates worry by exacerbating the "what if . . ." thinking style (Ladouceur et al., 1997; Dugas et al., 1998b)
Biased information-processing, related to exaggerated perception of threat	Attention is focused on a wide variety of threatening cues and on detecting threat in numerous situations (MacLeod et al., 1986)
	A wide variety of ambiguous stimuli and information are interpreted as threatening (Mogg et al., 1994)
	Memory for all threat-related information is better (biased) (Butler and Mathews, 1983; Mathews et al., 1989)
Low self-efficacy, poor problem orientation	GAD is associated with the belief that one is unable to exercise control over events (Kent and Gibbons, 1987); there may be lack of confidence in one's ability to cope with problems (Ladouceur et al., 1998); core beliefs of self-doubt are present (Davey and Levy, 1998)

Table 3–11. Psychodynamic Conceptualization of Anxiety in Generalized Anxiety Disorder

	Automatic Anxiety	Signal Anxiety
Key features	1. Predominance of physical symptoms of anxiety 2. Anxiety experienced as highly disruptive	Predominance of anxious anticipation, worry, and/or "free-floating" anxiety
Explanatory model	Failure of the mothering figure to provide protection, sense of security, and love in the pre-Oedipal phase results in the inability to tolerate or endure anxiety and in the experience of anxiety in its "raw" (predominantly physical) form	1. Anxiety serves as a "signal" to the ego to strengthen its defenses against sexual or aggressive drives 2. Anxiety indicates the presence of unconscious, unresolved intrapsychic conflicts 3. The origin of anxiety is in the Oedipal phase
Manifestations of anxiety	1. Fear of annihilation 2. Fear of losing one's identity through a merger with another person 3. Fear of separation 4. Fear of losing love	1. Fear of castration (fear of injury to one's physical integrity) 2. Fear of superego (fear of conscientiousness, punishment)

families (see Chapter 2). Hence, the notion that there are specific developmental antecedents to GAD lacks sufficient support. There appears to be a broad predisposition to a range of anxiety and other psychiatric disorders based on childhood experiences.

Life Events Research

Life events research in GAD has suggested that the onset of GAD may be preceded by stressful or traumatic experiences more often than expected (e.g., Nisita et al., 1990). This appears to be the case more with persons in whom GAD occurs in the third decade of life or later. More typically, the onset of GAD is gradual, and stressful events are more likely to precipitate exacerbations in the course of GAD than the very onset of GAD.

The link between relatively minor stress and exacerbation of GAD symptoms (Brantley et al., 1999) may suggest that patients with GAD have generally low tolerance for stress and that they easily decompensate in response to even minor stressors.

Generalized Anxiety Disorder as a Personality-Level Disturbance

There is a long tradition of considering some types of anxiety, particularly chronic anxiety, more "characterological" in nature, hence the concepts of "trait anxiety" (versus "state anxiety") and "anxious personality disorder" (as it most recently appeared in the *ICD-10*). This is analogous to the states of chronic depression often being referred to as "characterological depression" and "depressive personality."

Several characteristics of GAD make it look like a personality disorder. First, in many cases, GAD starts early, in childhood or adolescence. Second, the onset of GAD is usually gradual, with more than 80% of persons with GAD not being able to recall its precise onset (Rapee, 1985). Third, the course of GAD is usually chronic, its manifestations are persistent, and its pattern is pervasive. Fourth, the anxiety in GAD has a strong characterological "flavor" in that all aspects of personality seem to be affected by it. Is GAD then a personality disorder?

The fact that GAD may also first manifest itself later in life, after personality development has for the most part been completed, suggests that there are perhaps two conditions subsumed under the current concept of GAD (Table 3–12). As proposed by Brown et al. (1994), there may be a type of GAD with an early and gradual onset, which resembles a personality disorder; this type is more frequent and appears to be associated with behavioral inhibition, childhood anxiety disorders, and/or childhood fears. The late-onset type of GAD is less frequent, has a more acute onset in the third decade of life or later (usually after some stressful event), and resembles an anxiety disorder. In comparison with an early-onset type, the late-onset type of GAD may have a less chronic course and may be less likely to be associated with depression, other psychiatric conditions, and personality disorders. This dichotomy in the conceptualization of GAD has not been investigated further, but clinical observation has supported it to some extent.

The pathogenesis of the personality disorder-like GAD remains to be elucidated. Because of the close relationship between GAD and certain personality dimensions that are believed to be largely inherited (e.g., neuroticism, negative affectivity, and harm avoidance), it is possible that GAD is at the extreme end of these dimensions. If so, GAD may not necessarily be a distinct personality disorder but rather a temperament-based, nonspecific vulnerability or predisposition for the development of a range of anxiety and mood disorders (e.g., Nisita et al., 1990; Brown, 1997; Akiskal, 1998).

There are certain aspects of the relationship between GAD and personality disorders which suggest that GAD may be related to personality disturbance. In comparison with panic disorder, GAD was more often found to be associated with more severe character pathology, including antisocial traits, mistrust, suspiciousness, hostility, and irritability as well

Table 3–12. The Two Types of Generalized Anxiety Disorder

Criteria for Differentiation	Personality Disorder Type	Anxiety Disorder Type
Age of onset	Childhood or adolescence	Third decade and later
Mode of onset	Gradual	Relatively acute
Stressful event(s) preceding the onset	No	Yes
Course	More chronic	Less chronic
Association with behavioral inhibition, anxiety disorders in childhood, and/or childhood fears	Yes	No
Association with depression, other psychiatric conditions, and personality disorders	Yes	No
Frequency of occurrence	More frequent	Less frequent

as paranoid, schizotypal, obsessive-compulsive, and passive-aggressive personality disorders (Blashfield et al., 1994). Also, it has been suggested that severe character pathology might be a risk factor for developing GAD but not a risk factor for developing panic disorder (Nisita et al., 1990). Personality traits such as lack of self-confidence, insecurity, hypervigilance, and heightened sensitivity, and dependent and avoidant personality disorders are often found among GAD patients, but they seem nonspecifically associated with other anxiety disorders and depression as well.

TREATMENT

As with other anxiety disorders, early treatment of GAD is more likely to be effective than treatment that starts later in the course of GAD. Many persons with GAD often tolerate their anxiety and distress for years, believing that it is in their "nature" to worry and that there is little that can be done to change that. As a result, they often seek help and treatment when the disorder has become more severe and/or when they have developed complications. Therefore, by the time GAD patients present for treatment, they are likely to need a long-term treatment strategy that would also address any co-occurring psychiatric conditions.

PHARMACOLOGICAL TREATMENT

The main goal of pharmacological treatment in GAD is a significant decrease in tension and general anxiety (encompassing both its somatic symptoms and cognitive symptoms, i.e., worry or apprehensive expectation). Other goals of pharmacotherapy include treatment of co-occurring depression, other anxiety disorders and symptoms such as insomnia, and improvement in functioning. Medications may not be able to target all the components of GAD equally well, and they differ in terms of their ability to exert effects on specific symptoms of anxiety (see Table 3–13).

Many GAD patients take anxiolytic medications, usually benzodiazepines, on an as-needed (prn) basis. When they start visiting their primary care physicians more often or feel that they need to see a mental health professional, it usually means that they have greater difficulty tolerating their chronic anxiety, worries, and tension or that they have developed a complication of GAD (e.g., depression). It is often at that point that GAD patients are offered regular pharmacological treatment.

There are several relatively specific considerations in the pharmacological treatment of GAD (Table 3–13). Antidepressants have largely replaced benzodiazepines as medications of choice in the treatment of GAD, which is somewhat paradoxical, because benzodiazepines had been considered a gold standard for pharmacological treatment of GAD. In fact, panic

Table 3–13. Pharmacological Treatment Considerations for Generalized Anxiety Disorder

Issues and Factors	Clinical Implications
Close relationship between GAD and depression	Antidepressants should be given preference to treat GAD
In clinical setting, GAD is usually accompanied by another condition, most commonly depression; patients with GAD are also more likely to develop depression	Optimal medication for use in GAD is the one that is also likely to be effective in treatment of depression—an antidepressant
Benzodiazepines seem to be more efficacious for somatic anxiety symptoms, and autonomic hyperarousal in particular (Rickels et al., 1982; Hoehn-Saric et al.,1988; Rocca et al., 1997), which may not be very prominent in GAD; antidepressants appear to be more efficacious for cognitive anxiety symptoms (e.g., worry), which may be more characteristic of GAD	Antidepressants may offer specific advantages over benzodiazepines in treatment of GAD to the extent that cognitive anxiety symptoms predominate over the somatic anxiety symptoms
In comparison with panic disorder, there is usually a less prominent sense of urgency to obtain relief from somatic anxiety symptoms in GAD	Medications that act quickly (e.g., benzodiazepines) may be less often needed in GAD

disorder and GAD were initially distinguished from each other on the basis of the former responding to an antidepressant, imipramine, and the latter responding to benzodiazepines. What has changed?

The modern concept of GAD is quite different from that of its historical precursor, anxiety neurosis, and its diagnostic criteria have been changing significantly. Generalized anxiety disorder is now recognized as a chronic condition, and in some important ways, more closely related to depression than to the other anxiety disorders. The symptoms of GAD may be more cognitive than somatic in nature, although this continues to be debated. In clinical practice, GAD is more likely to be encountered with another disorder, such as depression. Furthermore, antidepressants may be more efficacious than benzodiazepines in the long-term treatment of GAD (e.g., Kahn et al., 1986; Rickels et al., 1993; Casacalenda and Boulenger, 1998). One systematic review did not find benzodiazepines definitively superior to placebo even in the short-term treatment of GAD, although the results were somewhat equivocal (Martin et al., 2007). All this makes antidepressants a more suitable pharmacological option than benzodiazepines. Table 3–14 lists current recommendations for pharmacotherapy of GAD.

Several selective serotonin reuptake inhibitors (SSRIs), venlafaxine (in its extended-release [XR] formulation), duloxetine, tricyclic antidepressants (TCAs), and pregabalin have all demonstrated convincing efficacy in the treatment of GAD. Although there are some differences in efficacy among these medications, they are not of a magnitude that would favor one over the other solely on that basis. Mainly because of their better tolerability and greater safety in overdose (see Chapter 2), SSRIs are considered first-line pharmacological treatment.

Medications are usually initiated in the lowest dose; the dose is then gradually increased until remission is achieved. Table 3–15 shows the usual dosages of antidepressants and other medications used in treatment of GAD. There is some evidence that early improvement, after 2 weeks of

Table 3–14. Choice of Medication in Treatment of Generalized Anxiety Disorder

Rank	Medication(s)
First-line	a. SSRIs (especially escitalopram, paroxetine, and sertraline)
	b. SSRI + BDZ (short term)
Second-line	a. Venlafaxine XR or duloxetine
	b. Venlafaxine XR or duloxetine + BDZ (short term)
Third-line	a. TCAs (imipramine)
	b. TCA + BDZ (short term)
Fourth-line	Pregabalin

SSRI, selective serotonin reuptake inhibitor; Venlafaxine XR, venlafaxine extended-release; TCA, tricyclic antidepressant; BDZ, benzodiazepine.

treatment, strongly predicts a favorable outcome of pharmacotherapy of GAD (Rynn et al., 2006; Pollack et al., 2008b).

Antidepressants in Treatment of Generalized Anxiety Disorder

All antidepressants start showing efficacy in GAD after at least 1–4 weeks of continuous treatment. If somatic anxiety symptoms or agitation are prominent, an antidepressant should be commenced at a very low dose, as if starting to treat panic disorder. Benzodiazepines can be administered with antidepressants at the beginning of treatment with the goals of accelerating the onset of anxiolytic action and/or alleviating antidepressant-induced anxiety or agitation.

Selective Serotonin Reuptake Inhibitors

Among the SSRIs, there is evidence of efficacy in GAD for escitalopram (Davidson et al., 2004a; Goodman et al., 2005; Allgulander et al., 2006; Baldwin et al., 2006; Bose et al., 2008), paroxetine (Rocca et al., 1997; Pollack et al., 2001; Rickels et al., 2003; Stocchi et al., 2003), and sertraline (Allgulander et al., 2004a; Brawman-Mintzer et al., 2006). When escitalopram was compared with paroxetine (Bielski et al., 2005; Baldwin et al., 2006) and paroxetine with sertraline (Ball et al., 2005), there was generally no difference in efficacy, although paroxetine was equivalent to escitalopram in efficacy only when used in a higher dose (up to 50 mg/day) (Bielski et al., 2005). In terms of tolerability, no difference was found between

Table 3–15. Medication Dosages Efficacious for Treatment of Generalized Anxiety Disorder

Medication	Dose Range
Selective Serotonin Reuptake Inhibitors	
Escitalopram	10–20 mg/day
Paroxetine	20–50 mg/day
Sertraline	50–200 mg/day
Other Antidepressants	
Venlafaxine extended-release	75–225 mg/day
Duloxetine	60–120 mg/day
Imipramine	75–200 mg/day
Benzodiazepines	
Diazepam	5–30 mg/day
Lorazepam	2–6 mg/day
Pregabalin	150–600 mg/day

paroxetine (20–40 mg/day) and sertraline (50–100 mg/day) (Ball et al., 2005), whereas escitalopram (10–20 mg/day) was better tolerated than paroxetine (20–50 mg/day) (Bielski et al., 2005), with the main side effects of paroxetine being insomnia, constipation, weight gain, and sexual dysfunction.

Insomnia is not only a common symptom among patients with GAD but also a potential side effect of SSRIs. Patients with insomnia and GAD treated with SSRIs may receive a hypnotic medication on a short-term basis to improve their sleep. One placebo-controlled study has shown that escitalopram-treated patients with insomnia and GAD who for 8 weeks also received eszopiclone, a nonbenzodiazepine hypnotic, significantly improved not only in terms of their sleep but also with regard to their levels of anxiety, mood, and daytime functioning (Pollack et al., 2008a).

In patients with GAD, higher doses may need to be used for SSRIs to be efficacious: escitalopram in the dose of 20 mg/day may be better than 10 mg/day (Baldwin et al., 2006), paroxetine in the dose of 40 mg/day may show better results than 20 mg/day (Rickels et al., 2003), and the mean dose of sertraline in one trial was fairly high—149 mg/day (Brawman-Mintzer et al., 2006). Because higher doses of escitalopram are associated with greater frequency of side effects in the treatment of GAD, it has been suggested that treatment should commence with 10 mg/day and increased to 20 mg/day if there is no response after 4 weeks of treatment (Baldwin et al., 2006). Furthermore, higher doses of escitalopram may be associated with greater likelihood of some discontinuation symptoms (Baldwin et al., 2006), although more symptoms consistently arise in the course of paroxetine taper and discontinuation than after discontinuation of escitalopram (e.g., Bielski et al., 2005; Baldwin et al., 2006). Other issues surrounding the use of SSRIs and factors assisting in the choice of SSRIs are discussed in Chapter 2.

Venlafaxine Extended-Release

Several studies have established the efficacy of venlafaxine XR, a serotonin and noradrenaline reuptake inhibitor, in short-term treatment of GAD (Davidson et al., 1999; Rickels et al., 2000; Nimatoudis et al., 2004). Venlafaxine XR was as efficacious for GAD as duloxetine (Hartford et al., 2007; Allgulander et al., 2008; Nicolini et al., 2009) and pregabalin (Montgomery et al., 2006). There is evidence that venlafaxine XR may in some respects be more efficacious than escitalopram, but the latter medication is better tolerated (Bose et al., 2008). The principles of treatment with venlafaxine XR, its side effects, and reasons for its status as the second-line pharmacotherapy option are discussed in Chapter 2. Venlafaxine XR has been found to be efficacious across a range of low to moderate doses (75–225 mg/day), with the starting dose of 75 mg/day. Some research suggests that the greatest improvements in GAD may be obtained with higher doses (225 mg/day) of venlafaxine XR (Rickels et al., 2000).

Duloxetine

Duloxetine is another serotonin and noradrenaline reuptake inhibitor. It was initially developed for use in depression but was subsequently found to be efficacious in the treatment of GAD (Hartford et al., 2007; Koponen et al., 2007; Rynn et al., 2008). As noted above, there was no difference in efficacy in GAD between duloxetine and venlafaxine XR. These findings have made duloxetine suitable as the second-line pharmacotherapy option for GAD because there is much less experience with its use in GAD than there is with SSRIs. The relatively common side effects of duloxetine include nausea, diarrhea, insomnia, sedation, sweating, and sexual dysfunction. In comparison with venlafaxine XR, duloxetine may have a lower propensity to cause hypertension and to be associated with severe discontinuation symptoms. Because duloxetine inhibits the metabolism of several drugs, including TCAs, it can raise levels of TCAs to toxic levels, which calls for caution when switching from a TCA to duloxetine (or vice versa). The initial dose is 60 mg/day, which is also the usual therapeutic dose; in some cases it is prudent to commence treatment with 30 mg/day. Unlike venlafaxine XR, duloxetine exhibits both the serotonin and noradrenaline reuptake blockade at this low dose. Some GAD patients may need a higher dose, up to 120 mg/day.

Tricyclic Antidepressants

Imipramine has also been efficacious in the treatment of GAD (Hoehn-Saric et al., 1988; Rickels et al., 1993). Sedative properties of imipramine and other side effects typically associated with TCAs (see Chapter 2) limit the use of this medication in GAD. Patients with prominent insomnia and restlessness, however, may benefit from imipramine.

Benzodiazepines

Although benzodiazepines are no longer the pharmacological treatment of choice, they continue to play a role in the treatment of GAD. They are useful for treating insomnia, symptoms of tension (especially muscle tension), and manifestations of autonomic hyperactivity. As already noted, benzodiazepines can be combined with antidepressants, and because of their quick onset of action they can accelerate pharmacological response and alleviate distress. In such a combination, benzodiazepines should preferably be used on a short-term basis, for several (4–8) weeks. A benzodiazepine can then be ceased gradually, while the treatment with an antidepressant continues.

Benzodiazepines can be administered as the only pharmacotherapy for GAD, and many studies have demonstrated their overall efficacy (e.g., Mitte et al., 2005), particularly for diazepam (e.g., Feighner et al., 1982; Rickels et al., 1982, 1993, 1997; Elie and Lamontagne, 1984; Boyer and

Feighner, 1993), alprazolam (e.g., Elie and Lamontagne, 1984; Hoehn-Saric et al., 1988; Lydiard et al., 1997, Rickels et al., 2005), and lorazepam (Feltner et al., 2003; Pande et al., 2003). In the long-term, however, this is not the optimal pharmacological strategy. Apart from the issue of dependence, the main reasons for this are a lack of effect of benzodiazepines on the cognitive symptoms of anxiety and on the symptoms of depression; the former symptoms are often prominent in GAD whereas the latter are important because of the frequent occurrence of depression in patients with GAD. As already noted, there has been some doubt about the efficacy of benzodiazepines not only in long-term but also in short-term treatment of GAD.

In long-term treatment, benzodiazepines with a longer half-life (e.g., diazepam) may be more suitable, because it is easier to administer them and they are less likely to be associated with significant discontinuation problems (see Chapter 2). When benzodiazepines need to be ceased after prolonged use, they should be carefully tapered to avoid withdrawal symptoms, as outlined in Chapter 2. In the absence of current and past drug and alcohol abuse or dependence, GAD patients are just as unlikely as patients with panic disorder to escalate the dose of a benzodiazepine or to abuse it.

Benzodiazepines can be taken on an as-needed (prn) basis, for example, in relatively mild cases of GAD or after treatment with an antidepressant has resulted in sustained remission and regular pharmacotherapy has been ceased. The benefit of such practice has not been investigated.

Pregabalin

In terms of its mechanism of action, pregabalin is unique among the pharmacological agents for GAD. It has been referred to as a "calcium channel modulator" because it binds to the $\alpha_2\delta$ subunit of voltage-gated calcium channels; this reduces calcium flow and decreases the release of several neurotransmitters, including glutamate, noradrenaline, and substance P, thereby producing anxiolytic and other effects. Pregabalin was developed first as an anticonvulsant and a drug for neuropathic pain. The efficacy of pregabalin in GAD was demonstrated in several short-term (4–6 weeks) placebo-controlled studies (Feltner et al., 2003; Pande et al., 2003; Pohl et al., 2005; Rickels et al., 2005; Montgomery et al., 2006). When compared with venlafaxine (Montgomery et al., 2006), lorazepam (Feltner et al., 2003; Pande et al., 2003), and alprazolam (Rickels et al., 2005), it was equally efficacious for GAD. One placebo-controlled, relapse-prevention study demonstrated a long-term (24 weeks) efficacy of pregabalin; for reasons that are not well understood, a fairly large proportion (36%) of patients discontinued pregabalin in this study (Feltner et al., 2008).

These trials have found several clinically relevant advantages of pregabalin. The drug showed an early onset of therapeutic action, after 1 week of treatment (Feltner et al., 2003; Pande et al., 2003; Pohl et al., 2005;

Montgomery et al., 2006). It had significant effects on both somatic and cognitive anxiety symptoms (Pohl et al., 2005; Montgomery et al., 2006) and decreased the co-occurring symptoms of depression (Pohl et al., 2005; Montgomery et al., 2006; Stein DJ et al., 2008). Pregabalin was not associated with significant withdrawal symptoms upon discontinuation (Feltner et al., 2003; Pande et al., 2003; Pohl et al., 2005), even after 32 weeks of treatment (Feltner et al., 2008). Importantly, the medication is not regarded to have a significant abuse potential (Feltner et al., 2008).

In terms of the side effects of pregabalin, it appeared less likely to cause sexual dysfunction (Feltner et al., 2003), and in the course of both short- and long-term treatment, pregabalin was reported to be well tolerated (Feltner et al., 2003, 2008; Pande et al., 2003; Pohl et al., 2005; Rickels et al., 2005). Its most common side effects are dizziness, sedation, and headache; other side effects include various gastrointestinal disturbances, weight gain, blurred vision, ataxia, and changes in cognitive functioning.

Despite these promising findings, pregabalin is not widely available and has not been licensed for GAD in most countries. It continues to be referred to as "an alternative treatment option for GAD" (e.g., Stein DJ et al., 2008). At present, therefore, pregabalin cannot be endorsed in the treatment of GAD before ascertaining whether a patient responds to one or more antidepressants with an established efficacy in GAD.

Alternative Pharmacotherapy Options for Generalized Anxiety Disorder

Buspirone and hydroxyzine have been used in GAD with some success. Their efficacy has been inconsistent or partial (i.e., only for some manifestations of GAD). These medications can be used as an alternative pharmacotherapy option, before the stage of treatment resistance has been reached, for example, when SSRIs, venlafaxine XR, duloxetine, or pregabalin are not tolerated or not available, and TCAs are contraindicated. They can also be helpful in treatment-resistant GAD (Table 3–16).

Buspirone

Buspirone is a nonbenzodiazepine, azapirone anxiolytic, which acts as a partial agonist on serotonin 1_A receptors. It was found to be efficacious for GAD in controlled studied (Pollack et al., 1997; Davidson et al., 1999) and as efficacious as benzodiazepines (e.g., Feighner et al., 1982; Rickels et al., 1982; Mitte et al., 2005). When compared with venlafaxine XR (Davidson et al., 1999) and hydroxyzine (Lader and Scotto, 1998), however, buspirone proved to be less efficacious.

In addition to these inconsistent reports from clinical trials, many clinicians have an impression that buspirone generally does not perform well in GAD. Some of this impression may be a consequence of an

Table 3–16. Alternative Pharmacotherapy Options and Options for Treatment-Resistant Generalized Anxiety Disorder

Alternative Pharmacotherapy Options, Before the Stage of Treatment Resistance Has Been Reached

Monotherapy with buspirone
Monotherapy with hydroxyzine

Lack of Response to First-, Second-, Third-, or Fourth-Line Pharmacotherapy

Monotherapy options
  Buspirone
  Hydroxyzine
  Antidepressants

    Trazodone
    Bupropion

  Antipsychotics

    Quetiapine
    Trifluoperazine

  Anticonvulsants

    Valproate
    Tiagabine

Partial Response to First-, Second-, or Third-Line Pharmacotherapy

Continue treatment for 2–3 months
Augmentation strategies

  Beta-adrenergic blockers (propranolol, atenolol)
  Clonidine
  Tiagabine
  Second-generation antipsychotics (risperidone, olanzapine, quetiapine)

---

apparent interference with the efficacy of buspirone by the previous use of benzodiazepines (Schweizer et al., 1986). Buspirone may still be efficacious if the previously administered benzodiazepine was discontinued very gradually (Delle Chiaie et al., 1995) or if a benzodiazepine has not been taken 1 month prior to commencing treatment with buspirone (DeMartinis et al., 2000). Therefore, to maximize the benefit of buspirone in GAD patients previously treated with benzodiazepines, a benzodiazepine needs to be discontinued very slowly and patients may need to go through a benzodiazepine-free period. This may not be practical and may be met with resistance.

Buspirone has several advantages: it does not cause sedation, it is not associated with dependence, and it is apparently efficacious in alleviating cognitive symptoms of anxiety (Rickels et al., 1982). Disadvantages of buspirone include a slow onset of therapeutic action (2–3 weeks after starting treatment), lack of efficacy in treating depression, and side effects (nausea, insomnia, headache, agitation, dizziness) that some patients find difficult to tolerate. One meta-analytic review has found that GAD patients are less compliant with buspirone than with benzodiazepines (Mitte et al., 2005). Buspirone might be a good choice for nondepressed GAD patients, those who have not been previously exposed to benzodiazepines, and patients who should not be prescribed benzodiazepines because of dependence or abuse issues. The treatment usually starts with 5 mg three times a day, and the dose may be increased to 60 mg/day, depending on the patient's response and side effects.

Hydroxyzine

Hydroxyzine is the histamine H_1 receptor antagonist that can be useful as monotherapy in the short-term treatment of GAD (Darcis et al., 1995; Lader and Scotto, 1998; Llorca et al., 2002). It may be particularly suitable for the symptoms of tension and insomnia, and in this regard, it could represent a viable alternative to benzodiazepines. Hydroxyzine appears to exhibit the onset of action fairly quickly (within 1 week), but in one study, a significant anxiolytic effect occurred only after 4 weeks of treatment (Darcis et al., 1995). Hydroxyzine can be very sedating and it has no effects on the cognitive anxiety and depressive symptoms, which limits its use in GAD. The optimal dosage of hydroxyzine for GAD has not been established, as it has been reported to be efficacious in a small dose (50 mg/day) and a fairly high dose (300–400 mg/day).

Long-Term Pharmacological Treatment

It is not clear how long pharmacotherapy of GAD should last after remission. In view of the chronic nature of GAD and its significant relationship with depression, it seems reasonable to administer medications for at least 12–24 months. Several placebo-controlled, relapse prevention studies in GAD have shown efficacy for escitalopram (Allgulander et al., 2006), paroxetine (Stocchi et al., 2003), and pregabalin (Feltner et al., 2008). Venlafaxine XR was not efficacious at relapse prevention (Montgomery et al., 2002), but other studies suggest that it may be efficacious over a long term (6 months) (Gelenberg et al., 2000; Allgulander et al., 2001). Use of benzodiazepines in long-term treatment of GAD is not recommended. Other issues in long-term pharmacotherapy of GAD are similar to those in long-term pharmacotherapy of panic disorder and are discussed in Chapter 2.

When the decision to cease pharmacotherapy is made, medication should be discontinued gradually. As with other anxiety disorders, the cessation of pharmacotherapy is associated with a high risk of relapse of symptoms of GAD. Perhaps this risk can be decreased somewhat by using psychological treatments or some of their techniques (e.g., relaxation), but there is no evidence to clearly support this.

Pharmacotherapy of Treatment-Resistant Generalized Anxiety Disorder

What constitutes an adequate medication trial for GAD and at what point a GAD patient can be considered treatment resistant are not well established. However, it is reasonable to assume that 4–8 weeks of treatment with one of the standard medications for GAD, given in the maximum recommended or tolerated dose, is sufficient to establish whether that medication is effective. Under circumstances of relative urgency, perhaps there is no need to wait for 4 weeks to see whether a patient will respond, as some research suggests that a lack of any improvement after only 2 weeks of treatment indicates a low likelihood of response after a full-length course of pharmacotherapy with that agent (e.g., Rynn et al., 2006; Pollack et al., 2008b).

From a clinical practice perspective, a GAD patient is resistant to pharmacotherapy if he or she has not responded to one of the SSRIs, venlafaxine XR or duloxetine, imipramine, and pregabalin. Some patients are deemed treatment resistant because one or more of these agents, as well as benzodiazepines, cannot be prescribed to them or they are unable to tolerate their side effects. As already noted, drugs such as buspirone and hydroxyzine could be used both as an alternative monotherapy for GAD and as monotherapy for treatment-resistant GAD patients (Table 3–16). A possibility of adding CBT or other psychological treatments in treatment-resistant cases should also be considered.

If there has been no response at all to treatment with a first-, second-, third-, and fourth-line medication for GAD, monotherapy with several other medications could also be considered. These include trazodone, quetiapine, valproate, bupropion, tiagabine, and trifluoperazine (Table 3–16).

The efficacy in GAD of trazodone, a serotonin 2_A receptor antagonist and a less potent serotonin reuptake inhibitor, was established in one controlled trial (Rickels et al., 1993). The main drawback of this agent is its sedative effect. However, GAD patients who are particularly troubled by insomnia and restlessness can benefit from the calming effects of trazodone.

Quetiapine, a second-generation antipsychotic, is another pharmacotherapy option for treatment-resistant patients, and it may well become standard pharmacotherapy for GAD. Quetiapine in its extended-release formulation as monotherapy for GAD was superior to placebo and as efficacious as paroxetine in one large study (Bandelow et al., 2007). The doses of quetiapine efficacious in GAD—50 mg/day and 150 mg/day—are much lower than those used in the treatment of schizophrenia and bipolar disorder. A possible advantage of quetiapine may be its early onset of action (after 4 days of treatment), while its sedative properties represent the main disadvantage of this medication.

There is some preliminary evidence from controlled, small, open-label, or pilot studies that anticonvulsants valproate (Aliyev and Aliyev, 2008) and tiagabine and antidepressant bupropion might be effective in GAD.

However, results from three controlled studies generally failed to support the efficacy of tiagabine in patients with GAD (Pollack et al., 2008c). The first-generation antipsychotic trifluoperazine was efficacious in one controlled trial but was poorly tolerated (Mendels et al., 1986).

If there has been a partial response to treatment with a first-, second-, or third-line medication for GAD, it may be worthwhile to continue treatment with it for another 2 or 3 months, as patients may show incremental response over the subsequent several months and achieve remission after 5 or 6 months of treatment. Alternatively, augmentation strategies can be considered. These include addition of a β-adrenergic blocker, clonidine, tiagabine, or a second-generation antipsychotic (Table 3–16).

Beta-adrenergic blockers (propranolol, atenolol) can be used to suppress physical symptoms caused by noradrenergic stimulation (e.g., tachycardia, palpitations, and tremor) if these symptoms are particularly prominent or distressing in GAD. Beta-adrenergic blockers are not effective for other manifestations of GAD and in the treatment of GAD as monotherapy (Meibach et al., 1987). They exhibit a therapeutic effect fairly quickly and can be taken continuously or on an as-needed (prn) basis. Beta-adrenergic blockers are contraindicated in patients with asthma, bradycardia, heart failure, and certain arrhythmias. Caution is required when administering some β-adrenergic blockers (especially propranolol) to patients with a history of depression, as they can precipitate another depressive episode.

Clonidine, a centrally acting α-2 adrenergic receptor agonist, may be used in the treatment of GAD with the goal of decreasing autonomic arousal symptoms. It was found to be efficacious in one study (Hoehn-Saric et al., 1981), but side effects (sedation, hypotension, dizziness, constipation, dry mouth), a tendency for it to lose therapeutic effect over time, and frequent discontinuation problems preclude its use in GAD as monotherapy.

Tiagabine, an anticonvulsant acting as a selective GABA reuptake inhibitor, has shown some efficacy as augmentation therapy for GAD and other anxiety disorders. Two second-generation antipsychotics—risperidone (Brawman-Mintzer et al., 2005) and olanzapine (Pollack et al., 2006)—have been used in controlled studies with some success to augment response to a standard pharmacological treatment for GAD. When used as augmentation therapy, quetiapine may also be effective for treatment-refractory patients.

PSYCHOLOGICAL TREATMENT

Cognitive, Behavior and Cognitive-Behavioral Therapy

Pathological worry as the main target of cognitive-behavioral therapy (CBT) in GAD has been more elusive than behaviors such as avoidance as the main target of CBT in many other anxiety disorders. Perhaps this is the main reason that CBT for GAD is still largely a "work in progress." The process of developing and refining CBT approaches to GAD is occurring alongside conceptual developments in pathological worry and GAD. As a result, various CBT "packages" have emerged for GAD, with many of them combining psychoeducation, cognitive, and behavior therapy techniques.

Cognitive Therapy

Cognitive therapy of GAD generally proceeds through the same stages as cognitive therapy of other anxiety disorders: *(1)* identification of appraisals of threat and beliefs that are associated with worries, *(2)* challenging of these appraisals and beliefs through evidence-seeking and introduction of alternatives, and *(3)* replacement of dysfunctional appraisals and beliefs with rational alternatives. In addition, the use of cognitive therapy in GAD is based on various assumptions about how pathological worry is maintained: by avoidance of autonomic arousal and other unpleasant emotions (Borkovec et al., 1991; 1998), by beliefs that worry is beneficial (Rapee, 1991; Freeston et al., 1994), and/or by intolerance of uncertainty (Ladouceur et al., 1997; Dugas et al., 1998b). Therefore, one of the main tasks of cognitive therapy is to decrease strength of the factors that maintain pathological worry, with the ultimate goal of alleviating pathological worry.

In the text that follows, several cognitive therapy procedures specific for use in GAD are briefly described (see also Table 3–17).

Distinguishing Between the Two Types of Worries   The first step is to distinguish between the two types of worries: *(1)* worries that pertain to the "here-and-now" situation and that have some basis in reality (e.g., worry about current marital problems and its consequences), and *(2)* worries that pertain to a relatively remote future and are of a hypothetical nature (e.g., worry about prolonged suffering from cancer at some point in the future). This distinction is believed to be important because of the different treatment strategies used for these two types of worries (Ladouceur et al., 1993). Improving "problem orientation" is more helpful for addressing worries

Table 3–17. Cognitive Therapy Techniques and Procedures for Use in Generalized Anxiety Disorder

- Distinguishing between Type 1 worries (which pertain to the current situation or issues and have some basis in reality) and Type 2 worries (which pertain to a relatively remote future and are of a hypothetical nature)

- Type 1 worries: improving problem orientation (reviewing and correcting steps in the decision-making and problem-solving processes, and helping patients cope with uncertainty)

- Type 2 worries: using cognitive exposure (imagery exposure to the content of worries)

- Identification of specific beliefs about the benefit of worrying, followed by direct and indirect challenging of these beliefs about current and relatively realistic issues, whereas "cognitive exposure" is used in the treatment of worries about remote and hypothetical issues.

Improving Problem Orientation and Addressing Intolerance of Uncertainty It has been hypothesized that patients with GAD often have poor problem orientation, which is suggested to be different from poor problem solving (Dugas et al., 1998b; Ladouceur et al., 1998). That is, GAD patients tend to have difficulties in understanding problems (poor problem perception, appraisal, and attribution) and perceive themselves as lacking the ability to deal effectively with problems. As a result, they cannot use their problem-solving skills effectively. This is manifested clinically through excessive need for information and reassurance and poor management of time in the problem-solving process, procrastination, indecisiveness, and feeling "paralyzed" by worries. Dugas et al. (1998a, 1998b) believe that poor problem orientation is largely due to intolerance of uncertainty, so that improving patients' "management" of uncertainty would lead to a more effective problem orientation.

Therefore, improving problem orientation involves reviewing and correcting steps in the decision-making and problem-solving processes, and helping patients cope with uncertainty. The latter is facilitated if patients are systematically encouraged to make decisions and deal with problems in the presence of ambiguity and relative lack of information. Patients may come to terms with uncertainty if it is demonstrated to them that absolute certainty is both unrealistic and unnecessary. Patients are also asked to set limits by prioritizing issues that they take into consideration while making decisions and dealing with problems; furthermore, they need to set deadlines to avert procrastination. Patients will be able to exercise more control over their worries if they can give up the indecisiveness-producing and time-consuming quest for certainty. Worries will also seem less "necessary" if there is less need for certainty.

Cognitive Exposure (worry exposure) Cognitive exposure or worry exposure is a good example of blending cognitive and behavioral therapy techniques. It rests on the assumption that avoiding concentration on worries and experiencing them as too vague and abstract (cognitive avoidance) is what maintains worries. Therefore, patients are asked to transform their worries into concrete images and then process these images. In other words, the patients' task is to regularly visualize in as much detail as possible and under a "worst case scenario" what they worry about (Craske et al., 1992; Brown et al., 1993).

The more accurate characterization of this procedure is imagery exposure to the content of worries—rather than exposure to worries themselves. The rationale for using the technique is twofold. First, it enables the worries to be processed via worry-related images, so that worries can become more concrete; second, the rationale is the same as that for the behavioral technique of exposure to phobic situations and objects—habituation to worry and the underlying anxiety, as represented by the corresponding images.

Challenging Beliefs About Worry   Challenging the content of worry (i.e., trying to persuade patients that it is unreasonable to worry about matters such as finances or health) may not be helpful, as the content of worry per se is rarely pathological. Therefore, the focus of challenging should be on the reasons for worry and, more specifically, on any beliefs about benefits of worrying. A successful use of this technique first requires identification of specific beliefs about the benefit of worrying (see Table 3–10). Does the patient believe that worrying prevents the occurrence of the catastrophe that he or she worries about? Or is it that the patient believes that worrying will allow better coping with the problem? The patient may also believe that worrying makes the disappointment less likely.

Whatever the underlying belief is, it should be challenged both directly and indirectly, through behavioral experiments. In the latter case, patients are encouraged to be as "indifferent" as possible about a matter that is otherwise in the focus of their worry. The goal is to demonstrate to patients that a decrease in worry does not make the feared events more likely or the problem-solving process less efficient.

Behavior Therapy

The use of behavior therapy in GAD is based on the hypothesis that pathological anxiety and worry are maintained by symptoms of tension, particularly muscle tension. Therefore, a significant decrease in muscle tension, usually by means of muscle relaxation, leads to a decrease in anxiety in general. Stated otherwise, the goal of behavior therapy in GAD is to achieve good symptom control and, more specifically, control over symptoms of tension.

The rationale for using muscle relaxation is the postulated incompatibility between the state of muscle relaxation on one hand and physiological arousal, tension, and anxiety on the other. Techniques of muscle relaxation have been used in various anxiety disorders; hence, they are not GAD-specific. Relaxation techniques have generally been efficacious in controlling tension and other somatic symptoms of anxiety and may be useful for GAD, especially when combined with cognitive therapy techniques.

The original relaxation technique, called "progressive muscle relaxation," was introduced by Jacobson (1938). It was subsequently modified by Wolpe and Lazarus (1966) and Bernstein and Borkovec (1973), and these modifications have largely been incorporated into the "applied relaxation" program (Öst, 1987a). Irrespective of which version of muscle relaxation technique is used, it rests on alternate tensing and relaxing of each muscle group in a certain order. This procedure helps patients to become better aware of muscle tension as they induce muscle tension and contrast it with muscle relaxation; it also allows patients to exercise control over this tension through relaxation. Furthermore, the effects of muscle relaxation become more obvious if it is preceded by the induced muscle tension. Once patients have learned the basic muscle relaxation technique, they can use it quickly and in various situations, relaxing several muscle groups in a well-coordinated fashion.

The use of relaxation can sometimes lead to a paradoxical increase in anxiety because the anxiety-related cognitions have been disinhibited. This should not necessarily be regarded as an adverse effect of relaxation. Indeed, patients should not use relaxation as a way to avoid thinking about the content of their worries. According to cognitive theorists and therapists, this use of relaxation would be just another safety device, designed to shift the attention away from the "dangerous" worries, thereby perpetuating the erroneous notion that these worries represent a threat.

Muscle relaxation is not the only way of controlling anxiety symptoms. If GAD patients already have the knowledge of meditation techniques, yoga, or tai chi and practice these with some success, there is no reason to insist that they use muscle relaxation instead of these techniques. It is important, though, that patients use them in a way that would maximize the benefits.

Efficacy of Cognitive and Behavioral Treatments

Some studies indicate that CBT of GAD is superior to behavior therapy alone (e.g., Butler et al., 1991; Durham et al., 1994). Other studies reported no advantage of CBT over either behavior therapy or cognitive therapy alone (e.g., Barlow et al., 1992; Borkovec and Costello, 1993), with some advantage of CBT over behavior therapy alone being evident only 12 months after the end of treatment (Borkovec and Costello, 1993). When CBT with greater emphasis on an earlier version of cognitive therapy was compared with behavior therapy (applied relaxation) alone, the two appeared equally efficacious in treating GAD (Öst and Breitholtz, 2000; Arntz, 2003).

Studies of the efficacy of earlier versions of CBT have suggested that a large proportion of GAD patients do not improve with this treatment. For example, at 6-month follow-up after the end of CBT, 58% of patients did not show a clinically significant change in one study (Butler et al., 1991), and 40%–50% were not considered recovered in another study (Fisher and Durham, 1999). The recovery rate at 6-month follow-up after treatment of GAD with an earlier version of cognitive therapy alone and applied relaxation alone was not higher than 55% (Arntz, 2003). These findings have contributed to a search for more effective treatments for GAD—perhaps treatments that are based on newer concepts of pathological worry and include "worry management" strategies and other, more specific cognitive techniques.

One study has demonstrated efficacy of CBT with a substantial cognitive component targeting poor problem orientation, intolerance of uncertainty, erroneous beliefs about worry, and cognitive avoidance (Ladouceur et al., 2000). Treatment gains in this study were maintained at 12-month follow-up. The same type of CBT, administered in a group format over 14 sessions, has also been efficacious in treating GAD patients (Dugas et al., 2003). It is not clear, however, whether this treatment approach is superior to other CBT packages.

Supportive Psychotherapy

This type of psychotherapy relies on nonspecific techniques and procedures. Many GAD patients have trouble tolerating stress and report that stressful events often precede exacerbations of GAD. Therefore, the focus of supportive psychotherapy is often on improving strategies of coping with stress. Some patients need much help and encouragement as they face stressful situations and events, especially if they perceive themselves as lacking the confidence and appropriate skills to manage stress.

Psychodynamic Psychotherapy and Psychoanalysis

It is unusual these days to use psychodynamic psychotherapy and psycho-analysis in the treatment of GAD, unless GAD is accompanied by significant character pathology. Because modern psychodynamic thinking tends to emphasize "positive" aspects of anxiety in terms of its facilitating role in accessing intrapsychic conflicts, the goal of psychodynamic psychotherapy in the treatment of GAD is not necessarily a disappearance of anxiety; rather, the goal is to increase patients' ability to tolerate anxiety.

Other specific treatment goals in the psychodynamic psychotherapy depend on the origin of anxiety (Table 3–11). For example, if the fear of punishment (or superego) is the main "driving force" behind the anxiety in GAD, the focus of treatment is on the softening of the rigid, harsh, and punitive superego, which would allow patients to realistically appraise the threats associated with "forbidden" and repressed urges.

A brief psychodynamic psychotherapy—"supportive-expressive psychotherapy"—has been specifically developed for GAD, and its efficacy was preliminarily tested in one study (Crits-Christoph et al., 1996). This type of treatment is based on psychodynamic assumptions about the role of ambivalent, conflictual attachments and relationships in the development of GAD—not unlike the presumed role of the same factors in the development of panic disorder (see Chapter 2). Within this conceptual framework, an incomplete processing of the trauma(s) is also believed to play an important role in the development of GAD.

COMBINED TREATMENTS

Even more than in other anxiety disorders, there appears to be a discrepancy in GAD between an apparently widespread use of combined (pharmacological and psychological) treatments in clinical practice and very few studies that might support this practice. One study which compared efficacy of the combination of CBT and diazepam, CBT alone, and diazepam alone in patients with GAD reported no differences in outcome between combined treatment and CBT alone, whereas combined treatment was superior to diazepam alone (Power et al., 1990). These findings were interpreted as suggesting both that combining CBT and benzodiazepines is not detrimental and that adding a benzodiazepine to CBT might be superfluous.

As noted in Chapter 2, combining CBT with pharmacotherapy is contentious, with strong views often being expressed about the advantages of CBT alone and the disadvantages of combined treatment. Many of the issues regarding combined treatment of panic disorder and discussed in Chapter 2, also pertain to combined treatment of GAD. Possible indications for using combined treatment in panic disorder (Table 2-30) and the sequencing of treatments in combined treatment of panic disorder (Table 2-31) can be applied to combined treatment of GAD.

The pragmatic and clinically sound approach is to adapt treatment to the specific characteristics of patients and clinical situations. This may entail initial use of pharmacotherapy followed by CBT, which appears to be the usual sequence of combining these treatments in GAD. Pharmacotherapy may also be instituted after CBT in case of a partial response to CBT or in the presence of depression. Although the least common approach, commencing CBT and pharmacotherapy at the same time may be reasonable on clinical grounds.

OUTLOOK FOR THE FUTURE

There may be no future for GAD if the profession cannot agree on *what is* GAD. We can no longer afford to have too discrepant views on GAD and have one "version" of GAD for use by clinical psychologists and the other for use by psychiatrists. It is an embarrassing paradox that GAD is apparently one of the most common psychiatric disorders in the general population, while being recognized relatively infrequently and diagnosed rarely without the presence of other psychopathology. This can only mean that the current diagnostic concept of GAD is seriously flawed.

If GAD continues to be conceptualized as a constellation of more or less nonspecific features, its perception as a somewhat artificial construct will not change and it will not be taken seriously. If GAD exists, at the very minimum it should be clearly defined, so that it can be recognized. And recognizing GAD will be possible insofar as its specific characteristics are emphasized in the conceptualization. At the same time, it is important to promote longitudinal diagnostic assessment, which would treat GAD and related disorders as cross-sectional "snapshots," while recording changes in clinical presentation and psychopathology over time.

Once we have an unambiguous, research- and consensus-derived description of GAD, it will be possible to gradually address some of the most salient issues. These include the relationship between pathological worry and GAD, types of chronic anxiety, and links between GAD, depression, personality disturbance, and other anxiety disorders. It is likely that GAD will be classified along with depression and outside of the group of anxiety (or fear) disorders. This, however, would not necessarily mean that GAD is equated with depression. Our currently fragmented understanding of the pathogenesis of GAD will improve through a greater dialogue between researchers of neurobiological and cognitive mechanisms that lead to GAD.

We cannot be satisfied with treatment results in GAD using our currently available pharmacological and psychological interventions. There is a need for developing new pharmacological agents for GAD because the effectiveness of current medications for GAD seems to have reached a plateau. Novel targets for pharmacological treatment of anxiety may include certain neuropeptides, especially corticotropin-releasing factor receptors antagonists. In addition to being effective and generally well tolerated, novel medications for GAD would specifically need to be able to target both somatic and cognitive anxiety symptoms, as well as symptoms of depression; other requirements for these medications are to work quickly, not to be habit-forming, and not to be associated with significant withdrawal symptoms upon discontinuation. The challenge for psychological treatment of GAD will be to make the most use of the worry- and tension-targeted approaches, focus on further identification of the most effective ingredients of CBT packages, and better address the underlying personality issues, while also developing novel strategies.

4

Social Anxiety Disorder
(Social Phobia)

Social anxiety disorder (SAD) is conceptualized as an excessive and/or unreasonable fear of situations in which the person's behavior or appearance might be scrutinized and evaluated. This fear is a consequence of the person's expectation to be judged negatively, which might lead to embarrassment or humiliation. Typical examples of feared and usually avoided social situations are giving a talk in public, performing other tasks in front of others, and interacting with people in general.

Although the existence of SAD as a psychopathological entity has been known for at least 100 years, it was only relatively recently, with the publication of *DSM-III* in 1980, that SAD (or social phobia) acquired the status of an "official" psychiatric diagnosis. The term *social anxiety disorder* has been increasingly used instead of *social phobia*, because it is felt that the use of the former term conveys more strongly the pervasiveness and impairment associated with the condition and that this term will promote better recognition of the disorder and contribute to better differentiation from specific phobia (Liebowitz et al., 2000).

KEY ISSUES

Like generalized anxiety disorder, social anxiety disorder is common and controversial. Unlike generalized anxiety disorder, which is described in different ways by different diagnostic criteria and different researchers and clinicians, SAD does not suffer from a "description problem." It is not particularly difficult to recognize features of SAD; what may be difficult is making sense of these features. Main issues associated with SAD are listed below.

1. Where are the boundaries of SAD? How well is SAD distinguished from "normal" social anxiety and shyness on one hand, and from severe psychopathology on the other?

2. Is there a danger of "pathologizing" intense social anxiety by labeling it a psychiatric disorder? How can the distress and suffering of people with high levels of social anxiety be acknowledged if they are not given the corresponding diagnostic label?
3. Is SAD a bona fide mental disorder?
4. Can the subtyping scheme (nongeneralized vs. generalized SAD) be supported?
5. Is there a spectrum of social anxiety disorders?
6. Should a full-blown (generalized) form of SAD be better conceptualized as a personality disturbance? What is the relationship between SAD and avoidant personality disorder?
7. What is the optimal way of addressing a significant relationship between SAD and alcohol or other substance use problems?
8. Are there specific pathophysiological mechanisms that lead to SAD? How specific for SAD are the postulated dysfunctional appraisals, beliefs, and information-processing mechanisms?
9. What is the optimal pharmacotherapeutic approach to SAD? Administering medications that broadly affect symptoms of anxiety and depression (e.g., selective serotonin reuptake inhibitors, benzodiazepines), or drugs that may have a more specific effect on SAD (e.g., classical monoamine oxidase inhibitors)?
10. How can insights of the cognitive theoretical model of SAD be "translated" to make the corresponding treatment approaches more convincingly effective?

CLINICAL FEATURES

Features of SAD range from very mild, when patients feel apprehensive about one or a few performance-type situations, to quite severe and incapacitating, when patients are socially isolated and impaired in virtually all domains of functioning. Two main features characterize SAD: excessive and persistent fear of social situations and avoidance of these situations (Figure 4–1). Social situations are mainly of two kinds. One type is the

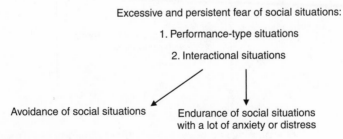

Excessive and persistent fear of social situations:

1. Performance-type situations

2. Interactional situations

Avoidance of social situations   Endurance of social situations with a lot of anxiety or distress

Figure 4–1. Clinical features of social anxiety disorder.

situations that involve "doing something" (i.e., performing) in the presence of others, and they are referred to as performance-type situations. Examples include speaking in public and eating, drinking, writing, working, and using public toilets in the presence of others (or while others are watching). The other type of situations involves informal and formal interactions with other people, and these are referred to as "interactional situations." Although avoidance of these situations is the most common way of coping with social anxiety, not all patients with SAD resort to avoidance. Some may endure social situations with a lot of anxiety or distress.

What are Patients with Social Anxiety Disorder Afraid of?

Very broadly, patients with SAD are afraid of negative evaluation by others; this is usually considered to be the core feature of SAD. However, there may be at least two reasons for the expected negative evaluation, especially in performance-type situations (Starcevic et al., 1994b): patients anticipate that they will make a mistake (or generally perform poorly), or they anticipate having visible physical symptoms (such as blushing and trembling) that would reveal their anxiety. Physical symptoms such as trembling may also affect performance, so that these two reasons for fearing negative evaluation may be interrelated (Figure 4–2).

A related type of basic fear, which can be found in fears of both types of social situations, is a fear of being under scrutiny (or sometimes, at the center of attention). Patients then anticipate that they will be judged negatively only because others are looking at them, regardless of what they do and whether they do anything at all. In other words, exposure to the scrutiny of others automatically leads to negative evaluation. The reasons for such fears do vary, but they often have to do with patients' beliefs about being defective or aberrant in some way. If patients also believe that others are able to "read their mind," a belief that may be quasi-delusional in

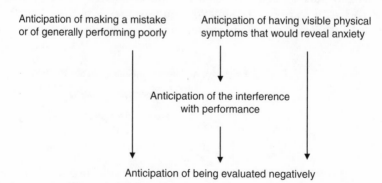

Figure 4–2. Underpinnings of the fear of negative evaluation in performance-type situations.

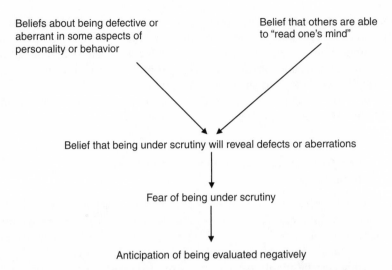

Figure 4–3. Underpinnings of the fear of negative evaluation in relation to the fear of being under scrutiny.

nature, they may end up believing that being under scrutiny reveals these defects or aberrations to others (Figure 4–3). Such a complex belief system may suggest a more severe underlying psychopathology.

The structure of the fear of interactional situations may be more complex, although the same personality characteristics—feelings of insecurity, low self-esteem, and poor self-confidence—may underlie its various manifestations (Figure 4–4). Sometimes the fear of interactional situations boils down to a fear of performing poorly in a particular social interaction, and ultimately, to a fear of negative evaluation of such performance by others. For example, patients may feel that they lack the skill of initiating,

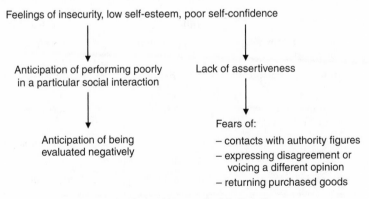

Figure 4–4. Structure of the fear of interactional situations.

maintaining, or terminating conversations, that they are "clumsy" when meeting new people, or that they do not know how to talk over the telephone with someone whom they have never met before. In other situations, the underlying fears of interactional situations may have to do more with patients' lack of assertiveness. Examples of such situations include talking to people in positions of authority, expression of disagreement, and returning purchased goods because they are defective.

Subtypes: Generalized and Nongeneralized Social Anxiety Disorder

Social anxiety disorder encompasses two subtypes—generalized and nongeneralized (also referred to as focal, isolated, limited, discrete, circumscribed, and specific). *Generalized SAD* is the term used to characterize fear of numerous social situations, which include both interactional and performance-type situations; *nongeneralized SAD* pertains to fear of one or just a few such situations, and these are usually (though not invariably) performance-type situations.

The subtypes of nongeneralized and generalized SAD can be conceptualized on a continuum of severity and features associated with severity (Table 4–1). Stated otherwise, the differences between these subtypes of SAD are mainly quantitative in nature, with increasing numbers of fears of social situations being associated with increasing severity of the disorder and greater disability (Stein MB et al., 2000; Ruscio et al., 2008). The relatively few nonquantitative differences (Table 4–2) and unclear boundaries

Table 4–1. Dimensional Conceptualization of Subtypes of Social Anxiety Disorder

Characteristics	Nongeneralized SAD	Generalized SAD
Intensity or severity	Mild	Moderate to severe
Co-occurrence with other psychiatric disorders	Less frequent	More frequent
Co-occurrence with personality disorders	Less frequent	More frequent
Complicated by depression or alcohol abuse or dependence	Less often	More often
Functioning	Less impaired	More impaired
Prognosis	Good	Guarded
Treatment	Relatively simple	More complex

Table 4–2. Contrasting Characteristics of Nongeneralized and Generalized Social Anxiety Disorder

Characteristics	Nongeneralized SAD	Generalized SAD
Age of onset	Variable, not unusual after adolescence	Usually in childhood or adolescence
Mode of onset	Variable, can be sudden	Gradual, can also be sudden
Genetic basis	Weaker	Stronger
Frequency in the community	More frequent	Less frequent
Frequency in clinical setting	Less frequent	More frequent
Gender distribution in clinical setting	About the same in women and men	More frequent among men

between the two subtypes in many cases have cast some doubt on the rationale for subtyping SAD.

In clinical samples, generalized SAD is encountered more frequently than nongeneralized SAD, but their prevalence seems to be different in the community, with the ratio of generalized to nongeneralized SAD being 1:2 (Wittchen et al., 1999; Furmark et al., 2000). The main reason for this difference between clinical and epidemiological samples is the greater severity of the generalized form of SAD; its sufferers are more likely to seek professional help. While the prevalence of nongeneralized SAD in clinical setting is similar among women and men, there are apparently more men than women with generalized SAD in the same setting.

The onset of generalized SAD is usually gradual and dates back to patients' adolescence or childhood. Patients typically say that they have always been shy or anxious in social situations. In the nongeneralized subtype of SAD, the onset after adolescence is not unusual and it may be relatively abrupt—for example, after an unpleasant event, such as suddenly blushing, quivering, losing one's voice, or even having a panic attack while giving a talk. There is some indication, however, that sudden onset of SAD may occur in both of its subtypes (Kristensen et al., 2008).

A genetic link seems to be stronger for generalized SAD. Patients with generalized SAD were significantly more likely to have a first-degree relative with generalized SAD than were those in the control group. In contrast, the frequency of first-degree relatives with SAD was similar among patients with nongeneralized SAD and control group subjects (Mannuzza et al., 1995; Stemberger et al., 1995; Stein MB et al., 1998a).

Fear of Performance-Type Situations

One of the hallmarks of the fear of performance-type situations is the absence of problems when patients perform alone or in front of one or only a few persons whom they know well and trust. This suggests that the fear of performance-type situations is generally less about performance itself and more about the performance being watched and judged by the unsympathetic others.

Fear of Speaking in Public

Fear of speaking in public is a typical example of the fear of performance-type situations. It is one of the most frequently reported fears in the general population: according to one epidemiological survey in the United States, 30.2% of the population reported ever having this fear (Kessler et al., 1998). Of course, only a small portion of these people—those who avoid public-speaking situations persistently or endure them with inordinate anxiety or distress and are impaired or significantly distressed because of this fear and its consequences—qualify for the diagnosis of SAD. The public-speaking fear is the most common type of fear in both subtypes of SAD. Because it is so widespread and more often accompanied by high autonomic arousal, the public-speaking phobia has been considered as representing a distinct and separate type of SAD (Stein MB et al., 1994). However, many patients with a fear of public speaking are afraid of other social situations as well.

Patients with fear of public speaking may have various underlying concerns: they may be afraid of certain visible symptoms during the talk (e.g., blushing, shortness of breath) or of being under scrutiny by others. These patients are particularly concerned about their performance and often expect to make a mistake, say "stupid" things, or do something embarrassing during the talk. The end result is an expectation that they would be humiliated or ridiculed because of poor performance.

Fear of Taking Tests and Being Examined

A related fear is that of taking tests and being examined, especially when patients are examined orally or while they are performing a certain task as part of their examination. The reactions to tests and examinations may be quite severe, both in the preparation stages and while patients are actually being examined. Just before the exam or in the weeks preceding the exam, patients may have symptoms such as diarrhea, headache, insomnia, and loss of appetite. The symptoms may be so severe that patients decide against taking the exam. During the exam itself, patients may feel that they are about to lose bladder control and have to go to the toilet immediately; sometimes, they become short of breath, experience rapid heart beat, have severe tremor, or develop a full-blown panic attack. Any of these symptoms may be the reason for them to give up. With such severe physical symptoms, patients may end up fearing them more than the negative evaluation by their examiners.

Fear of Eating, Drinking, and Writing in the Presence of Others

Patients who are afraid of eating or drinking in the presence of others are usually concerned that a symptom, such as trembling, would reveal that they are anxious. The fear of trembling is also prominent among patients who are afraid of writing in front of others, such as when they are signing a receipt or another document. These fears are usually accompanied by other social fears. Patients may resort to extensive avoidance of the corresponding situations, which may be quite distressing for them.

Fear of Performing Work Duties Under Observation

Some patients are particularly distressed when they have to perform their job under observation by other people. They are usually concerned that under such circumstances, their work-related performance would suffer (e.g., because of poor concentration and/or a greater likelihood of making a mistake). Patients often feel that, in turn, this might have serious consequences, such as losing a job.

Fear of Using Public Toilets in the Presence of Others

Fear of using public toilets in the presence of others or, more precisely, fear of not being able to urinate in public toilets or when other people are aware that the person is urinating is not very common but can be quite disabling. It is encountered more often in men and is also referred to as "shy bladder syndrome" or paruresis. The underlying fear of being under scrutiny by others may lead to an inhibition of urination, even when the urinary bladder is full. The sufferers usually avoid public toilets and structure their daily routine around this avoidance. There is a frequent co-occurrence of paruresis and fears of other performance-type situations, and many sufferers of paruresis are also depressed (Vythilingum et al., 2002). It has been argued that paruresis is an anxiety disorder distinct from SAD (e.g., Boschen, 2008).

Fears of Other Performance-Type Situations

Some patients with SAD have a particularly strong fear of entering a room or hall in which people are in a meeting, already seated, and/or are attending a concert, a lecture, or other public performance. These patients are particularly concerned that they will suddenly become the center of attention in this situation and be judged with disapproval or in some other negative way. Patients typically say that the stare of so many eyes at the same time is deeply disturbing. Although this is not a prototype of the performance-type situation, sufferers often feel that they are "supposed to act" (i.e., perform) in a certain, prescribed manner. As a consequence of this fear, patients may miss meetings and other important activities or may be unable to attend classes regularly and maintain their jobs.

Fear of Interactional Situations

As already noted, the fear of interactional situations encompasses various fears. In a very broad sense, patients with these fears are concerned about any situation in which they are expected to communicate with others. These situations include simple interactions, such as asking a passerby for directions, as well as more complex interactions, like socializing at a party. The underlying theme in many of these fears is patients' general feeling that they lack basic social skills. The consequences of interactions are likely to be feared more when patients are in contact with someone known to them; in this situation, patients are particularly concerned about the impression they make.

Some fears of interactional situations pertain predominantly to certain people and certain situations. This is particularly the case with situations in which patients are expected to demonstrate some assertiveness. Typical examples include making a complaint about poor service, returning defective items to the store in which they were purchased, or expressing an opinion about an issue that is being discussed, particularly if it is contrary to the prevailing opinion. The corresponding avoidance may be distressing, because it prevents patients from "getting things done" or from showing their "true personality." The fear may be in stark contrast to patients' relative calm in "ordinary" social situations in which their insecurity and lack of assertiveness are hidden beneath a well-learned use of social conventions.

Fears of visible and "revealing" physical symptoms that might occur during interpersonal interactions may be so strong that they become the main reason for avoidance of interactional situations or some aspects of these situations. For example, some patients are so terrified about blushing that this particular fear, sometimes referred to as "erythrophobia," drives them to avoid most social contacts. In other cases, patients avoid hand-shaking because of "showing" that their hands are clammy, or have a fear of talking because they are concerned that they might start stuttering.

Cultural Variants of Social Anxiety Disorder

Considering that social fears do not occur in social isolation, it is understandable that social and cultural factors influence the way social fears are experienced and manifested. With the exception of some Asian countries, however, the social context of SAD has received surprisingly little attention.

A specific form of SAD has been described in Japan. There has been some confusion regarding the name and meaning of this condition, when translated from Japanese. Taijin-Kyofu (meaning "fear vis-à-vis other people") was postulated to have a "tension" subtype and a "conviction" subtype (e.g., Kasahara, 2005), with the former roughly corresponding to the Western concept of SAD (Kinoshita et al., 2008). The "conviction" subtype refers to both a strong belief and fear that a person is offending others by blushing, trembling, emitting unpleasant bodily odors, having loud bowel sounds, exhibiting odd facial expression, or having other anxiety symptoms; this belief and fear then lead to avoidance of social situations. This type of social anxiety is very different from its Western counterpart and appears to be related to the specific characteristics of the Japanese society: the sufferers are not preoccupied with the impact of the anxiety on themselves, but they worry about the possible discomfort that they cause in others by their anxiety.

Taijin-Kyofu-Sho (meaning a "syndrome of the fear vis-à-vis other people") has been listed among culture-bound syndromes in *DSM-IV*, referred to as an "offensive subtype" of SAD and presumed to be a synonym for the conviction subtype of Taijin-Kyofu. It has been proposed, however, that offensiveness should be conceptualized on a continuum of belief, with only those cases exhibiting a firm belief corresponding to the conviction subtype of Taijin-Kyofu (Kinoshita et al., 2008). Not surprisingly, this subtype is often diagnosed as a delusional disorder outside of Japan. There has also been some discussion as to whether the conviction subtype of Taijin-Kyofu and Taijin-Kyofu-Sho (or offensive subtype of SAD) should continue to be regarded as culture-bound syndromes (Suzuki et al., 2003), considering that they have been encountered in the Western settings (e.g., Clarvit et al., 1996).

Stage Fright, Shyness, and Social Anxiety Disorder

"Normal" forms of social anxiety—stage fright and shyness—have an important relationship with SAD. Stage fright is related to the fear of performance-type situations, whereas shyness is related to generalized SAD. Unlike SAD, neither stage fright nor shyness is associated with impairment in functioning. Assessment of the effects on functioning, however, may be difficult in people who have adjusted their lifestyles to their social anxiety and do not feel that this anxiety interferes significantly with their lives. Moreover, the relationship between shyness and SAD is more complex, as discussed below.

The Yerkes-Dodson bell-shaped curve (Yerkes and Dodson, 1908) can help us understand the relationship between the stage fright and phobic fear of performance-type situations. This curve represents a relationship between the degree of anxiety and the quality of performance; whereas mild to moderate anxiety is often stimulating and contributes to better performance, moderate to severe anxiety tends to interfere with performance. Up to a certain point, stage fright may enhance performance; hence the saying that only a bad actor is completely free from stage fright. At the top of the curve (after which the performance declines with increasing anxiety) is a sometimes-imperceptible boundary between stage fright and SAD.

Unlike stage fright, the phobic fear of performance-type situations is characterized by excessive preoccupation with fear. Although there may be an element of reality in the patients' expectation that their performance will not be good, the performance is not necessarily impaired by the phobia. However, patients avoid "testing" themselves in performance situations, especially if they were disappointed with their performance in the past. Of course, this only perpetuates the phobia, as patients do not have an opportunity to see for themselves what their performance would be like.

Shyness and SAD have numerous similarities in terms of their physical, anxiety-related symptoms (e.g., sweating, trembling, tachycardia, blushing), cognitive distortions, and behavioral responses to distressing social situations (Turner et al., 1990). The differences between shyness and generalized SAD are believed to pertain mainly to the intensity, frequency, and/or duration of these variables.

Thus, generalized SAD can be distinguished from shyness on the basis of the severity of anxiety. That means that people who are very shy are far more likely to have generalized SAD than those who are moderately or minimally shy; this notion is supported by the finding that most shy persons do not have SAD (Heiser et al., 2003). However, severe shyness and generalized SAD still seem to be distinct, as there are people who are very shy but do not qualify for a diagnosis of generalized SAD (Chavira et al., 2002). Also, it does not seem that shyness is necessary for the development of generalized SAD (Beidel and Turner, 1999). The link between shyness and phobia of performance-type situations is not strong, as people with this type of SAD are often not shy at all. Some research suggests that shyness is a very broad construct that is associated not only with SAD but also with various anxiety and mood disorders, as well as personality disorders, especially avoidant personality disorder (Heiser et al., 2003).

Other data also suggest that there are differences between shyness and SAD. For example, general population surveys support a very broad conceptualization of shyness, with at least 40% of survey respondents stating that they are shy (e.g., Pilkonis and Zimbardo, 1979). By comparison, lifetime prevalence rates of SAD are estimated to be much lower, between 0.5% and 16% (see Epidemiology, below). Another distinction between shyness and SAD is important and often clinically useful. Shy persons feel anxious about performance and other social interactions before entering these situations, but once they have been engaged socially, their anxiety levels drop considerably. In contrast, people with SAD do not experience this relief after the beginning of performance or social interaction, and their anxiety levels remain consistently high throughout the performance or interaction. This may be a consequence of shy persons' greater attentiveness to cues from others about their appearance, performance, and behavior, and higher likelihood of responding favorably to positive feedback (Stopa and Clark, 1993).

RELATIONSHIP BETWEEN SOCIAL ANXIETY DISORDER AND OTHER DISORDERS

Social anxiety disorder, particularly its generalized subtype, very often co-occurs with other psychiatric disorders. In the general population, the lifetime rate of the co-occurrence of SAD with any psychiatric disorder has been estimated to range between 69% and 81% (Schneier et al., 1992; Magee et al., 1996). Social anxiety disorder often co-occurs with depression, other anxiety disorders, alcohol abuse and dependence, and personality disorders. Clinical implications of the co-occurrence with depression, alcohol-related problems, and personality disorders are summarized in Table 4–3.

Social Anxiety Disorder and Depression

The presence of SAD increases the risk of major depression (Nelson et al., 2000; Stein MB et al., 2001; Beesdo et al., 2007). In the community, 17%–37% of persons with SAD have major depression during their lifetime (Schneier et al., 1992; Magee et al., 1996); in clinical samples, this association is even stronger, with 60%–70% of SAD patients being affected by depression (Stein MB et al., 1990b; Van Ameringen et al., 1991). Social anxiety disorder seems to be associated not only with major depressive disorder but also with other mood disorders, including dysthymia and bipolar disorder (Kessler et al., 1999b; Grant et al., 2005b).

Although the sequence may vary, depression usually follows SAD (e.g., Beesdo et al., 2007). According to the "demoralization hypothesis," the chronic and often relentless course of SAD makes patients feel less and less able to "cope with life," so that they become helpless and hopeless and thus prone to developing depression. There may also be a genetic link between SAD and depression, with an increased frequency of depression among first-degree relatives of individuals with SAD.

Generalized SAD bears a similarity with the construct of atypical depression, as they both share heightened interpersonal sensitivity and, in particular, hypersensitivity to criticism and rejection. Some support for this association comes from the efficacy of classical, irreversible monoamine

Table 4–3. Clinical Implications of Relationship Between Social Anxiety Disorder and Depression, Alcohol-Related Problems, and Personality Disturbance

Social Anxiety Disorder and Depression

- Depression frequently co-occurs with SAD, particularly in clinical settings
- The presence of SAD increases the risk of major depression
- Depression usually occurs after the onset of SAD
- Clinical features are more severe when SAD co-occurs with depression and patients are then more likely to seek help
- Patients are more likely to be suicidal if depression co-occurs with SAD
- There may be an overlap between generalized SAD and atypical depression, which may account for the efficacy of classical, irreversible monoamine oxidase inhibitors in the treatment of SAD
- When patients treated with cognitive-behavioral therapy for SAD become depressed, addition of an antidepressant should be considered

Social Anxiety Disorder and Alcohol Abuse and Dependence

- A specific link exists between SAD and alcohol dependence
- Many patients with SAD have alcohol-related problems. Excessive use of alcohol usually results from patients' attempts to alleviate social anxiety and improve performance
- Social anxiety disorder usually precedes alcoholism and generally represents a risk factor for alcoholism. The risk is greater if patients are female, if they have generalized SAD and/or avoidant personality disorder, and if the onset of SAD was early
- Some patients are recognized as suffering from primary SAD only after they have developed a significant alcohol problem
- Opinions differ on the issue of whether alcohol-related problems should be treated first or whether they should be treated at the same time as SAD. However, abstinence from alcohol is needed to make treatment of SAD effective
- Benzodiazepines should be avoided in the treatment of SAD complicated by excessive use of alcohol

Social Anxiety Disorder and Personality Disorders

- Personality disorders are far more likely to accompany the generalized type than the nongeneralized type of SAD
- Avoidant, obsessive-compulsive, and dependent personality disorders tend to be most frequently associated with SAD
- There is a significant overlap between generalized SAD and avoidant personality disorder, with the latter condition often being considered a more severe variant of the same psychopathology
- The presence of a personality disorder in patients with SAD generally implies chronicity and poorer outcome

oxidase inhibitors in the treatment of both atypical depression (Zisook et al., 1985; Liebowitz et al., 1988; Quitkin et al., 1991) and generalized SAD (Gelernter et al., 1991; Liebowitz et al., 1992; Versiani et al., 1992; Heimberg et al., 1998).

Patients with an early onset of SAD (before age 15) are more likely to develop depression (Lecrubier and Weiller, 1997). When accompanied by depression, SAD is associated with greater severity of clinical presentation, and patients are then more likely to be suicidal (Schneier et al., 1992; Davidson et al., 1993a; Nelson et al., 2000), develop alcohol-related problems (Nelson et al., 2000), and seek help (Lecrubier and Weiller, 1997). Likewise, major depressive disorder and other mood disorders co-occurring with SAD tend to be more severe and have a more chronic course and poorer prognosis (e.g., Kessler et al., 1999b; Stein MB et al., 2001; Beesdo et al., 2007).

Social Anxiety Disorder and Alcohol and Other Substance Abuse and Dependence

Data from the U.S. National Comorbidity Survey suggest that almost 24% of persons with SAD develop alcohol dependence in their lifetime, with the corresponding rate for any substance abuse or dependence being almost 40% (Magee et al., 1996). Another epidemiological survey from the United States reported that 48% of persons with a lifetime diagnosis of SAD also met criteria for a lifetime diagnosis of an alcohol use disorder (Grant et al., 2005b). Rates of alcohol abuse and dependence in other epidemiological and clinical samples of people with SAD have ranged from 15% to 36% (Schneier et al., 1989; Van Ameringen et al., 1991; Davidson et al., 1993a; Weiller et al., 1996). There may also be a significant proportion (16%–25%) of patients with alcohol abuse or dependence who have an underlying and often unrecognized SAD (Mullaney and Trippett, 1979; Smail et al., 1984; Thomas et al., 1999). Some patients are identified as suffering from primary SAD only after they have developed a significant alcohol problem.

Social anxiety disorder has been associated specifically with alcohol dependence, but not alcohol abuse (Buckner et al., 2008), and it usually precedes alcohol-related problems (Schneier et al., 1992; Lampe et al., 2003; Buckner et al., 2008). In one longitudinal study, SAD emerged as a unique and significant risk factor (relative to other anxiety disorders and mood disorders) for both alcohol dependence and cannabis dependence (Buckner et al., 2008). Alcohol and cannabis may be preferred over some of the other psychotropic substances because of their calming, anxiolytic, and/or disinhibiting properties. Use of alcohol is also more likely because of its accessibility and social tolerance of its moderate use in most Western countries.

Several models have been proposed to explain the relationship between SAD and alcohol-related problems; of these, the most influential has been the self-medication hypothesis (e.g., Khantzian, 1985; Carrigan and Randall, 2003). This hypothesis assumes that SAD precedes excessive alcohol use and that people with social anxiety drink increasing amounts of alcohol, because alcohol reduces their anxiety and brings about some relief.

A greater risk of alcoholism in patients with SAD has been associated with female gender, early onset, generalized subtype of the condition, and co-occurrence of avoidant personality disorder (Stravynski et al., 1986; Schneier et al., 1989; Morgenstern et al., 1997; Lecrubier, 1998; Regier et al., 1998). People with SAD and alcohol dependence are more impaired across a variety of domains than those with SAD and no alcohol dependence (Buckner et al., 2008).

Patients with SAD and alcohol-related problems cannot benefit from treatment of SAD if they continue drinking. Opinions vary on whether these patients need to be treated for alcoholism first or undergo treatment for SAD and alcohol abuse or dependence at the same time. An integrated, simultaneously administered treatment for both conditions might be theoretically most suitable, but such programs are not always readily available. Because patients who have achieved abstinence from alcohol can be engaged much better in psychological interventions for SAD, addressing alcohol-related problems first is also a logical strategy. The administration of paroxetine can be useful in the treatment of both SAD and alcoholism (Randall et al., 2001; Book et al., 2008). In contrast, benzodiazepines should be avoided in SAD patients who have a history of alcohol or other substance abuse or dependence.

Social Anxiety Disorder and Personality Disorders

Personality disorders are far more likely to accompany the generalized type than the nongeneralized type of SAD. Avoidant personality disorder is the most common form of personality disturbance associated with SAD, followed by other *DSM* Cluster C personality disorders—obsessive-compulsive and dependent (e.g., Alnaes and Torgersen, 1988; Turner et al., 1991; Lampe et al., 2003; Grant et al., 2005b). Much less often, SAD patients have *DSM* Cluster B personality disorders such as histrionic, borderline, and antisocial. This is understandable, because SAD may be conceived of as an antithesis of the externalizing, risk-taking behaviors and histrionic behavioral style: whereas histrionic persons seek attention, SAD patients prefer anonymity and would do anything not to be noticed and not to be in the center of attention.

Patients with SAD are more likely to exhibit insecurity, lack of self-confidence, low self-esteem, extreme sensitivity to criticism, feelings of inferiority, unassertiveness, shyness, and tendency toward social withdrawal. Depending on how prominent and pervasive these personality traits are, a diagnosis of avoidant personality disorder may be warranted.

The relationship between avoidant personality disorder and generalized SAD has attracted much attention because of their substantial overlap. There appear to be few significant differences between avoidant personality disorder and generalized SAD, with either the former condition being considered more severe (Herbert et al., 1992; Holt et al., 1992; Turner et al., 1992; van Velzen et al., 2000; Chambless et al., 2008) or avoidant personality disorder and generalized SAD representing merely different ways of conceptualizing the same underlying condition (Reich, 2000; Ralevski et al., 2005). One study has reported that genetic risk factors for these disorders appear to be identical in women, while different types of life events may predispose to one or the other condition (Reichborn-Kjennerud et al., 2007). The rates of avoidant personality disorder among patients with generalized SAD vary significantly (from 22% to 89%) (Schneier et al., 1991; Turner et al., 1991), which is a consequence of the different diagnostic criteria and various methodological issues.

Patients with SAD may exhibit traits of other personality disorders. When their perfectionist tendencies are particularly strong and when they exhibit a marked preoccupation with control and rigid attitudes as to what is socially desirable, expected, and allowed, patients may have an obsessive-compulsive personality disorder. Others are passive, extremely afraid of being rejected or abandoned with an excessive need to please others, reluctant to express their own opinion or any disagreement, and unable to make even simple decisions, thus exhibiting features of dependent personality disorder.

Schizoid personality disorder may be encountered in patients with SAD who have largely withdrawn from the outside world, possibly because of the disappointing interactions with other people and fear that such interactions might be harmful. Patients with paranoid personality disorder and SAD are hypervigilant and suspicious about other people's intentions, deeply mistrustful of them, and constantly expecting that others will ridicule them and/or take advantage of them.

The presence of personality disturbance in SAD patients, especially avoidant personality disorder, generally implies a more chronic course of SAD and poorer prognosis (e.g., Massion et al., 2002). The presence of avoidant personality disorder, however, does not necessarily predict the outcome of treatment of generalized SAD (e.g., Brown EJ et al., 1995).

Social Anxiety Disorder and Other Anxiety Disorders

Social anxiety disorder can co-occur with other anxiety disorders, most commonly with specific phobias, panic disorder with or without agoraphobia, and generalized anxiety disorder. The rates of co-occurrence with these disorders tend to vary, depending on the nature of the sample, instruments used in the study, and diagnostic criteria. Approximately a third of patients with SAD may have a co-occurring panic disorder with or without agoraphobia, whereas the rates for specific phobias may be higher.

The relationship between generalized anxiety disorder and SAD is discussed in Chapter 3. Generalized anxiety disorder may be seen in 33% of patients with the principal diagnosis of SAD (Turner et al., 1991) and is significantly related to it (Grant et al., 2005b). In one study, patients with SAD and co-occurring generalized anxiety disorder were found to have a more severe illness than patients with SAD and no generalized anxiety disorder (Mennin et al., 2000). Despite this, the response to cognitive-behavioral group therapy of SAD was not affected by the presence of generalized anxiety disorder.

ASSESSMENT

Diagnostic and Conceptual Issues

The diagnosis of SAD can be made on the basis of the same general criteria used to diagnose other phobic disorders (Table 4–4). As with other phobic disorders, the clinical significance criterion is the most difficult one because it is most elusive. This is also the criterion most responsible for drawing the boundary between "normal" social anxiety and SAD and includes distress caused by social anxiety and/or effects of social anxiety on functioning. Usually, the impairment caused by social anxiety affects relationships, social activities, academic and occupational performance, and/or family functioning. Sometimes the impairment is more evident in certain areas of functioning. For example, students with a paralyzing phobia of examinations may give up their studies, but function fairly well in other social situations.

Table 4–4. General Characteristics of Phobic Disorders

1. There is a fear of *known* objects, situations, activities, or phenomena ("phobic stimuli")

2. Phobic stimuli generally *do not pose a realistic threat*; if they do, the anxiety response is irrational or excessive

3. An *insight* exists that the fear is irrational or excessive

4. Exposure to phobic stimuli *elicits an immediate anxiety response*, which may be in the form of a (situationally bound) panic attack

5. Behavior is characterized either by *avoidance* of phobic stimuli *or endurance* of phobic stimuli with great distress and/or anxiety

6. There is impaired functioning or significant distress about having the fear

In *DSM-IV-TR*, the diagnosis of SAD cannot be made if the anxiety in social situations is a consequence of other disorders, such as stuttering and squinting. Likewise, the diagnosis of SAD is not to be made if some symptoms often found in SAD—for example, tremor—are a consequence of another illness, such as Parkinson's disease. Some of these propositions are debatable, as it is not clear, for example, why the anxiety of people who stutter should be attributed only to (fear of) stuttering.

In *ICD-10*, attention is drawn to the relationship between SAD and an underlying psychotic disorder. This is relevant for clinical practice, as some patients who are labeled "socially phobic" feel anxious because of delusions of reference (e.g., they are afraid of some people because of a delusional belief that these people talk about them in a derogatory manner and ridicule them). The *ICD-10* concept of SAD also emphasizes the presence of somatic symptoms that are relatively characteristic of social anxiety disorder (e.g., blushing, tremor, sweating).

The diagnosis of SAD is based on information elicited from patients and clinical observation. Patients should be asked questions relevant to all phobic situations, and not just those that they mention spontaneously. When patients with SAD are seen for an assessment, they typically lack spontaneity and look inhibited, anxious, and/or tense. Sometimes they shake or blush, and their hands are often clammy. Being interviewed may seem like a major effort for them. They often avoid eye contact and seem as if the end of an interview cannot come soon enough. However, the appearance and behavior of other patients may be quite different from this stereotype. For example, some SAD patients may be very talkative and difficult to interrupt, usually because they have trouble tolerating silence and prefer talking to the silence-producing tension. Other patients may seem detached, as they attempt to decrease their discomfort in an interpersonal situation. This may be interpreted as lack of interest in other people or aloofness.

Although many attempts have been made to raise the awareness of SAD and improve its detection, it is still often overlooked and neglected (e.g., Sheeran and Zimmerman, 2002). This seems to be the case particularly when SAD is overshadowed by depression, alcoholism, or personality disturbance. Also, it appears that many cases of SAD are dismissed as "shyness" and are not taken seriously.

Indeed, shyness continues to be equated with SAD. The concept of SAD has been criticized on the grounds that it has "medicalized" or "pathologized" shyness and turned a variant of normal behavior or temperament into a psychiatric illness (e.g., Wakefield et al., 2005; Lane, 2008). This criticism ignores a body of research suggesting that there are important differences between shyness and SAD and that SAD is not merely and not necessarily, an extreme form of shyness (see Stage Fright, Shyness, and Social Anxiety Disorder, above). The controversy largely boils down to the unclear boundary between "normality" and psychopathology and highlights the problematic lack of the clear definition of mental disorder.

Another issue of interest is the proposed spectrum of social anxiety disorders (Muller et al., 2004). This is similar to obsessive-compulsive spectrum disorders (see Chapter 6), with the suggestion that besides SAD, there may be several groups of conditions that overlap with SAD or are related to it and can be conceptualized dimensionally along several spectra. These include the spectrum of social discomfort (shyness, nongeneralized SAD, generalized SAD, avoidant personality disorder), the spectrum of social fears related to body image concerns (general medical conditions, eating disorders, body dysmorphic disorder, olfactory reference syndrome, etc.), the spectrum of increased social awareness and need for social contact (SAD, avoidant personality disorder) versus social deficit (schizoid personality disorder, autism, and related conditions), the spectrum of social inhibition versus disinhibition, and so on. As with similar proposals for other anxiety disorders, the spectrum concept of social anxiety disorders and their dimensional assessment require further study; at present, their clinical usefulness is uncertain.

Assessment Instruments

The Liebowitz Social Anxiety Scale (Liebowitz, 1987) is a clinician-administered instrument used to measure the severity of SAD in terms of both the fear and avoidance of performance-type and interactional situations. Thus, it yields separate scores for fear and avoidance of performance and social interactional situations. This instrument is useful for monitoring treatment-related changes in the severity of various aspects of SAD.

The Social Phobia and Anxiety Inventory (Turner et al., 1989) is a self-report measure of the severity of psychological and somatic symptoms associated with social situations and avoidance or escape related to social situations. The instrument also yields a total score. The Social Phobia and Anxiety Inventory assesses SAD comprehensively and has excellent psychometric properties, but because of its length and cumbersome scoring, it is not ideal for routine use.

The Fear Questionnaire (Marks and Mathews, 1979), which is also a self-report instrument, is very simple to administer because it has only five items on a subscale for SAD (and 5 items each on subscales for agoraphobia and blood-injection-injury phobia). It can be used to assess the severity of SAD, but this measure is crude and is entirely based on avoidance behavior. The Fear Questionnaire is suitable for screening purposes.

Differential Diagnosis

In terms of differential diagnosis, SAD should be distinguished from shyness and "normal" social anxiety, other anxiety disorders (especially agoraphobia), body dysmorphic disorder, some types of personality disturbance (e.g., avoidant personality disorder), depression, and psychotic

Table 4–5. Differential Diagnosis of Social Anxiety Disorder

- Shyness, "normal" social anxiety
- Other anxiety disorders (especially agoraphobia)
- Body dysmorphic disorder
- Personality disorders (especially avoidant, schizoid, and paranoid personality disorders)
- Depression
- Psychotic illness (e.g., schizophrenia, delusional disorder)

illness (Table 4–5). The differentiation between SAD, shyness, and avoidant personality disorder is discussed in Clinical Features and Relationship Between Social Anxiety Disorder and Other Disorders, above.

Other Anxiety Disorders

The differentiation between SAD and some of the other anxiety disorders may sometimes pose problems. For example, patients with agoraphobia may have concerns that are similar to worries of patients with SAD: they may be afraid of crowded places not only because of the possibility of having a panic attack and of not being able to escape but also because of the embarrassment and shame they would experience if a panic attack occurred. Although agoraphobia and SAD may co-occur, it is important to ascertain whether features of one disorder are, in fact, a part of the other, as both diagnoses are not warranted in these cases.

The structure of fear in agoraphobia is quite different from that in SAD (Table 4–6). Patients with agoraphobia are typically concerned about being helpless and alone in case of a panic attack, whereas patients with SAD are

Table 4–6. Distinguishing Between Social Anxiety Disorder and Agoraphobia

Characteristics	Social Anxiety Disorder	Agoraphobia
Main underlying concerns	Scrutiny and harsh judgment by others	Having a panic attack in specific situations
Fear of being alone	Generally rare	Generally frequent
Fear of large crowds	Generally rare	Very common
Anonymity seeking	Present	Usually absent
Type of symptoms in phobic situations	Blushing, sweating trembling, muscle spasms	Dizziness, lightheadedness, choking feelings

not at all troubled by being alone because it is the scrutiny by others that is most troublesome to them. Therefore, situations that provide anonymity and in which there is no expectation to perform, with low likelihood of being under scrutiny (e.g., being in crowded places) generally do not represent a problem for patients with SAD. This is in contrast to small groups, where SAD patients may be expected to perform and may easily be observed. Also, when in a phobic situation, patients with SAD tend to have different physical symptoms from those experienced by patients with agoraphobia (and panic disorder). The former are more likely to blush, sweat, tremble, and have dry mouth and muscle spasms, whereas the latter are more likely to feel dizzy and lightheaded and have palpitations, chest pain or discomfort, and choking feelings (Amies et al., 1983; Reich et al., 1988).

Unlike unexpected panic attacks that occur in panic disorder (without agoraphobia), panic attacks associated with SAD have an obvious relationship with the feared social situations. Patients with panic disorder may avoid certain social situations not because they fear that they will be under scrutiny from others but because they feel embarrassed about the possibility of experiencing a panic attack in such situations and then having an urge to escape.

Body Dysmorphic Disorder

Body dysmorphic disorder may sometimes resemble SAD, and the two conditions may also co-occur. However, the reason for social discomfort and anxiety in body dysmorphic disorder pertains to the imagined bodily defect to which other people are expected to respond negatively, and which the person also finds unacceptable and often repugnant.

Depression

Sometimes it is difficult to differentiate between SAD and depression, as both are characterized by social withdrawal. However, the underlying reason for social withdrawal is what distinguishes these two conditions: in depression, social withdrawal is a consequence of the generalized loss of interest, whereas in SAD (not complicated by depression), social withdrawal results from active and specific avoidance of social situations. As already noted, depression and SAD also co-occur frequently.

Psychosis

Patients with SAD may present in a way that is difficult to distinguish from psychotic illness. In these cases, patients often express fears of other people and attribute to them malicious intentions, sometimes worrying about their own safety. Patients are typically concerned that others are "singling" them out, paying special attention to them, taking every notice of them, talking about them, making derogatory comments, and/or ridiculing them. Beneath such concerns there may be paranoid (persecutory) delusions, delusions of reference, delusional misinterpretations, or delusions that others are able to read one's mind. These phenomena suggest a delusional disorder with a strong paranoid component or paranoid schizophrenia. Interestingly, social anxiety and persecutory ideation have been reported to have much in common, with various perceptual abnormalities being the only distinct predictor of the development of persecutory ideation (Freeman et al., 2008).

EPIDEMIOLOGY

Highlights of the epidemiology of SAD are presented in Table 4–7. Social anxiety disorder is a common condition in the community, but the estimate of its prevalence has been a matter of some controversy. In the United States, the lifetime prevalence rate of SAD was only 2.7% in the Epidemiologic Catchment Area Study, based on the *DSM-III* diagnostic criteria (Robins and Regier, 1991). The National Comorbidity Survey, using the *DSM-III-R* diagnostic criteria, put the lifetime prevalence rate of SAD at 13.3% (Kessler et al., 1994; Magee et al., 1996), and the National

Table 4–7. Epidemiological Data for Social Anxiety Disorder

- Lifetime prevalence in the United States: 2.7% (*DSM-III* criteria, Epidemiologic Catchment Area Study), 13.3% (*DSM-III-R* criteria, National Comorbidity Survey), 12.1% (*DSM-IV* criteria, National Comorbidity Survey Replication), 5.0% (*DSM-IV* criteria, National Epidemiologic Survey on Alcohol and Related Conditions)

- Lifetime prevalence in various countries, according to various diagnostic criteria: 0.5%–16%

- Best-estimate lifetime prevalence rate across the world: 3.6%

- More women than men have SAD in the community (ratio 1.5:1), but the frequency of women and men with SAD is approximately the same in clinical samples

- Persons with SAD are more likely to be single, unemployed, in the lower socioeconomic group, and with lower levels of education

- Age of onset usually in adolescence (mid-teens to the early twenties); mean age of onset: 15–16 years

- Characteristic help-seeking patterns: most persons with SAD do not seek help at all; usual period between onset and time of seeking help is more than 10 years, with help often being sought for complications of SAD (e.g., depression, excessive use of alcohol) or in the context of some important life change; help is initially sought from psychotherapists, psychologists, and school counselors rather than from primary care physicians

Comorbidity Survey Replication, based on the *DSM-IV* diagnostic criteria, reported a lifetime prevalence rate of SAD of 12.1% (Kessler et al., 2005; Ruscio et al., 2008). In the National Comorbidity Survey, one third of individuals with SAD in the community had a phobia of public speaking, another third had a fear of at least one other social situation, and the remaining third had fears of multiple social situations (Magee et al., 1996). According to both the National Comorbidity Survey and National Comorbidity Survey Replication, SAD is one of the most common psychiatric disorders, after major depressive disorder, alcohol abuse, and specific phobia. This underscores the public health importance of SAD.

The striking difference in prevalence rates in the United States between the Epidemiologic Catchment Area Study and the two epidemiological studies conducted later reflects different diagnostic criteria, different instruments used to diagnose SAD, and different research methodology. Also, there is an issue of the threshold at which the diagnosis of SAD is made. One study addressed this problem by counting as "positive" only those cases of psychiatric disorders that were deemed clinically significant (Narrow et al., 2002). With this approach, a 1-year prevalence rate for SAD was estimated to be 3.2%, down from the 7.4% rate that was reported in the National Comorbidity Survey (corrected lifetime prevalence rates were not reported). Another study conducted in the United States, National Epidemiologic Survey on Alcohol and Related Conditions, which used the *DSM-IV* criteria, estimated that the lifetime prevalence rate of SAD was 5.0% (Grant et al., 2005b). Thus, the "true" frequency with which SAD is encountered in the community remains to be established, but regardless of the figures, there is a broad agreement that SAD is a common condition.

The variability of prevalence rates of SAD is even larger when results of epidemiological studies conducted in different countries are compared. The lifetime prevalence rates range from 0.5% in Korea (Lee et al., 1990) to 16% in Switzerland (Wacker et al., 1992). The best-estimate lifetime prevalence rate for SAD across epidemiological studies published between 1980 and 2004 and conducted in various countries was 3.6% (Somers et al., 2006). The striking differences in prevalence rates can be accounted for by the different diagnostic criteria, different diagnostic instruments used in different studies, and cultural differences in the presentation of SAD. Not only are there important differences between Western and Eastern cultures in the concept of SAD (see Cultural Variants of Social Anxiety Disorder, above), but there may also be differences between ethnic groups and various countries within Western cultures.

There are more women than men (the approximate ratio of 1.5:1) with SAD in the community (Bourdon et al., 1988; Schneier et al., 1992; Somers et al., 2006). In samples of patients with SAD, however, the number of women and men tends to be the same, and sometimes there are even more men than women in clinical settings (e.g., Boyd et al.,

1990; Degonda and Angst, 1993). This difference may result from several factors. First, women may endure SAD without seeking help or may adapt to it more easily, because features of SAD are not as incompatible with traditional social roles and expectations for women as they are with the corresponding roles and expectations for men (e.g., a requirement to be assertive). In other words, a failure to fulfill traditional social roles and meet traditional social expectations may be a strong motivating factor for men with SAD to seek professional help. Second, the prevalence of SAD among men in the community may be underestimated because SAD is often hidden behind its complications, especially alcohol abuse. Finally, men may have a greater tendency to have a more severe form of SAD, prompting them to seek help more readily than women.

People with SAD tend to be single, marry less often, and have fewer social contacts and fewer friends than comparable groups without SAD (Schneier et al., 1992; Wittchen et al., 1999). They are also more likely to remain living with their parents well into their adulthood. As a result of the handicapping effects of SAD on their ability to attend school, look for jobs, maintain employment, and advance in their careers, people with SAD are more likely to have lower education, feel frustrated about their professional achievements, be unemployed and financially dependent, rely on social support and welfare agencies, and be in the lower socioeconomic group (Schneier et al., 1992; Wittchen et al., 1999). Their work productivity is often decreased and work performance impaired (Wittchen et al., 2000b).

It may be difficult to precisely determine the onset of SAD, especially in the generalized type. As already noted in Clinical Features (above), nongeneralized and generalized forms of SAD may differ in terms of the age and mode of onset. A sudden onset of SAD may be a consequence of a panic attack in a social situation ("post-panic SAD"), and SAD that starts suddenly also occurs later than SAD that starts more gradually (Kristensen et al., 2008). The typical onset of SAD is in adolescence, with the mean age of onset being between 15 and 16 years (Schneier et al., 1992; Grant et al., 2005b). It is unusual for SAD to first manifest itself after the age of 25 (Schneier et al., 1992; Magee et al., 1996). Because SAD starts so early in life, it affects adversely the development of children and adolescents. Their academic performance may be well below their intellectual level, they do not develop adequate interpersonal and social skills, their interactions with peers are quite limited, and they often have problems in intimate relationships.

Most people with SAD (72%–87%) do not seek professional help and receive no treatment (Magee et al., 1996; Grant et al., 2005b). When they do seek help, the time lag between onset of the disorder and onset of treatment is often longer than 10 years, so that the treatment usually commences when patients are in their late twenties or thirties. It has been estimated that the mean age at first treatment for SAD is 27.2 years (Grant et al., 2005b). There are many reasons for this delay: people with SAD often feel embarrassed about their fears and are reluctant to disclose them. They may also "adapt" themselves to their fears and accept to a certain extent limitations imposed by SAD. Some believe that SAD is a part of their personality and that nothing can be done about it.

When SAD sufferers seek professional help, more often than not they do this because of complications of SAD (e.g., depression, excessive use of alcohol) or in the context of some important life change. For example, a new job that demands assertiveness and effective interpersonal communication makes it very difficult for the person with a hidden SAD to continue avoiding certain social activities. Unlike patients with panic disorder and generalized anxiety disorder, those with SAD are more likely to initially seek help from psychotherapists, psychologists, and school counselors than from primary care physicians (Wittchen et al., 1999).

COURSE AND PROGNOSIS

Most patients with generalized SAD have a chronic course, with few, if any, fluctuations in its intensity, creating an impression that it is a lifelong condition. The course of nongeneralized SAD may show some variations, related to the frequency with which patients have to be in social situations and their ability to avoid such situations.

Data on the duration of SAD confirm the chronicity of this condition. In two studies, 9%–15% of patients had the illness for most of their lives; almost one third of patients suffered from SAD for at least 15 years, and the remainder had SAD for at least 6 years (Heimberg et al., 1990a; Schneier et al., 1992). A median duration of SAD was estimated to be 25 years in one study (DeWit et al., 1999), whereas another study reported the mean duration of 16.3 years (Grant et al., 2005b).

As already noted, the prognosis of generalized SAD is worse than that of nongeneralized SAD. This is largely a consequence of the difference in severity between these subtypes. Factors suggesting a poor prognosis of SAD (Table 4–8) include an onset in childhood and longer duration of SAD,

Table 4–8. Factors Suggesting a Poor Prognosis of Social Anxiety Disorder

Onset in childhood (before age 7–11 years)

Longer duration

Greater initial severity, greater number of symptoms

Co-occurring psychiatric disorders

Presence of depression

Presence of health problems

Lower education level

greater initial severity with greater number of symptoms, presence of other psychiatric disorders, especially depression, various health problems, and lower education (Davidson et al., 1993a; DeWit et al., 1999).

Independent functioning may be very difficult for patients with severe SAD, as they perceive every novel social situation as highly distressing. The impairment and disability associated with SAD can be quite severe (e.g., Stein MB and Kean, 2000), as noted in Epidemiology (above). It has been reported that SAD patients may be as impaired as those with debilitating medical conditions, such as multiple sclerosis and chronic renal failure (Antony et al., 1998).

Do patients with SAD ever recover? It appears that some do, but they are a minority (e.g., Reich et al., 1994; Chartier et al., 1998). Still, recovery may occur after many years of the continuing presence of illness; one study has reported that about one half of patients recovered after 25 years of SAD (DeWit et al., 1999).

ETIOLOGY AND PATHOGENESIS

Many etiological factors contribute to the development of SAD. No etiological model can explain by itself all the cases and all the manifestations of this condition. It appears that there are several biological and psychological pathways that lead to SAD. The models reviewed below shed some light on these pathways.

BIOLOGICAL MODELS

Genetic Factors

Social anxiety disorder may run in some families. It has been found more often among first-degree relatives of patients with SAD than among first-degree relatives of patients with panic disorder and control subjects without mental disorder (Reich and Yates, 1988; Fyer et al., 1993, 1995; Mannuzza et al., 1995; Stein MB et al., 1998a). The genetic component seems to be stronger in the generalized type of SAD (see Clinical Features, above).

Results of twin studies of shyness and social anxiety have been conflicting (Torgersen, 1983; Kendler et al., 1992c; Skre et al., 1993). One twin study estimated the contribution of genetic factors to the development of SAD at 40%–60% (Kendler et al., 1999), while another twin study among female adolescents estimated the heritability of SAD at 28% (Nelson et al., 2000).

Although family and twin studies suggest that there is a heritable component in SAD, nongenetic patterns of transmission of social fears within certain families (e.g., through modeling) can play an important role. A large part of what is inherited in SAD may be a nonspecific, general vulnerability to anxiety disorders (Andrews et al., 1990) or depression (Nelson et al., 2000).

Neuroanatomy and Pathophysiological Mechanisms

Little is known about brain structures and pathophysiological mechanisms involved *specifically* in the pathogenesis of SAD. Research has yet to determine whether there are any neurobiological differences between the generalized and nongeneralized forms of SAD and which pathophysiological mechanisms play a role in the pathogenesis of SAD, as opposed to being just the correlates of SAD.

Neuroimaging Studies

Functional magnetic resonance imaging studies have examined responses to human facial expressions (either photographic or schematic) and to other people's comments in patients with SAD. Several brain regions, especially the amygdala, medial prefrontal cortex, and anterior cingulate, seem to be involved in these responses (e.g., Birbaumer et al., 1998; Stein MB et al., 2002a; Amir et al., 2005; Straube et al., 2005; Phan et al., 2006; Blair et al., 2008a; Evans et al., 2008). The types of stimuli that elicited increased activity (especially in the amygdala) varied from one study to another: although most human facial expressions were negative (e.g., angry, contemptuous, fearful, or disgusting), some were neutral or positive (e.g., happy), suggesting that the processing of facial expression in SAD may not be altered only for negative, social anxiety-inducing facial expressions. In contrast, only negative comments referring to patients with SAD produced increased responses in one functional magnetic resonance imaging study (Blair et al., 2008b).

Neurotransmitter Systems

The serotonin, noradrenaline, gamma-aminobutyric acid (GABA), and dopamine neurotransmitter systems have been implicated in the pathogenesis of SAD. However, data pointing to abnormalities in these systems have been inconsistent. Hypotheses about the involvement of dopamine and serotonin systems have been partly derived from findings of the efficacy in SAD of classical, irreversible monoamine oxidase inhibitors and selective serotonin reuptake inhibitors, respectively.

Patients with prominent performance-type social anxiety may have an underlying noradrenaline dysfunction so that they are either hypersensitive to normal noradrenergic stimulation or they exhibit central and peripheral noradrenergic hyperactivity. This hypothesis is supported by the symptoms (palpitations, tremor, sweating, blushing) that typically occur in performance situations and by the efficacy of β-adrenergic blockers in the treatment of the performance/nongeneralized type of SAD.

The central dopamine deficiency hypothesis in generalized SAD (Liebowitz et al., 1987) is of some interest, as the classical, irreversible monoamine oxidase inhibitors are presumed to prevent degradation of dopamine. The convincing efficacy of these medications in generalized

SAD is rather unique among the anxiety disorders. Furthermore, a substantial number of patients with Parkinson's disease, which is characterized by dopamine deficiency, do have SAD prior to the onset of Parkinson's disease (Stein MB et al., 1990a). Patients with Tourette's disorder, by contrast, were observed to develop SAD following treatment with haloperidol, a dopamine antagonist (Mikkelson et al., 1981). The dopamine deficiency hypothesis has also received further support (e.g., Schneier et al., 2000).

Biological "Preparedness" for Social Anxiety (Preparedness Conditioning Theories)

Humans may be biologically "prepared" to fear certain stimuli in the environment, with this "preparedness" having a survival value and contributing to the preservation of the species (Seligman, 1971; McNally, 1987). Studies have shown that people are very sensitive to facial expressions of others and are afraid of angry and threatening faces, but only if these facial expressions are directed at them (Öhman, 1986). People respond to such facial expressions in a way that helps them adjust to various interpersonal situations and decrease danger implied by these expressions. If the person is too sensitive to these facial and other interpersonal and social stimuli so that the fear response appears automatically even when there is no real threat, or if the fear response is excessive, the person may develop SAD. This perspective on SAD is interesting in view of the poor eye contact exhibited by many patients with SAD and their strong fear of being observed.

PSYCHOBIOLOGICAL MODEL—BEHAVIORAL INHIBITION

The behavioral inhibition to the unfamiliar (Kagan et al., 1984, 1987, 1988) was conceptualized as a temporally stable component of inborn temperament that represents a biological basis for shyness. As such, behavioral inhibition has been conceived of as one of the major factors in the pathogenesis of anxiety disorders in general and SAD in particular.

Manifestations of behavioral inhibition to the unfamiliar are observable during the first year of life: children of that age have difficulty sleeping in unfamiliar surroundings and often exhibit irritability in novel situations. By 2 years of age, such children tend to avoid contacts with unfamiliar people, places, and objects, and prefer to cling to their mothers (or other main caregivers). They respond to novel situations with fear, cessation of exploratory and playful activity, and somatic symptoms that are similar to those seen in anxious adults upon exposure to the feared stimuli. This behavioral and physiological pattern at age 2 is predictive of behavioral inhibition at age 7.

In the course of further development, these children often exhibit extreme caution in a range of situations, appear introverted and shy, find themselves at the periphery of social activities, and are likely to become even more isolated. They seem physiologically "overprepared" for danger, as their heart rate is elevated at rest, with further disproportionate increase in heart rate upon exposure to even mild stressors. These children also tend to have elevated blood levels of cortisol and catecholamines.

Behavioral inhibition does not have a unique relationship with SAD, but it is most consistently linked with SAD (e.g., Mick and Telch, 1998; Cooper and Eke, 1999) and, to a somewhat lesser degree, with panic disorder and agoraphobia (e.g., Rosenbaum et al., 1988). In comparison with uninhibited children, those with behavioral inhibition seem to have a higher risk of developing phobic disorders, including SAD (Kagan et al., 1988). When parents of children with and without behavioral inhibition were compared, the former were more likely to have SAD or other anxiety disorders, and more often reported anxiety-related problems and anxiety disorders in their own childhood (Rosenbaum et al., 1991). In comparison with children of normal or depressed parents, many more children of parents with panic disorder were behaviorally inhibited (Rosenbaum et al., 1988).

PSYCHOLOGICAL MODELS

Behavioral and Cognitive Approaches

Aversive Conditioning Model

Traumatic conditioning may play some role in the development of SAD, especially the nongeneralized subtype (Stemberger et al., 1995). For example, a sudden blushing or loss of voice during a performance may lead to the perception of a particular social situation as being embarrassing, humiliating, and therefore dangerous. According to one estimate, more than one half of patients may be able to identify an unpleasant incident that preceded the onset of SAD (e.g., Öst and Hugdahl, 1981). It appears that such a traumatic incident precipitates SAD in the context of a specific predisposition, for example, if the person is excessively shy or carries relevant genetic vulnerability. Without a specific predisposition, aversive (traumatic) experiences are rarely sufficient for the development of SAD, especially its generalized subtype. According to this model, SAD is primarily maintained by the avoidance of relevant social situations, in a fashion similar to the maintenance of other phobias through avoidance.

Cognitive Models

According to cognitive models, patients with SAD generally underestimate their social performance, overestimate the probability of poor performance or other adverse social outcome, and overestimate dire consequences of such an outcome (Beck et al., 1985; Lucock and Salkovskis, 1988; Rapee and Lim, 1992). Also, patients overestimate the likelihood of the occurrence of

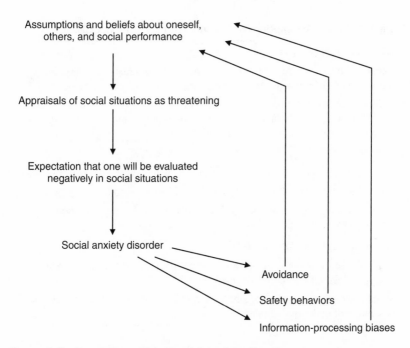

Figure 4–5. Cognitive model of social anxiety disorder.

anxiety symptoms, their visibility, and attention paid to them by others, which leads them to believe that they come across "negatively" to others.

Two similar cognitive models of SAD have been formulated (Clark and Wells, 1995; Rapee and Heimberg, 1997) (Figure 4–5). They are based on the idea that the fundamental issue in SAD is the fear of negative evaluation by others and that SAD results from the expectation that one will be evaluated negatively in social situations. This expectation is regarded as a consequence of certain assumptions and beliefs that SAD patients have about themselves, others, and social situations (Table 4–9), which then lead to appraisals of social situations as threatening. Such assumptions, beliefs, and appraisals are maintained through avoidance of social situations, use of various safety behaviors, and biases in information processing.

Several biases in information processing may be somewhat specific for SAD (Table 4–10). A particularly salient aspect of information processing in SAD appears to be a combination of decreased attention to external social and interpersonal information with increased focusing on oneself. Largely as a result of the latter, patients with SAD become preoccupied with their physical symptoms and believe that these symptoms are "responsible" for how they appear to other people. In other words, because they blush or tremble, patients assume that others see them as a failure. This assumption is then difficult to disconfirm because patients generally pay much less

Table 4–9. Typical Assumptions of Patients With Social Anxiety Disorder

Assumptions About Oneself

- Negative, social situation-specific beliefs about oneself (e.g., "I am stupid," "I am weak," "I am worthless," "I am boring")
- Beliefs about oneself in social interactions and as an object of social evaluation (e.g., "If I have to give a talk and appear anxious, I will humiliate myself," "If I don't do it right, they will laugh at me")

Assumptions About Others

- Others pay close attention to one's appearance, behavior, and/or performance
- Others have knowledge of one's thoughts and/or feelings
- Others are likely to be harsh and judgmental and quick to reject anyone who makes mistakes or appears inept

Assumptions About Social Performance

- Standards of social performance must be strictly adhered to in order to avoid disappointment, humiliation, or rejection
- Social performance must be of a high, perfectionist standard to minimize the possibility of making a mistake

attention to external social information, and they particularly tend to disregard any positive feedback about themselves. The disconfirmation is also made difficult by the inherent ambiguity of social interactions so that patients can never be *completely* sure how they are perceived by others. Another potential consequence of preoccupation with oneself is neglect and undermining of the actual social performance (e.g., Woody, 1996). In this case, one's fears about poor performance may to some extent be validated.

Another cognitive mechanism in SAD involves expectations of anxiety, discomfort, and physical symptoms in social situations. These expectations make it more likely for anxiety, discomfort, and physical symptoms to indeed occur in such situations, thereby strengthening the fear and driving patients to continue avoiding social situations.

Social Skills Deficits Model

A lack of social skills may be observed in SAD patients who report a long-standing lack of understanding of some very basic and simple rules of social communication and interaction (e.g., not knowing what the sequence of steps is when purchasing or ordering something). These patients usually did not have adequate opportunities to learn social skills or have felt extremely inhibited in their exploratory behavior since early childhood.

Table 4–10. Information Processing Bias in Social Anxiety Disorder

Attention bias	Increased self-focused attention, heightened "public self-consciousness" (Fenigstein et al., 1975; Hope and Heimberg, 1988; Mellings and Alden, 2000)
	Decreased attention to external social situation or information (Chen et al., 2002)
Interpretation bias	Interpretation of physical symptoms as an indication that one appears negatively to others, e.g., as anxious, insecure, or weak (McEwan and Devins, 1983; Amir et al., 1998; Mansell and Clark, 1999; Mulkens et al., 1999; Mellings and Alden, 2000; Roth et al., 2001; Wells and Papageorgiou, 2001)
	Tendency to be more rigid when interpreting one's own anxiety symptoms than when interpreting the same symptoms in others (Amir et al., 1998; Roth et al., 2001)
	Interpretation of ambiguous, self-relevant social situations and events as negative (Amir et al., 1998; Stopa and Clark, 2000)
	Catastrophic interpretation of mildly negative, but quite innocuous, self-relevant social situations and events (Stopa and Clark, 2000)
Biased self-imagery	Tendency to perceive oneself negatively from an "observer's perspective" rather than watching oneself "with one's own eyes" (Clark and Wells, 1995; Hackmann et al., 1998; Wells and Papageorgiou, 1999)
Memory bias	Defective memory for certain aspects of social situations, interpersonal information, or interactions (Kimble and Zehr, 1982; Hope et al., 1990; Mellings and Alden, 2000)
	Memory bias for socially threatening information (Amir et al., 2000)
Biased appraisal	Negative expectations from accomplishment and future success (e.g., social success will lead to more social demand and pressure; Wallace and Alden, 1997)

Many patients with SAD do not have a genuine social skills deficit, and their anxiety may only interfere with the use of their social skills. The social awkwardness and ineptness of some SAD patients may be more a result of their need to make a certain impression on others, coupled with their insecurity and doubt about being able to do so. This proposition is at the core of the self-presentation theory of social anxiety (Schlenker and Leary, 1982).

Psychodynamic Approaches

A comprehensive psychoanalytic/psychodynamic account of SAD is lacking, mainly because SAD tends to be regarded by psychoanalysts as part of a character organization and not a psychopathological entity per se. Certain psychoanalytic views, however, may be relevant for clinical practice.

Some psychoanalysts relate SAD to the feeling of shame and fear of superego. The feeling of shame and anticipation of humiliation may be a consequence of the projection of harsh, critical, or punitive parental intro-jects onto others, with the consequent expectation that others treat patients harshly (Gabbard, 1992). The presumed underlying conflict is between a need to compete, achieve, and succeed on one hand, and the fear of success on the other. The success is feared because it is unconsciously equated with "Oedipal victory" and the consequent punishment. In other words, the person is not "allowed" to compete and succeed. Unable to resolve this conflict and striving to avoid the feeling of shame, the person withdraws from social interactions, thereby developing SAD.

Another psychodynamic perspective on SAD invokes problems in the process of separation-individuation, usually as a result of serious distur-bances in attachment and early object relations (Gabbard, 1992; Cloitre and Shear, 1995). In this case, the presumed conflict is between striving toward independence and self-affirmation on one hand, and fears of the loss of love, rejection, and abandonment by primary objects (parents), on the other, as a punishment for such independence. Persons who develop SAD give up their pursuit of independence and withdraw from social interactions to appease the primary objects.

In the psychoanalytic literature, SAD has also been related to exhibitio-nistic urges or narcissistic need to make a "perfect" impression of oneself. A fear of being unable to make such an impression leads the person to anticipate narcissistic injury; to avoid this injury, the person withdraws from social interactions. This account can help explain narcissistic traits in some SAD patients.

Role of Developmental and Childhood Factors

Patients with SAD have an increased tendency to perceive their par-ents as overprotective and rejecting (e.g., Lieb et al., 2000). If parents are indeed overprotective, critical, harsh, and/or rejecting, that may contribute to the patients' sense of insecurity and inability to rely on themselves in social interactions. Although such a perception of par-ents is not specific for SAD, it may help account for the development of SAD in children who are predisposed to it genetically or through behavioral inhibition.

TREATMENT

Despite greater attention paid to SAD over the past several decades, there is evidence that it continues to be undertreated or treated inadequately

(Wittchen et al., 1999; Lecrubier et al., 2000), and that paradoxically, individuals with the most fears of social situations are least likely to receive treatment for SAD (Ruscio et al., 2008).

The treatment of some forms of nongeneralized, performance-type SAD may be relatively simple and result in quick improvement, even if only temporarily. Treatment of the generalized subtype of SAD, by contrast, tends to be challenging. It is in many ways akin to the treatment of personality disturbance because of the negative effects that SAD has on virtually all aspects of personality development. The analogy with treatment of personality disorders also means that more often than not, the treatment lasts longer, with its outcome in many cases being precarious.

Several effective treatment modalities are available for both nongeneralized and generalized SAD. They include pharmacotherapy and various forms of cognitive-behavioral therapy (CBT). Supportive and psychodynamic psychotherapy can also be helpful to patients with generalized SAD. A combination of pharmacological and psychological treatment may be used as well.

Comparisons of efficacy between medications and CBT for generalized SAD have found different patterns of treatment response, depending on the duration of treatment. In the short term-treatment, pharmacotherapy and CBT have been either equally efficacious (Otto et al., 2000; Furmark et al., 2002; Davidson et al., 2004b), or medications have been somewhat superior to CBT (Heimberg et al., 1998) and worked faster. In long-term treatment, however, relapses may be more frequent with pharmacotherapy and treatment gains are maintained longer with CBT (Liebowitz et al., 1999).

PHARMACOLOGICAL TREATMENT

There are several specific aspects of the pharmacological treatment of SAD (Table 4–11). First, pharmacological interventions for generalized SAD are quite different from those for the nongeneralized subtype. In the latter, pharmacotherapy is distinctly used for fear of performance-type situations, particularly when the feared situations are occasional and for the most part predictable. Second, generalized SAD is unique among the anxiety disorders in terms of the classical irreversible monoamine oxidase inhibitors being consistently effective in its treatment and tricyclic antidepressants showing no efficacy. Finally, benzodiazepines are not well suited for long-term treatment of SAD because there is a higher risk of alcohol and other substance abuse (including benzodiazepines) in patients with SAD than in patients with other anxiety disorders. Therefore, great caution should be exercised when benzodiazepines are administered for prolonged periods of time to these patients.

Table 4–11. Aspects of Pharmacological Treatment Specific for Social Anxiety Disorder

- The pharmacological approach depends on whether the patient has a nongeneralized or generalized type of SAD

- In relation to other anxiety disorders, classical irreversible monoamine oxidase inhibitors have a unique, convincingly demonstrated efficacy in treating generalized SAD

- Unlike in panic disorder, generalized anxiety disorder, obsessive-compulsive disorder, and posttraumatic stress disorder, no tricyclic antidepressant showed efficacy in the treatment of generalized SAD

- Great caution should be exercised if benzodiazepines are administered on a long-term basis to patients with SAD, as there is a higher risk for alcohol and other substance abuse (including benzodiazepines) in these patients than in patients with other anxiety disorders

Pharmacotherapy of Nongeneralized Social Anxiety Disorder (Performance Anxiety)

The goal of pharmacological treatment of nongeneralized SAD is a substantial decrease in or disappearance of specific physical symptoms that patients find unpleasant or distressing during a particular task or performance. Most commonly, such symptoms are a manifestation of hyperactivity of the sympathetic nervous system: tremor, palpitations, tachycardia, and sweating. Hence, the use of β-adrenergic blockers has been popular for this purpose, and there is some empirical support for it (e.g., Brantigan et al., 1982; Neftel et al., 1982; Hartley et al., 1983). In one survey of musicians, 27% admitted to occasionally using β-blockers before giving a performance, and 96% believed that these medications were helpful (Fishbein et al., 1988). The use of β-adrenergic blockers for fear of performance-type situations is largely based on the assumption that anxiety occurs as a consequence of experiencing certain physical symptoms. Propranolol (10–40 mg) can be taken 30–60 minutes prior to a performance situation (e.g., giving a lecture or playing at a concert). Some patients take atenolol (50–100 mg), a more selective β-blocker. Issues surrounding the use of β-blockers (e.g., precautions and contraindications) are discussed in Chapter 3.

The alternative pharmacological treatment of nongeneralized SAD, especially if β-adrenergic blockers are contraindicated, is an as-needed (prn) use of benzodiazepines prior to a performance situation. Usually, a short-acting benzodiazepine (e.g., alprazolam, lorazepam) is taken for that purpose. When benzodiazepines are administered in this context, there are two important issues. First, benzodiazepines may be sedating, may impair movement coordination, and may interfere with the process of remembering material learned after the medication has been taken, which in turn could adversely affect performance. Second, benzodiazepines may have a disinhibiting effect on some individuals, which could also interfere with their performance.

Pharmacotherapy of Generalized Social Anxiety Disorder

Because of the chronic nature of the disorder, relentless anxiety, frequent presence of issues rooted in personality, frequent co-occurrence with other psychiatric disorders, and substantial disability, pharmacological treatment of generalized SAD is much more complex than that of nongeneralized SAD. Psychological intervention is often needed in addition to pharmacotherapy. The goal of pharmacological treatment of generalized SAD is to substantially decrease symptoms and behaviors associated with this disorder. In practical terms, the goals of treatment are to help patients feel less distressed in a range of socially difficult situations, decrease or eliminate symptoms of autonomic hyperarousal upon exposure to these situations, and minimize or eliminate socially driven avoidance. All of these changes lead to an improvement in overall functioning.

On the whole, pharmacological treatment has been moderately successful in achieving these goals; usually a long-term administration of medications is required. Although pharmacological treatment does not address the underlying pervasive, negative self-perception and fear of negative evaluation by others, it may help patients perceive themselves more favorably by improving their performance, strengthening a sense of security in social situations, and boosting their self-confidence. Pharmacotherapy may also be useful in terms of helping patients react with certain indifference to their otherwise distressing thoughts about how they appear to others.

Pharmacotherapy is usually indicated for the more severe and disabling forms of generalized SAD. It may also be useful for patients with co-occurring depression or other psychiatric conditions and for those who have a preponderance of distressing somatic symptoms of anxiety in various social situations.

The following medications have shown efficacy in the treatment of generalized SAD: selective serotonin reuptake inhibitors (SSRIs), venlafaxine (in its extended-release [XR] formulation), classical irreversible monoamine oxidase inhibitors (MAOIs), and benzodiazepines. There are some differences in efficacy between these agents, but the choice of medication is usually made on the basis of tolerability and other pharmacological properties. Because of their more favorable side effect profile, no need for a tyramine-free diet, and fewer interactions with other medications, SSRIs and venlafaxine XR are preferred over classical MAOIs (Table 4–12).

Table 4–12. Choice of Medication in Treatment of Generalized Social Anxiety Disorder

Rank	Medication
First-line	a. SSRIs (especially paroxetine, sertraline, escitalopram, and fluvoxamine)
	b. SSRI + BDZ (short term)
Second-line	a. Venlafaxine XR
	b. Venlafaxine XR + BDZ (short term)
Third-line	Classical, irreversible MAOIs
Fourth-line	BDZs (clonazepam), with caution

SSRI, selective serotonin reuptake inhibitor; BDZ, benzodiazepine; Venlafaxine XR, venlafaxine extended-release; MAOIs, monoamine oxidase inhibitors.

Antidepressants in Treatment of Generalized Social Anxiety Disorder

Selective Serotonin Reuptake Inhibitors

Of the SSRIs, evidence of efficacy in generalized SAD exists for paroxetine (Stein MB et al., 1998b; Allgulander, 1999, 2004b; Baldwin et al., 1999; Liebowitz et al., 2002, 2005a; Lepola et al., 2004), sertraline (Katzelnick et al., 1995; Blomhoff et al., 2001; Van Ameringen et al., 2001; Liebowitz et al., 2003), escitalopram (Lader et al., 2004; Kasper et al., 2005), fluvoxamine (van Vliet et al., 1994; Stein MB et al., 1999b; Davidson et al., 2004c; Westenberg et al., 2004; Asakura et al., 2007), and citalopram (Furmark et al., 2005). The results for fluoxetine were mixed: while it was more efficacious than placebo in one study (Davidson et al., 2004b), in two other controlled studies it did not show efficacy (Kobak et al., 2002; Clark et al., 2003). Response rates to SSRIs in these trials ranged from 40% to 72%. When escitalopram (20 mg/day) and paroxetine (20 mg/day) were compared in a controlled study, escitalopram showed some advantage, but this could be due to a relatively lower dose of paroxetine (Lader et al., 2004). In similar comparison studies, paroxetine and venlafaxine XR were equally efficacious (Allgulander et al., 2004b; Liebowitz et al., 2005a). In two small, controlled studies, paroxetine had beneficial effects on both SAD and co-occurring alcohol use problems (Randall et al., 2001; Book et al., 2008).

As in the treatment of panic disorder and generalized anxiety disorder, benzodiazepines are often used initially and on a short-term basis in conjunction with SSRIs or venlafaxine XR to treat generalized SAD. The goals of this combination are to achieve a faster response and better tolerability of SSRIs and venlafaxine XR. Although it is apparently popular, such practice has been underinvestigated. When paroxetine in combination with clona-zepam was compared with paroxetine plus placebo in patients with gen-eralized SAD, this combination did not show a faster response but was associated with better outcome (Seedat and Stein, 2004).

The initial dosage of an SSRI is the same as in the treatment of depres-sion, unless there is a co-occurring panic disorder or presence of severe physical symptoms of anxiety. Some patients with generalized SAD need higher doses of SSRIs (Table 4–13). More than 25% of patients who did not respond after 8 weeks of treatment with paroxetine, responded after 12 weeks (Stein DJ et al., 2002b). This suggests that the longer treatment with an SSRI might bring about a response (with the optimal duration of a trial with an SSRI perhaps being around 12 weeks). Issues related to the use of SSRIs in general, and in the anxiety disorders in particular, are discussed in more detail in Chapter 2.

Venlafaxine Extended Release

Several controlled studies (Allgulander et al., 2004b; Rickels et al., 2004; Liebowitz et al., 2005a, 2005b) have demonstrated efficacy of venlafaxine XR, a serotonin and noradrenaline reuptake inhibitor, for generalized SAD. Response rates ranged from 44% to 69%. Venlafaxine XR also proved to be superior to placebo during a long-term (6-month) study (Stein MB et al., 2005), with improvement unlikely to occur in patients who have not responded by the first 12 weeks of treatment. When compared with parox-etine (20–50 mg/day), venlafaxine XR (75–225 mg/day) was equally

Table 4–13. Medication Dosages Efficacious for Treatment of Generalized Social Anxiety Disorder

Medication	Dose Range
Selective Serotonin Reuptake Inhibitors	
Paroxetine	20–50 mg/day
Sertraline	50–200 mg/day
Escitalopram	10–20 mg/day
Fluvoxamine	100–300 mg/day
Citalopram	20–40 mg/day
Venlafaxine Extended-Release	75–225 mg/day
Classical, Irreversible Monoamine Oxidase Inhibitors	
Phenelzine	45–90 mg/day
Benzodiazepines	
Clonazepam	1.5–8 mg/day

efficacious for generalized SAD and showed a somewhat faster onset of therapeutic effect (Allgulander et al., 2004b; Liebowitz et al., 2005a). The more frequent side effects and higher dropout rates in the first week of treatment prompted a suggestion to initially use low doses, e.g., 37.5 mg/ day (Stein MB et al., 2005). The noradrenaline reuptake blockade of venlafaxine XR may not be essential for efficacy in the treatment of generalized SAD, because its lower and higher doses were equally efficacious (Stein MB et al., 2005). Side effects of venlafaxine XR and issues surrounding its use are discussed in more detail in Chapter 2.

Classical Irreversible Monoamine Oxidase Inhibitors

The efficacy of phenelzine, a classical, irreversible and nonselective MAOI, in the treatment of SAD has been established by several studies (Gelernter et al., 1991; Liebowitz et al., 1992; Versiani et al., 1992; Heimberg et al., 1998). Phenelzine is regarded by many as the most powerful pharmacological agent for SAD; it was more efficacious than benzodiazepines (Gelernter et al., 1991) and a β-blocker (Liebowitz et al., 1992), and in some aspects even superior to CBT (Gelernter et al., 1991; Heimberg et al., 1998). In one study, as many as 91% of SAD patients were classified as responders to phenelzine (Versiani et al., 1992). A substantial number of patients improve significantly after 8–12 weeks of treatment, and efficacy is maintained over prolonged periods of time. Tranylcypromine, another classical MAOI, may also be effective in treating patients with generalized SAD (Versiani et al., 1988), but controlled studies are lacking.

The use of classical MAOIs is limited by their unfavorable side-effect profile (hypotension, insomnia, agitation, weight gain, sexual dysfunction), significant interactions with numerous medications (various sympathomimetic amines and dextromethorphan that are contained in many cold and cough over-the-counter medicines, adrenaline, psychostimulants, opioid analgesics, anesthetics, isoproterenol), and need to avoid all food that contains tyramine (e.g., many types of cheese) to prevent an abrupt and large increase in blood pressure. When switching a patient's treatment from an SSRI to a classical MAOI or vice versa, a washout period must be strictly observed (at least 2 weeks for all SSRIs except for fluoxetine, in which case the washout should last at least 5 weeks). Under no circumstances should an SSRI be combined with a classical MAOI because of the risk of serotonin syndrome.

Considering that phenelzine is efficacious in both generalized SAD and atypical depression (see Relationship Between Social Anxiety Disorder and Other Disorders, above), it might be a pharmacological treatment of choice when atypical depression co-occurs with generalized SAD.

Benzodiazepines   As already noted, benzodiazepines can be used very cautiously as the pharmacological monotherapy for long-term treatment of generalized SAD. These medications may be administered in the absence of a co-occurring depression and history of alcohol or other substance abuse, but even then, their use requires careful and ongoing monitoring. Clonazepam is the only benzodiazepine for which efficacy in SAD has been demonstrated (Davidson et al., 1993b). The doses of clonazepam efficacious in the treatment of generalized SAD may be somewhat higher than those used in the treatment of panic disorder (Table 4–13). Issues related to long-term use of benzodiazepines are discussed in more detail in Chapter 2.

Long-Term Pharmacological Treatment

Generalized SAD is a chronic condition that requires long-term treatment. Although the optimal duration of pharmacotherapy has not been established, it should probably last for at least 1–2 years following remission, with the goal of maintaining treatment gains and decreasing the likelihood of relapse. Placebo-controlled, relapse-prevention studies have demonstrated efficacy over 24-week treatment following a response to acute treatment with paroxetine (Stein DJ et al., 2002c), sertraline (Walker et al., 2000), escitalopram (Montgomery et al., 2005), and venlafaxine XR (Stein MB et al., 2005). In other trials, long-term efficacy in generalized SAD has been found for sertraline (Blomhoff et al., 2001), escitalopram (Lader et al., 2004), and phenelzine (Versiani et al., 1992). Long-term treatment of generalized SAD with benzodiazepines is not optimal, but in some, carefully selected cases, it may be beneficial. Other issues in long-term pharmacotherapy are similar to those in long-term pharmacotherapy of panic disorder and are discussed in Chapter 2.

As with other anxiety disorders, discontinuation of medication for generalized SAD is associated with an increased risk of relapse; addition of a psychological treatment, especially CBT, might decrease this risk. A medication should be discontinued gradually and carefully.

Pharmacotherapy of Treatment-Resistant Generalized Social Anxiety Disorder

Opinions differ in terms of what constitutes an adequate pharmacological trial in generalized SAD. In light of the available evidence (e.g., Stein DJ et al., 2002b), such a trial would probably comprise about 12 weeks of treatment with a medication administered in its maximum recommended or tolerated dose.

Treatment resistance has not been well defined for generalized SAD. While all patients for whom pharmacotherapy is contemplated should be treated with at least one SSRI and then venlafaxine XR (unless contraindicated), a good proportion may be unwilling to take a classical MAOI. In other patients, long-term treatment with a benzodiazepine is unsuitable. Therefore, the stage of treatment resistance may be reached without exposure to classical MAOIs and benzodiazepines. Cognitive-behavioral

Table 4–14. Pharmacological Options for Treatment-Resistant Generalized Social Anxiety Disorder

Lack of Response to First-, Second-, and Perhaps Third- and Fourth-Line Pharmacotherapy

Monotherapy options
  Moclobemide
  Anticonvulsants

    Gabapentin
    Pregabalin
    Tiagabine
    Topiramate
    Levetiracetam

  Mirtazapine
  Olanzapine

Partial Response to First-, Second-, Third-, or Fourth-Line Pharmacotherapy

Continue treatment for several months
Augmentation strategies
  SSRI + buspirone

SSRI, selective serotonin reuptake inhibitor.

therapy and several medications, administered as monotherapy, can be considered as options for patients with generalized SAD who have had no response at all to the first-, second-, and perhaps third- and fourth-line pharmacotherapy (Table 4–14). These include moclobemide, gabapentin, several other anticonvulsants, mirtazapine, and olanzapine. Because there are no guidelines that would assist in making a choice between various options for treatment-resistant patients, a physician has to rely on clinical judgment and consideration of individual patient circumstances.

Moclobemide, a reversible and selective MAO-A inhibitor, initially showed promise for treatment of generalized SAD (e.g., Versiani et al., 1992). The drug is better tolerated than classical MAOIs and its use is not associated with other problems (e.g., a need to have a tyramine-free diet) that make classical MAOIs troublesome in routine clinical practice. However, results of later efficacy studies were inconsistent. While some studies showed superiority of moclobemide over placebo (IMCTGMSP, 1997; Stein DJ et al., 2002a), others did not confirm efficacy of moclobemide for generalized SAD (Noyes et al., 1997; Schneier et al., 1998). This has diminished the initial expectation that moclobemide might be an adequate substitute for classical MAOIs. If moclobemide is effective in short-term treatment, it might also work over the long term (24–36 weeks), as suggested by the results of two studies (Versiani et al., 1992; Stein DJ et al., 2002a). The dose of moclobemide for SAD is 300–600 mg/day.

The anticonvulsant gabapentin (600–3600 mg/day) offers some promise in the treatment of generalized SAD, as its efficacy has been demonstrated in one controlled study (Pande et al., 1999). Pregabalin was also efficacious in one controlled study (Pande et al., 2004), but it is not clear whether this agent may be as useful for generalized SAD as it appears to be for generalized anxiety disorder (see Chapter 3). The efficacy of several other anticonvulsants—topiramate, levetiracetam, and tiagabine—has been reported in a preliminary way. Mirtazapine, a noradrenergic and specific serotonergic antidepressant, has also demonstrated efficacy in one controlled study (Muehlbacher et al., 2005). The second-generation antipsychotic olanzapine was superior to placebo in a very small, pilot study.

If the patient responds only with some improvement to an adequate trial of one of the standard pharmacological agents for generalized SAD, further improvement may be observed with continued pharmacological treatment or with the addition of CBT. The other strategy (Table 4–14) is to augment a primary agent with another medication, but this has hardly been studied. Good outcome has been reported when buspirone was added to patients partially responsive to an SSRI (Van Ameringen et al., 1996).

PSYCHOLOGICAL TREATMENT

Various techniques of CBT have been successfully used in SAD. Social skills training is a form of psychological therapy related to CBT and used to treat some patients with SAD. Psychodynamic psychotherapies also play a role in the treatment of SAD, but there is little empirical support for their use.

Cognitive-Behavioral Therapy

Cognitive-behavioral therapy for SAD can be delivered in a group or individual format and is available in three main forms: exposure-based therapy, cognitive therapy, and a combination of exposure and cognitive techniques. The recommendations summarized in Table 4–15 are based on research findings and clinical experience. Thus, exposure-based therapy has been most consistently efficacious and should be included in any treatment package for SAD. Cognitive therapy can be added with the goal of directly changing social anxiety-relevant appraisals and beliefs. If the patient has a marked deficit in social skills, it is reasonable to also use social skills training, usually before commencing CBT.

Exposure-Based Therapy

Exposure to feared social situations in the treatment of SAD is based on the same principles as those of exposure-based treatments for other anxiety disorders (see Chapters 2 and 5). Exposure is conducted gradually, in accordance with the hierarchy of phobic situations, so that patients first

Table 4–15. Indications for Use and/or Goals of Treatment for Various Techniques of Cognitive-Behavioral Therapy (CBT) and Social Skills Training in Social Anxiety Disorder

Indications for Use and/or Goals of Treatment	Technique(s)
Technique that should always be used, because of its efficacy, as part of any CBT program	Exposure
Technique that should be used with the goal of directly making relevant cognitive changes	Cognitive therapy
Technique that may be used if there is a marked deficit in social skills	Social skills training
Multiple treatment goals and/or enhancement of treatment effects	Exposure + cognitive therapy
	Exposure + social skills training
	Exposure + cognitive therapy + social skills training

conduct exposure to the least anxiety-provoking situations. They move up the hierarchy of phobic situations as soon as they have habituated themselves to the previously practiced situation and have been able to remain in the situation without feeling too anxious. The outcome of exposure-based therapy depends largely on patients' motivation and persistence with the homework, self-directed exposure between sessions with the therapist. There are also some specific aspects of exposure in SAD (Table 4–16).

First, in-session exposure is often helpful to prepare patients for self-directed exposure in vivo. These exposure exercises involve role-playing with the therapist, whereby the therapist takes on a role of the person with whom the patient feels anxious and/or has difficulty interacting. The simulation of the real-life social situation allows the therapist to observe patients' behavior firsthand. The therapist can then give feedback to

Table 4–16. Aspects of Exposure-Based Therapy that are Relatively Specific for Social Anxiety Disorder

- In-session (therapist-assisted) exposure usually needs to be used before in vivo (self-directed) exposure
- Role-playing by the therapist is very helpful
- In vivo (self-directed) exposure should be gradual
- Exposure should well reflect the reality of social situations, which are often unpredictable and not under patients' control
- More exposure sessions may be needed for successful outcome

patients and discuss with them all the relevant aspects of that situation. This is also an opportunity for patients to talk about their feelings and thoughts during the exposure. Some of these thoughts may be challenged by the therapist, who thereby adds a cognitive technique.

Second, conducting exposure-based therapy is more difficult in SAD than in agoraphobia or specific phobias because of the dynamic nature and unpredictability of many social situations; neither the therapist nor the patients have much control over them. This unpredictability is particularly anxiety-provoking to SAD patients and calls for a more spontaneous approach when devising specific exposure tasks. For example, patients should plan to attend a meeting as part of their exposure, regardless of whom they might see there, whether they might be called to participate actively in the discussion, how long the meeting would last, and what else might happen. The rationale is to conduct exposure in a way that reflects well patients' encounters with real-life social situations.

Exposure-based therapy for SAD has demonstrated efficacy (e.g., Butler et al., 1984; Turner et al., 1994; Mersch, 1995; Salaberria and Echeburua, 1998; Hofmann et al., 2004), but further treatment gains might be made with the addition of cognitive techniques (see below). Improvement that occurs in the course of exposure treatment tends to be maintained over periods of up to 18 months (e.g., Butler et al., 1984; Mersch, 1995; Salaberria and Echeburua, 1998). Some data (e.g., Scholing and Emmelkamp, 1996) suggest that successful exposure therapy for SAD may require more sessions (up to 16), but the number of sessions needed to bring about a significant improvement varies from one patient to another. In addition to habituation and extinction that are usually implicated as the main mechanisms of change during exposure-based therapy, exposure may work by bringing about relevant cognitive changes (e.g., Mattick and Peters, 1988; Newman et al., 1994; Mersch, 1995; Salaberria and Echeburua, 1998; Hofmann, 2004).

Cognitive Therapy

Cognitive therapy is based on the cognitive model of SAD (see Etiology and Pathogenesis, above), which emphasizes the key role of faulty appraisals of oneself (as weak, inadequate, etc.), others (as powerful, negative assessors of the patient), and social interactions and situations (as being inherently dangerous). Therefore, the goal of cognitive therapy is to correct these appraisals and replace them with more accurate alternatives. Cognitive therapy may also aim to change some of the patients' core beliefs and self-concepts. Its main components are identification of the underlying appraisals and beliefs, challenging of their validity, and their replacement with realistic alternatives.

Identification of appraisals and beliefs proceeds by asking patients to imagine typical social situations that they are afraid of and then to

Table 4–17. Typical Appraisals and Beliefs of Patients With Social Anxiety Disorder

Assumptions of What Patients Might Do or What Might Happen to Them

- "I will embarrass myself"
- "I won't know what I'm doing"
- "I will talk nonsense"
- "I will lose control"
- "I will start shaking"
- "I will blush"
- "I will lose my voice"
- "I won't be able to say what I wanted"

Assumptions of How Others Will Respond or What Others Might Think

- "Everyone will laugh at me"
- "They will think I am stupid"
- "They will think I am a fool"
- "They will see that I am anxious"
- "They will think something is seriously wrong with me"

verbalize or record the thoughts that occur in their mind as they contemplate entering a social situation or as they find themselves in one. More detailed information about appraisals and beliefs can be obtained through patients' diaries, and this information is also useful for understanding what SAD patients are really afraid of (Table 4–17). It is also important for the therapist to have a good grasp of various expectations, predictions, and concerns that patients may have about themselves and others. Patients' grossly unrealistic expectations and anticipation of catastrophic consequences of their performance or other behaviors in social situations should be the focus of treatment.

The core aspect of cognitive therapy is challenging the validity of patients' appraisals and beliefs. This can be done in various ways (Table 4–18): by listing the evidence in support of and against appraisals and beliefs (and in support of and against everything that they imply), by identifying cognitive errors that patients are making (e.g., catastrophizing, mind-reading, personalization, "all-or-nothing" thinking [Butler and Wells, 1995]), by conducting behavioral experiments, and, sometimes, by using paradoxical interventions. The goal of the challenging exercises is for patients to understand the basis of their irrational thinking, which would then make it possible for them to change it.

The final component of cognitive therapy is introducing and exploring alternative, more rational ways through which patients might perceive themselves and others and understand social situations more realistically. Alternative interpretations, views, and understanding should be subjected to validation in the same way that dysfunctional appraisals and beliefs are.

Table 4–18. Procedures Used to Challenge Validity of Appraisals and Beliefs in Social Anxiety Disorder

Procedures	Components or Examples of the Procedures
Listing the evidence in support of and against appraisals and beliefs (and in support of and against everything that they imply)	Questions that patients need to ask: – How do I know that they will laugh at me? – Why do I think that I will embarrass myself? – What will happen if I do come across as awkward?
Identifying and challenging cognitive errors: • Catastrophizing • Mind-reading • Personalization • "All-or-nothing" thinking	Questions that patients need to ask: – What will happen if I make a mistake? – How do others know how I feel? – Why do I think that it all has to do with me? – What will happen if I don't do it the right way? Will I lose it completely?
Behavioral experiments	Asking for directions and finding out that no one is giving the patient a "strange look"
Paradoxical procedures	Being deliberately clumsy and realizing that nothing catastrophic happens as a result

Table 4–19. Example of Replacing Dysfunctional Appraisals and Beliefs in Social Anxiety Disorder with Realistic, "Normalizing" Alternatives

Previous Assumption	Alternatives
I will look stupid because I don't know how to ask to buy tickets correctly	• There is no "correct" way of asking for tickets • Even if I ask in a way that is unusual, I will still get the tickets • If I worry too much about how I look to others, I may not get things done • Looking clumsy or inexperienced is not the same as looking stupid • I can live with the thought that I may look stupid to some, because I know I am not stupid • I will not worry about people who judge others on the basis of their behavior in ordinary or trivial situations • I will not worry too much about how I appear to others

Only if the alternatives pass this test and patients are satisfied with their validity will they be fully accepted. An example of this part of cognitive therapy is given in Table 4–19.

There is generally less evidence of efficacy of "pure" cognitive therapy for SAD. It mainly comes from one study in which individually delivered cognitive therapy based on the model of SAD postulated by Clark and Wells (1995) was significantly more efficacious than both fluoxetine plus self-exposure and placebo plus self-exposure (Clark et al., 2003). Other treatment strategies closely related to cognitive therapy have also been successfully used in SAD—for example, rational-emotive therapy (Mersch, 1995).

Combined Exposure and Cognitive Techniques

Although exposure-based therapy has proved valuable and essential for the treatment of SAD, it does not address directly the underlying dysfunctional beliefs, patients' self-perception, appraisals, and issues such as fear of negative evaluation. Likewise, pure cognitive therapy may be less successful than exposure in reducing avoidance of social situations. Therefore, it appears logical to combine behavioral (exposure-based) and cognitive treatment approaches—a strategy first espoused by Butler et al. (1984) and subsequently supported by reports of the superiority of the combined treatment over exposure alone (Mattick and Peters, 1988; Mattick et al., 1989).

Another view, derived mainly from meta-analytic studies, stipulates that adding cognitive therapy to exposure-based therapy for SAD does not produce results better than those of exposure therapy alone (e.g., Feske and Chambless, 1995; Taylor, 1996). Also, if the cognitive change produced by exposure therapy is sufficient, using cognitive therapy might be superfluous.

On balance, a combined (cognitive-behavioral) approach to the treatment of SAD is reasonable, appears complementary, and is widely used in clinical practice. Gains with CBT are maintained over prolonged periods of time (e.g., Turner et al., 1995).

Group Therapy

Cognitive-behavioral therapy for SAD may be conducted in a group setting, as it offers some advantages over individual treatment. These advantages include simulation of various social situations, greater opportunities for social exposure and different forms of role-play, support from other members of the group, learning through observation of other group members, the giving and receiving of feedback about social performance, and modification of one's own attitudes and views as a result of direct participation in observed interactions.

Group therapy may also have some disadvantages. For example, many patients with SAD initially find groups intimidating. In group therapy, there is less opportunity for individual members to work through their own, relatively specific problems. Some patients may not be suitable for group therapy programs because their personality characteristics (e.g., argumentativeness, hostility) might have an adverse effect on group dynamics. A compromise solution for some patients may be to offer them individual therapy first (which might focus on building social skills or on the more personal, specific issues), and then enroll them in a group.

A decision as to whether to use individual or group treatment in SAD should be based on the specific circumstances of each patient. With regard to cognitive therapy, individual treatment was somewhat superior to the group one (Stangier et al., 2003). One meta-analysis has found that individual treatments for SAD, irrespective of treatment type, are more efficacious and have lower attrition rates than group treatments (Aderka, 2009).

Cognitive-behavioral group therapy for SAD, as developed by Heimberg and colleagues, is a highly structured treatment program, consisting of 12 sessions held once a week and conducted by two therapists in a group of six patients. This treatment package incorporates most of the ingredients of cognitive therapy and exposure therapy discussed above for SAD and has established itself as the standard psychological treatment of SAD. It was also found to be efficacious (Heimberg et al., 1990a, 1993, 1998). Furthermore, significant clinical improvement was reported to persist for 5 years following cessation of cognitive-behavioral group therapy (Heimberg et al., 1993).

Social Skills Training

Social skills training is derived from the social skills deficits model of SAD and based on the assumption that SAD patients have a basic deficiency in social skills (see Etiology and Pathogenesis, above). A "true" deficit in social skills does not characterize all patients with SAD, but those who are grossly socially inept may benefit from social skills training (Trower et al., 1978).

Social skills training is used with the purpose of helping patients acquire skills that would be useful in various social situations. There are several components of a typical social skills training program:

1. Providing patients with information on what constitutes successful and effective social behavior
2. Giving instructions to patients on how to learn verbal and nonverbal communication skills
3. Role-playing and modeling, so that the therapist first shows to patients how to negotiate a specific situation, subsequently asking patients to do the same
4. Giving corrective feedback to patients on how they performed
5. Patients practicing a particular skill in the presence of the therapist (rehearsal)
6. Patients practicing the same skill in real-life situations (homework)

Most social skills, particularly basic and advanced communication skills, can be learned using this sequential approach. If an emphasis is on learning assertive behavior (i.e., how to say "no," how to deal with authority figures, or how to be more effective in a leadership role), the program is sometimes referred to as "assertiveness training." It can be conducted in both an individual and group format.

While social skills training has been useful in terms of alleviating some manifestations of SAD and improving certain aspects of patients' functioning, it has often been insufficient to significantly decrease avoidance behavior and modify patients' core fears and beliefs (e.g., Marzillier et al., 1976; Trower et al., 1978; Stravynski et al., 1982). Research findings have been inconsistent: while there is some evidence that efficacy of social skills training may be comparable to that of exposure and cognitive therapy (Mersch et al., 1989, 1991; Wlazlo et al., 1990), other reports suggest that social skills training may not be more efficacious than placebo or that it may fail to maintain treatment gains over time (Juster and Heimberg, 1995; Taylor, 1996). Consequently, the role of social skills training in the treatment armamentarium for SAD remains somewhat unclear. Perhaps it can optimally be used in conjunction with CBT or some of its techniques; this is suggested by a study in which group CBT augmented with social skills training produced substantially better results than group CBT alone (Herbert et al., 2005).

Psychodynamic Psychotherapy

The aim of psychodynamic psychotherapy in SAD is to uncover and work through the specific, underlying conflicts and issues. There is no single type of unconscious conflict that characterizes all or most patients with SAD, as this condition may have different developmental antecedents (see Etiology and Pathogenesis, above). The conflicts are uncovered and worked through primarily by means of transference and interpretation. The relatively specific issues in the course of the psychodynamic psychotherapy of SAD include addressing patients' expectations to be judged negatively and harshly by the therapist, mistrust toward the therapist, patients' feelings of shame for wanting to succeed or win, and various narcissistic problems, such as pursuit of perfection and needs for praise and admiration.

COMBINED TREATMENTS

As with other anxiety disorders, combining medications and CBT for SAD seems to be common in clinical practice. It is unclear, however, how these treatment modalities should be optimally combined—for example, what the sequence of their administration should be. One form of treatment is usually started first, and then another treatment is added, particularly if there has been an insufficient response to the initial treatment or if the goal is to enhance the response to the initial treatment by adding another one. Issues arising in the course of combining pharmacotherapy and CBT are discussed in Chapter 2.

There have been few studies examining the efficacy of combined treatments in SAD. Their results generally suggest that in the short term, efficacy of combined treatment (sertraline plus exposure or fluoxetine plus group CBT) is comparable to that of CBT alone (exposure or group CBT) or pharmacotherapy alone (sertraline or fluoxetine) (Blomhoff et al., 2001; Davidson et al., 2004b). In a study by Blomhoff et al. (2001), however, exposure alone was not superior to placebo, whereas treatments with sertraline plus exposure and sertraline alone were more efficacious than placebo. In an extension of this study, patients treated with exposure alone continued to improve after cessation of treatment, whereas those treated with sertraline exhibited a tendency toward deterioration (Haug et al., 2003). The authors concluded that in the long term, exposure alone was more efficacious than a combination of exposure and sertraline, a finding similar to the long-term effects of combined pharmacotherapy and CBT in panic disorder (see Chapter 2).

Perhaps the effects of combined treatment depend on the type of medication and version of CBT that is used. This is suggested by the finding that after short-term treatment and at follow-up, phenelzine plus self-exposure fared somewhat better than alprazolam plus self-exposure and that it was also superior to placebo plus self-exposure and group CBT alone (Gelernter et al., 1991). When individual cognitive therapy was compared to fluoxetine plus self-exposure and placebo plus self-exposure, it was superior to both (Clark et al., 2003).

These discrepant and inconclusive findings call for more research, with the hope that such research would also reflect more accurately the reality of clinical practice.

Administration of a fear extinction enhancer D-cycloserine before exposure therapy sessions may be a novel, potentially promising way of combining pharmacotherapy and exposure-based treatment. Two controlled studies have reported this combination to be efficacious in the treatment of SAD (Hofmann et al., 2006; Guastella et al., 2008). Augmentation of exposure therapy with D-cycloserine is discussed in more detail in Chapter 5.

OUTLOOK FOR THE FUTURE

Social anxiety disorder is still often considered to be just another term for "too much" shyness. There is little appreciation that SAD and shyness differ in more than degree of severity. Therefore, the concept of SAD will be useful to the extent that it is clearly delineated from shyness and other forms of normal social anxiety, and further efforts need to be made to draw a practical, not only academic, demarcation line between SAD and shyness.

This task is closely related to the way mental disorder in general will be defined—a task of gigantic proportions, but great significance for the profession.

While the construct validity of SAD remains to be established, just like the validity of most psychiatric diagnoses, the imperative of clinical practice is to take seriously people with SAD. This is because they are often impaired in various areas of functioning and because SAD may represent only a tip of the iceberg of the overall psychopathology. Thus, there is a need to promote awareness of the seriousness of SAD, so that it would be taken accordingly, diagnosed promptly, and treated early. Doing so does not run a risk of "pathologizing" something normal, and it would prevent complications (especially alcohol and other substance use disorders and depression) and reduce disability associated with SAD.

A research agenda for SAD includes a need to ascertain whether there are any specific neurobiological underpinnings of SAD (e.g., central dopamine deficiency) and whether any of the appraisals, beliefs, and information-processing aberrations (e.g., increased self-focused attention along with decreased attention to external information) might be considered truly unique for SAD. One way to achieve this is to compare children at risk for SAD with those at risk for other anxiety disorders and follow them prospectively.

Treatment approaches to the generalized SAD are likely to benefit from a view that this condition is often akin to a personality disorder because of its pervasive nature and the way it affects personality development. Therapists cannot afford to ignore the disordered personality matrix of many patients with SAD, expecting that patterns of personality functioning will improve as a result of the improvement in manifestations of SAD. Thus, future treatments of SAD should target its "surface" features as well as its "deep-seated" personality structure. This will call for greater flexibility in planning and conducting treatment and means that treatments may need to last longer and that they should not be confined to a single theoretical model. Likewise, psychotherapy approaches to SAD need to rely more on those ingredients of CBT packages that further research identifies as most effective. Within this framework there is room for pharmacotherapy, especially insofar as it is able to affect the relevant underlying pathophysiological processes.

5

Specific Phobias

Specific phobias (also referred to as simple phobias and isolated phobias) represent a heterogeneous group of disorders characterized by excessive and/or irrational fear of one of relatively few and usually related objects, situations, places, phenomena, or activities (phobic stimuli). The phobic stimuli are either avoided or endured with intense anxiety or discomfort. People with specific phobias are aware that their fear is unreasonable, but this does not diminish the intensity of the fear. Rather, they are quite distressed about being afraid or feel handicapped by their phobia. Specific phobias are frequently encountered in the general population, but they are relatively uncommon in the clinical setting. Most phobias have a remarkable tendency to persist, prompting an assumption that they cannot be easily extinguished because of their "purpose" to protect against danger.

KEY ISSUES

Specific phobias are deceptively simple, as they are easy to describe and recognize but often difficult to understand. There are several conceptual problems and a number of issues associated with specific phobias:

1. Where are the boundaries of specific phobias? How can we develop better criteria on the basis of which specific phobia could be distinguished as a psychiatric disorder from fears and avoidance considered to be within the realm of "normality?"
2. How can specific phobias be taken seriously by *both* the sufferers and clinicians?
3. In view of the considerable differences between various types of specific phobias, should they continue to be grouped together?
4. Should specific phobias be grouped on the basis of whether they are driven by fear or disgust?
5. In view of its unique features, should the blood-injection-injury type of specific phobia be given a separate psychopathological, diagnostic, and nosological status?

6. Considering a significant overlap between situational phobias and agoraphobia, should they be grouped together, along a hypothetical situational phobia/agoraphobia spectrum?

7. What is the relationship between specific phobias and other psychopathology? Are they relatively isolated from other disorders, both cross-sectionally and longitudinally, or should they more appropriately be conceptualized as a predisposition to or a risk factor for some psychiatric conditions?

8. How specific are pathways that lead to specific phobias?

9. Has the dominant treatment model for specific phobias, based on exposure therapy, exhausted its potential? Is the tendency for specific phobias to persist adequately addressed by treatments derived from learning theory?

CLINICAL FEATURES

As with other phobic disorders (agoraphobia and social anxiety disorder), main features of specific phobias are excessive, persistent, and irrational fear of certain phobic stimuli and avoidance of these stimuli as much as possible. In contrast to agoraphobia and social anxiety disorder, the nature of phobic stimuli is different; patients with specific phobias are fearful of certain animals, heights, the sight of blood, flying, and so on. Also, reasons for the fear of phobic stimuli are usually different from those for the phobic fear in agoraphobia and social anxiety disorder (Table 5–1).

One reason has to do with some aspects of the phobic stimulus that may represent a real danger under certain circumstances. For example, people can be bitten by venomous snakes, one can fall from a high-rise building, and planes do crash occasionally. Patients with phobias of snakes, heights, and flying, however, grossly exaggerate the likelihood of any of this happening to them.

Another reason for fearing certain phobic stimuli in specific phobias is related to the reasons given by patients with agoraphobia and by some with social anxiety disorder. That is, some patients with a specific phobia may be afraid of certain symptoms that they expect upon exposure to a phobic

---

Table 5–1. Reasons for Fear and Avoidance in Specific Phobias

- Some aspects of the phobic stimuli represent a real threat under certain circumstances

- Fear of certain symptoms and their anticipated consequences (e.g., loss of control), which might occur upon exposure to a phobic stimulus

- Phobic stimuli elicit a strong feeling of disgust

stimulus. They may also be afraid of the anticipated consequences of these symptoms, for example, loss of control or some somatic catastrophe. Thus, patients with claustrophobia often worry that they will not have enough air and will then suffocate and die in enclosed places. Patients with a phobia of having blood drawn are often afraid that they will faint and "make a scene" in corresponding situations.

Yet another reason underlying some specific phobias is a feeling of disgust. Some patients may be afraid of spiders not so much because they are potentially dangerous but because they elicit a strong feeling of disgust. Sometimes it is difficult to ascertain whether the primary emotion is fear or disgust, or whether both are present.

Two or more reasons for fearing phobic stimuli may be present in patients with a particular specific phobia. For example, patients may be afraid of heights both because they might fall and because they might feel lightheaded and dizzy in high places, and then lose control and fall. Likewise, a patient with a phobia of having blood drawn may anticipate feeling disgusted at the sight of blood, fear the pain involved, and be afraid of fainting. It is important to understand the underlying reasons for any particular phobia because successful treatment largely depends on this understanding.

Although persistent fear of phobic stimuli is a feature of specific phobias, the intensity of fear varies depending on whether patients are in contact or expect to be in contact with their phobic stimuli. Panic attacks are not rare if the contact with phobic stimuli cannot be prevented and if patients are unable to escape situations in which these contacts occur. The phobia will not represent a clinical problem as long as its sufferers are able to avoid phobic stimuli without a cost to their functioning. The phobia turns into a psychiatric disorder only when the fear becomes too distressing, avoidance is no longer possible, and/or avoidance starts to interfere significantly with functioning. For example, a person with a long-standing fear of flying and avoidance of air travel who has recently received a job promotion and is now expected to make frequent business trips by plane can no longer resort to avoidance. The person finds it very difficult to cope with the demands of the new situation and seeks professional help for the phobia.

There are several subtypes of specific phobias that were originally proposed on the basis of the nature of phobic stimuli. According to *DSM-IV-TR*, these subtypes are as follows: phobias of animals, phobias of stimuli (e.g., water, heights) that occur in the natural environment, blood-injection-injury phobia, situational phobias, and other types of phobias (e.g., choking phobia). Besides the differences pertaining to their object, these subtypes of specific phobias may also be differentiated on the basis of the usual age of onset, female-to-male ratio, presence of unexpected panic attacks, dominant underlying themes, problems, or issues, degree to which a familial component is present, and other characteristics (Table 5–2).

Table 5–2. Characteristics of the Subtypes of Specific Phobias

	Animal Phobias	Natural Environment Subtype	Blood-Injection-Injury Phobia	Situational Phobias
Onset	Childhood	Variable	Childhood	Adolescence, early 20s
Female-male ratio	Women > men	Women > men	Women = men	Women > men
Presence of unexpected panic attacks	No	No	No	Yes
Dominant theme, problem, or issue	Disgust, exaggerated appraisal of danger	Exaggerated appraisal of danger	Disgust, concern about fainting	Fear of physical symptoms or a panic attack, exaggerated appraisal of danger
Familial component	Less prominent	Less prominent	More prominent	Less prominent
Unique pathophysiology	No	No	Yes	No

Phobias of Animals

While the reason for fearing certain animals lies in their dangerousness (e.g., sharks, lions, crocodiles), many dangerous animals are not objects of an animal phobia. This is because most people afraid of these animals are not impaired by such fear (e.g., they simply avoid places where they might encounter dangerous animals). Indeed, patients with animal phobia are usually afraid of animals such as snakes, dogs, cats, spiders and other insects, rats, and mice. Only a minority of these animals is dangerous, so factors other than danger seem to be more important in determining whether particular animals will be feared and avoided to the extent characteristic of a phobia. The most important of these factors is a feeling of disgust elicited by some animals (e.g., Tolin et al., 1997; Lipsitz et al., 2002). It has been argued that with animals such as spiders, the main underlying issue is a feeling of disgust rather than a perception of danger, considering that only 0.1% of all the varieties of spiders are dangerous to humans (McNally, 2002).

The universal nature of the feeling of disgust probably accounts for the finding that disgust-relevant animals (e.g., spiders, cockroaches, worms) are feared to the same or very similar extent in different countries (e.g., Davey et al. 1998), even countries where contacts with some of these animals are unlikely. Animal phobias typically have an onset in childhood and are more common among women.

Phobia of Elements in the Natural Environment

This is a heterogeneous group of phobias, which includes phobias of heights (acrophobia), water, storms, and thunder and/or lightning. It appears that in many patients with phobias from this group, particularly patients with phobias of heights and water, there is no history of contact or traumatic experience with the phobic stimuli prior to the onset of the phobia. This finding suggests that such phobias may have an "innate," survival-relevant character (see Etiology and Pathogenesis, below).

The age of onset of natural environment phobias varies, but in many cases it is early. The main underlying theme in this subtype of phobia is the danger associated with phobic stimuli (Lipsitz et al., 2002). That is, patients with the phobia of heights are typically afraid of falling off, whereas those with the water phobia are afraid of drowning.

Blood-Injection-Injury Phobia

This is a unique type of specific phobia. Unlike all other phobias, it is characterized by a pathophysiological reaction to the phobic stimulus which has two phases: after initial and short-lasting tachycardia, there is a parasympathetic activation and vasovagal response, with bradycardia and hypotension, which very often—in more that 75% of cases—leads to fainting (vasovagal syncope). Many patients feel embarrassed about fainting and sometimes resort to extensive avoidance because of that. Their health may be jeopardized because they refuse to undergo the necessary medical procedures.

A feeling of disgust (at the sight of blood or needle penetrating a person's skin) has been reported as the main underlying problem (Page, 1994; Tolin et al., 1997; Lipsitz et al., 2002). Therefore, blood-injection-injury phobia appears to be one of the disgust-driven phobias. Blood-injection-injury phobia has a stronger familial component than other subtypes of specific phobias (e.g., Marks, 1988; Fyer et al., 1990), and unlike other subtypes, the proportion of women and men with this phobia is about the same. Most cases have an onset in childhood.

Situational Phobias

These phobias denote a fear of certain situations. Most common forms of situational phobias are claustrophobia, fear of flying, and phobia of driving. This subtype generally has a later onset than others. There is some disagreement as to what the main underlying concern or problem is for patients with situational phobias; some suggest that it is the fear of physical symptoms and panic-like sensations (Craske and Sipsas, 1992), while others report that the main issue for these patients is an expectation of danger in the situations they are afraid of (Lipsitz et al., 2002). Unexpected panic attacks seem to occur more often in situational phobias than in other subtypes of specific phobias (Ehlers et al., 1994; Lipsitz et al., 2002), so patients' fear of panic and its symptoms is understandable.

There is an overlap between situational phobias and agoraphobia, and the two may co-occur; similarities and differences between situational phobias and agoraphobia are reviewed in Relationship Between Specific Phobias and Other Disorders (below).

A typical example of the situational phobia is claustrophobia—fear of small, enclosed places. Being in an elevator is a prototypical claustrophobic situation, but patients with claustrophobia are often afraid of other places and situations, such as long tunnels, underground passages, subways, cellars, caves, mines, and even airplanes. The essence of claustrophobia is a fear of being confined to a small place from which escape is difficult or impossible. Patients with claustrophobia typically state that they are afraid of being "stuck" or "trapped"; some have frightening images of being "buried alive" in case of an underground accident. They may also voice a concern that there would be no one to help them in a claustrophobic situation. Patients with claustrophobia are often afraid of not having enough air and of choking in a claustrophobic situation. If they have a panic attack in such a situation, their respiratory symptoms (shortness of breath, choking sensations) may be particularly prominent or paid attention to.

Fear of flying is a unique type of situational phobia in that there may be different reasons underlying this fear: *(1)* confinement, as in claustrophobia; *(2)* being high above the ground, as in fear of heights; *(3)* possibility of having a panic attack, as in agoraphobia; and *(4)* possibility of an accident (plane crash), as in "true" phobia of flying. Sometimes there is more than one reason behind the fear of flying in a particular patient.

Fear of driving or travel is another phobia in which it is very important to establish the underlying reason for fear. Patients may be afraid of having a panic attack while being in a car, train, or other vehicle (in which case, this fear may be a part of agoraphobia), or they are preoccupied with a possibility of having an accident. This phobia may precede the onset of agoraphobia.

Other Types of Specific Phobias

Phobia of Choking

This type of phobia is less common and is characterized by the fear of swallowing. The fear is usually a result of the belief that swallowing food or drinking fluids may lead to choking and it typically follows accidental choking on food. In the most severe cases, patients may appear malnourished or become dehydrated because they do not have an adequate intake of food or fluids. In less severe and more typical cases, patients have trouble swallowing large pills, are extremely cautious and slow while eating or drinking, and may refuse certain types of food because of the concern that they might choke while trying to swallow it.

Disease Phobia

Disease phobia is characterized by excessive fear of getting a serious, life-threatening disease. It is directly related to the perception of diseases; the greater the perception of the disease as dangerous or incurable, the higher the likelihood that it will become the focus of a phobia. This helps explain the widespread phobic fear of tuberculosis, syphilis, and other incurable bacterial infections a century ago, and the frequency of AIDS phobia and cancer phobia today. Patients with a disease phobia tend to avoid all situations, people, objects, or other stimuli related to the dreaded disease. This avoidance is rarely incapacitating but may at times adversely affect treatment-seeking behavior.

Dental Phobia

Dental phobia usually denotes fear of various dental procedures. However, it is a heterogeneous condition, and upon detailed analysis, it may point to one or more of the following underlying problems: *(1)* fear of needles, blood, and/or specific dental interventions, which may be indistinguishable from the blood-injection-injury phobia (and include fainting); (2) fear of pain; (3) fear of local anesthesia, which may entail fear of an allergic reaction and/or fear of losing control; (4) fear of becoming infected with a disease, such as HIV/AIDS; (5) fear of being confined to the dentist's chair, which may be a form of situational phobia or a part of agoraphobia (in the latter case, there is a prominent fear that a panic attack might occur while the patient is seated in the dentist's chair); and (6) fear of choking during dental intervention.

It is important to understand the nature of the underlying fear and plan treatment accordingly. The avoidance associated with dental phobia may lead to a serious neglect of dental health, thereby making later dental interventions more complicated.

RELATIONSHIP BETWEEN SPECIFIC PHOBIAS AND OTHER DISORDERS

The overall relationship between specific phobias and other psychiatric disorders is not clear. Clinical impression suggests that specific phobias are relatively "isolated" from other psychopathology and that in this regard, they are different from most other anxiety disorders. Epidemiological studies contradict this clinical impression, as they report that specific phobias co-occur frequently with other anxiety disorders (e.g., Magee et al., 1996; Kessler et al., 2005; Stinson et al., 2007) and also, with mood, personality, and substance use disorders (e.g., Stinson et al., 2007). The most common co-occurring disorders are agoraphobia and social anxiety disorder.

Specific phobias are frequently diagnosed as a co-occurring condition when the principal disorder for which help is being sought is another anxiety disorder (de Ruiter et al., 1989; Sanderson et al., 1990; Starcevic et al., 1992b). This suggests that specific phobias may be complicated by other anxiety disorders, especially since in most cases of co-occurrence, specific phobias tend to precede the onset of other anxiety disorders. Alternatively, specific phobias may be overdiagnosed in the context of another anxiety disorder. A diagnosis of specific phobia co-occurring with another principal anxiety disorder rarely has significant clinical implications.

Specific Phobias and Agoraphobia

An important relationship exists between claustrophobia and agoraphobia (Table 5-3). The situations feared and avoided by patients with claustrophobia and agoraphobia (e.g., elevators, tunnels, planes, other enclosed places) are often very similar and pertain to confinement. Patients may mention a similar reason for avoidance—fear of certain physical symptoms or panic attack occurring in the phobic situations. Both claustrophobia and

Table 5–3. Similarities and Differences Between Claustrophobia and Agoraphobia

Similarities
Type of situations feared and avoided (confinement-type situations)
Reason for avoidance: fear of certain physical symptoms and/or fear of a panic attack occurring in the phobic situations
More common in women
Onset at approximately the same age (early 20s)

Differences		
Criteria for Differentiation	Claustrophobia	Agoraphobia
Range of situations avoided	More constricted	Wider, including non-claustrophobic situations
Symptoms upon exposure to phobic situations	Breathing difficulties, "air hunger," choking-like sensations	Unsteadiness, dizziness, fainting feelings
Catastrophic cognitions	Choking	Fainting, losing consciousness
Intensity of phobic fear over time	More constant	More often tends to fluctuate

agoraphobia are more common in women and have an onset at approximately the same age (early twenties).

There are also important differences between claustrophobia and agoraphobia. Patients with agoraphobia typically avoid a wider range of situations (in addition to those typical of claustrophobia), and they are more likely to report unsteadiness, dizziness, and fainting feelings upon exposure to phobic stimuli. In contrast, patients with claustrophobia are more troubled by breathing problems, "air hunger," and choking-like sensations in claustrophobic situations. Largely as a result of the different symptoms experienced and/or anticipated, patients with claustrophobia and agoraphobia have different catastrophic cognitions: claustrophobic patients are more likely to expect and be concerned about suffocation in a phobic situation, whereas those with agoraphobia more often worry about the possibility of fainting or losing consciousness.

Claustrophobic fears are sometimes viewed as part of agoraphobia because the latter is a broader psychopathological entity. Claustrophobia may sometimes precede the onset of agoraphobia.

Other types of situational phobias may also co-occur with agoraphobia, and in these cases it is important to ascertain, on the basis of the reason given for fear and avoidance, whether they should be regarded as part of agoraphobia or as disorders in their own right. When patients are afraid of driving, travel, or flying because they are excessively concerned about accidents and the possibility of having panic attacks (and then not being able to escape from a car, bus, train, boat, or plane), they qualify for diagnoses of both specific phobia and agoraphobia. If one of these reasons for fear and avoidance is much more prominent, only one diagnosis should be given.

The phobia of heights may co-occur with agoraphobia as well. In this type of phobia, the main underlying problem is fear of falling. This fear is strengthened by the expectation of having a panic attack in that situation, which is more characteristic of agoraphobia. Both diagnoses are warranted if both reasons for fear and avoidance of heights are given; the diagnosis of agoraphobia is more appropriate if, in addition to heights, there are fears of other, more typical agoraphobic situations.

ASSESSMENT

Diagnostic and Conceptual Issues

A diagnosis of specific phobia is made on the basis of the criteria used for diagnosing phobic disorders in general (see Table 4–4). The most difficult diagnostic criterion is the one pertaining to the impairment in functioning (or interference with functioning) as a result of a phobia. This criterion also marks the boundary between normal fears and specific phobia as a psychiatric disorder. For example, while the fear of flying is common and cannot by itself be considered an illness, refusal of an attractive job by a person with a severe fear of flying because that job would involve frequent airplane travel suggests that this person suffers from a phobic disorder. In clinical practice, it is not always easy to determine whether functioning is impaired because of the phobia. Considering the relatively circumscribed nature of phobic stimuli and greater ease with which they are avoided, the impairment in specific phobias is usually not as generalized as it is in agoraphobia and social anxiety disorder; that is, only certain areas of functioning tend to be affected by specific phobias.

When the person is not clearly impaired by the phobia, a diagnosis can be made only if he or she is distressed by the fear and/or avoidance. The wider context of fear and avoidance and the likelihood of exposure to a phobic stimulus also play a role in determining whether any given fear qualifies for a diagnosis of specific phobia—and even when the diagnosis is made, whether it is of *real* importance. For example, a phobia of snakes is not clinically significant if the sufferer is unlikely to come in contact with snakes because of the place where he or she resides, his or her lifestyle, and/or type of job.

The diagnostic criteria for specific phobias are essentially the same in *DSM-IV-TR* and *ICD-10*. During the assessment, it is good practice to inquire whether patients have fears other than those that they report spontaneously; many patients have fears of several stimuli within the same subtype of specific phobias. For example, patients with a phobia of elevators often have phobic fears of many other situations and places from which escape might be difficult. Patients may also have fears from different specific phobia subtypes (e.g., Hofmann et al., 1997; Curtis et al., 1998). In fact, over 70% of individuals with specific phobias were found to have multiple fears in one study (Stinson et al., 2007).

In an interview situation, patients with specific phobias usually do not seem anxious or troubled as long as they do not have to talk about the objects of their phobias and as long as they do not have to face the phobic stimuli. When facing these stimuli, patients have typical physiological and behavioral fear responses, including panic attacks, avoidance, and escape. This contrast in the patients' appearance and behavior, depending on whether they have to face phobic stimuli, may be quite striking.

Counterphobic behavior may suggest presence of a phobic disorder. It denotes excessive confrontation with danger and sources of fear and its purpose is to deny any danger and fear.

A diagnosis of specific phobia should not be made if the phobic features can be better accounted for by another, more broadly conceptualized psychiatric condition, such as obsessive-compulsive disorder, agoraphobia, posttraumatic stress disorder, social anxiety disorder, separation anxiety disorder, or even a psychotic disorder.

There are two main issues challenging the concept of specific phobias. The first is the problem of the boundary between specific phobia and normality. The current criteria for making this distinction are not always useful on theoretical grounds and in clinical practice. The second problem is the heterogeneity of specific phobias, along with the possibility that some subtypes are more related to other anxiety disorders than to other subtypes within specific phobias. In addition, it remains to be ascertained whether the differences between disgust-driven and fear-driven phobias are sufficient to require their separate categorization.

Assessment Instruments

Numerous instruments are used to ascertain the presence of various fears and specific phobias, assess the severity of fear and/or avoidance, and monitor changes during treatment. The most comprehensive is the Fear Survey Schedule (Wolpe and Lang, 1964), but because of its length, it is not particularly suitable for routine use in clinical practice. Several modifications of the Fear Survey Schedule have been developed since its original publication.

Instruments that measure the severity of fear and/or avoidance in certain types of specific phobia may be more useful in clinical practice. An example of such an instrument is the commonly used self-report Fear Questionnaire (Marks and Mathews, 1979), which assesses avoidance associated with agoraphobia, social anxiety disorder, and blood-injury phobia. Another instrument that specifically assesses various aspects of the blood-injection-injury phobia is the Blood-Injection Symptom Scale (Page et al., 1997).

Differential Diagnosis

The most common disorders for consideration in the differential diagnosis of specific phobias include agoraphobia, obsessive-compulsive disorder, and hypochondriasis. The relationship between specific phobias and agoraphobia and criteria for making a diagnostic distinction between the two are presented in Relationship Between Specific Phobias and Other Disorders (above).

Obsessive-compulsive disorder may sometimes resemble a phobic disorder, especially when prominent avoidance is part of its clinical presentation. The differentiation between the two is based mainly on reasons for fear and avoidance. For example, patients who are afraid of heights because they might have an urge to jump off probably suffer from obsessive-compulsive disorder, not a phobia of heights. The same consideration applies to patients who are afraid of driving because they have disturbing images of running off the road, patients who fear needles and all sharp objects because these could be used to hurt someone, and patients who have distressing thoughts about contamination and infectious diseases and therefore avoid using public toilets and payphones. In these cases, patients are unlikely to have a "simple" driving phobia, blood-injection-injury phobia, or disease/contamination phobia, respectively.

Hypochondriasis occasionally needs to be differentiated from disease phobia. While patients with hypochondriasis are usually afraid that they already have a serious physical disease, patients with disease phobia fear that they will become a victim of such a disease in the future. In addition, patients with disease phobia are more likely to avoid various disease-related situations, activities, and stimuli (e.g., hospitals, doctors, conversations about health and illness), whereas patients with hypochondriasis make numerous visits to doctors, undergo many investigations, and show much interest in all matters related to health and illness. Unlike patients with hypochondriasis, those with disease phobia typically do not seek reassurance (that they are not ill) and tend to have good insight into the excessive and/or unreasonable nature of their fears.

Table 5–4. Epidemiological Data for Specific Phobias

- Lifetime prevalence in the United States: 11.2%–12.5% (*DSM-III* criteria, Epidemiologic Catchment Area Study), 11.3% (*DSM-III-R* criteria, National Comorbidity Survey), 12.5% (*DSM-IV* criteria, National Comorbidity Survey Replication), 9.4% (*DSM-IV* criteria, National Epidemiologic Survey on Alcohol and Related Conditions)

- Lifetime prevalence in various countries, according to various diagnostic criteria: 0.6%–12.5%

- Best-estimate lifetime prevalence rate across the world: 5.3%

- The frequency of different subtypes of specific phobias appears to vary, depending on the setting (general vs. clinical population) and cultural and social factors. For example, animal phobia is the most frequent subtype among adults in the community but the least common subtype in clinical settings

- Generally more common among women, with a ratio of 2–2.5:1 (except for blood-injection-injury phobia)

- Usual age of onset depends on the subtype:
  - Animal phobias: (early) childhood
  - Blood-injection-injury phobia: (later) childhood
  - Situational phobias: adolescence, early 20s
  - Natural environment subtype: variable

- Help-seeking patterns: very few persons with specific phobias seek professional help; help may be sought after a change in one's life circumstances has made avoidance of phobic stimuli very difficult or impossible; it is not likely for help to be sought from primary care physicians

EPIDEMIOLOGY

The main epidemiological data on specific phobias are presented in Table 5–4. Community surveys suggest that specific phobias are among the most common psychiatric disorders. The lifetime prevalence figures for specific phobias in the United States have shown only minor fluctuations over the years. In the Epidemiologic Catchment Area study, based on the *DSM-III* diagnostic criteria, lifetime prevalence was reported to be 11.2% (Robins and Regier, 1991) or 12.5% (Regier et al., 1988). In the National Comorbidity Survey, which used the *DSM-III-R* criteria, the lifetime prevalence rate of specific phobias was 11.3% (Kessler et al., 1994; Magee et al., 1996), and in the National Comorbidity Survey Replication, based on the *DSM-IV* diagnostic criteria, a figure reflecting this rate was 12.5% (Kessler et al., 2005). Another study conducted in the United States, the National Epidemiologic Survey on Alcohol and Related Conditions, reported a somewhat lower lifetime prevalence of *DSM-IV* specific phobias of 9.4% (Stinson et al., 2007).

The prevalence rates for specific phobias in the United States are higher or much higher than the corresponding rates in other countries. The lifetime prevalence rates range from 0.6% in Italy (Faravelli et al., 1989) to 12.5% in the United States (Regier et al., 1988; Kessler et al., 2005). The best-estimate lifetime prevalence rate for specific phobias across epidemiological studies published between 1980 and 2004 and conducted in various countries was 5.3% (Somers et al., 2006). The large differences in prevalence figures are a consequence of the influence of cultural factors on the patterning of phobias (e.g., Raguram and Bhide, 1985; Chambers et al., 1986) and methodological issues, especially different thresholds for the diagnosis of specific phobia (i.e., levels of impairment or distress needed to make the diagnosis). Although it appears that specific phobias are common in the community, the severity of the disorder and its clinical significance seem to vary substantially.

Animal phobia is the most frequent subtype of specific phobias among adults in the community (Eaton et al., 1991; Becker et al., 2007; Stinson et al., 2007). The phobia of heights is also commonly encountered in the general population, followed by the phobia of flying and claustrophobia in some studies (e.g., Stinson et al., 2007) and blood phobia in others (e.g., Becker et al., 2007). Phobias of water and storms are less common in the community (Eaton et al., 1991; Stinson et al., 2007).

In adult clinical populations, the most frequent subtype of specific phobias is situational phobia, followed by the natural environment, blood-injection-injury, and animal subtypes (American Psychiatric Association, 2000). Within these subtypes, claustrophobia, phobia of driving or flying, phobia of heights, and spider phobia are commonly seen in clinical practice. Dental phobia is not rare in clinical populations. The differences between the prevalence of various subtypes of specific phobias in the community and clinical settings are likely due to different levels of impairment or distress associated with these subtypes. For example, animal phobias generally seem to lead to less impairment or to be experienced with less distress, which accounts for lower proportions of people with animal phobias in clinical populations than in the community. The same explanation can be invoked for the much lower frequency of specific phobias than that of agoraphobia and social anxiety disorder in clinical settings, as opposed to the community.

All subtypes of specific phobias, except for blood-injection-injury phobia, are more commonly seen among women, with the female-to-male ratio being approximately 2–2.5:1 (Bourdon et al., 1988; Fredrikson et al., 1996; Magee et al., 1996; Stinson et al., 2007). The prevalence of blood-injection-injury phobia is approximately the same in women and men (Agras et al., 1969; Himle et al., 1989; Fredrikson et al., 1996). Women were also found to be more likely to have several types of specific phobias at the same time (Fredrikson et al., 1996). A greater prevalence of phobic fears among women is usually considered a consequence of social and cultural factors; that is, the expression of fear tends to be more socially acceptable in women than it is in men, and there are fewer expectations from women to perform fearlessly.

The age of onset of specific phobias depends on the subtype. Phobias of animals and blood-injection-injury phobia usually appear in childhood, while the situational phobias occur later, in adolescence or early 20s (Öst, 1987b; Himle et al., 1989; Starcevic and Bogojevic, 1997; Lipsitz et al., 2002; Becker et al., 2007). The mean ages of onset for various types of specific phobias were reported in one study to be as follows: for animal phobia, 7 years; for blood-injection-injury phobia, 9 years; for dental phobia, 12 years; and for claustrophobia, 20 years (Öst, 1987b). The age of onset of phobias encompassed by the natural environment subtype appears to vary.

It has been estimated that less than 1% of all persons with specific phobias seek treatment (Agras et al., 1969; Regier et al., 1990). More recent data put this figure slightly higher, at 8% (Stinson et al., 2007). Persons with specific phobias seem unlikely to seek professional help from primary care physicians and may be more prone to contacting clinical psychologists or other mental health professionals for this purpose.

COURSE AND PROGNOSIS

The course of specific phobias ranges from spontaneous remission to chronicity. Some children with specific phobias seem to grow out of their phobia and experience remission without any treatment. In fact, many children with specific phobias develop no psychopathology in adulthood (Biederman et al., 2007). On the other hand, the condition seems to be characterized by remarkable longitudinal stability, as adults with specific phobias usually have histories of specific phobias in childhood (Gregory et al., 2007). Indeed, it has been consistently reported that specific phobias have a chronic, unremitting course (e.g., Becker et al., 2007; Stinson et al., 2007).

It is not clear whether any particular type of phobia is more likely to disappear spontaneously, but it has been speculated that this may be the case more with phobias of animals, darkness, thunder, and water. One study showed that practically all persons with specific phobias younger than 20 were improved at follow-up, whereas improvement was reported by less than one half of adults with specific phobias (Agras et al., 1972). If a phobia in adults has continuously been present from childhood, its spontaneous disappearance is uncommon and may occur in only 20% of cases.

The course of specific phobias may depend on the mode of onset, presence of avoidance, and the nature of the main underlying emotion. Thus, phobias that appeared after traumatic events may be more chronic than phobias that developed as a result of the transmission of information or observational learning (see Etiology and Pathogenesis, below). The most persistent course may be seen in those phobias that were apparently not learned (e.g., some cases of phobia of heights, water, or spiders); the fact that it is difficult for these phobias to be extinguished may suggest that they have survival value. As for the effects of avoidance on the course of specific phobias, the longer the avoidance of phobic stimuli, the more likely it is for the phobia to be maintained for long periods of time. Disgust-driven phobias (e.g., many cases of blood-injection-injury phobia and spider phobia) may be more difficult to extinguish and more likely to have a chronic course.

The course of specific phobias may be less likely to be complicated by conditions such as depression or substance use disorder than the course of most other anxiety disorders. Specific phobias precede other anxiety disorders more often and their presence may be considered a risk factor for developing other anxiety disorders. Some situational phobias (particularly claustrophobia and phobia of driving or traveling) may predispose to agoraphobia.

Although specific phobias in adults often have a chronic course and are unlikely to disappear without treatment, their prognosis may generally be better than that of other anxiety disorders. This is controversial, however, because estimates of impairment related to specific phobias do vary, and some studies suggest that specific phobias may be associated with substantial disability (Becker et al., 2007; Stinson et al., 2007).

ETIOLOGY AND PATHOGENESIS

Specific phobias are a heterogeneous group of disorders unlikely to have common etiology and pathogenesis. Moreover, there are often several etiological and pathogenetic factors operating within the same type of phobia. For example, phobias of certain animals may be innate, have a hereditary component, or appear as a result of traumatic experience, observational learning, and/or transmission of relevant information.

BIOLOGICAL MODELS

Genetic Factors

One family study (Fyer et al., 1990) has found that the first-degree relatives of patients with specific phobia have a three times higher risk for specific phobia than the first-degree relatives of control subjects without any psychiatric disorder. However, this tendency for specific phobias to run in families may be more a consequence of shared environment (and interactions among various family members) than a consequence of hereditary transmission, as suggested by the results of twin studies (Kendler et al., 1992c; Skre et al., 1993). There is some indication that blood-injection-injury phobia has a stronger hereditary component than other types of specific phobias (e.g., Marks, 1988; Fyer et al., 1990).

Neurobiological Factors

Relatively few neuroimaging studies have been conducted in patients with specific phobias and it is not possible to draw definite conclusions about cerebral structures and pathophysiological mechanisms that may be involved. Most studies used functional magnetic resonance imaging in patients with spider phobia and reported an increased activation in the amygdala and insula in response to the relevant stimuli (e.g., Straube et al., 2006; Goossens et al., 2007). This change disappeared after exposure therapy (Goossens et al., 2007). In patients with blood-injection-injury phobia, one neuroimaging study found a decreased medial prefrontal cortex activity in response to the corresponding stimuli (Hermann et al., 2007).

Nonassociative Theory

Although this theory (Menzies and Clarke, 1995) has emerged from psychological studies of etiological factors in specific phobias, it implicitly suggests some biological mechanism in the causation of certain types of specific phobias. The theory proposes that these phobias are not learned but are inborn and its central tenet is that at least some phobias are not acquired through associative learning. That is, for a phobia to occur, it is not necessary that the association be made between the initially neutral stimulus and perception of danger. This link is presumed to be automatic, that is, innate. What is there to support this theory?

In many instances of phobias, there is no recollection or report of a traumatic or any other contact with the phobic stimulus before the onset of phobia; patients with such phobias or their parents typically state that the phobia has "always" been present or that it has existed from the very first, nontraumatic contact with the stimulus. This pattern was observed in some instances of water phobia, phobia of heights, and spider phobia (Menzies and Clarke, 1993a, 1993b, 1995), but was extended to other types of fear, such as "stranger anxiety" and separation anxiety in infants, and fears of pain, strong noise, and sudden loss of physical balance. The underlying hypothesis invokes the concepts of natural selection, survival, and preservation of the species, assuming that our ancestors developed fears of naturally occurring dangers; these fears were then incorporated into a human genetic code and became part of the transgenerationally transmitted genetic material. As a result, the human infant is innately equipped to protect itself from dangers, and therefore avoids potentially dangerous stimuli without previously being in contact with them.

Although humans are "prepared" to fear and avoid stimuli such as water, heights, and the like, most do not develop a phobia because of habituation, that is, repeated nontraumatic exposure to the potentially phobic stimuli. Those who develop phobias as adults do so because of incomplete habituation, because their fears have been reinforced by their parents, or as a result of "dishabituation" in the context of stress (Menzies and Clarke, 1995).

PSYCHOLOGICAL MODELS

There are two main psychological models of the origin of specific phobias: the first encompasses various accounts derived from learning theory, whereas the second is the psychoanalytic account of phobias. The first model has been much more useful for clinical practice. The psychoanalytic model is included for historical reasons and has limited clinical relevance.

Models Derived From Learning Theory

Stated very broadly, all models of specific phobias derived from learning theory postulate that phobic manifestations are a consequence of learning. Another characteristic common to these models is a distinction between the factors that give rise to phobias and factors that are responsible for their maintenance. Phobic fears can be acquired through classical (traumatic) conditioning, vicariously (by observing emotional reactions and behavior of others), and by transmission of relevant information (Rachman, 1991). Phobias are maintained through avoidance by means of operant (instrumental) conditioning.

Classical (Pavlovian, Aversive, Traumatic) Conditioning

This is the oldest learning-theory account of the development of phobias. In essence, it conceptualizes phobia as a conditioned reflex. This was demonstrated through the case of "little Albert" by Watson and Rayner (1920). Albert was an 11-month-old boy who developed a phobia of white rats (initially a neutral, not an anxiety-provoking stimulus) after he had been repeatedly exposed to a white rat together with a loud noise (an aversive, unconditioned stimulus). Because the loud noise elicited an automatic, unconditioned fear response, its pairing with exposure to a white rat made Albert learn to fear white rats through association of the two. This fear then became a conditioned fear response to a newly conditioned stimulus (white rat). Albert not only showed fear every time he saw a white rat (without hearing a loud noise at the same time) but also had a fear reaction to other objects that resembled white rats, such as white rabbits and white fur coats. The latter phenomenon came to be known as the *generalization* of the phobic stimuli.

Many people develop phobias after classical conditioning, which is often traumatic in nature. A typical example is a phobia of dogs that develops after a dog attack. Likewise, a person who was stuck in an elevator may develop a phobia of elevators, and the person who had a sudden panic attack while driving may develop a phobia of driving. Phobias that occur as a result of traumatic conditioning tend to have an abrupt onset and are usually more severe; unlike phobias that appear through other mechanisms, these phobias occur at any age.

As demonstrated by one study among people who had had a traumatic experience with dogs, the number of those who did and did not develop a phobia of dogs was approximately the same (DiNardo et al., 1988). This suggests that other factors (e.g., genetic vulnerability, aspects of personality such as neuroticism, negative appraisals of the traumatic situation and/or of one's skills of coping with such a situation) may also contribute to the development of phobias.

Preparedness "Variant" of the Conditioning Theory

Proponents of the classical conditioning model had difficulty explaining the fact that out of the vast pool of potential phobic stimuli, only relatively few become the focus of phobias. In an attempt to overcome this limitation, Seligman (1971) suggested that phobic stimuli were not subject to random selection in the process of conditioning: humans are "prepared" to fear certain objects and/or situations because these stimuli indicated physical danger and a threat to survival to our ancestors (even though they do not necessarily represent such a threat today). Because phobias have a survival value, they are difficult to extinguish. This is the essence of the *preparedness theory* of fear acquisition. Its main tenets, however, have not been supported (e.g., McNally, 1987).

Vicarious (Observational) Learning

Phobias may be acquired through observation of another person's fearful behavior in a particular situation and the corresponding nonverbal cues. This is particularly common with children, who can learn from their parents to be afraid of certain animals or situations. Although parents do not tell their children that they have particular fears, children observe that their parents are afraid and adopt the same fear and fear-related behavior (e.g., avoidance) through imitation of or identification with their parents. Phobias that develop through this mechanism are usually less severe and are more easily subject to extinction than phobias acquired through traumatic conditioning.

Learning Through Transmission of Relevant Information

Phobias may also develop through direct transmission of information about the dangerousness of certain objects, situations, or phenomena. For example, many children are not afraid of dogs before their parents tell them that dogs are dangerous. Phobias that develop in this way tend to be less severe than phobias acquired through traumatic conditioning. The fear can be relatively easily dismissed with the acquisition of new information and maturation.

Operant (Instrumental) Conditioning

As already noted, operant conditioning explains the maintenance of phobias. According to a *two-factor theory* (Mowrer, 1960), fear initially develops
as a result of classical conditioning; in the second phase, fear is temporarily
reduced or eliminated by avoidance of the feared stimulus, and the phobia
is thereby maintained (operant conditioning). That is, the fear motivates a
person to look for means to reduce fear, and every behavior (e.g., avoidance) that succeeds in reducing fear is reinforced. However, phobic fear can
persist even in the absence of avoidance behavior. In these cases, factors that
perpetuate phobic fear include secondary gain, cognitive biases, and specific meaning or significance attached to the phobic stimuli.

Cognitive Factors in the Etiology and Pathogenesis of Specific Phobias

Similar to other anxiety disorders, specific phobias have been found to be
associated with biases in information processing, particularly biases in
attention and reasoning. Certain beliefs about phobic stimuli (e.g., beliefs
about their dangerousness as a consequence of the exaggerated perception
of threat) and beliefs that phobic individuals have about themselves (e.g.,
beliefs that they are not capable of coping with anxiety when facing their
phobic stimuli) may play an important role in maintaining phobias (e.g.,
Thorpe and Salkovskis, 1995). It is important to identify these beliefs and
challenge them in the course of treatment.

Psychoanalytic Approaches

The main tenet of the psychoanalytic theory of phobias is that there is some
fundamental anxiety behind every fear. Therefore, the therapist's task is to
uncover this fundamental anxiety and the associated intrapsychic conflicts;
without such an uncovering, the understanding of phobias is only super-
ficial. Moreover, if the conflicts are not resolved, the treatment may lead to a
replacement of one type of phobia with another ("symptom substitution"), a
claim that has generally not been supported by studies and clinical practice.

Freud (1909/1955a) illustrated the psychoanalytic approach to phobias
with the case of "little Hans." Freud proposed that Hans, who was frightened of horses, had, in fact, castration anxiety and was afraid of his father
because of the unconscious sexual longings for his mother. Thus, the unresolved Oedipal conflict was behind Hans' phobia of horses. Freud also
postulated specific defense mechanisms—displacement, symbolization,
and avoidance—that are used by people with phobia, with the goal of
defending the ego against the unacceptable sexual urges. Displacement
refers to transfer of the conflictual material to a neutral object, which has
no obvious relationship with the conflict but becomes a focus of the phobia.
The true nature of the person's anxiety is disguised through displacement.
The underlying issues are less concealed by the use of symbolization,

because some aspects of the phobic object or situation symbolize the original conflict.

Post-Freudian psychoanalysis considered some phobias to be related to conflicts originating from different developmental stages (e.g., pre-Oedipal) or to reflect superego anxiety. However, the original idea—that there is something "more fundamental" behind every phobia—has remained, despite the general lack of support for it. This idea has hindered, rather than fostered, further development of the psychoanalytic theory of phobia. Not surprisingly, patients with specific phobias as their main or sole problem are unlikely to be treated by psychoanalysts or psychodynamically oriented psychotherapists.

TREATMENT

It is practically impossible to treat specific phobias without some form of exposure. This is why behavior therapy has such an important role in treatment. Even Freud considered exposure necessary in the treatment of phobias, but exposure therapy has never been integrated with psychoanalysis or psychodynamic therapy.

The treatment of specific phobias to some extent depends on the type of phobia. It relies very much on patients' motivation, as patients may be more tempted than those with other disorders to give up treatment and return to their previous pattern of avoidance and phobia-constricted lifestyles. The main goals of treatment are alleviation of fear, disappearance of avoidance, and the consequent improvement in functioning.

BEHAVIORAL TREATMENTS

Main behavior therapy techniques for specific phobias have been systematic desensitization and exposure-based treatments (Table 5–5).

Table 5–5. Characteristics of Systematic Desensitization and Exposure-Based Treatments Used in Specific Phobias

Behavioral Techniques	Nature of Exposure	Rate of Exposure	Use of Relaxation
Systematic desensitization	Imaginal	Gradual	Yes
Standard exposure	In vivo, sometimes combined with imaginal, rarely imaginal alone	Gradual	No
Flooding	In vivo	Massive	No
Implosion therapy	Imaginal	Massive	No

Exposure in vivo appears to produce better results than imaginal and other exposure (e.g., Marks et al., 1971; Bourque and Ladouceur, 1980; Wolitzky-Taylor et al., 2008). Modifications of exposure-based treatments have been developed for use in certain types of phobias and/or for patients who cannot comply with the requirements of standard exposure. After the course of behavior therapy, treatment gains may be maintained, especially if patients continue to practice self-exposure. Long-term outcome of behavior therapy is less certain, as there may be a relatively high risk of relapse in specific phobias.

Systematic Desensitization

This technique, introduced by Wolpe (1958), was the first efficacious behavioral technique but is rarely used today. It consists of imaginal exposure to the phobic stimulus (i.e., active visualization of the phobic stimulus) while the patient is undergoing progressive muscle relaxation. Exposure is simultaneously combined with relaxation because of the presumed mechanism of reciprocal inhibition: fear-induced hyperactivity of the sympathetic nervous system is inhibited by activation of the parasympathetic nervous system through muscle relaxation. The repeated coupling of imaginal exposure and muscle relaxation leads to counterconditioning, so that the phobic stimulus elicits progressively less fear.

Systematic desensitization uses a hierarchy of phobic stimuli (see Chapter 2, Exposure-Based Therapy for Agoraphobia). The treatment starts with imaginal exposure to the phobic stimulus (or an aspect of the phobic stimulus) that is anticipated to produce the least amount of anxiety, and this exposure continues until the anxiety subsides substantially. The treatment then proceeds with imaginal exposure to the stimuli (or certain aspects of the stimuli) that are anticipated to elicit progressively more anxiety. This gradual approach to exposure, with the prior construction of a hierarchy of phobic stimuli, has been incorporated into various exposure-based treatments.

Exposure-Based Treatments

The type of exposure therapy used most commonly in the treatment of specific phobias is gradual exposure in vivo. It is performed in a manner very similar to that used in the treatment of agoraphobia and described in more detail in Chapter 2. Imaginal exposure sometimes precedes exposure in vivo or is conducted at the same time as exposure in vivo. Progressive muscle relaxation is usually not used during exposure in vivo, unless patients develop severe physical symptoms. Patients are exposed to various components of phobic stimuli in the gradual, hierarchy-based sequence. For example, patients with a dog phobia can be exposed to tapes of barking dogs and/or slides and videos in which dogs are presented in situations of increasing threat.

Exposure therapy is often combined with modeling, which requires the therapist to demonstrate to the patient how to make contact with the phobic stimulus (e.g., a spider) and then ask the patient to do the same. This procedure is often referred to as "therapist-directed exposure."

There has been a tendency to shorten exposure-based treatment without sacrificing its efficacy. For example, a single prolonged session (2–3 hours) of therapist-directed exposure, whether conducted individually (Öst, 1989) or in a group setting (Öst, 1996), was found to be as efficacious as self-exposure conducted over a longer period (Hellström and Öst, 1995). However, one meta-analysis has reported that multiple sessions of exposure therapy yield better results than one session, especially in the long run (Wolitzky-Taylor et al., 2008).

Massive, ungraded exposure therapy can be conducted in vivo (flooding) or through imagination (implosion therapy). Patients undergo exposure to the phobic stimulus (or aspect of the phobic stimulus) that elicits high levels of anxiety, usually in the presence of the therapist. These forms of exposure therapy are relatively rarely used because they tend to be poorly tolerated.

Avoidance prevents the person from learning that the phobic stimuli need not be feared because the anticipated, harmful outcomes do not occur. Exposure to the phobic stimuli is essential for habituation and other changes to take place, with the goal of extinguishing phobic fear and eliminating phobic avoidance (see Chapter 2 for discussion of mechanisms of change in the course of exposure therapy).

Modifications of Exposure Therapy for Specific Phobias

Exposure-based treatment has been modified for certain types of specific phobias. For example, in blood-injection-injury phobia, patients often fear fainting during exposure as much as they fear the actual phobic stimulus. To minimize the possibility of fainting during exposure, "applied tension" has been used: it requires patients to induce muscle tension during exposure because fainting is incompatible with the physiological correlates of tension (Öst and Sterner, 1987).

If the main underlying emotion is disgust rather than fear, treatment with exposure may not be sufficient because it takes longer for disgust to diminish (Smits et al., 2002; Olatunji et al., 2007). Adding other techniques (e.g., cognitive therapy) may be necessary in these cases.

Interoceptive exposure (described in Chapter 2) can be efficacious in treating claustrophobia (e.g., Booth and Rachman, 1992) because it targets fears of the anxiety symptoms (e.g., shortness of breath, dizziness, palpitations) that are often prominent in this type of phobia.

Virtual reality exposure therapy has been efficacious for phobias of flying (e.g., Rothbaum et al., 2000) and heights (e.g., Emmelkamp et al.,

2002), but this modification of exposure therapy needs further testing of efficacy and technical refinement to improve its delivery. Virtual reality exposure therapy might be a suitable option for patients who are reluctant to engage in exposure in vivo.

COGNITIVE THERAPY

Cognitive therapy techniques have been used less often to treat specific phobias than other anxiety disorders, perhaps because exposure-based treatment is so convincingly effective. Cognitive therapy may be more suitable for certain types of specific phobias, particularly those in which there is a prominent fear of anxiety symptoms. When used alone, cognitive therapy may be beneficial in treatment of claustrophobia (e.g., Booth and Rachman, 1992), and perhaps dental phobia (e.g., De Jongh et al., 1995). When added to exposure in vivo for claustrophobia, it may improve treatment outcome (Craske et al., 1995).

OTHER FORMS OF PSYCHOLOGICAL TREATMENT

Although exposure therapy is quite efficacious in the treatment of specific phobias (with response rates of up to 80%–90%), some patients find it too demanding, fail to maintain motivation for treatment, and/or are unable to complete the course of therapy. It is estimated that as many as 25%–50% of patients drop out of behavioral treatment of specific phobias (e.g., Prochaska, 1991). For patients who fail behavior therapy or are not sufficiently motivated for it, exploring other treatment options is worthwhile. These include supportive psychotherapy, hypnotherapy, eye movement desensitization and reprocessing (described in Chapter 7), and psychodynamic psychotherapy.

Supportive psychotherapy entails use of nonspecific measures to improve coping (e.g., provision of support and encouragement) as well as some nonsystematic use of the elements of exposure therapy. Results of hypnotherapy in the treatment of dental phobia have been mixed. A potential drawback of hypnotherapy is a tendency for treatment gains not to be maintained over time. The efficacy of eye movement desensitization and reprocessing in comparison with exposure in vivo has been questioned, but it may suit some patients with specific phobias.

As already noted, psychoanalysis and psychodynamic psychotherapy are rarely used in the treatment of specific phobias. The goal of these therapies is to uncover the underlying, unconscious problems and resolve the corresponding intrapsychic conflicts. Not only is there lack of evidence that these psychotherapies are efficacious for specific phobias, but they also do not appear to be a rational treatment choice for a relatively circumscribed problem for which brief, well-focused, and effective treatments exist.

PHARMACOLOGICAL AND COMBINED TREATMENT

Pharmacotherapy alone is not the treatment of choice for specific phobias. It may be used if patients cannot tolerate exposure-based treatments, if they are not motivated for behavioral therapy or other types of psychological therapy, or if these forms of treatment are not available. Pharmacotherapy may be useful in the treatment of patients with specific phobias who also have panic attacks. Medications with a fast onset of action, such as benzo-diazepines, may be used on an as-needed basis, usually before patients come in contact with the phobic stimulus. For example, patients with a phobia of flying can take a benzodiazepine before going to the airport or before boarding the plane. However, when used in this fashion, medica-tions are not to be taken frequently (e.g., several times during an episode of being in contact with the phobic stimulus or every time before exposure). In addition, patients should bear in mind that effects of such pharma-cotherapy are only short term.

Even when combined with behavioral therapy, benzodiazepines may not be particularly useful and fail to have long-term effects. Many behavior therapists advise against this combination, for reasons discussed elsewhere in this volume (see Chapter 2). However, benzodiazepines may be admi-nistered very cautiously during the initial phases of exposure treatment, with the goal of alleviating anxiety and facilitating exposure.

A novel way of combining behavioral therapy and medication in the treatment of specific phobias is through administration of D-cycloserine (DCS) 1–4 hours before exposure therapy sessions. Unlike benzodiazepines and antidepressants that have direct anxiolytic effects, DCS does not affect symptoms of anxiety and acts as a partial agonist at the N-methyl-D-aspartate (NMDA) glutamatergic receptor, which is believed to be critically involved in associative learning and memory. By doing so, DCS is thought to accelerate emotional learning and enhance the extinction of fear, which occurs during exposure therapy. Therefore, DCS may improve exposure therapy by both making it work faster and making it more effective. One controlled study found a combination of DCS and exposure therapy to be more efficacious than placebo combined with exposure for the phobia of heights (Ressler et al., 2004); another study, however, did not show super-iority of this combination in treating spider phobia (Guastella et al., 2007). There is a need for more research that would not only ascertain the useful-ness of this combination strategy but also clarify practical issues such as the optimal dose of DCS and the timing of its administration (i.e., how long before exposure).

OUTLOOK FOR THE FUTURE

While specific phobias are common in the general population, they are relatively rarely encountered in clinical settings. One way of interpreting this discrepancy is to assume that specific phobias represent a minor form of psychopathology, because most sufferers can apparently live without seeking help for it. The other interpretation is that people with specific phobias may feel embarrassed to seek help or that there are other impediments to their treatment. Regardless of the interpretation, there is a need to change the conceptualization of specific phobias.

One task here is to "legitimize" specific phobias by tightening the boundary with normal fears. Perhaps this can be done by using a diagnostic designation only for cases with *severe* phobic fear, *extensive* avoidance, and evidence of *substantial* distress or impairment caused by fear and/or avoidance. The other task is making an effort toward eliminating trivialization of the suffering and impaired functioning of people with specific phobias. A successful completion of these tasks would make it possible for both the sufferers and clinicians to take specific phobias seriously. And if they are taken seriously, they will no longer be relatively neglected by researchers.

Addressing the heterogeneity within specific phobias should receive priority because various types of phobias differ too much to be classified together. Understanding better the psychopathology and pathogenesis of various phobias would illuminate the relationships between them. Efforts to do this are already under way, for example, through research aimed at elucidating the role of disgust in some types of phobias. The putative dichotomy between disgust-driven and fear-driven phobias is not the only one; all distinctions that seem conceptually and clinically meaningful should be considered.

Exposure-based treatments for specific phobias are generally effective, but they need to become more accessible to sufferers. This implies greater use of the computer, Internet, and other modern technology. Treatments should also be adapted with the goal of improving compliance and minimizing dropout rates. Tendencies to shorten the therapy and pressure for treatments to be more cost-effective need to be balanced against evidence of efficacy of ultrabrief treatments and needs of many patients for a slower pace and greater attention to detail throughout treatment. Maintaining treatment gains is particularly important for phobias that are not likely to abate without treatment, and in these cases greater emphasis should be placed on ensuring the long-term benefit of exposure therapy and preventing relapse. Finally, exposure therapy needs to be modified for phobias that are more resistant to treatment; it remains to be ascertained whether adding cognitive or other techniques or pharmacotherapy in these situations would result in greater improvement.

6

Obsessive-Compulsive Disorder

As its name implies, the main characteristics of obsessive-compulsive disorder (OCD) are obsessions and/or compulsions. Different types of obsessions and compulsions make OCD a heterogeneous condition. Also, OCD exists on a continuum from mild cases to those with extremely severe and incapacitating manifestations generally not seen in other anxiety disorders. Clinical manifestations of OCD are striking and leave few people who observe them unimpressed. This is arguably due to the seriousness with which persons with OCD take their own obsessions and compulsions along with concurrent realization that these same obsessions and compulsions are senseless and should be gotten rid of. Indeed, there are few other examples in psychopathology where insight and deficiency of insight stand together, and where espousing and fighting the absurd are so intertwined. For all these reasons, OCD is often portrayed as a puzzling or intriguing disorder; in addition, it often represents a treatment challenge.

KEY ISSUES

Obsessive-compulsive disorder is probably the least controversial condition within the anxiety disorders because its clinical features are well described and relatively easily recognized and because hardly anyone doubts its existence as a psychopathological entity. What is controversial about OCD, however, is where it belongs and how it should be classified. This is a consequence of a number of features of OCD that make it look different from other anxiety disorders and of the close relationship that OCD has with some conditions outside of the realm of anxiety disorders. Listed below are a number of key questions about OCD.

1. In view of its different clinical features and the vastly different severity of these features, should OCD be considered a unitary condition or divided into subtypes?

2. If OCD is to be divided into subtypes, on the basis of what criteria should it be done? Types of obsessions and compulsions, reasons for performing compulsions, severity of illness, degree of insight, age of onset, or something else?
3. Should neutralizing responses other than compulsions be given a more prominent role in the description and conceptualization of OCD?
4. How does insight contribute to the conceptualization of OCD?
5. What are the core features of OCD? Is OCD primarily an affective disorder, is it characterized by a primary disturbance in thinking, or is it essentially a disorder of repetitive behaviors?
6. Is OCD an anxiety disorder or should it be classified as one of the obsessive-compulsive spectrum disorders?
7. Why is there a discrepancy between the advances in understanding of the neurobiological underpinnings of OCD and unsatisfactory effectiveness of biological treatments for OCD? How can specific anti-obsessional drugs be developed?
8. How can the cognitive and behavioral models of OCD be more effectively integrated with cognitive and behavioral treatments?
9. Considering a poor or partial response to treatment of many OCD patients, what is the way for results of treatment, both pharmacological and psychological, to be improved?

CLINICAL FEATURES

Typical clinical features of OCD include obsessions and overt (behavioral) compulsions. In addition to overt compulsions, patients with OCD may exhibit a range of other behaviors (e.g., avoidance and reassurance seeking) as well as use covert (mental, cognitive) compulsions in response to obsessions. All these behaviors and mental compulsions that appear in response to obsessions have been encompassed by the term *neutralization*. The purpose of neutralization is to alleviate anxiety or distress, "undo" obsessions, and/or prevent harm associated with obsessions. Thus, it would perhaps be more accurate to rename OCD as "obsessive-neutralizing disorder." The components of OCD are schematically presented in Figure 6–1.

Obsessions

Obsessions are usually defined as recurrent thoughts, impulses, and/or images that are experienced as uncontrollable. Also, they are not just excessive worries about real-life problems, and they cause marked anxiety or distress, so that a person feels compelled to "do something" with them, for example, attempt to ignore, suppress, or neutralize them or resist them in some other way. The other reason for this urge to do something with obsessions is that they are usually, though not invariably, experienced by the person as alien, intrusive, strange, "crazy," senseless, or inappropriate (ego-dystonic

Obsessions

- Causing anxiety or distress and/or
- Experienced as alien and/or harm-portending

↓

Neutralization

- Alleviating anxiety or distress and/or
- "Undoing" obsessions and/or
- Preventing harm associated with obsessions

↓   ↓

BEHAVIORAL   MENTAL (COGNITIVE)

1. Overt compulsions (rituals)   1. Covert (mental, cognitive) compulsions
2. Avoidance   (rituals)
3. Reassurance seeking

Figure 6–1. Components of obsessive-compulsive disorder.

obsessions). The person experiencing ego-dystonic obsessions is regarded as having good insight. Poor insight is exhibited by individuals who do not experience and recognize obsessions as unacceptable, senseless, or unreasonable (ego-syntonic obsessions). In such cases, it should be ascertained whether beliefs related to these phenomena are overvalued ideas or even delusions. The characteristics of obsessions are summarized in Table 6–1.

Table 6–1. Characteristics of Obsessions

- Thoughts, impulses, and/or images
- Recurrent
- Uncontrollable
- Not just excessive worries about real-life problems
- Cause marked anxiety or distress
- Usually (though not invariably) experienced or recognized by the person as alien, intrusive, strange, "crazy," senseless, or inappropriate ("ego-dystonic") and portending harm
- The person feels compelled to "do something" with obsessions—attempt to ignore, suppress, or neutralize them or resist them in some other way—to achieve one or more of the following goals:

  1. Alleviate anxiety or distress
  2. "Undo" obsessions because of their alien or "dangerous" nature
  3. Prevent harm associated with obsessions

It is important to distinguish between obsessions, normal intrusive thoughts, mental compulsions, worries (such as those found in generalized anxiety disorder), ruminations (e.g., ruminations encountered in depressed persons), other types of intrusive thoughts (e.g., trauma-related intrusions in posttraumatic stress disorder), overvalued ideas (e.g., those seen in hypochondriasis, body dysmorphic disorder, or anorexia nervosa), and delusions (as part of a psychotic illness). These phenomena are often repetitive; some are experienced as intrusive, uncontrollable, and/or distressing whereas others are associated with an urge to do something in response to their content or as a result of the way in which they are experienced. The features of other phenomena that distinguish them from obsessions are shown in Table 6–2.

Compulsions

Compulsions are defined as repetitive behaviors (overt compulsions) or unobservable mental acts (covert, mental, or cognitive compulsions) that are performed in response to an obsession and often according to strict rules; the purpose of compulsions is to alleviate anxiety or distress, "undo" obsessions, and/or prevent harm associated with obsessions. Although compulsions usually produce some relief, they have to be performed over and over again because this relief does not last very long. Over time, the person may start believing that a dreaded event has not happened because he or she is performing the compulsion. In such cases, the person may adopt a belief that a failure to perform a compulsion would have disastrous consequences, and this belief may then become the main reason for performing the compulsion.

Patients with OCD typically report that they feel driven to perform compulsions, but this urge is subjective and patients do not really "have" to perform them. Stated otherwise, unlike obsessions that are intrusive and thus not a product of free will, compulsions are initiated and performed voluntarily and are under patients' control (although on casual inspection it may not seem like that). The term *ritual* is often used interchangeably with compulsion, but more precisely, the ritual refers to a stereotyped act (whether overt or covert) that is performed in accordance with strict and rigid rules. Characteristics of compulsions are summarized in Table 6–3.

A distinction should be made between "classical," obsession-driven compulsions and compulsions driven by the "sensory phenomena" ("not-just-right experiences" and sense of incompleteness; Miguel et al., 2000; Coles et al., 2003), sometimes referred to as "impulsions" (Shapiro and Shapiro, 1992), and impulsive behavior (Table 6–4).

Mental (covert) compulsions are frequently encountered among patients with OCD, but they may be difficult to recognize because they are unobservable, "invisible" mental acts; hence, the term *covert compulsions*. Examples include silent counting in a certain way, performing of other operations with numbers, imagining a particular situation, repeating a thought a certain

Table 6–2. Distinguishing Between Obsessions and Related Phenomena

Normal Intrusive Thoughts

- Not interpreted in a harm-portending or catastrophic way (i.e., not assuming that they make certain fearful events more likely or suggesting something very negative about the person experiencing them) and no particular meaning is attached to them (e.g., that the person is responsible for having these thoughts and for any consequences that may arise from them should he or she fail to take action to neutralize them)

- No attempt to ignore, suppress, or neutralize them; usually not resisted

Mental Compulsions

- Initiated voluntarily and, thus, under the person's control

- Occur in response to obsessions, with the purpose of alleviating anxiety or distress caused by obsessions, "undoing" obsessions, and/or preventing harm

Pathological Worry

- Content pertains to real-life problems, without reference to something abhorrent or shameful and one's personal responsibility for worrying; usually future-oriented

- Not experienced as alien, "crazy," senseless, or inappropriate

Depressive Ruminations

- Content pertains to themes of loss or personal failure; usually past-oriented

- Not experienced as alien, "crazy," senseless, or inappropriate

- No attempt to ignore, suppress, or neutralize them; usually not resisted

Trauma-Related Intrusions (as in posttraumatic stress disorder)

- Monothematic and highly specific: content pertains to a particular traumatic event

- Not experienced as alien, "crazy," senseless, or inappropriate

Overvalued Ideas

- Held with relatively strong conviction, but can be shakable

- Not held on the basis of delusional evidence (explanation for having these ideas may be plausible)

- Not experienced as alien, "crazy," senseless, or inappropriate

- No attempt to ignore, suppress, or neutralize them; usually not resisted

Delusions

- Fixed, unshakable beliefs, without the person experiencing uncertainty and doubt about their validity

- Often held on the basis of delusional evidence (explanation for having delusions is not plausible and suggests loss of reality testing)

- Not experienced as alien, "crazy," senseless, or inappropriate

- No attempt to ignore, suppress, or neutralize them; usually not resisted

Table 6–3. Characteristics of Compulsions

- Overt behaviors or unobservable mental acts (covert compulsions, mental compulsions, cognitive compulsions) that the person feels driven to perform in response to an obsession and often according to strict rules
- Repetitive
- The purpose of compulsions is one or more of the following:

  1. Alleviation of anxiety or distress caused by obsession (but compulsions are performed excessively and repeatedly without achieving this goal in the long run)

  2. "Undoing" of obsession (although compulsions cannot realistically do that)

  3. Prevention of harm associated with the obsession (although compulsions cannot realistically do that)

Table 6–4. Distinguishing Between Compulsions, "Impulsions," and Impulsive Acts

"Impulsions" (compulsions driven by "not-just-right experiences" and sense of incompleteness)
- Occur in response to a sensation or an urge (not in response to a clear-cut obsession)
- Performed with the purpose of achieving a sense of completion, relief, or satisfaction and until the person feels "just right" or satisfied

Impulsive Acts
- Performed in response to an urge or tension
- Performed to provide relief, pleasure, or gratification (reward-seeking behaviors)

number of times, recalling the "right" thought, and praying. If patients do not mention spontaneously that they perform mental compulsions, it is useful to ask how they cope with a particular obsession (which they previously had volunteered to reveal) or what they do to alleviate their distress about having such an obsession. The common feature of mental compulsions is their purpose to alleviate obsession-induced anxiety or distress, "undo" obsession, and/or prevent harm by nonbehavioral means.

As is the case with overt compulsions, it is important to understand the purpose of covert compulsions by asking patients why they are performing them. Prevention of harm in the future is a common reason for the use of covert compulsions. For example, a patient with an obsession that her parents would die every time she saw vehicle license plates with digits that added up to an even number "had" to look for license plates where the corresponding sum was an odd number. The purpose of this concealed compulsive activity was to "prevent" her parents' death.

Avoidance

Avoidance is commonly used for coping with some obsessions, as it is for coping with phobic fears; this is achieved through a temporary alleviation of anxiety. Unlike compulsions, avoidance cannot "undo" an obsession and except in relatively few circumstances (e.g., avoidance of driving for fear of having an urge to drive the car off the road), it is not bestowed with the power of preventing some dreadful event in the future. Therefore, avoidance is often used as a first-line response to obsessions that are not experienced as threatening to the extent that further measures need to be taken against them, at least initially. For example, a regular churchgoing patient with an obsession involving an image of him shouting blasphemous sentences in church avoided church services. When he had to attend a service and could not resort to avoidance, he was compelled to come up with other means of coping with his obsession and developed a covert compulsion.

Reassurance Seeking

Reassurance seeking is also a commonly used measure against obsessions and serves the purpose of alleviating anxiety, albeit temporarily. Like avoidance, it cannot prevent harm, and is often used in a way analogous to that in which avoidance is used. However, obtaining reassurance may "undo" the reassurance-related obsession, at least temporarily. Another difference is that reassurance seeking depends on someone else—the person willing to provide reassurance—whereas avoidance is independent of others.

Reassurance seeking is often related to checking compulsions and may be resorted to instead of checking or alternatively with checking. Whereas checking can be both past- and future-oriented and thus used in a variety of situations and serve different purposes (see Pathological Doubt, Checking, and Reassurance Seeking, below), reassurance seeking is more restricted in its scope and effects in that it is mainly past-oriented (i.e., reassurance is sought about something that has or has not occurred in the past, for example, whether the patient hit a pedestrian while driving or whether he or she was infected with HIV).

Insight

As already noted, a realization by patients with OCD that their obsessions are alien, intrusive, strange, "crazy," senseless, irrational, or inappropriate is referred to as "insight." Only patients who have good insight will have a need to ignore, suppress, neutralize, or resist their obsessions. Patients with OCD who do not experience their obsessions as alien, "crazy," senseless, irrational, or inappropriate and therefore do not resist them, and who have certain beliefs attached to their obsessions or compulsions, may, in fact, exhibit overvalued ideas in addition to obsessions (see Table 6–2). For example, a patient with obsessions about someone breaking into his house who believed that he had to check the locks on the doors and windows in a certain sequence to ensure that his home would not be broken into did not resist checking at all. He could be characterized as having poor insight. He acknowledged, however, that his belief was "unusual," while not finding it unreasonable or senseless, because he thought that his checking compulsion actually prevented burglary. Labeling this clinical presentation as poor-insight OCD does not refer to any OCD-related beliefs that may be held with varying degrees of insight.

It is now widely accepted that the presence of insight in OCD is a matter of degree, with some OCD patients having very good insight on one side of the continuum, and others, at the other extreme, having no insight at all (Insel and Akiskal, 1986; Kozak and Foa, 1994). This distribution of insight in OCD patients has been highlighted by a study that found excellent insight in 48% of patients, good insight in 21.5%, moderate insight in 15.5%, poor insight in 10%, and no insight in 5% (Marazziti et al., 2002).

While the continuum conceptualization of insight takes into account the multidimensional nature of the construct of insight, it does not resolve the conceptual problem of OCD with poor insight. For example, do OCD patients with poor insight represent a distinct subgroup that differs from OCD patients with good insight in respects other than insight? Some studies (e.g., Marazziti et al., 2002) have reported that this is not the case, whereas others suggest that OCD with poor insight is more likely to be associated with certain types of obsessions and compulsions—for example, hoarding (Frost et al., 1996). Moreover, does OCD with poor insight predict a response to treatment? Again, the answers are equivocal: while hoarding (as a typical representative of poor-insight OCD) generally implies a poorer response to treatment (e.g., Black et al., 1998; Winsberg et al., 1999), no relationship between the degree of insight and treatment outcome was reported in another study (Eisen et al., 2001). Clinical experience does suggest, however, that the treatment of poor-insight patients tends to be more complex, often requiring modifications to standard treatment of OCD. Finally, is OCD with poor insight associated with psychotic illness? While OCD patients with co-occurring psychotic illness often have poor insight with regard to OCD, poor-insight OCD is not necessarily associated with psychosis nor with any history of psychotic symptoms (e.g., Marazziti et al., 2002). These issues need to be resolved to clarify the role of insight in qualifying OCD.

Types of Obsessions and Compulsions

The most common types of obsessions and compulsions are listed in Table 6-5. Patients with OCD usually have both obsessions and compulsions, although one or the other component of OCD may predominate at any point in time, giving an impression that a person is experiencing obsessions only or exhibiting only compulsions. In fact, OCD with "pure" obsessions (without compulsions) and OCD with "pure" compulsions (without obsessions) seem to be rare, with the frequency of the former being 8.5% and frequency of the latter being 0.5% in one sample of OCD patients (Foa and Kozak, 1995).

The themes of obsessions and the types of compulsions may vary over time, a pattern reported by 60% of OCD patients in one long-term, follow-up study (Skoog and Skoog, 1999). Sometimes these changing obsessions and compulsions appear to be related; for example, there seemed to be an underlying theme of perfectionism in a patient who presented with doubting obsessions and indecisiveness at one time, and repetitive rituals of rearranging objects so that they would "look right" at another time. Studies have shown that over time, adult patients tend to maintain symptoms within the same subtype, that is, with similar obsessions and/or compulsions (Mataix-Cols et al., 2002a; Rufer et al., 2005).

Multiple obsessions and compulsions are very common (Table 6–5). Some patients with this presentation may seem to have only one type of obsession and/or compulsion because that is the most troubling one to them; they do not mention spontaneously other obsessions or compulsions if they are not asked about them.

Attempts have been made to classify obsessions and compulsions in several groups on the basis of their theme or content and other characteristics. Phenomenological or symptom subtypes of OCD have been proposed, with these subtypes also having in common other features and distinct patterns of response to treatment. There has

Table 6–5. Common Types of Obsessions and Compulsions

Obsessions	Frequency* (%)	Compulsions	Frequency* (%)
Multiple obsessions	72	Checking	61
Contamination	50	Multiple compulsions	58
Pathological doubt	42	Washing, cleaning	50
Somatic	33	Counting	36
Need for symmetry	32	Need to ask or confess	34
Aggressive	31	Need for symmetry or precision, rearranging objects	28
Sexual	24	Hoarding	18

*Frequency data are from Rasmussen and Eisen (1992).

been a mixed support for these attempts at classification, partly because many OCD patients have obsessions and compulsions from various putative subtypes and also because the underlying psycho-pathological mechanisms are often the same regardless of the subtype. Still, various types of obsessions and compulsions seem to be associated with certain specific features (Table 6–6). The most common obsessions and compulsions are described and their relative specificities reviewed in the text below.

Contamination, Washing, and Cleaning

Contamination obsessions are among the most frequent in patients with OCD. Their main underlying theme is a fear of being contaminated through germs, dirt, bodily secretions and excretions, or in some other way. Contamination fears may be connected with fears of certain diseases, particularly infectious illnesses, because of the way they spread. These fears may also be related to a strong feeling of disgust about human secretions and excretions or potentially contaminated objects.

Patients with contamination obsessions are preoccupied with distressing and frightening thoughts or images of being infected or dirty as a result of having been in contact with supposedly contaminated objects or people. Because of these obsessions, patients become hypervigilant about any possibility of contamination and may first attempt to avoid and prevent every contact with the perceived sources of contamination. Thus, they may try to open the doorknob with gloves on their hands or by using elbows rather than hands; other examples are placing a handkerchief over a pay phone while using it or avoiding a handshake. Patients may involve other people in their "preventative measures," for example, by asking them to first wash their hands when they come for a visit or by requesting that their children follow a strict code of hygiene.

If patients feel that they have inadvertently been in contact with the contaminated object or person, they will feel even more distress, often because of an underlying assumption "once in contact, always in contact." The urge to wash or clean serves the purpose of "getting rid" of the contaminating material, but this material may spread and always "remain around." Many patients are very distressed about this uncertainty of the extent of contamination and have the corresponding doubts ("what else might be contaminated?"). The ultimate goal of washing or cleaning is to prevent harm, that is, not becoming sick through contamination or preventing an illness from spreading. This is a "classic" contamination-decontamination type of OCD (Feinstein et al., 2003) in which contamination obsessions are associated with harm (e.g., becoming sick or spreading an illness), and washing or cleaning compulsions serve the purpose of preventing that harm (in addition to alleviating distress or anxiety). The washing and cleaning compulsions need to be performed for as long as patients feel contaminated or dirty, and this may take

Table 6–6. Characteristics Associated With Various Types of Obsessions and Compulsions

Types of Obsessions and Compulsions	Characteristics
Contamination obsessions, washing and cleaning compulsions	– Excessive fear of diseases
	– Extreme washing can lead to dermatitis
	– Washing and cleaning compulsions are usually performed with the purpose of preventing harm
	– Washing and cleaning compulsions may also be performed to reduce distress about feeling contaminated, and these are usually related to excessive feeling of disgust
Doubting obsessions, checking, and reassurance seeking	– Perhaps "generic" features of OCD (present in various types of obsessions and compulsions)
	– Often associated with inflated responsibility for potentially catastrophic outcomes, exaggerated appraisal of harm, intolerance of uncertainty, and memory distrust
Symmetry, ordering, and arranging obsessions and compulsions (including touching, tapping, counting, and repeating)	– Compulsions are usually driven by "sensory phenomena" ("not-just-right experiences" and sense of incompleteness)
	– Related to perfectionist tendencies or obsessions
	– Often associated with "obsessional slowness"
	– Often experienced as ego-syntonic
	– Early onset
	– Frequent co-occurrence with Tourette's disorder and chronic tic disorder
	– Treatment outcome less favorable
Sexual, aggressive, and religious obsessions and compulsions	– Main underlying theme: fear of losing control over one's behavior and thus revealing a shameful or abhorrent content of obsessions
	– Overt compulsions less likely (and hence the frequent but erroneous term "pure obsessions")
	– Often associated with the relatively specific appraisals of and/or beliefs about obsessions
Hoarding	– Often performed automatically (without a clear purpose)
	– Associated with poor insight, more personality disturbance (including schizotypal personality disorder), and greater severity of OCD
	– Tends to respond poorly to standard treatments for OCD and to have poorer prognosis
	– Separate psychopathological entity from OCD?

a very long time (e.g., several hours). Episodes of washing may also be relatively brief, but have to be repeated many times throughout the day.

In another "type" of OCD with contamination obsessions and washing or cleaning compulsions, there is mainly a discomfort or distress about feeling contaminated or not clean (Feinstein et al., 2003). Patients then engage in excessive cleaning or washing to reduce the feeling of contamination and not to prevent any particular contamination-related harm. These patients seem to have strong feelings of disgust (Tsao and McKay, 2004).

To ensure getting clean, some patients use strong and obviously inappropriate cleaning devices while washing their hands, such as detergents or bleach; others rub their hands or other body parts so much that they damage the skin, sometimes creating severe lesions and causing dermatitis. In the latter case, it is important to ascertain whether washing compulsions have an additional purpose, for example, self-punishment for imagined or real wrongdoing. Sometimes washing has a symbolic meaning, as an expression of the need to atone for aggressive, sexually unacceptable, or other inappropriate acts, or to "undo" such acts, regardless of whether these have been committed in fantasy or reality. Harsh and very concrete washing and cleaning rituals (e.g., cleaning completely, until the skin starts bleeding) often indicate the presence of a significant underlying psychopathology, such as severe personality disturbance or even psychosis.

Although washing and cleaning compulsions are usually related to contamination obsessions, they may subsequently run their own course or be unrelated to such obsessions even from the onset of OCD. Thus, patients may develop a compulsion to wash a certain number of times not necessarily because that would cleanse them from germs but because that number has a special significance for them and patients fear the consequences of not only washing less but also of washing more. Magical thinking is the basis for such ritualized compulsions, and compulsions then serve the purpose of preventing a dreaded, noncontamination-related catastrophe.

Pathological Doubt (Doubting Obsessions), Checking, and Reassurance Seeking

Checking compulsions are often associated not only with pathological doubt and doubting obsessions but also with a range of other OCD phenomena. For example, patients with contamination fears commonly check whether their surroundings have been contaminated. Likewise, pathological doubt is commonly present in patients with other manifestations of OCD. These patients are rarely sure about anything and it is easy for a seed of doubt to be planted in their mind, regardless of whether their primary concern is contamination, sexual obsessions, or something else. Thus, pathological doubt and checking compulsions can be considered to be "generic" features of OCD, which characterize a variety of its putative subtypes.

In very broad terms, obsessional self-doubt pertains to a person's recurrent and tormenting feeling that something about him or her is "not right." This feeling may refer to various aspects of the person's personality, behavior, thinking, physical appearance, or health. Self-doubt is often associated with uncertainty as to whether the person has done something or not. This uncertainty and inflated sense of responsibility often lead to checking compulsions. They may serve several purposes: alleviating distress or anxiety, "making sure" that there is no reason for further doubting, abolishing uncertainty, and reassuring oneself that one will not be held responsible in case of an accident or other mishap. The latter is particularly evident when checking is future-oriented. For example, if a burglary occurs after the person has checked five times that all the doors and windows are locked, the expectation is that the person will be less likely to hold himself or herself responsible; likewise, in case of fire, the person who has made sure that all the electrical and gas appliances have been turned off and unplugged would feel safe in that he or she has not made the fire more likely. When performed ritualistically and driven by magical thinking, future-oriented checking compulsions serve the purpose of preventing future harm or "undoing" the corresponding obsession.

Checking compulsions that are more past-oriented are related to excessive reassurance seeking and serve the purpose of alleviating anxiety and diminishing the burden of responsibility for something that patients suspect they have or have not done. Sometimes, this checking and reassurance have the effect of temporarily "undoing" the underlying obsession. For example, patients who are uncertain in a quasi-delusional way as to whether they have committed a crime will constantly check and/or ask for reassurance that they did not do that. They are relieved when they find out or are told that nothing dreadful happened and may feel that the underlying obsessional doubt has been abolished; however, these effects of checking and reassurance do not last very long. Another example of pathological doubt, intolerance of uncertainty, reassurance seeking, and checking compulsions can be found among some patients with somatic obsessions and hypochondriasis, as their doubts and uncertainty pertain to their health.

Like washing and cleaning compulsions, checking compulsions may become increasingly complex over time so that they must be performed in a certain, strictly specified way and/or a certain number of times. Because of the prominent magical thinking behind such checking, any deviation from the rules of the ritual is then believed to have some dreaded consequence. This makes the patient feel even more responsible for precise, ritualistic performance of the compulsion.

Checking compulsions have been associated with several abnormalities in the domain of appraisals, beliefs, and other cognitive phenomena and processes (see Etiology and Pathogenesis, below). These include inflated responsibility for potentially catastrophic outcomes (Salkovskis, 1985), exaggerated appraisal of harm (Rachman, 2002), intolerance of uncertainty (Tolin et al., 2003), and memory distrust (van den Hout and Kindt, 2003a).

Need for Symmetry, Rearranging Objects, and Perfectionism (Symmetry, Ordering, and Arranging Obsessions and Compulsions)

The dominant clinical manifestation of some patients with OCD is a preoccupation with rearranging objects so that they follow a certain pattern, usually a symmetrical or balancing one (for example, balancing the shape and color of objects). The compulsion to rearrange objects occurs in response to an obsession about objects having to be arranged in a certain pattern, order, or sequence. This compulsion is usually preceded by discomfort and tension about objects not being arranged in the "right" way and is therefore performed with the purpose of alleviating discomfort and tension (Rasmussen and Eisen, 1991). Typically, patients state that they have an urge to move objects not because they attempt to prevent some harm but because the way in which objects are arranged "just doesn't feel right" or creates a sense of incompleteness (Summerfeldt, 2004). In other words, their compulsions are driven by "sensory phenomena" ("not-just-right experiences" and sense of incompleteness; Miguel et al., 2000; Coles et al., 2003). Accordingly, patients continue moving and rearranging objects until they are arranged in a way that "feels right." Therefore, these compulsions often resemble "impulsions" or may be indistinguishable from them (see Compulsions, above). A related type of compulsion is doing something (typically touching, tapping, or counting) or repeating one's movements in a specific pattern.

It is often difficult to understand what constitutes a pattern that is "just right." One possibility is that it reflects a peculiar and highly idiosyncratic tendency toward perfectionism or obsessions related to perfectionism. This is supported by clinical observations that, like perfection, finding the "right" pattern is very hard, with patients spending a lot of time trying to find one with which they would be satisfied. When this type of compulsion is combined with pathological doubt and checking, it may be almost impossible to complete tasks. Patients then appear extremely slow, a phenomenon referred to as "primary obsessional slowness" (Rachman and Hodgson, 1980).

Patients with symmetry, ordering, and arranging obsessions and compulsions tend to experience their obsessions and compulsions as more egosyntonic (Eisen et al., 2006) and seek help less often (Mayerovitch et al., 2003). The onset of OCD is usually earlier in these patients (e.g., Mataix-Cols et al., 1999; Rosario-Campos et al., 2001). This is the type of OCD that more frequently co-occurs with Tourette's disorder and chronic tic disorder (Baer, 1994; Leckman et al., 1994; Miguel et al., 1995; Mataix-Cols et al., 1999). The primary obsessional slowness has been associated with poor response to both pharmacotherapy and behavior therapy, and the presence of symmetry, ordering, and arranging obsessions and compulsions generally indicates a less favorable treatment outcome (e.g., Starcevic and

Brakoulias, 2008). Less often, when compulsions of rearranging objects are connected through magical thinking with some imagined catastrophic outcome, they are performed with the purpose of preventing harm. This is done in a ritualized manner and a strictly specified sequence for fear of harmful consequences if the compulsion is performed incorrectly. In these situations, patients also have an inflated sense of responsibility for preventing the feared catastrophe.

Sexual, Aggressive, and Religious Obsessions and Compulsions

Sexual and aggressive obsessions are probably the most unpleasant and most frightening of all obsessions. Patients with these obsessions are usually afraid that they might behave in a sexually inappropriate manner or hurt and even kill their family members, friends, co-workers, or mere bystanders. Patients with sexual obsessions are typically concerned that they might become sexually disinhibited, behave in a sexually "perverted" manner and have sex with a family member or someone outside marriage, or have a sexual relationship not consistent with their sexual orientation. The feared aggressive behavior might be only verbal, so that patients are concerned that they might swear at someone or shout. Sometimes, patients are obsessively preoccupied with thoughts or images of harming or killing themselves.

The main theme underlying sexual and aggressive obsessions is a fear of losing control over one's behavior; a possibility of losing control makes sexual and aggressive obsessions even more distressing. Since patients are plagued by doubt as to whether they will remain in control, they often take measures to prevent the dreaded sexual or aggressive act. They usually do so by avoiding people with whom they might have a sexual encounter or by removing from their home all objects that could be used as weapons (typically all sharp objects such as knives and scissors). These patients are less likely to exhibit overt compulsions but may respond to their obsessions with covert compulsions (serving the purpose of preventing harm, that is, loss of control). Therefore, the term *pure obsessions*, often used to refer to this type of OCD, is not a correct designation.

It is even more troublesome when patients have sexual or aggressive obsessions that they have already committed a crime (e.g., robbed a bank, killed someone, or sexually molested a child), had an extramarital affair, or behaved otherwise in a sexually inappropriate manner. These patients repeatedly ask for reassurance that this did not happen or check whether it did happen. In more severe cases, patients are plagued by guilt and a need to be punished and may confess their "wrongdoing" to their close friend or turn themselves in to the police, admitting their crime. This type of obsession may be associated with beliefs that seem delusional in quality.

Because of the abhorrent nature of sexual and aggressive obsessions and the fact that themes of most of them are socially unacceptable, patients with these obsessions often feel guilty for having them. The guilt can also drive patients to come up with compulsions (usually covert) that would "undo" obsessions: this elimination of obsessions liberates patients from guilt, albeit temporarily. For example, a patient with an obsession about exposing himself sexually developed a mental compulsion that consisted of imagining himself dead; his understanding of this compulsion was as follows: "If I am dead, I can't have these terrible thoughts. Therefore, such thoughts do not exist."

Religious obsessions are related to sexual and aggressive obsessions in that they are usually embarrassing or shameful and embody the notion of the threatened loss of control. Patients with religious obsessions are often concerned that they might utter something blasphemous in public situations and places of worship or during religious ceremonies. The reasons for having these obsessions may or may not pertain to the person's attitudes toward religion and related matters. Compulsions that appear in response to religious obsessions often serve the purpose of "undoing" these obsessions and thereby preventing harm. Such compulsions are not necessarily religious in nature.

Religious compulsions may be difficult to recognize when they resemble sanctioned religious rituals. A clinician should have good understanding of the religious beliefs and rituals to be able to separate what is "normal" from what is a manifestation of OCD. Religious compulsions are usually excessive, often far above and beyond everything that institutionalized religions prescribe; also, they tend to be performed in ways that are unusual, even for the most devout worshipers. Religious compulsions are performed for various reasons: their purpose may be to alleviate distress as well as "undo" the underlying obsession and prevent the imagined harm.

The cognitive model of OCD has shed some light on aggressive, sexual, and religious obsessions (see Etiology and Pathogenesis, below). These obsessions have been associated with appraisals or beliefs that intrusive thoughts are important and with catastrophic appraisals of a failure to control such thoughts (Freeston et al., 1996; Obsessive Compulsive Cognitions Working Group, 1997). In addition, aggressive, sexual, and religious obsessions may be even more distressing if they are associated with beliefs that having unacceptable or immoral thoughts is morally wrong or that having some thoughts increases the likelihood that certain frightening events will occur (Shafran et al., 1996).

Hoarding

Hoarding is characterized by excessive collection and storage of objects that do not have any market or personal (sentimental or otherwise) value. Persons who hoard are usually unable to discard such objects. As with many other manifestations of OCD, hoarding is encountered on a spectrum from very mild to extreme, when the person seems completely preoccupied with the hoarding activity. In the most severe cases, there is no room to store any more objects and the home of the affected person is extremely unkempt.

Hoarding is an unusual compulsion in that it is often not preceded by or associated with corresponding obsessions. Also, the act of hoarding does not bring about an obvious decrease in anxiety and discomfort, although attempts to prevent hoarding are usually met with resistance. Unlike some other compulsions, hoarding rarely seems to have a symbolic meaning and is not performed with the purpose of averting some catastrophe. The reason for hoarding can sometimes be found in the belief that the collected items will have value in the future or be important in some other way (e.g., in case of shortages). However, many patients who hoard are unable to explain why they do it, other than stating that they "just have to do it." Therefore, hoarding often appears to be an automatic activity.

Hoarding is usually accompanied by poor insight (Frost et al., 2000; Samuels et al., 2007) and, therefore, patients do not tend to resist it and are generally less motivated for treatment. Hoarding is commonly associated with personality disturbance, including schizotypal personality disorder, and greater overall severity of OCD (Frost et al., 2000; Samuels et al., 2007).

Hoarding is a less frequent manifestation of OCD and may also be seen in persons with obsessive-compulsive personality disorder and other conditions (e.g., some psychotic and "organic" mental disorders). It is not always easy to determine whether hoarding is a part of OCD or obsessive-compulsive personality disorder. In OCD, there are usually other obsessions and/or compulsions and hoarding directly interferes with functioning, whereas hoarding as part of obsessive-compulsive personality disorder does not contribute significantly to the overall impairment associated with that condition.

Hoarding in OCD appears to have unfavorable treatment implications as it tends to respond poorly to selective serotonin reuptake inhibitors, clomipramine, various forms of cognitive-behavior therapy, and combinations of these treatments (e.g., Starcevic and Brakoulias, 2008). Animal models have shown that the dopaminergic system may play an important role in hoarding (Stein DJ et al., 1999), which supports augmentation of a selective serotonin reuptake inhibitor or clomipramine with antipsychotic drugs (acting as dopamine receptor antagonists) in the treatment of OCD patients with hoarding.

The status of hoarding in the classification of mental disorders remains uncertain. It is recognized that hoarding differs in important ways from most other manifestations of OCD, but the proposed options for its conceptualization and classification are somewhat divergent. While in some instances, hoarding may be a symptom subtype of OCD, in others it may be a separate syndrome, which could be classified as one of the putative obsessive-compulsive spectrum disorders (Pertusa et al., 2008). Other research has not found evidence of a specific relationship between hoarding and OCD, calling into question the notion that hoarding is a specific manifestation of OCD and suggesting that hoarding should be regarded more broadly, as a set of behaviors that appears in conjunction with OCD and other disorders (Abramowitz et al., 2008).

RELATIONSHIP BETWEEN OBSESSIVE-COMPULSIVE DISORDER AND OTHER DISORDERS

Obsessive-compulsive disorder tends to co-occur or be associated with several other disorders. The relationship with depression and psychotic illness is particularly important because of the implications for clinical practice. In addition, OCD may co-occur with tic disorders, personality disturbance, and several other anxiety disorders. The concept of obsessive-compulsive spectrum disorders was proposed to emphasize the similarities between OCD and a number of other conditions. Clinical implications of the relationship between OCD and other disorders are summarized in Table 6–7.

Obsessive-Compulsive Disorder and Depression

Obsessive-compulsive disorder and depression commonly occur together. One study showed that 67% of patients with OCD had a lifetime diagnosis of major depression, whereas 31% were currently depressed (Rasmussen and Eisen, 1988). In most patients, depression seems to follow OCD, perhaps as a result of the demoralizing effects of long-lasting OCD. Consequently, patients with an early onset and chronic course of OCD may be more likely to develop depression.

The relationship between OCD and depression may be quite complex. Obsessions and compulsions may become more or less prominent during a major depressive episode. Depressive ruminations sometimes resemble obsessions, and it is important to distinguish between the two (Table 6–2). Co-occurring major depression does not necessarily have a negative impact on the pharmacotherapy (Denys et al., 2003a) and behavior therapy (Foa et al., 1984; Basoglu et al., 1988; O'Sullivan et al., 1991) of OCD. A more severe depression, however, is likely to interfere with behavior therapy of OCD (Foa et al., 1981, 1983; Keijsers et al., 1994; Abramowitz et al., 2000).

Obsessive-Compulsive Disorder and Psychotic Illness

An important relationship exists between OCD and psychotic illness. This link appears particularly strong in adolescents who initially present with OCD or an OCD-like picture but then go on to develop a psychosis. It comes as no surprise, then, that it was believed that OCD might be a prodrome of schizophrenia; however, comparisons with the general population and long-itudinal studies have shown that people with OCD do not have a higher risk than others of developing schizophrenia (Goodwin et al., 1969; Black, 1974).

Table 6–7. Clinical Implications of the Relationship Between Obsessive-Compulsive Disorder and Other Disorders

Obsessive-Compulsive Disorder and Depression

- Depression often co-occurs with OCD
- Depressive ruminations should be distinguished from obsessions
- Features of OCD may become more or less prominent during an episode of depression
- Co-occurring depression does not necessarily have a negative impact on the outcome of treatment of OCD; a more severe depression is likely to interfere with behavior therapy of OCD
- When OCD patients treated only with behavior therapy or cognitive-behavioral therapy become depressed, adding an antidepressant should be considered

Obsessive-Compulsive Disorder and Psychotic Illness

- Some patients with OCD eventually develop psychosis or already have an underlying psychotic illness
- It is important to identify OCD patients who have an underlying psychotic illness or who are prone to developing one (some patients with poor insight and complex or bizarre obsessions and/or compulsions?)
- Beliefs related to OCD, overvalued ideas, and delusions need to be distinguished
- It is important to distinguish between "delusional OCD" or "obsessive-compulsive psychosis" on one hand, and OCD that co-occurs with schizophrenia and schizotypal personality disorder on the other; the former may have better prognosis than the latter

Obsessive-Compulsive Disorder and Tic Disorders

- Some patients with OCD have a tic disorder and a sizable proportion of patients with tic disorders also have OCD or obsessions and compulsions
- Clinicians should look for tic disorders especially in OCD patients with symmetry, ordering, and arranging obsessions and compulsions and in those with hoarding because they are more likely to have tic disorders
- Patients with OCD and Tourette's disorder have more family members with both OCD and Tourette's disorder, and an earlier onset of OCD
- OCD patients with a co-occurring Tourette's disorder are more likely to respond to a combination of a selective serotonin reuptake inhibitor or clomipramine and antipsychotic medication

Obsessive-Compulsive Disorder and Personality Disturbance

- Although there is some overlap between OCD and obsessive-compulsive personality disorder, the relationship between them is not unique
- Presence of severe personality disturbance, especially schizotypal personality disorder, suggests poorer prognosis and poorer response to treatment

Patients with psychosis-related OCD ("delusional OCD" or "obsessive-compulsive psychosis") may have poor insight, that is, they may not think that their obsessions and/or compulsions are irrational. Some types of obsessions and compulsions have a strong "flavor" of psychosis, especially when they seem too complex or bizarre. Obsessive-compulsive disorder may be accompanied by delusional beliefs related, at least initially, to the obsessions and/or compulsions. For example, a patient with obsessions about having committed a crime developed a delusional belief that he is guilty and repeatedly requested to be punished.

In one study, psychotic symptoms were found in 14% of OCD patients; almost one half of these patients had delusional OCD whereas the remainder received diagnoses of schizophrenia, schizotypal personality disorder, and delusional disorder (Eisen and Rasmussen, 1993). A distinction between delusional OCD on one hand and OCD that co-occurs with psychotic disorders and schizotypal personality disorder on the other may be important because the former may have a better prognosis than the latter. Co-occurring schizotypal personality disorder (believed to be related to schizophrenia) was clearly identified as indicating poor prognosis in OCD (Jenike et al., 1986; Minichiello et al., 1987; Baer et al., 1992; Ravizza et al., 1995; Moritz et al., 2004; Catapano et al., 2006). Schizophrenia co-occurring with OCD also appears to be associated with a generally poorer response to treatment of OCD.

Obsessions and compulsions may be seen among patients with a primary diagnosis of schizophrenia. The proportion of these patients varies, with 8%–41% of schizophrenic patients having symptoms of OCD or meeting the diagnostic criteria for OCD (Fenton and McGlashan, 1986; Eisen et al., 1997). When these patients were compared with schizophrenic patients who had no obsessions and compulsions, they were more likely to have a more chronic course and greater impairment (Fenton and McGlashan, 1986). It has been suggested that OCD co-occurring with schizophrenia ("schizo-obsessive disorder," Zohar, 1997) may be a distinct subtype of schizophrenia with unique clinical characteristics (Rajkumar et al., 2008).

Obsessive-Compulsive Disorder and Tic Disorders

Tic disorders and OCD have an interesting relationship. The focus has been mainly on Tourette's disorder, a condition with prominent motor and vocal tics. There is a similarity between OCD and Tourette's disorder in that both are characterized by repetitive behavior; tics in Tourette's disorder are involuntary only to a certain degree and are often performed to provide relief and until patients "feel right" (Leckman et al., 1994). There are several other important aspects of the relationship between OCD and Tourette's disorder.

First, OCD occurs in a significant proportion of patients with Tourette's disorder; symptoms of OCD and/or a full-blown OCD have been reported in 30%–40% of patients with Tourette's disorder (Leckman et al., 1993).

Conversely, 20% of OCD patients had a lifetime history of multiple tics, and 5%–10% of OCD patients had a lifetime history of Tourette's disorder (Leckman et al., 1994). Second, OCD patients with Tourette's disorder have more family members with both OCD and Tourette's disorder and an earlier onset of OCD (Pauls et al., 1995). Third, OCD patients with symmetry obsessions and compulsions involving ordering, arranging, and hoarding are more likely to have Tourette's disorder (Baer, 1994; Leckman et al., 1994; Miguel et al., 1995; Mataix-Cols et al., 1999). Finally, OCD patients with Tourette's disorder are more likely to respond to a combination of a selective serotonin reuptake inhibitor or clomipramine and antipsychotic medication.

Obsessive-Compulsive Disorder and Personality Disturbance

Obsessive-compulsive disorder was considered to have a unique relationship with obsessive-compulsive personality disorder. It was believed that obsessive-compulsive personality disorder predisposes to OCD, that personality attributes associated with OCD are invariably those of obsessive-compulsive personality disorder, and/or that in comparison with obsessive-compulsive personality disorder, OCD is just a more severe variant of the same underlying psychopathology. These beliefs about the relationship between OCD and obsessive-compulsive personality disorder have not been confirmed. In fact, one study found obsessive-compulsive personality disorder in a small number (6%) of OCD patients, whereas dependent and histrionic personality disorders were more common (Baer et al., 1990).

Nevertheless, the relationship between OCD and obsessive-compulsive personality disorder remains important, especially considering some overlapping features such as perfectionist tendencies, pathological indecisiveness, hoarding behavior, and preoccupation with control. Developmental pathways to OCD and obsessive-compulsive personality disorder may to some extent be common to both, but then they diverge (see Etiology and Pathogenesis, below).

The presence of severe personality disturbance is associated with poorer prognosis and a less favorable outcome of treatment of OCD. As already noted, this has been clearly shown for schizotypal personality disorder.

Obsessive-Compulsive Disorder and Anxiety Disorders

Obsessive-compulsive disorder co-occurs less frequently with anxiety disorders than with depression and the co-occurrence with anxiety disorders seems to have fewer implications for clinical practice than that with depression. Among patients with the principal diagnosis of OCD, the lifetime rates of specific phobia, social anxiety disorder, and panic disorder have been reported to be 22%, 18%, and 12%, respectively (Rasmussen and Eisen, 1988). The frequency of current OCD in patients with panic disorder was

17% (Breier et al., 1986). This co-occurrence of OCD with several other anxiety disorders suggests that there may be a common diathesis among some individuals to develop OCD and/or another anxiety disorder.

Obsessive-Compulsive Spectrum Disorders

The concept of obsessive-compulsive spectrum disorders (Hollander, 1993; Hollander and Wong, 1995) arose from observations of certain similarities between OCD and other disorders. These similarities pertain to some aspects of clinical presentation (e.g., intrusive thoughts, irresistible urges to perform certain acts, repetitive behaviors), patterns of co-occurrence with other disorders, age of onset, course, family history of OCD or disorders related to OCD, neurobiological underpinnings, and treatment response (especially a favorable response to selective serotonin reuptake inhibitors). The conditions that are usually subsumed under obsessive-compulsive spectrum disorders include a preoccupation with appearance and/or with presumed body defect (body dysmorphic disorder), fears and/or beliefs of having a serious illness (hypochondriasis), some eating disorders (e.g., anorexia nervosa), impulse control disorders (e.g., trichotillomania), "behavioral addictions" (e.g., "sexual addiction," compulsive buying, "Internet addiction"), neurological disorders with repetitive behaviors (e.g., Tourette's disorder), some personality disorders (e.g., obsessive-compulsive personality disorder), and others (Table 6–8).

A lack of ability to delay or inhibit repetitive behaviors (Hollander and Benzaquen, 1997) has been proposed as the key common feature of the very diverse conditions postulated to constitute obsessive-compulsive spectrum disorders. These disorders can be conceptualized to lie on a continuum from compulsivity (or overestimation of harm and risk avoidance) to impulsivity (or underestimation of harm and risk-taking). Some research findings along with a view that OCD is not an anxiety disorder (see Diagnostic and Conceptual Issues, below) have led to a proposal to remove OCD from the group of anxiety disorders and to create obsessive-compulsive spectrum disorders as a nosologically separate group. The proposed criteria for membership in this group are listed in Table 6–9.

The concept of obsessive-compulsive spectrum disorders has not been accepted by all and is still being debated. It has been criticized on grounds that there are important differences between the conditions included in the spectrum and between OCD and some of these conditions and that many of the spectrum disorders have a broader relationship with anxiety and depressive disorders in general, rather than with OCD in particular (e.g., Rasmussen, 1994; Crino, 1999). If the group of obsessive-compulsive spectrum disorders is introduced, it is not clear what it will encompass. A consensus seems to be emerging, however, that the spectrum should be kept relatively narrow and that it should probably not include autism,

Table 6-8. Disorders Often Included in the Obsessive-Compulsive Spectrum Disorders

Somatoform Disorders (as per DSM-IV-TR)
Body dysmorphic disorder
Hypochondriasis
Somatization disorder

Eating Disorders
Anorexia nervosa
Bulimia nervosa
Binge eating disorder

Impulse Control Disorders (including "behavioral addictions")
Trichotillomania
Onychophagia (nail-biting)
Pathological gambling
Kleptomania
Compulsive buying
Pyromania
Intermittent explosive disorder
"Internet addiction"

Sexual Disorders
Nonparaphilic compulsive sexual behaviors ("sexual addiction," "sexual compulsions," "hypersexuality")
Paraphilias

Neuropsychiatric Disorders: Tic Disorders and Other Movement Disorders
Tourette's disorder
Sydenham's chorea

Pervasive Developmental Disorders
Autistic disorder
Asperger's disorder

Repetitive Self-Injurious Behaviors (self-mutilation)

Personality Disorders
Obsessive-compulsive personality disorder
Borderline personality disorder

Dissociative Disorders
Depersonalization disorder

Dermatological Conditions
Dermatitis artefacta
Psychogenic excoriation (compulsive skin-picking)

Table 6–9. Proposed Criteria for Membership in Obsessive-Compulsive Spectrum Disorders (Hollander et al., 2008)

At least 3 of the following 5 criteria must be present for a disorder to belong to the obsessive-compulsive spectrum disorders; of these 3, 1 must be a prominent family history of OCD or OCD-related disorders, or fronto-striatal (cortico-striatal-thalamic-cortical) brain circuitry dysfunction (i.e., caudate hyperactivity):

1. Clinical similarities with OCD (in terms of course and the presence of obsessions or obsession-like phenomena and/or compulsions or compulsion-like acts)
2. Pattern of co-occurrence with other disorders similar to that seen in OCD
3. Prominent family history of OCD or OCD-related disorders
4. Fronto-striatal brain circuitry dysfunction (i.e., caudate hyperactivity)
5. Treatment response similar to that seen in OCD

eating disorders, most impulse control disorders, depersonalization disorder, and obsessive-compulsive personality disorder (Jaisoorya et al., 2003; Mataix-Cols et al., 2007; McKay et al., 2008).

What may be included in the putative obsessive-compulsive spectrum disorders? The least controversial candidate for inclusion seems to be body dysmorphic disorder (Jaisoorya et al., 2003; Mataix-Cols et al., 2007; Hollander et al., 2008; McKay et al., 2008). Other likely candidates are hypochondriasis (Jaisoorya et al., 2003; McKay et al., 2008), Tourette's disorder or tic disorders more broadly (Jaisoorya et al., 2003; Mataix-Cols et al., 2007; Hollander et al., 2008), and trichotillomania (Jaisoorya et al., 2003; Mataix-Cols et al., 2007). Table 6–10 shows the relationship between OCD and these candidate spectrum disorders, except for tic disorders, whose relationship with OCD is discussed in the Relationship Between OCD and Other Disorders (above) and summarized in Table 6–7.

ASSESSMENT

Diagnostic and Conceptual Issues

The key aspect of the diagnosis of OCD is the presence of obsessions and compulsions. The *DSM-IV-TR* and *ICD-10* diagnostic criteria for OCD contain the definitions of obsessions and compulsions that are presented with some modification in Clinical Features, above (see also Tables 6–1 and 6–3). The current diagnostic manual definitions of obsessions and compulsions could be expanded so that they further clarify these concepts and underscore the links between obsessions and all behaviors, not just compulsions, that appear in response to obsessions (see Figure 6–1).

Table 6–10. Similarities and Differences Between Obsessive-Compulsive Disorder, Body Dysmorphic Disorder, Hypochondriasis, and Trichotillomania

Disorder	Similarities with OCD	Differences
Body dysmorphic disorder	1. Checking in mirrors in BDD resembles checking compulsions in OCD 2. Intrusive thoughts about appearance and presumed body defects in BDD resemble obsessions in OCD 3. Response to exposure and response prevention and to serotonergic antidepressants may be similar	1. Anxiety can be worsened by checking in mirrors in BDD; compulsions in OCD usually decrease anxiety 2. Intrusive thoughts about appearance and presumed body defects in BDD can more often be characterized as over-valued ideas and are more often associated with delusional beliefs than are obsessions in OCD 3. Patients with BDD have generally less insight than those with OCD
Hypochondriasis	1. Health checking and reassurance seeking in HCH resemble checking compulsions in OCD 2. Intrusive thoughts about health and disease in HCH resemble obsessions in OCD 3. Response to exposure and response prevention and to serotonergic antidepressants may be similar	1. Intrusive thoughts about health and disease in HCH are ego-syntonic and often can be characterized as overvalued ideas; obsessions in OCD are usually ego-dystonic 2. Patients with HCH have generally less insight than those with OCD 3. Somatic symptoms are more prominent and levels of somatization are higher in HCH than in OCD
Trichotillomania	1. Perception of hair pulling in TTM as unreasonable, uncontrollable, and irresistible resembles the perception of compulsions in OCD 2. Both patients with TTM and OCD may respond to serotonergic antidepressants	1. Hair pulling in TTM often occurs automatically; compulsions in OCD occur in response to obsessions 2. Hair pulling in TTM is often pleasurable; compulsions in OCD are performed to decrease anxiety or prevent harm 3. Habit reversal is used to treat TTM; exposure and response prevention is used in treatment of OCD

BDD, body dysmorphic disorder; HCH, hypochondriasis; TTM, trichotillomania.

One of the main issues in the *DSM* conceptualization of OCD is a distinction between OCD with poor insight and "classical" (good-insight) OCD (see also Clinical Features, above). It is uncertain whether these OCD subtypes represent essentially different conditions. While insight and strength of beliefs are distributed dimensionally, it would be important to establish "cutoffs" on the corresponding dimensions and scales in order to ascertain more precisely at what point insight in OCD is to be deemed poor, and OCD-related beliefs become over-valued ideas and delusions. Efforts to clarify these issues conceptually and psychometrically (e.g., Eisen et al., 1998; Neziroglu et al., 1999) should continue.

In the *ICD* system, OCD is not formally grouped along with the other anxiety disorders, but *ICD-10* diagnostic criteria for OCD are similar to those in the *DSM* system. There are 2 subtypes of OCD in *ICD-10*: "pre-dominantly obsessional thoughts and ruminations" and "predominantly compulsive acts (obsessional rituals)." Considering that most OCD patients present with both obsessions and compulsions, this subtyping seems superfluous.

Unlike some of the other anxiety disorders (e.g., generalized anxiety disorder, social anxiety disorder, posttraumatic stress disorder), OCD has not been a controversial diagnostic category. The existence of OCD and the validity of the diagnosis of OCD are rarely disputed in the professional community, and OCD is also perceived as "real" by the lay public. A part of the reason for this status of OCD is the fact that it is a condition with a long history. As such, there is no risk of OCD being regarded as an artificial product of diagnostic and classification schemes or as voguish diagnosis. Furthermore, unlike many psychiatric disorders, OCD possesses a degree of longitudinal stability (e.g., Mataix-Cols et al., 2002a) that reinforces its perception as real. That is, OCD tends to persist for many years and tends to be present in diagnostically subthreshold forms in individuals who appear recovered.

Questions do remain about the very nature of OCD, its core fea-tures, heterogeneity, and classification. Thus, how should OCD be conceptualized—as a primary disorder of emotions, thinking, or beha-vior? In the *DSM* system, the core feature of OCD is the underlying emotion, that is, anxiety, but OCD may also be conceived of as a condition mainly characterized by disordered thinking or repetitive behavior. The *DSM* classification of OCD among the anxiety disorders may be adequate for types of OCD that are characterized by patholo-gical anxiety and resemble other anxiety disorders (e.g., many instances of contamination obsessions and fears and washing compul-sions). Other patients may have more in common with psychotic indi-viduals, while patients with tics and symmetry, arranging, and ordering obsessions and compulsions may have a neurological rather than a psychiatric condition. Moreover, hoarding may not remain within the concept of OCD.

Because of the heterogeneity within OCD, it would be simplistic to respond in either direction to the dilemma of whether OCD (as a whole) is an anxiety disorder. Some aspects or types of OCD make it look more like an anxiety disorder, whereas others favor placing OCD in the putative group of obsessive-compulsive spectrum disorders (Table 6–11). Therefore, the issue of the classification of OCD remains open.

Table 6–11. Reasons For and Against Retaining Obsessive-Compulsive Disorder Among the Anxiety Disorders (in the *DSM* system)

Reasons for OCD to Remain Classified Among the Anxiety Disorders	Reasons for OCD Not to Be Classified Among the Anxiety Disorders
Studies of the structure of psycho-pathology provide some support to the inclusion of OCD in the newly proposed group of "fear disorders," which will encompass core anxiety disorders (Watson, 2005; Slade and Watson, 2006)	Differences in gender distribution: OCD is the only current *DSM* anxiety disorder in which there is no convincing predominance of women (Zohar et al., 2007)
OCD and other anxiety disorders may crucially share catastrophic misinterpretation of objectively non-dangerous stimuli (one's own intrusive thoughts) and counterproductive attempts (through preoccupation with such thoughts, avoidance, reassurance seeking, compulsions) to deal with the resulting anxiety (Abramowitz and Deacon, 2005)	Differences in brain circuitry: OCD is characterized by the fronto-striatal circuitry abnormalities, whereas the circuitry in many anxiety disorders involves dysfunction of the amygdala (Stein DJ, 2007; Zohar et al., 2007)
OCD and other anxiety disorders also share underlying threat-related beliefs and safety-seeking behaviors that are responsible for maintaining the disorders and the corresponding fears (Storch et al., 2008)	Differences in pharmacological challenge results: unlike some other anxiety disorders, OCD does not respond with symptom worsening to challenges with carbon dioxide, yohimbine, caffeine, or cholecystokinin (Stein DJ, 2007; Zohar et al., 2007)
Like other anxiety disorders, OCD can be effectively treated by means of cognitive-behavioral therapy, using very similar principles as in the treatment of other anxiety disorders	Differences in response to pharma-cotherapy: unlike other anxiety disorders that respond to a variety of medications, OCD selectively responds to serotonergic agents (Stein DJ, 2007; Zohar et al., 2007)

Assessment Instruments

The Yale-Brown Obsessive Compulsive Scale (Y-BOCS; Goodman et al., 1989a) has been the most widely used instrument for measuring the severity of obsessions and compulsions in OCD already diagnosed by other means. It is administered by clinicians as a semistructured interview, and is quite comprehensive because it assesses obsessions and compulsions in terms of time spent on them, their interference with functioning, distress caused by obsessions and compulsions, resistance to them, and ability to control these features of OCD. The Y-BOCS has been used to monitor changes during the treatment of OCD and has therefore been important in treatment outcome studies, acquiring the status of a gold standard measure. It is not suitable for use as a screening instrument for OCD.

The Padua Inventory (Sanavio, 1988) is a comprehensive, 60-item, self-report instrument for measuring the severity of OCD and for monitoring changes during the treatment of OCD. Versions with 39 and 41 items have also been developed, but because of its length, this instrument is not particularly useful for screening purposes.

Another widely used self-report instrument, containing 30 true-false items, has been the Maudsley Obsessional Compulsive Inventory (Hodgson and Rachman, 1977). A revised and updated version of this instrument, called the Vancouver Obsessional Compulsive Inventory (Thordarson et al., 2004), has 55 items and assesses features of OCD more comprehensively on six subscales: contamination, checking, obsessions, hoarding, "just right," and indecisiveness.

Differential Diagnosis

In the differential diagnosis of OCD, the most important step is to distinguish between obsessions and compulsions on one hand, and phenomena and behaviors that may resemble obsessions and compulsions on the other (see Tables 6–2 and 6–4). Once obsessions are distinguished from depressive ruminations, overvalued ideas, delusions, and pathological worry (Table 6–2), the distinction between OCD and depression, hypochondriasis or body dysmorphic disorder, psychotic illness, and generalized anxiety disorder, respectively, will generally be easier. Likewise, if compulsions are distinguished from impulsive acts (Table 6–4), the distinction between OCD and various impulse control disorders will not be too difficult.

The questions that need to be asked in the differential diagnosis of OCD are as follows:

- What is the content of the obsession-like phenomenon?
- Is the obsession-like phenomenon experienced as ego-dystonic?

- Are there any beliefs attached to the obsession-like phenomena and compulsion-like acts?
- What are the behavioral responses to the obsession-like phenomenon, if any?
- How can the compulsion-like acts be described?
- Does the compulsion-like act appear in response to an obsession-like phenomenon or in response to a particular feeling or urge? Does it appear automatically, and not in response to any identifiable phenomenon?
- What is the goal or purpose of the compulsion-like acts?

Keeping in mind that OCD bears similarities with several other disorders and that it often co-occurs with them, Table 6–12 presents the most important criteria for distinguishing between OCD and these conditions.

There is also a need to differentiate OCD from "normal" obsession-like phenomena and compulsion-like acts (e.g., certain superstitious beliefs, checking behaviors, religious rituals). Although the demarcation line between OCD and "normality" sometimes seems to be very thin, useful criteria for making this distinction do exist. As long as the obsession-like phenomena are not taken too seriously by the person, as long as the compulsion-like acts are not too time-consuming, and as long as both the obsession-like phenomena and compulsion-like acts do not cause distress and do not interfere with functioning, they are likely to remain within the realm of normality.

EPIDEMIOLOGY

Highlights of the epidemiology of OCD are presented in Table 6–13. Obsessive-compulsive disorder is not as common as most of the other anxiety disorders. Lifetime prevalence figures in the United States have fluctuated somewhat, from 2.5% in the Epidemiologic Catchment Area Study, based on the *DSM-III* diagnostic criteria (Bourdon et al., 1992), to 1.6% in the National Comorbidity Survey Replication, based on the *DSM-IV* diagnostic criteria (Kessler et al., 2005). The prevalence rate of OCD in the Epidemiologic Catchment Area Study has been called into question, mainly because of the methodological issues (a diagnostic instrument used by lay interviewers) and the consequent possibility that the prevalence rate of OCD might have been overestimated (e.g., Stein MB et al., 1997a). Still, the prevalence rates of OCD in the two major epidemiological surveys in the United States have been similar, which reflects the stability of the concept of OCD and few changes that its diagnostic conceptualization has undergone over time (see Diagnostic and Conceptual Issues, above). When methodological considerations are taken into account, it is probably safe to assume that the lifetime prevalence rate of OCD in the United States is between 1.5% and 2%.

Table 6–12. Criteria for Distinguishing Between Obsessive-Compulsive Disorder and Other Disorders

Disorders	Criteria for Distinguishing
Psychosis (e.g., schizophrenia, delusional disorder)	– Loss of reality testing – Presence of delusions (obsession-like phenomena are espoused with firm conviction and are not experienced as ego-dystonic)
Depression	Obsession-like phenomena (depressive ruminations) are congruent with depressed mood and are not experienced as ego-dystonic
Hypochondriasis, body dysmorphic disorder, anorexia nervosa	Obsession-like phenomena (overvalued ideas) are held with a more firm belief, they are monothematic (preoccupation with health and disease, body image, weight and intake of food) and are not experienced as ego-dystonic
Generalized anxiety disorder	Obsession-like phenomenon (pathological worry) pertains to real-life problems and is not experienced as ego-dystonic
Specific phobia	Obsession-like phenomenon (preoccupation with specific fears) is not experienced as ego-dystonic and is responded to with avoidance, not compulsions
Impulse control disorders (e.g., trichotillomania, compulsive buying, compulsive sexual behaviors)	Compulsion-like acts (impulsive acts) are performed in response to an urge or tension (not in response to obsession), with the goal of obtaining relief, pleasure, or gratification (not with the goal of decreasing anxiety or preventing harm)
Tic disorders	Compulsion-like acts (tics) consist of relatively simple motor movements or vocalizations, which are not performed with the goal of decreasing anxiety or preventing harm
Stereotypic movement disorder	Compulsion-like acts (stereotyped movements) consist of a seemingly driven, purposeful motor behavior, which may be performed with the goal of obtaining self-stimulation (not with the goal of decreasing anxiety or preventing harm)
Obsessive-compulsive personality disorder	– Absence of obsessions and compulsions – Excessive devotion to work, frugality, stubbornness, rigidity, excessive need to control interpersonal situations, lack of warmth

Table 6–13. Epidemiological Data for Obsessive-Compulsive Disorder

- Lifetime prevalence in the United States: 2.5% (*DSM-III* criteria, Epidemiologic Catchment Area Study), 1.6% (*DSM-IV* criteria, National Comorbidity Survey Replication)
- Lifetime prevalence in various countries, according to various diagnostic criteria: 0.3%–3.2%
- Best-estimate lifetime prevalence rate across the world: 1.3%
- Prevalence rates in different countries vary less than prevalence rates of most other anxiety disorders
- Practically no difference in prevalence rates between women and men
- Males have an earlier age of onset and a generally worse prognosis
- OCD in children and adolescents is more common among males than females
- Less likely to be married
- Mean age of onset: 21–22 years (range: 18–24 years), with a substantial proportion having onset in childhood
- Onset is usually insidious, in some cases acute
- Characteristic help-seeking patterns: delayed help-seeking (average period between onset and time of seeking help: 7.5 years); help is often sought when the person is overwhelmed by manifestations of OCD and is no longer able to tolerate them; help may also be sought at the initiative of family members or significant others, or for psychiatric and nonpsychiatric complications of OCD; help is usually sought from primary care physicians, psychiatrists, clinical psychologists, or mental health services

Cross-cultural differences in prevalence have been smaller for OCD than for other anxiety disorders. The lifetime prevalence rates of OCD range from 0.3% in rural Taiwan (Hwu et al., 1989) to 3.2% in Puerto Rico (Canino et al., 1987), a difference that may seem large only because these represent extreme rates. One cross-national epidemiological survey reported very similar lifetime prevalence rates of OCD in different countries (except for Taiwan): 1.9%–2.5% (Weissman et al., 1994). The best-estimate lifetime prevalence rate for OCD across epidemiological studies published between 1980 and 2004 and conducted in various countries was 1.3% (Somers et al., 2006). These figures suggest that the prevalence of OCD is more independent from the social, cultural, and economic influences than the prevalence of some of the other anxiety disorders (e.g., social anxiety disorder). Nevertheless, the question of how cultural factors may shape the presentation of OCD and affect its frequency remains largely unanswered.

Obsessive-compulsive disorder is insignificantly more frequent among women than among men (e.g., Black, 1974; Rasmussen and Eisen, 1992; Foa and Kozak, 1995), but there are several differences between women and men with OCD. First, OCD in children and adolescents is more often encountered among males (Leonard et al., 1989), and it starts earlier in boys (Swedo et al., 1989a). Second, the onset of the adult form of OCD is also earlier in men (Rasmussen and Eisen, 1990). Third, men may be more likely to have a co-occurring psychotic disorder or schizotypal personality disorder (Eisen and Rasmussen, 1993). Finally, the prognosis of OCD may be generally worse in men, possibly because an earlier onset of OCD and co-occurrence of psychotic disorders and schizotypal personality disorder are associated with poor prognosis.

Demographic factors other than gender have not been consistently associated with OCD. Individuals with OCD may be less likely to marry (Rasmussen and Eisen, 1991) and tend to be impaired in various areas of functioning (social, occupational, academic). Direct and indirect costs of OCD to the society have been estimated to be very high (Hollander et al., 1996).

Obsessive-compulsive disorder often begins in childhood and adolescence, with more than 20% of patients reporting onset before age 14 (Rasmussen and Eisen, 1990). Many children exhibit superstitious behavior or have obsessions and compulsions but subsequently grow out of them. Only a minority of children with obsessions and compulsions actually develop OCD (Riddle et al., 1990). The prevalence of OCD among adolescents and adults appears to be the same (Flament et al., 1988). The disorder may continue into adulthood in a substantial number of children with OCD. The usual mean age of onset of the adult form of OCD is around 21–22 years, and ranges from 18 to 24 (e.g., Bland et al., 1988; Karno et al., 1988; Rasmussen and Eisen, 1992). Late onset of OCD is rare; one study reported that in less than 15% of individuals with OCD, the illness first manifested itself after age 35 (Rasmussen and Eisen, 1992).

The onset of OCD is usually insidious, with few, if any stressful or other events preceding it. A sudden onset of OCD has been reported among women during pregnancy (Neziroglu et al., 1992), in men after the birth of a child (Abramowitz et al., 2001), or in males and females after a streptococcal infection (Leonard and Swedo, 2001).

People with OCD often have the illness for a long time, an average of 7.5 years, before seeking help (Rasmussen and Tsuang, 1986). An important reason for waiting so long before seeking help is the shame and secrecy surrounding OCD. Many patients are puzzled by their obsessions and compulsions, often fear that they are "crazy," and go to great lengths to hide their symptoms. Professional help is usually sought when obsessions and/or compulsions become overwhelming or impossible to hide, or if they start interfering with functioning much more than before. Not infrequently, family members of OCD sufferers become alarmed and initiate contact with mental health care providers. In some cases, psychiatric (e.g., depression) or nonpsychiatric (e.g., infections or malnutrition in people with extreme hoarding) complications of OCD may prompt persons to present for treatment.

Problems with recognizing OCD also contribute to the time lag between the onset of OCD and its correct diagnosis. Obsessive-compulsive disorder may be missed when patients present to nonpsychiatric physicians for problems that are apparently unrelated to OCD. For example, patients who wash compulsively may develop dermatitis or eczema and seek help from primary care physicians or dermatologists. In fact, one study showed that almost 20% of patients in a dermatology outpatient clinic suffered from a clinically significant OCD, and almost all of these patients had not been previously diagnosed with OCD (Fineberg et al., 2003). It is important to continue raising the awareness of OCD and promote its early detection and accurate diagnosis. Another initiative is to educate primary care providers and mental health professionals about effective treatments for OCD because the data suggest that even patients who are correctly diagnosed do not receive adequate treatment for 6–7 years (Hollander and Wong, 1998).

COURSE AND PROGNOSIS

Data on the course of OCD are summarized in Table 6–14. It has been established that OCD is a chronic illness in most patients. The length of follow-up periods, description of chronicity, related terminology, and other methodological aspects have varied from one study to another, contributing to some discrepant findings regarding the course of OCD. It appears that three general types of chronicity occur in OCD:

- A fluctuating chronic course, in which there are exacerbations and periods of complete or partial remission, observed in 2% (Rasmussen and Tsuang, 1986; Rasmussen and Eisen, 1992), 25% (Kringlen, 1965), 37% (Demal et al., 1993), 46% (Ingram, 1961), and 35%–47% (Black, 1974) of patients.
- A steady (constant, continuing) chronic course, without significant fluctuations, observed in 15% (Ingram, 1961), 28% (Demal et al., 1993), 30% (Kringlen, 1965), 54%–61% (Black, 1974), 84% (Rasmussen and Tsuang, 1986), and 85% (Rasmussen and Eisen, 1992) of patients. The last two figures (84% and 85%) include patients who apparently also had some fluctuations.
- Progressive, deteriorating course, observed in 5% (Kringlen, 1965), 10% (Rasmussen and Eisen, 1992; Demal et al., 1993; Skoog and Skoog, 1999), and 14% (Rasmussen and Tsuang, 1986) of patients.

Spontaneous and enduring remissions of OCD occur rarely. The proportion of OCD patients who achieve a lasting remission (complete absence of symptoms) has been consistently small across studies, reaching 20% at the most (Skoog and Skoog, 1999; Steketee et al., 1999).

The longest (40 to 50 years) prospective follow-up study of patients with OCD reported that patients relapsed after being symptom-free for 10 or even 20 years (Skoog and Skoog, 1999). This suggests that OCD patients are

Table 6–14. Course of Obsessive-Compulsive Disorder

Course	Percentage of Patients
Lasting remission or recovery	Maximum 20%
Fluctuating chronic course, with exacerbations and periods of complete or partial remission	2%–47%
Steady (constant, continuing) chronic course, without significant fluctuations (no clear-cut exacerbations and remissions)	15%–61%
Progressive, deteriorating course	5%–14%

rarely permanently recovered. The same study reported that 83% of patients showed general improvement and 48% were "clinically recovered" after a 40 to 50 year follow-up, but 60%–67% of patients continued to experience symptoms of varying severity and 37% had a diagnosable OCD.

Exacerbations in the course of OCD often occur at times of stress but cannot be reliably predicted by stressful events. Some exacerbations are relatively mild, below the diagnostic threshold for OCD, and are not registered as true relapses.

Predictors of poor prognosis of OCD have been identified by several studies (Table 6–15). These include early age at onset, not being married,

Table 6–15. Predictors of Poor Prognosis of Obsessive-Compulsive Disorder

- Early age at onset (Skoog and Skoog, 1999; Rosario-Campos et al., 2001)
- Not being married (Steketee et al., 1999)
- Greater initial severity of illness (Steketee et al., 1999; Hollander et al., 2002)
- Longer duration of illness and chronicity (Skoog and Skoog, 1999; Hollander et al., 2002)
- Presence of both obsessions and compulsions (Skoog and Skoog, 1999)
- Prominent magical thinking (Skoog and Skoog, 1999)
- Poor insight (Kozak and Foa, 1994; Hollander et al., 2002)
- Presence of delusions (Hollander et al., 2002)
- Presence of severe personality disturbance, particularly schizotypal, paranoid, and borderline personality disorders (e.g., Jenike et al., 1986; Minichiello et al., 1987; Baer et al., 1992; Ravizza et al., 1995; Moritz et al., 2004; Catapano et al., 2006)
- Co-occurrence of bipolar disorder and eating disorder (Hollander et al., 2002)
- Co-occurrence of chronic tics (Leonard et al., 1993)
- Poor social adjustment and inadequate social skills (Skoog and Skoog, 1999)

greater initial severity of illness, longer duration of illness and chronicity, presence of both obsessions and compulsions, prominent magical thinking, poor insight, presence of delusions, presence of severe personality disturbance (particularly schizotypal, paranoid, and borderline personality disorders), co-occurrence of bipolar disorder, eating disorder and chronic tics, poor social adjustment, and inadequate social skills.

ETIOLOGY AND PATHOGENESIS

Obsessive-compulsive disorder has attracted the attention of researchers and clinicians of various backgrounds and theoretical orientations. Although we still do not have a comprehensive account of the causes and development of OCD, it is useful to look at the contributions of major schools of thought to our current understanding of this illness.

BIOLOGICAL MODELS

The past several decades have witnessed an explosion of research into biological origins of OCD. The results of this research activity do not point to any pathophysiological mechanism as being unique to OCD, suggesting that OCD is a heterogeneous condition with different etiological and pathogenetic factors involved. Nevertheless, we have a better understanding of some of the pathophysiological processes implicated in the etiology and pathogenesis of OCD and we know more about brain structures in which these processes take place. Table 6–16 presents findings of biological and neuroimaging studies that are relatively specific for OCD. The results of genetic, pathophysiological, pharmacological, brain imaging, and neuropsychological studies in OCD are summarized in the text below.

Genetic Factors

Family studies have demonstrated that there are more first-degree relatives with OCD among children with OCD and adults with an early onset of OCD than among adults with a later onset of OCD (e.g., Lenane et al., 1990; Riddle et al., 1990; Pauls et al., 1995; Nestadt et al., 2000). Patients with late-onset OCD may not differ from persons without OCD in terms of the proportion of first-degree relatives who have OCD. Therefore, it appears that childhood and early-onset adult OCD have a stronger genetic component than late-onset OCD. In those cases where the risk of developing OCD is inherited, OCD may start in childhood or adolescence. At this stage, however, it is unclear what is inherited in OCD. It is possible that certain variations in serotonin genes increase susceptibility to develop OCD (e.g., Hemmings and Stein, 2006).

Table 6–16. Findings of Biological and Neuroimaging Studies That Are Relatively Specific for Obsessive-Compulsive Disorder

- Dysfunction (partly specific, partly nonspecific?) of the serotonin neurotransmitter system
- Altered dopaminergic function in some OCD patients, particularly those with co-occurring Tourette's disorder
- Brain structures implicated in the etiology and pathogenesis of OCD:
  - Limbic system: orbitofrontal cortex, cingulate, amygdala, thalamus
  - Basal ganglia: striatum (caudate nuclei)
- Dysfunction in the cortico-striatal-thalamic-cortical (fronto-striatal) circuits
- Certain forms of OCD in childhood: autoimmune processes following an infection with group A β-hemolytic streptococci, with OCD occurring in conjunction with choreiform movements (Sydenham's chorea) or tics

A sizable number of patients with OCD and Tourette's disorder have more family members with both OCD and Tourette's disorder, and these patients also tend to have an earlier onset of OCD (Pauls et al., 1995). One study found higher frequency of certain obsessive-compulsive spectrum disorders (hypochondriasis, body dysmorphic disorder, and eating disorders) among the relatives of people with OCD (Bienvenu et al., 2000).

Neuroanatomy and Pathophysiological Mechanisms

Brain Structures Involved in Obsessive-Compulsive Disorder

Results of brain imaging and neuropsychological studies as well as experience with neurosurgical procedures have all suggested that certain brain structures are involved in OCD. These include the limbic system (orbitofrontal cortex, cingulate, amygdala, thalamus) and parts of the basal ganglia (striatum, and more specifically caudate nuclei) (e.g., Baxter et al., 1987; Swedo et al., 1989b; Rauch et al., 1994; Breiter et al., 1996; Rosenberg et al., 1997; Szeszko et al., 1999; Adler et al., 2000; Gilbert et al., 2000). It has been suggested that OCD symptoms are a consequence of functional alterations of the cortico-striatal-thalamic-cortical (or fronto-striatal) circuits. Disturbances in the pathways between the cortex and the thalamus have been implicated in the pathogenesis of obsessions and obsession-like phenomena, whereas abnormalities in the striatum may be involved in the pathogenesis of compulsions and repetitive motor acts (Insel, 1992; Rauch and Jenike, 1993).

Neuroimaging studies have also demonstrated functional changes in the orbitofrontal cortex, cingulate, and caudate nuclei in OCD patients who responded to serotonergic antidepressants or behavior therapy (e.g., Baxter et al., 1992; Perani et al., 1995; Schwartz et al., 1996; Rosenberg et al., 2000).

Neurotransmitter Systems

The serotonin hypothesis of OCD has been most influential, mainly because of the efficacy of serotonergic antidepressants in the treatment of OCD (and the striking lack of efficacy of noradrenergic antidepressants). Studies with agents that block or stimulate serotonin receptors have suggested a role for the serotonin neurotransmitter system abnormalities in the pathogenesis of OCD. The exact nature of serotonergic abnormalities in OCD remains elusive, and it is also unknown to what extent some of these may be specific for OCD. It appears that several pathophysiological mechanisms involving various serotonin receptors in various areas of the brain may lead to OCD.

In addition to dysfunction of the serotonin system, other neurotransmitters have been implicated in the pathogenesis of OCD. Of clinical relevance is altered dopaminergic function in some OCD patients (Goodman et al., 1990a; Denys et al., 2004a), particularly those with co-occurring Tourette's disorder. Antipsychotics block dopamine receptors and may be effective in OCD when combined with serotonergic antidepressants.

Other Neurobiological Aspects

Some types of OCD, particularly those that appear in childhood, may be caused by immunological mechanisms. For example, children with Sydenham's chorea (a disorder of the basal ganglia like Tourette's disorder) very often have symptoms of OCD, and some children with OCD exhibit choreiform movements (Swedo, 1994; Swedo et al., 1994). Because Sydenham's chorea is believed to be a consequence of autoimmune mechanisms following an infection with group A β-hemolytic streptococci, it has been speculated that childhood OCD with an abrupt onset may be a manifestation of the bacteria-induced autoimmune processes (e.g., Allen et al., 1995). This condition, characterized by OCD and/or neurological abnormalities in childhood, has been referred to as Pediatric Autoimmune Neuropsychiatric Disorder Associated with Streptococcal Infection or PANDAS (Swedo et al., 1998). A hypothesis about autoimmune etiology was supported by a magnetic resonance imaging finding of enlarged basal ganglia in children with OCD or tics who also had a streptococcal infection (Giedd et al., 2000).

PSYCHOLOGICAL MODELS

In view of the centrality of cognitive processes and certain behaviors in the clinical picture of OCD, cognitive and behavioral theories of OCD have attempted to give an account of why and how OCD patients find themselves so engaged in the specific, anxiety-laden patterns of thinking and reasoning and so driven to perform their compulsions. Although no longer as influential as in the heyday of psychoanalysis, the psychodynamic model of OCD has also contributed to an understanding of OCD, and it will be briefly presented in the text that follows.

Cognitive Model

The cognitive model of OCD (Salkovskis, 1985, 1989, 1999; Freeston et al., 1996; Obsessive Compulsive Cognitions Working Group, 1997; Rachman, 1997, 1998) broadly proposes that OCD occurs as a result of activation of certain dysfunctional appraisals of and/or beliefs about one's own thinking and coping with such thinking. These are postulated to include appraisals and/or beliefs that certain thoughts are dangerous because they suggest catastrophic scenarios; that these catastrophes might be prevented by the person who is experiencing such thoughts; that prevention of catastrophes involves further cognitive activity; that because such cognitive activity is not effective, it has to be augmented by harm-preventing behaviors (e.g., compulsions). Within this general cognitive framework of OCD, specific models have emerged. They fall into two general types: (1) dysfunctional appraisals of intrusions and (2) erroneous or maladaptive beliefs about intrusions and thinking processes, with prominence of certain cognitive patterns.

An example of the first type of cognitive accounts of OCD is the model put forward by Salkovskis (1985, 1989, 1999). He has proposed that intrusive thoughts involving unacceptable, disturbing, or repugnant urges are not by themselves pathological and lead to obsessions only if they are appraised in a specific way. For OCD to develop, this appraisal entails the person's exaggerated sense of responsibility for having intrusive thoughts, for harm associated with these thoughts, and/or for preventing harm. The origin of such responsibility appraisals can be found in strict upbringing and rigid codes of conduct required by schools or certain religious institutions (Salkovskis et al., 1999). A dysfunctional appraisal of intrusive thoughts may also occur as a result of selective attention paid to these thoughts (Clayton et al., 1999).

In the second type of cognitive accounts of OCD are those that emphasize erroneous or maladaptive beliefs about intrusive thoughts and thinking processes, as well as certain cognitive patterns (Purdon and Clark, 1994; Freeston et al., 1996; Shafran et al., 1996; Obsessive Compulsive Cognitions Working Group, 1997; Rachman, 1997, 1998). Some of these beliefs and patterns appear to be moderately to highly specific for OCD (exaggerated importance of thoughts, concern about control over one's thoughts), others are relatively specific for OCD (thought-action fusion, intolerance of uncertainty, perfectionist tendencies), and some are common to all anxiety disorders (exaggerated perception of threat, overestimation of danger). The beliefs and cognitive patterns that are relatively specific for OCD, along with corresponding examples, are shown in Table 6–17.

Table 6–17. Beliefs About Intrusive Thoughts and Thinking Processes and Cognitive Patterns That Are Relatively Specific for Obsessive-Compulsive Disorder

Beliefs and Cognitive Patterns	Examples of Beliefs or Patterns
Exaggerated importance of thoughts (Freeston et al., 1996; OCCWG 1997; Rachman, 1997, 1998)	"If I think about something, it has to be important, regardless of content"
Concern about inability to control one's own thoughts and the anticipated consequences of failed control, whereby such control is considered very important (Purdon and Clark, 1994; Freeston et al., 1996; OCCWG, 1997)	"I should always be in control over what goes through my mind. That I continue to have these crazy thoughts despite my efforts to get rid of them, will have some dire consequences"
Thought-action fusion (TAF) (Shafran et al., 1996)	"Having thoughts about doing something is the same as doing it"
A. Likelihood TAF (thinking about a disturbing event makes it more probable for the event to occur)	"It will happen just because I think about it"
B. Moral TAF (having a thought about something unacceptable or disturbing is the same as carrying out that unacceptable or disturbing act and suggests that one has some moral defects)	"Thinking about something so awful means that I am a bad person"
Overvaluing the need for certainty, intolerance of uncertainty (Freeston et al., 1996; OCCWG, 1997)	"I can't stand any uncertainty because it is dangerous"
Excessive need for perfectionism, tendencies toward perfectionism (Freeston et al., 1996; OCCWG, 1997)	"It has to be 100% good, otherwise there is no value in it"

OCCWG, Obsessive Compulsive Cognitions Working Group.

The cognitive model also postulates that OCD is maintained by various neutralizing activities: compulsions, avoidance, and reassurance seeking. According to Salkovskis (1996), neutralizing activities occur because of the patients' sense of responsibility for preventing harm. The effect of the neutralizing activities in terms of preventing harm and feeling safe is temporary, and patients repeatedly resort to neutralization. This, however, only increases the perception of threat.

The cognitive model of OCD also proposes that there may be memory biases toward specific themes and issues that are distressing to OCD patients (Radomsky and Rachman, 1999); for example, patients with contamination obsessions and washing compulsions may have better memory for objects and situations related to contamination. Another hypothesis postulates that patients with checking compulsions feel insecure about their own memory, which drives them to perform checking rituals again and again (Macdonald et al., 1997). This hypothesis has been elaborated with the proposition that patients with checking compulsions have an excessive need for certainty (e.g., Tolin et al., 2003) and critical attitude toward their own memory (van den Hout and Kindt, 2003). Both of these make these patients distrustful of their memory, which leads to checking. However, instead of decreasing memory distrust, repeated checking only increases it and thus creates a vicious circle.

The cognitive model of OCD has given important insights into some of the key aspects of the psychopathology of OCD. It is unclear, however, whether and to what extent the cognitive abnormalities contribute to the development of OCD or whether they may be better understood as correlates or consequences of OCD. Various aspects of the cognitive model have received empirical support but need further refinement. For example, it has been difficult to distinguish between appraisals and beliefs. The literature abounds with examples of an interchangeable use of the terms *appraisals* and *beliefs* (e.g., "inflated responsibility appraisals" and "inflated responsibility beliefs"). One possibility is to conceptualize appraisals as situation-specific interpretations and beliefs as situation-nonspecific, more enduring styles or patterns of thinking (e.g., Berle and Starcevic, 2005). Also, some beliefs may precede and lead to certain appraisals; for example, a belief that "one's own thoughts should always be taken seriously" could give rise to an appraisal of a violent intrusive thought as something that requires urgent attention to prevent violence. It remains to be ascertained whether appraisals of intrusive thoughts also appear without preceding beliefs and under what conditions certain beliefs lead to the corresponding appraisals of intrusive thoughts.

Behavioral Model

The behavioral model of OCD (Figure 6–2) may seem somewhat simplistic, but it has served as a foundation for an effective treatment, exposure with response prevention. The model is based on Mowrer's (1960) two-factor theory of fear acquisition and maintenance. According to this theory, obsessions are seen as unconditioned, fear-inducing stimuli, which are maintained by operant conditioning: by temporarily alleviating fear produced by obsessions, compulsions prevent habituation to obsessions and thereby maintain this fear, while at the same time reinforcing themselves as means of reducing fear. In other words, compulsions (as well as avoidance) are seen as a maladaptive behavioral response to obsessions. This response alleviates anxiety in the short term, but in the long term, its

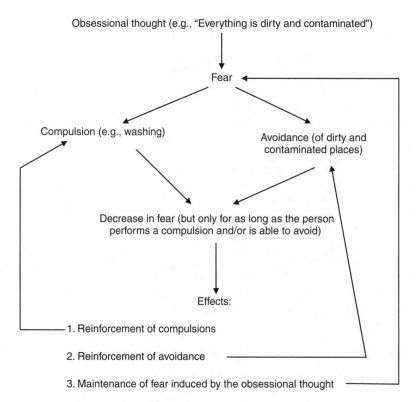

Figure 6–2. Behavioral model of obsessive-compulsive disorder.

anxiety-alleviating function maintains the compulsions, avoidance, and fear induced by obsessions.

Psychoanalytic Contributions

The central tenet of the psychoanalytic theory of OCD (Figure 6–3) is that OCD results from regression to the anal-sadistic stage of development (Freud, 1909/1955b; 1913/1958; Nemiah, 1988), as all the other features of OCD are a consequence of this regression.

The psychoanalytic theory of OCD is a coherent explanatory model that offers understanding of OCD on the basis of key psychoanalytic ideas. Although the concepts of conflicts, fixation points, and regression are currently less widely accepted, the lasting achievement of the psychoanalytic model is its contribution to an understanding of the aspects of OCD such as aggressive themes, ambivalence, doubting, indecisiveness, and magical thinking. The postulation that magical thinking plays an important

(Non)specific conflicts pertaining to aggression and sexuality

↓

Presence of the corresponding "fixation points"
(suggested by preoccupation with dirt and aggression)

↓

Defensive regression to the anal-sadistic stage of development

↓

Consequences of regression:

1. Fusion of sexual and aggressive drives characteristic of the anal-sadistic stage →
Simultaneous love and hatred (ambivalence) → Paralyzing indecisiveness,
doubting

2. Magical thinking ("omnipotence of thoughts")

3. Dominance of the rigid, punitive superego

↓

Use of the defense mechanisms against anxiety and conflicts pertaining to aggression
and sexuality, with the goals of decreasing anxiety and controlling aggressive and
sexual drives:

1. Isolation of affect

2. Undoing ("second line of defense," manifested in compulsions)

3. Reaction formation

Figure 6–3. Psychoanalytic account of obsessive-compulsive disorder.

role in the psychopathology and pathogenesis of OCD has been influential,
with its implicit suggestion that OCD involves disordered thinking processes. Although the cognitive model of OCD is derived from a different
theoretical framework, it is also to some extent an outgrowth of the concept
of magical thinking.

The psychoanalytic theory is also helpful in illuminating the similarities and differences between OCD and obsessive-compulsive personality disorder. As a comparison, the psychoanalytic account of obsessive-
compulsive personality disorder (Freud, 1908/1959; Abraham, 1921/
1942; Shapiro, 1965; Salzman, 1968) is schematically presented in
Figure 6–4.

TREATMENT

It is a truism that treatment of OCD is often difficult and challenging,
putting to test therapeutic skills, patience, and perseverance of many therapists. There is no place for therapeutic nihilism because efficacious treatments for OCD do exist. Unfortunately, current treatments for OCD rarely
bring about a complete and lasting disappearance of symptoms and a
substantial proportion of patients respond poorly or only partially to

(Non)specific disturbances in relations with primary objects
(e.g., "cold parents")

↓

Low self-esteem + conflicts pertaining to aggression:

↓

A. Consequences of low self-esteem:

1. Need to "conquer" superego → Tendencies toward perfectionism → Fear of making a mistake → Rigid and dogmatic cognitive style

2. Tendency to control others to prevent their loss

3. Difficulty with (fear of) interpersonal intimacy

B. Consequences of conflicts pertaining to aggression:

1. Fear of losing control

2. Ambivalence and indecisiveness

3. Use of the defense mechanisms (reaction formation, isolation of affect)

Figure 6–4. Psychoanalytic account of obsessive-compulsive personality disorder.

multiple treatment modalities. Still, with the more realistic goals of treatment of OCD—e.g., alleviation of symptoms and improvement in functioning—current treatments hold promise for many patients.

The comparative efficacy of pharmacotherapy (clomipramine and selective serotonin reuptake inhibitors) versus cognitive-behavioral therapy (CBT) or more precisely, exposure and response prevention (ERP), the most commonly used psychological treatment for OCD, continues to be debated. While some data suggest that these treatments show approximately equal efficacy (e.g., Abramowitz, 1997; Kobak et al., 1998), other research has reported ERP or a CBT package that includes other techniques besides ERP to be more efficacious than clomipramine and fluvoxamine, respectively, (e.g., Foa et al., 2005; O'Connor et al., 2006).

Although most treatment guidelines endorse both effective pharmacological agents and ERP in the treatment of OCD, they show some differences in terms of which treatment is recommended first. This seems to depend on the combination of four factors: severity of OCD, availability of ERP, willingness to undergo ERP, and efficacy of the previously administered ERP (Table 6–18). For mild cases of OCD, ERP tends to be recommended as the first-line treatment, if available and if patients are willing to undergo this treatment. For moderate and severe cases of OCD and for patients unwilling to undergo ERP or previously unresponsive to it, pharmacotherapy tends to be recommended. A combination of pharmacotherapy and ERP may be indicated for patients with severe OCD who are willing to undergo ERP.

Table 6–18. **General Treatment Recommendations for Obsessive-Compulsive Disorder**

Severity of OCD	Availability of ERP	Willingness to Undergo ERP	Efficacy of Prior ERP	Recommended Treatment(s)
Mild	Yes	Yes	–	ERP
Mild	Yes	No	–	Pharmacotherapy*
Mild	No	–	–	Pharmacotherapy*
Mild	Yes	Yes	No	Pharmacotherapy* or ERP
Moderate	Yes	Yes	–	ERP ± pharmacotherapy**
Moderate	Yes	No	–	Pharmacotherapy*
Moderate	No	–	–	Pharmacotherapy*
Moderate	Yes	Yes	No	Pharmacotherapy* or ERP
Severe	Yes	Yes	–	ERP + pharmacotherapy"***
Severe	Yes	No	–	Pharmacotherapy*
Severe	No	–	–	Pharmacotherapy*
Severe	Yes	Yes	No	Pharmacotherapy*

ERP, exposure and response prevention;
* Pharmacotherapy includes clomipramine or selective serotonin reuptake inhibitors (plus any pharmacological augmentation strategy, if applicable);
** Exposure and response prevention may or may not be combined with pharmacotherapy;
*** Exposure and response prevention should probably be combined with pharmacotherapy.

Pharmacological treatment and CBT for OCD are presented separately, followed by a discussion of combined treatments, mainly pharmacotherapy in conjunction with CBT. Other biological treatments for treatment-resistant OCD are also discussed.

PHARMACOLOGICAL TREATMENT

Aspects of pharmacological treatment that are specific for OCD are listed in Table 6–19. Obsessive-compulsive disorder was the first among the anxiety disorders for which selective serotonin reuptake inhibitors (SSRIs) demonstrated efficacy. Prior to that, clomipramine, a tricyclic antidepressant with predominant serotonergic activity (inhibition of serotonin reuptake), had established itself as a pharmacotherapy gold standard for OCD. Comparisons between medications with serotonin reuptake blocking properties and antidepressants that do not block serotonin reuptake, such as nortriptyline (Thoren et al., 1980), amitriptyline (Ananth et al., 1981), and

Table 6–19. Aspects of the Pharmacological Treatment Specific for Obsessive-Compulsive Disorder

- Medications that inhibit serotonin reuptake (SSRIs, clomipramine) have been more efficacious in OCD than medications targeting other neurotransmitter systems and having other mechanisms of action
- In comparison with OCD, other anxiety disorders and most other psychiatric conditions are treated with medications that have a greater variety of mechanisms of action
- Criteria for response to pharmacotherapy are less strict for OCD than for other anxiety disorders (e.g., a 25%–35% decrease in the score on a rating scale such as Y-BOCS); as a result, many responders to pharmacotherapy are still quite symptomatic
- Even with the less stringent criteria for response, only 40%–60% of patients with OCD respond to clomipramine or SSRIs
- Longer duration of treatment (at least 12 weeks) and higher doses of serotonergic antidepressants (usually higher than doses used in the treatment of depression) are needed for response to occur
- Slow and gradual response to pharmacological agents over weeks and months is often observed

SSRIs, selective serotonin reuptake inhibitors; Y-BOCS, Yale-Brown Obsessive Compulsive Scale.

desipramine (Leonard et al., 1989; Goodman et al., 1990b; Hoehn-Saric et al., 2000), showed that the former were superior in the treatment of OCD. These findings provided support to the hypothesis that OCD is specifically related to serotonin dysfunction (see Etiology and Pathogenesis, above) and that inhibition of serotonin reuptake is necessary for drugs to be effective in OCD.

Medications are used with the goals of alleviating clinical manifestations of OCD, decreasing severity of certain co-occurring conditions (e.g., depression, Tourette's disorder), decreasing impairment, and improving functioning. Pharmacotherapy can be used in almost all cases of OCD, but the more severe OCD is, the more likely it is to be treated with medications (Table 6–18). Besides overall severity of OCD, reasons for considering pharmacotherapy include a history of good response to a given medication in the past, patient preference or unwillingness to participate in psychological treatments (especially ERP), and unavailability of specialized psychological treatments for OCD (Table 6–18).

The clinical presentation is not a particularly useful indicator of the likelihood of response to pharmacotherapy in OCD, although it is often assumed that obsessions respond to medications better than compulsions. This assumption has received only partial support. While some studies suggest that obsessions in general are associated with a good response to pharmacotherapy (e.g., Ackerman et al., 1998), other research has found the opposite (Christensen et al., 1987). Likewise, the presence of sexual and religious obsessions predicted poorer response to pharmacotherapy in one study (Shetti et al., 2005), better outcome of pharmacotherapy in another study (Stein DJ et al., 2007a), and was not associated with the outcome of pharmacotherapy in three studies (Mataix-Cols et al., 1999; Erzegovesi et al., 2001; Denys et al., 2003a). There are more studies suggesting that the predominance or severity of compulsions in general predicts a poorer outcome of pharmacotherapy (Ravizza et al., 1995; Ackerman et al., 1998; Shetti et al., 2005; Catapano et al., 2006) than there are studies suggesting that there is no such relationship (DeVeaugh-Geiss et al., 1990; Ackerman et al., 1994). In terms of the types of compulsions, washing or cleaning predicted a poorer response to medications (Alarcon et al., 1993; Ravizza et al., 1995; Shetti et al., 2005; Stein DJ et al., 2007a), though not in all studies (Mataix-Cols et al., 1999; Erzegovesi et al., 2001).

Selective serotonin reuptake inhibitors and clomipramine continue to be the mainstay of pharmacotherapy of OCD. Because of their better tolerability, SSRIs are usually considered first- and second-line pharmacological treatment (Table 6–20). Unfortunately, about one half of patients are resistant to SSRIs and clomipramine. A few other medications have been efficacious as monotherapy for OCD, albeit inconsistently; in most cases, other drugs have been used to augment response to SSRIs or clomipramine.

Selective Serotonin Reuptake Inhibitors and Clomipramine in Treatment of Obsessive-Compulsive Disorder

Of the SSRIs, the efficacy in OCD has been demonstrated for fluvoxamine (Perse et al., 1987; Goodman et al., 1989b, 1996; Hohagen et al., 1998; Hollander et al., 2003a; Nakatani et al., 2005), fluoxetine (Montgomery et al., 1993; Tollefson et al., 1994), sertraline (Chouinard et al., 1990; Greist et al., 1995a; Kronig et al., 1999), paroxetine (Zohar and Judge, 1996; Hollander et al., 2003b; Stein DJ et al., 2007b), escitalopram (Stein DJ et al., 2007b), and citalopram (Montgomery et al., 2001). Clomipramine has shown efficacy in a number of controlled studies (Thoren et al., 1980;

Table 6–20. Choice of Medication in Treatment of Obsessive-Compulsive Disorder

Rank	Medication
First-line	First SSRI (any SSRI, but the strongest evidence of efficacy exists for fluvoxamine, fluoxetine, sertraline, and paroxetine)
Second-line	Another SSRI (if no response at all to the first SSRI)
Third-line	Clomipramine (if no response at all to the two SSRIs)

SSRI, selective serotonin reuptake inhibitor.

Ananth et al., 1981; Insel et al., 1983; Clomipramine Collaborative Study Group, 1991).

Several studies have suggested that clomipramine is more efficacious than SSRIs in treating OCD (Greist et al., 1995c; Piccinelli et al., 1995; Stein DJ et al., 1995; Abramowitz, 1997; Ackerman and Greenland, 2002; Eddy et al., 2004). This was speculated to be a consequence of clomipramine's additional effect of inhibiting the dopamine function (Austin et al., 1991; Denys et al., 2003b). However, there was no significant difference in efficacy when clomipramine was directly compared with fluvoxamine (Freeman et al., 1994; Koran et al., 1996; Milanfranchi et al., 1997; Mundo et al., 2000), fluoxetine (Pigott et al., 1990; Lopez-Ibor et al., 1996), sertraline (Bisserbe et al., 1997), and paroxetine (Zohar and Judge, 1996), but SSRIs were generally better tolerated. Therefore, the superiority of clomipramine over SSRIs in OCD is not entirely convincing, and the choice between SSRIs and clomipramine is usually based on the expected side-effect profiles and presence of any contraindications. The latter factors usually favor SSRIs.

As already noted, using one of the SSRIs as initial treatment is a reasonable choice (Table 6-20). It cannot be predicted whether a patient will respond to any given SSRI, and no SSRI has emerged as more effective for OCD. There has been only one direct comparison between SSRIs, which showed that escitalopram (20 mg/day) might have some, though not very convincing, advantage over paroxetine (40 mg/day) in terms of efficacy and tolerability (Stein DJ et al., 2007b). Apart from clinician preference and experience, the selection of an SSRI depends on factors such as past treatment response, side effects, likelihood of significant interactions with other drugs, likelihood of association with discontinuation symptoms, and ease of ceasing and switching it. These issues are discussed in more detail in Chapter 2.

If there is no response at all to the first SSRI used in treatment of OCD, another SSRI can be administered as the second-line pharmacotherapy (Table 6-20) because patients who do not respond to one SSRI may respond to another (e.g., Hollander et al., 2002). Also, some patients may not tolerate the first SSRI but experience few, if any side effects, with another SSRI.

Although clomipramine is usually considered a suitable pharmacotherapy option if there has been no response to two SSRIs (Table 6-20), it may also be used initially or after only one SSRI has failed. The main concerns with clomipramine are its tolerability and potential for dangerous adverse events. In addition to the anticholinergic and other side effects caused by all tricyclic antidepressants (see Chapter 2), clomipramine is associated with an increased likelihood of seizures in higher doses. The cardiotoxicity and death from overdose represent an additional risk. For these reasons, the maximum dose of clomipramine is set at 250 mg/day (Table 6-21), but many patients are unable to tolerate doses higher than 150 mg/day. The initial dose is 25 mg at bedtime; this dose can subsequently be increased by 25-50 mg every 4-7 days, as tolerated. Clomipramine is contraindicated in the presence of prostatic hypertrophy, closed-angle glaucoma, and cardiac arrhythmias. In case of other heart problems and a history of seizure disorder, clomipramine should be avoided or perhaps used only with utmost caution.

Two practical considerations are important in the treatment of OCD with SSRIs. First, the dosage of an SSRI needed to produce a response is often higher than the dosage used in depression, although some patients may respond to the usual antidepressant dosages of SSRIs. The evidence that OCD patients need higher doses of SSRIs to respond and that only higher doses of SSRIs are more efficacious than placebo is somewhat inconsistent (Montgomery et al., 1993; Tollefson et al., 1994; Greist et al., 1995b; Montgomery et al., 2001; Hollander et al., 2003b; Stein DJ et al., 2007b), but there is a consensus that clinicians should aim for higher doses. Therefore, after initiating treatment at standard antidepressant doses (e.g., 20 mg/day of fluoxetine), the doses should be increased fairly quickly, depending on tolerability and response. Higher doses of SSRIs may also be needed to prevent relapse (e.g., Romano et al., 2001). The doses of SSRIs and clomipramine used in OCD are shown in Table 6–21. In some cases, doses of SSRIs higher than the maximum recommended ones can be used.

The second practical consideration pertains to the pattern of response of OCD to pharmacotherapy. Although OCD patients may respond to medication early in the course of treatment, a slow and gradual response over weeks and months is often observed (e.g., de Haan et al., 1997; Stein DJ et al., 2007b). A 12-week course of treatment is often considered necessary to determine whether patients respond to pharmacotherapy. If the symptoms of OCD have been only slightly alleviated after 12 weeks of treatment at the highest dose of medication, further improvement over the subsequent several months is still possible. Depending on the circumstances of individual patients, they may then be encouraged to continue taking the medication rather than advised to change it or add another drug. The uncertainty as to whether there will be further treatment gains after 3, 4,

Table 6–21. Dosages of Selective Serotonin Reuptake Inhibitors and Clomipramine in Obsessive-Compulsive Disorder

Medication	Starting Doses	Minimum Therapeutic Doses	Highest Recommended Doses
Fluvoxamine	50 mg/day	100 mg/day	300 mg/day
Fluoxetine	20 mg/day	20 mg/day	80 mg/day
Sertraline	50 mg/day	50 mg/day	200 mg/day
Paroxetine	20 mg/day	40 mg/day	60 mg/day
Escitalopram	10 mg/day	10 mg/day	40 mg/day
Citalopram	20 mg/day	20 mg/day	80 mg/day
Clomipramine	25 mg/day	75 mg/day	250 mg/day

or 6 months of drug treatment without changing either the medication or its dose makes it difficult to establish more precisely the end point of a pharmacological trial in OCD.

Long-Term Pharmacological Treatment

Obsessive-compulsive disorder is usually a chronic condition and needs to be treated for a long time. Several controlled, long-term (up to 1 year) studies have demonstrated the efficacy of fluoxetine (Romano et al., 2001), sertraline (Greist et al., 1995b; Koran et al., 2002), paroxetine (Hollander et al., 2003b), and escitalopram (Fineberg et al., 2007) in preventing relapse of OCD after acute treatment (in most studies lasting up to 16 weeks). In one controlled, long-term study, clomipramine was as efficacious 1 year after the beginning of treatment as it was during short-term treatment (Katz et al., 1990). These findings suggest that the long-term treatment with SSRIs and clomipramine may prevent relapse and maintain efficacy over many months and perhaps years (e.g., Rasmussen et al., 1997). The maintenance dosage of SSRIs and clomipramine should probably be the same as the one with which response was attained during short-term treatment. It is reasonable to continue pharmacotherapy for at least 1–2 years after achieving response. General issues in long-term pharmacotherapy are discussed in Chapter 2.

There is a substantial risk of relapse—up to 90% (Pato et al., 1988; Leonard et al., 1991)—when the medication is discontinued. This means that especially for severe and disabling OCD that responded to pharmacotherapy, medication(s) should be used for a very long time, perhaps even indefinitely. If cessation of pharmacotherapy is contemplated at all, it should be done very carefully and gradually. The risk of relapse can perhaps be decreased by the use of psychological treatment, especially CBT. In case of relapse, the medication to which the patient responded previously should be administered, but it is uncertain whether a response to it will be achieved again.

Pharmacotherapy of Treatment-Resistant Obsessive-Compulsive Disorder

As already noted, the proportion of OCD patients who do not respond to standard pharmacological agents, SSRIs and clomipramine, or who respond only partially tends to be high. Therefore, further treatment of these patients is a frequent and important issue in clinical practice.

An adequate trial of pharmacotherapy for OCD consists of at least 12 weeks of treatment with an SSRI or clomipramine at a maximum recommended or tolerated dose. However, the duration of a pharmacological trial in OCD should be flexible because of the tendency of some patients to show further treatment gains beyond the initial 12 weeks of treatment. Therefore, some clinicians continue to administer medication for another 6–12 weeks (or longer) before deciding that a patient has had an adequate trial. The duration of a pharmacological trial depends on the circumstances of individual patients and is likely to vary from one case to another.

Analogous to an imprecise definition of an adequate pharmacotherapy trial in OCD, it may be difficult to establish what constitutes resistance to pharmacotherapy in OCD. Most clinicians, however, probably do not regard patients as treatment resistant unless they have had adequate trials with at least 2 SSRIs and clomipramine. Some clinicians consider patients resistant if they have had only partial response to these drugs. Patients may also reach the stage of treatment resistance through intolerance of SSRIs or clomipramine, or if some of these agents are contraindicated. In view of the potentially different meanings of treatment resistance, it is important to stipulate what the term refers to whenever it is used.

Pharmacotherapy Options in Case of a Lack of Response to Standard Medications for Obsessive-Compulsive Disorder

If patients with OCD exhibit no response at all to two SSRIs and clomipramine, several monotherapy options can be considered (Table 6–22). The first one is venlafaxine, a serotonin and noradrenaline reuptake inhibitor. The evidence of efficacy of venlafaxine in OCD has been inconsistent, and large double-blind, placebo-controlled trials of this drug are lacking. One small controlled study with methodological problems did not find venlafaxine superior to placebo (Yaryura-Tobias and Neziroglu, 1996). In a randomized, single-blind comparison of venlafaxine and clomipramine, the response rate was nonsignificantly lower in patients treated with venlafaxine (Albert et al., 2002). One double-blind comparison study of venlafaxine (in its extended-release formulation) and paroxetine found no difference in efficacy between the two drugs (Denys et al., 2003b). In a double-blind switching study involving the same drugs, there were significantly more venlafaxine-nonresponders who responded to paroxetine than there were paroxetine-nonresponders who responded to venlafaxine (Denys et al., 2004b). A range of doses of venlafaxine, from 150 mg/day to 375 mg/day, has been used without a clear benefit of the higher doses. Therefore, the dual action of venlafaxine (serotonin and noradrenaline reuptake inhibition associated with its higher doses) has not been superior to the serotonin reuptake inhibition of SSRIs, clomipramine, and venlafaxine in lower doses.

Other monotherapy options for treatment-resistant OCD patients (Table 6–22) include mirtazapine, a noradrenergic and specific serotonergic antidepressant (Koran et al., 2005), and phenelzine, a classical, irreversible monoamine oxidase inhibitor (Vallejo et al., 1992; Jenike et al., 1997). The evidence of efficacy of these drugs, however, has been insufficient, unconvincing, or inconsistent.

Table 6–22. Pharmacological Options for Treatment-Resistant Obsessive-Compulsive Disorder

Lack of Response to First-, Second-, and Third-Line Pharmacotherapy
Monotherapy options

  Venlafaxine
  Mirtazapine
  Phenelzine

Lack of Response to Clomipramine
Intravenous clomipramine

Partial Response to First-, Second-, or Third-Line Pharmacotherapy (or loosely defined "treatment resistance")
Continue treatment for several months without changing the dose
Continue treatment for several months with a higher dose (applicable only to SSRIs)
Intravenous clomipramine (applicable only to clomipramine)
Augmentation strategies

  SSRI or clomipramine + first-generation antipsychotic (haloperidol)
  SSRI or clomipramine + second-generation antipsychotic (risperidone, quetiapine, olanzapine)
  SSRI or clomipramine + other medications (clonazepam, buspirone, pindolol, L-tryptophan, lithium, gabapentin, topiramate, reboxetine, memantine, riluzole, inositol, etc.)
  SSRI + clomipramine

SSRI, selective serotonin reuptake inhibitor.

Yet another possibility is to administer clomipramine intravenously to OCD patients who do not respond to oral clomipramine (or who respond to it only partially) because a significant proportion of patients may then become responders (or respond better) (Fallon et al., 1998). This treatment is administered through daily infusions for a period of about 2 weeks, with the doses of clomipramine reaching and even exceeding 300 mg/day (Koran et al., 1997). Intravenous clomipramine may not be readily available, and there are concerns about its side effects and toxicity in such high doses.

Pharmacotherapy Options in Case of Partial Response to Standard Medications for Obsessive-Compulsive Disorder

It is difficult to precisely characterize partial response to pharmacotherapy because the response in pharmacological studies of OCD is usually defined as a relatively small decrease (25%–35%) in the score on the Y-BOCS. If the clinician were to adhere to these standards, then a partial response would mean that there has been only a 10%–20% improvement in symptoms. Most physicians do not have time to administer lengthy instruments such as the Y-BOCS, and their conclusions as to whether a patient has responded partially are likely to be based on global impression. Hence, it is understandable that the symptomatic status of OCD patients who are deemed partial responders varies from one clinical setting to another, and that some clinicians consider them simply as "treatment resistant" or "nonresponders."

If there has been a partial response to an SSRI or clomipramine in the highest recommended or tolerated dose after 12 weeks of treatment, one strategy, as noted previously, is to continue treatment with the same dose because of the possibility of incremental improvement over the subsequent weeks and months. The other option is to further increase the dose, if tolerated, and also continue treatment for several months (Table 6–22). There is some support for the latter strategy. In one controlled study, OCD patients who failed to respond to the highest recommended dose of sertraline (200 mg/day) after 16 weeks of treatment and were then treated with very high doses of sertraline (250-400 mg/day) improved significantly more than those who continued treatment with 200 mg/day (Ninan et al., 2006). Likewise, patients who did not respond to escitalopram 20 mg/day in an open-label study improved when the dose was increased to 50 mg/day (Rabinowitz et al., 2008). Intravenous clomipramine may also improve response to the previously administered oral clomipramine.

Numerous augmentation strategies have been tested for OCD patients who responded partially to SSRIs or clomipramine or who were otherwise considered treatment resistant. Thus, antipsychotic drugs, clonazepam, buspirone, pindolol, L-tryptophan, lithium, gabapentin, topiramate, reboxetine, memantine, riluzole, inositol, and others have all been added to an SSRI or clomipramine. Except for the augmentation with antipsychotics, these strategies either failed to produce consistent results or their results (favorable or unfavorable) were only preliminary.

Adding antipsychotic drugs to an SSRI or clomipramine has become a popular strategy in the treatment of OCD. It is used not only to augment partial response to an SSRI or clomipramine but in many complex cases of OCD, in the presence of psychotic symptoms, and for several other reasons. The latter include the presence of a co-occurring Tourette's disorder (McDougle et al., 1994, 2000) and schizotypal personality disorder (McDougle et al., 1990; Bogetto et al., 2000), severe obsessions (Denys et al., 2004c), and OCD with poor insight (Hollander et al., 2003c). In these cases, antipsychotics can perhaps be used from the very beginning of treatment, before OCD becomes treatment resistant.

Of the first-generation antipsychotics, evidence of efficacy from a controlled study exists for augmentation of fluvoxamine with haloperidol (McDougle et al., 1994). Haloperidol is usually administered in low doses (up to 5 mg/day). This strategy seemed to be particularly beneficial for

OCD patients with a co-occurring tic disorder (McDougle et al., 1994) or schizotypal personality disorder (McDougle et al., 1990).

Several second-generation antipsychotics, which act as serotonin-dopamine antagonists, have been used to augment SSRIs or clomipramine in the treatment of refractory OCD. In controlled trials, the combinations of risperidone (McDougle et al., 2000; Hollander et al., 2003c; Erzegovesi et al., 2005), quetiapine (Denys et al., 2004c), and olanzapine (Bystritsky et al., 2004) with SSRIs or clomipramine proved to be more efficacious for treatment-resistant OCD patients than SSRIs or clomipramine alone. The previously refractory patients tended to respond to these combinations, with response rates ranging from 40% to 55%. One meta-analysis has found that only one third of treatment-resistant OCD patients respond to antipsychotic augmentation (Bloch et al., 2006). Patients who do not respond to one antipsychotic augmentation strategy may respond to another. The optimal doses of the augmenting second-generation antipsychotics remain to be established, but they may be in the low to medium range (e.g., risperidone 1–3 mg/day, quetiapine 300–400 mg/day, olanzapine 2.5–10 mg/day).

Many findings regarding the antipsychotic augmentation of SSRIs or clomipramine are inconsistent and call for further studies. For example, in two meta-analyses, risperidone and haloperidol seemed to be more efficacious as augmenting agents than quetiapine and olanzapine (Bloch et al., 2006; Skapinakis et al., 2007). In contrast, when the risperidone augmentation strategy was compared to the olanzapine one, there was no significant difference in the percentage of patients who responded (Maina et al., 2008). A meta-analysis of controlled trials in which quetiapine was used to augment treatment with SSRIs or clomipramine showed efficacy of this combination (Fineberg et al., 2006). Response to antipsychotic augmentation may also depend on which primary medication for OCD is used and in what dose, as there was a greater response to quetiapine augmentation when clomipramine, fluoxetine, and fluvoxamine were used in lower doses (Denys et al., 2007).

Results of studies of the antipsychotic augmentation strategies also have implications for understanding of the neurobiological underpinnings of OCD. It appears that in addition to the serotonin system dysfunction, changes in the dopamine function occur in some types of OCD (see Etiology and Pathogenesis, above). This is most obvious in patients with a co-occurring Tourette's disorder, because they respond most readily to a combination of an antipsychotic drug and SSRI or clomipramine (Bloch et al., 2006). Interestingly, no success has been reported when using antipsychotics alone in the treatment of OCD, and there are occasional reports of either the worsening of OCD or of the appearance of its symptoms in the course of monotherapy with antipsychotic agents.

Perhaps the ultimate augmentation strategy is a combination of an SSRI and clomipramine, with clomipramine usually being added to an SSRI in patients who have responded to it only partially (Szegedi et al., 1996). This combination requires caution, however, because plasma levels of clomipramine can be raised to the toxic range, with an increased risk of seizures and cardiac problems. Fluoxetine, paroxetine, and fluvoxamine increase plasma clomipramine levels through inhibition of the hepatic enzymes. When combining an SSRI with clomipramine, the patient's electrocardiogram, other indicators of cardiovascular status, and plasma levels of clomipramine and its metabolite should be monitored carefully, and the lowest possible dose of clomipramine should be administered, usually not more than 100 mg/day (Szegedi et al., 1996).

The treatment-refractory and disabled OCD patient who has failed to respond to all or most of the aforementioned monotherapy and augmentation strategies, as well as to psychological interventions, should be referred to a highly specialized center for diagnostic reevaluation and consideration of further treatment options. In terms of biological treatment, these options include electroconvulsive therapy, transcranial magnetic stimulation, and, when available and indicated, neurosurgery.

OTHER BIOLOGICAL TREATMENTS

Electroconvulsive Therapy

There is no evidence that electroconvulsive therapy is effective for treatment-resistant OCD. However, it may be used for conditions co-occurring with OCD, such as severe depression, for which the efficacy of electroconvulsive therapy is well established.

Transcranial Magnetic Stimulation

Transcranial magnetic stimulation produces a magnetic field, which induces electric current in the brain and stimulates it. This noninvasive technique has been used to treat a variety of psychiatric conditions, particularly depression. Studies evaluating the efficacy of transcranial magnetic stimulation in OCD have produced inconsistent results. While some have reported benefit of transcranial magnetic stimulation (Sachdev et al., 2001; Mantovani et al., 2006), others could not confirm it (e.g., Alonso et al., 2001b). Future studies need to refine procedural aspects—for example, the frequency with which this technique is used, brain location for application, and duration of treatment.

Neurosurgery

Ablative neurosurgery has shown some success in treatment of the most severe and treatment-resistant patients with OCD. Between 25% and 84% of patients have been reported as improved up to 17 years after neurosurgery (Jenike et al., 1991; Baer et al., 1995; Dougherty et al., 2002; Rück et al., 2008).

However, many patients who have undergone surgical intervention still need ongoing pharmacotherapy and/or CBT for OCD.

Most surgical procedures disrupt connections between the basal ganglia and frontal cortex. Although the techniques have been improved, it is uncertain which procedure may be most effective, while carrying the lowest risk of adverse effects. Anterior cingulotomy has apparently been the preferred procedure, followed by various capsulotomy techniques (thermocapsulotomy, gammacapsulotomy or gamma knife radiosurgery), subcaudate tractotomy, and limbic leucotomy. These procedures differ with regard to the structures involved and size of the lesions; some also need to be performed more than once.

Follow-up studies suggest that ablative neurosurgery for OCD is associated with the substantial risk of adverse effects. Some of these may be transient, whereas others are long term or permanent. They include weight gain, seizures, hydrocephalus, headache, personality changes, various cognitive and executive functioning problems, lack of initiative, apathy, disinhibition, impulsive and aggressive behavior, and suicide (e.g., Jenike et al., 1991; Sachdev and Hay, 1995; Dougherty et al., 2002; Rück et al., 2008). The potential adverse effects of neurosurgery need to be weighed very carefully against its possible benefits. In addition, the public perception of neurosurgery for psychiatric disorders has generally been very negative, and clinicians considering this management option should be well prepared to address this perception and the associated legal and ethical issues.

Because of the controversial status of ablative neurosurgery in the treatment of OCD and its use as the last resort, indications for it should be strict. A minimum of 5 years of treatment with little or no response has been suggested as necessary for consideration of neurosurgery (Jenike, 1998). This treatment has to include trials of all SSRIs and clomipramine, augmentation with antipsychotics and other agents, and behavior therapy.

A less invasive alternative to ablative neurosurgery is deep brain stimulation, which is a reversible and adjustable neurosurgical procedure involving the insertion of a device that generates electrical signals to stimulate certain structures deep within the brain. Various parts of the internal capsule are the usual targets of this intervention, but other brain structures may also be targeted. There is some preliminary and some conflicting evidence regarding the efficacy of deep brain stimulation for treatment-resistant OCD (e.g., Nuttin et al., 2003; Abelson et al., 2005; Greenberg et al., 2006). Subthalamic nucleus stimulation was found to significantly reduce OCD symptoms, but it was also associated with a high risk of serious adverse events, including intracerebral hemorrhage (Mallet et al., 2008).

PSYCHOLOGICAL TREATMENTS

Various psychotherapeutic approaches have been used in OCD, including psychoanalysis, psychodynamic psychotherapy, supportive psychotherapy, and CBT. Of these, evidence of efficacy exists only for CBT. Other types of psychotherapy may play a limited role in the treatment of some OCD patients and in certain clinical settings, but they cannot be recommended as the standard or sole treatment for OCD.

Cognitive-Behavioral Therapy

Cognitive-behavioral therapy encompasses various combinations of the techniques of behavior and cognitive therapy. The two basic modalities are ERP, also referred to as "exposure and ritual prevention" or "behavior therapy," and cognitive therapy or cognitive restructuring. Both can be administered in an individual and group format. One meta-analysis did not find significant differences in efficacy between ERP, cognitive therapy, and a combination of the two (Rosa-Alcázar et al., 2008). Considering that a large body of research demonstrated the efficacy of ERP, whereas efficacy of cognitive therapy was based on fewer studies, ERP was endorsed as the psychological treatment of choice (Rosa-Alcázar et al., 2008). The same recommendation has been made by several treatment guidelines.

Behavior Therapy—Exposure and Response Prevention

Exposure and response prevention (Table 6–23) is based on the behavioral model of OCD (see Etiology and Pathogenesis, above) and general principles of behavior therapy. It was introduced in the 1960s and quickly became the most widely used psychological treatment for OCD.

The technique has two components: *(1)* exposure (used more to alleviate obsessions) and *(2)* response prevention (used more with the goal of removing compulsions). Patients expose themselves to the feared, obsession-related situations that provoke or intensify anxiety or discomfort, and then refrain from performing a compulsion that they would have otherwise performed to decrease anxiety or discomfort. For example, patients with contamination obsessions and washing compulsions are instructed to touch objects that they consider "dirty" or contaminated (e.g., pieces of clothes that were in contact with the seat on the bus), and then they are asked to refrain from washing their hands. With repeated exposure, the obsession elicits less and less anxiety as a result of habituation; this decrease in anxiety level also leads to a decrease in the patients' need to perform compulsions. Response prevention demonstrates to patients that an urge to perform a compulsion can be successfully resisted, which boosts their sense of self-efficacy. There are different ways in which ERP can be delivered, and over the years the technique has undergone various modifications.

Psychoeducation The use of ERP depends crucially on educating patients about OCD and on explaining to them why ERP is used and how it should be used. Before ERP commences, it is also important to explain what constitutes normative behavior and standards in those realms affected by

Table 6–23. Aspects of Behavior Therapy for Obsessive-Compulsive Disorder

Exposure

• Use of both in vivo exposure and imaginal exposure is preferable.

• Gradual exposure is much better tolerated than flooding.

• There is a greater degree of therapist participation, with use of modeling during therapist-assisted exposure sessions.

• Therapist-assisted exposure sessions should be prolonged (1–2 hours per session) and frequent (preferably conducted more than once a week). Intensive (at least 1 hour per day) and frequent (daily) self-exposure plays an important role.

• Assistance from family members, partners, or friends in conducting exposure is very important.

Response Prevention

• Response prevention is not time limited and continues as long as possible after the end of an exposure session.

• The therapist must carefully monitor whether the patient is using any type of concealed neutralizing activity (e.g., mental compulsions) to decrease anxiety or distress.

• Response prevention should never be carried out through coercion or physical prevention of a compulsion by the therapist or someone else.

• Assistance from family members, partners, or friends in conducting response prevention is very important.

OCD (e.g., it is sufficient to take a shower once or twice a day, unless it is a very hot day, and the person perspires a lot). The patients' strict standards of cleanliness or safety or their rigid moral attitudes often obfuscate their understanding of what is normal, sufficient, and appropriate.

Exposure   In vivo exposure to fearful stimuli may be combined with imaginal exposure, depending on the nature of obsessions. In fact, in vivo exposure combined with imaginal exposure tends to fare better than exposure in vivo alone (Abramowitz, 1996; Rosa-Alcázar et al., 2008). Imaginal exposure is usually used for obsessions with aggressive and sexual themes and involves activation of the corresponding imagery (i.e., visualization), often with therapist-assisted manipulation of the feared outcomes. Gradual exposure is better tolerated than flooding and can be conducted in a way similar to that used in the treatment of agoraphobia and other phobias (see Chapters 2 and 5). This involves the construction of hierarchies of situations and stimuli to which patients are gradually but progressively exposed, starting from the situations that elicit the least amount of anxiety.

In comparison with exposure therapy for other anxiety disorders, there is usually a greater degree of therapist participation in the course of exposure for OCD. Therapist-assisted (therapist-guided) exposure often produces better results than self-exposure, with or without therapist assistance (Abramowitz, 1996; Rosa-Alcázar et al., 2008). Thus, in-session, therapist-assisted exposure, which relies on modeling, is used. Taking as an example contamination obsessions and washing compulsions, modeling is provided by the therapist who touches his or her shoes without washing the hands afterwards, and then asks the patient to do the same in his or her presence.

The number of therapist-assisted exposure sessions depends on the time that patients need to habituate to the feared situation and thus experience a substantial decrease in anxiety or distress. These exposure sessions usually last 1–2 hours; the frequency of more than once a week may produce better results. For therapist-assisted exposure to be efficacious in the treatment of OCD, it should be intensive—prolonged, repeated, and frequent.

Patients should engage in self-exposure and response prevention exercises between therapist-assisted sessions; these homework exercises should be conducted daily and should last at least 1 hour per day. They should be recorded in terms of the level of anxiety and distress experienced and the feelings and thoughts that appeared in the course of these exercises. Partners and family members can play a vital role in this portion of treatment, and their support should be sought whenever possible.

Response Prevention The response prevention component is often described imprecisely and understood partially by patients. It also relies heavily on patients' motivation and self-discipline to refrain from performing a compulsion when they feel the greatest urge to do so. In addition, response prevention continues as long as possible after the end of exposure. That means that patients are expected to refrain from performing the compulsion not only during and immediately after the exposure but also for prolonged periods after the exposure. The therapist has two main tasks. The first is to support patients as they make an effort not to succumb to an urge to perform compulsion. Second, the therapist must monitor patients to check whether they are using any concealed neutralizing activity (e.g., mental compulsions) to decrease anxiety or distress. Using such neutralizations might defeat the purpose of response prevention, as one type of neutralizing activity would be substituted for another.

Response prevention will not be effective if it is attempted through coercion or physical prevention of a compulsion by the therapist or someone else—for example, if a family member locks the bathroom and thereby attempts to prevent excessive washing. This is only likely to increase patients' resistance. Family members, partners, or friends are often key players in conducting response prevention. Their cooperation with the therapist may be crucial for the outcome of treatment; for example, they can help by consistently refusing to be involved in patients' compulsions or provide unnecessary, repetitious reassurance.

Problems Encountered During Treatment   Difficulties in the course of ERP usually arise from provocation of anxiety and distress and prevention of relief that would have been obtained from a compulsion or other neutralizing acts. Being unable to perform compulsion is particularly frightening to patients who strongly believe that this will lead to something dreadful. Patients can fully engage in ERP only if they trust their therapist, if the therapist has succeeded in enlisting patients' collaboration, and if they are continuously supported by the therapist and all others who are involved in treatment.

Patients need to be highly motivated to succeed in ERP. Not surprisingly, about 25% of OCD patients refuse this treatment (Foa et al., 1983; Greist, 1994), 20% drop out (Rachman and Hodgson, 1980), and 25% fail to adhere to it (Foa et al., 1985). Making ERP more "user-friendly" and improving adherence to it is difficult. Therapists should be flexible and responsive to their patients' needs, which may require some modifications of ERP, if necessary and appropriate. For example, OCD patients may respond well to a step-by-step approach in managing compulsions. This involves setting limits on compulsions, so that patients initially spend a certain maximum amount of time performing compulsions (e.g., no more than 2 hours/day) or agree to a maximum number of compulsive acts allowed (e.g., washing not more than two times per episode or washing not more than 20 times a day). These limits should always be negotiated with patients and they become increasingly stricter during treatment.

Efficacy   Keeping in mind that complete and permanent recovery from OCD is rare, ERP has proved to be efficacious for this condition. This was documented in numerous controlled studies (e.g., Marks et al., 1975, 1988; Boersma et al., 1976; Foa and Goldstein, 1978; Foa et al., 1984, 2005; Emmelkamp et al., 1989; Lindsay et al., 1997). One early review (Foa et al., 1985) reported that 90% of patients responded to ERP, with response being defined as more than 30% reduction in symptoms. A decade later (Foa and Kozak, 1996), 83% of patients across a number of studies were found to be responders to ERP immediately after completion of treatment. In a more recent, large study (Foa et al., 2005), more than 80% of patients treated with ERP were classified as responders. Across the studies, ERP has been found to produce an improvement in 75% of patients and recovery in more than 60% of patients (Fisher and Wells, 2005), with an average reduction in OCD symptoms of 48% (Abramowitz et al., 2002). However, only 25% of patients treated with ERP may be without OCD symptoms at the end of treatment (Fisher and Wells, 2005).

A significant advantage of ERP appears to be the maintenance of treatment gains over time: in long-term outcome studies, 76% of patients remained treatment responders over a mean period of almost

2½ years (Foa and Kozak, 1996). Despite this, OCD patients have a tendency to relapse, and booster sessions of ERP and maintenance, relapse-prevention programs based on ERP (e.g., McKay, 1997) may be very helpful.

Predictors of Outcome and Indications for Exposure and Response Prevention   Predictors of outcome of ERP (whether administered alone or in conjunction with medications) have been identified by many studies (Table 6–24). To some extent, these studies have been helpful in guiding treatment decisions in OCD. Thus, ERP does not seem to be a suitable or sufficient treatment option for patients with severe forms of OCD and for those with severe depression, severe personality disturbance, hoarding, and obsessions (especially sexual and religious) in the absence of overt compulsions. By contrast, the presence of co-occurring mild to moderate depression does not affect the outcome of ERP (Foa et al., 1984; Basoglu et al., 1988; O'Sullivan et al., 1991). Likewise, the presence of personality disorders does

Table 6–24. Predictors of Outcome of Behavior Therapy (Exposure and Response Prevention) of Obsessive-Compulsive Disorder

More Consistently or More Strongly Shown to Be Predictors of Poor Outcome
- Greater severity of OCD symptoms (Keijsers et al., 1994; de Haan et al., 1997; Franklin et al., 2000; Mataix-Cols et al., 2002b)
- Presence of severe depression (Foa et al., 1981, 1983; Keijsers et al., 1994; Abramowitz et al., 2000)
- Presence of severe personality disturbance, especially schizotypal personality disorder (Minichiello et al., 1987; de Haan et al., 1997; Moritz et al., 2004)
- Hoarding (Mataix-Cols et al., 2002b; Abramowitz et al., 2003)
- Sexual and religious obsessions in the absence of overt compulsions (Alonso et al., 2001a; Mataix-Cols et al., 2002b)
- Absence of overt compulsions in general (Christensen et al., 1987; Buchanan et al., 1996)
- Prominent avoidance of the feared stimuli (Foa et al., 1983; Cottraux et al., 1993)
- Unemployment (Castle et al., 1994; Buchanan et al., 1996)
- Living alone (Castle et al., 1994; Buchanan et al., 1996)
- Lack of compliance with exposure homework during the first week of therapy (de Araujo et al., 1996)

Less Consistently or Less Strongly Shown to Be Predictors of Poor Outcome
- Longer duration of OCD symptoms (Keijsers et al., 1994)
- Checking compulsions (Basoglu et al., 1988)
- Excessive arousal in the presence of feared stimuli (Foa et al., 1983)
- Previous (unsuccessful) attempts to treat OCD (Buchanan et al., 1996)

not necessarily have a negative effect on the outcome of ERP (Dreessen et al., 1997) and there is some indication of possible beneficial effects of ERP on the co-occurring personality disturbance (McKay et al., 1996).

Unfavorable results of ERP in the treatment of hoarding have been attributed to patients' poor motivation, lack of compliance with ERP, and premature termination of treatment (Mataix et al., 2002a). As a result, a modified treatment approach has been developed for patients with hoarding (Steketee and Frost, 2006); this includes motivational inter-viewing, learning skills for better attention-focusing, organizing, decision making and problem solving, and longer duration of treatment (26 sessions).

In the treatment of obsessions (sexual, religious) without overt compul-sions, ERP can be combined with cognitive therapy techniques. The latter may be better suited to target the appraisals and beliefs often associated with this type of OCD. The presence of contamination fears (Buchanan et al., 1996), washing and checking compulsions (Foa and Goldstein, 1978; Mataix et al., 2002a; Abramowitz et al., 2003), and compulsions in general (Buchanan et al., 1996; Alonso et al., 2001a) has been associated with good results of ERP. However, the outcome of ERP may be influenced more by the purpose of compulsions and presence of any beliefs attached to com-pulsions than by the type of obsessions and compulsions. It appears that ERP works better when compulsions mainly serve the purpose of alle-viating anxiety produced by the obsessions, whereas ERP may be less effective if compulsions are performed more automatically (to achieve a sense of completeness or to "feel just right") or if they are driven by needs to "undo" obsessions or prevent some catastrophe.

Presence of overvalued ideas and OCD with poor insight often imply a poor outcome of ERP (e.g., Foa, 1979; Kozak and Foa, 1994), but patients with fixed and bizarre beliefs may still respond to ERP (Lelliott et al., 1988). On balance, it seems that ERP needs to be modified for OCD patients with poor insight (e.g., as in hoarding) so that the underlying beliefs and magical thinking, if present, are addressed.

Cognitive Therapy and Integrated Cognitive-Behavioral Approaches

Cognitive therapy is based on the cognitive model of OCD (see Etiology and Pathogenesis, above), which proposes that modifications of appraisals and beliefs related to obsessions and compulsions are required for treat-ment outcome to be successful. Cognitive therapy may be particularly suitable for the treatment of obsessions. In clinical practice, cognitive therapy is often combined with ERT, which may be more effective for treating compulsions.

There are two goals of cognitive therapy: *(1)* to eliminate dysfunctional appraisals and beliefs related to intrusive thoughts (e.g., that these thoughts are important and should be taken seriously or that one is responsible for experiencing obsessions and preventing any harm attached to them) and (2) to eliminate neutralizing activities that arise in response to the inflated sense of responsibility and other appraisals and beliefs. Once patients feel that they no longer have to take their thoughts seriously, their sense of responsibility for having such thoughts is likely to diminish. In turn, this decreases a need for performing compulsions or other neutralizing activities. During cognitive therapy, other beliefs and thinking patterns relatively specific for OCD are also addressed: beliefs that lack of control over one's thoughts is dangerous and that having a thought about doing something is the same as doing it (thought-action fusion), intolerance of uncertainty, and perfectionist tendencies.

Cognitive therapy consists of identifying dysfunctional appraisals, beliefs, and thinking patterns; challenging them; using behavioral experiments; and providing alternative, more realistic appraisals. Identification of dysfunctional appraisals, beliefs, and thinking patterns requires that patients record every thought related to their obsessions. These thoughts are subsequently challenged by asking patients to give evidence "for and against." Behavioral experiments are set up with the goal of testing the validity of patients' appraisals and beliefs; for example, a belief that aggressive thoughts may kill a family member is challenged by asking a patient to deliberately have such a thought so that he or she can find out that this thought does not lead to anyone's death. Demonstrating to patients that their predictions are based on faulty reasoning or magical thinking makes it possible for the therapist to introduce rational alternatives. For example, an alternative appraisal of aggressive obsessions might be that they seem dangerous because patients link them with the highly unlikely, frightening outcomes.

Another component of cognitive therapy is addressing various "safety behaviors," that is, neutralizing activities. It is important for patients to understand how a range of behaviors and mental activities adopted in response to obsessions ultimately maintain these obsessions and feed the associated anxiety. This understanding of the neutralizing activities also makes it easier for patients to engage in response prevention.

As already noted, ERP remains the psychological treatment of choice for OCD, and cognitive therapy for OCD is to some extent still a "work in progress." There has been some uncertainty about the efficacy of cognitive therapy when compared with that of ERP (e.g., James and Blackburn, 1995). Opinion is divided on the issue of whether it is beneficial to add cognitive therapy to ERP or to use cognitive therapy alone in the treatment of OCD. It has been argued that ERP is "adaptable" to various manifestations of OCD (Clark, 2005), which may account for its general efficacy, while making cognitive therapy superfluous. Some research suggests that ERP may be as effective as cognitive therapy in changing OCD-related appraisals and beliefs (Whittal et al., 2005), raising a question about a need to add cognitive techniques to ERP. It has also been reported that effects on compulsions predict all treatment results in OCD better than effects on obsessions and that decreasing compulsions is the process through which both ERP and cognitive therapy produce change (Anholt et al., 2008). If so, the primary aim in the treatment of OCD should perhaps be a decrease in compulsions, for which ERP seems better suited.

In contrast to these reservations, other research has shown efficacy of cognitive therapy in treating OCD (Emmelkamp and Beens, 1991; van Oppen et al., 1995; Jones and Menzies, 1998; van Balkom et al., 1998; McLean et al., 2001; Whittal et al., 2008). The proportion of symptom-free patients at the end of treatment was reported to be very similar when using ERP and cognitive therapy (25% vs. 21%; Fisher and Wells, 2005). Other comparisons of cognitive therapy and ERP showed no differences in effi-cacy and long-term effects (i.e., about 50% of responders to acute treatment were considered recovered at a 2-year follow-up), with the potential advan-tage of cognitive therapy being its better tolerability and lower dropout rates (Whittal et al., 2008). There is much overlap between cognitive therapy and ERP, and their creative integration is likely to improve treatment out-comes, including adherence to treatment. Efforts have been under way to combine the active ingredients of cognitive therapy and ERP in a way that would maximize the benefits (e.g., Freeston et al., 1997; Cordioli et al., 2003; Vogel et al., 2004; Fineberg et al., 2005).

Supportive Psychotherapy

There is little that may be specific for supportive psychotherapy of OCD. General supportive measures used in the treatment of other anxiety dis-orders and, for that matter, other psychiatric disorders may be applied to the treatment of OCD, regardless of whether the primary treatment mod-ality is pharmacotherapy or CBT. Examples of these supportive measures are psychoeducation, help in coping with stressors that may exacerbate clinical features of OCD, and attention to OCD-related family dynamics.

Psychoanalysis and Psychodynamic Psychotherapy

Psychoanalysis and psychodynamic psychotherapy are rarely used to treat OCD because they have generally been unable to alleviate obsessions and eliminate compulsions. Some of the insights of the psychoanalytic theory of OCD now seem more applicable to the treatment of obsessive-compulsive personality disorder, insofar as there are shared features between these two conditions (see Figures 6–3 and 6–4).

COMBINED TREATMENTS

The reasons for combining pharmacotherapy with ERP or CBT (ERP plus cognitive therapy) in the treatment of OCD seem compelling because pharmacotherapy alone and CBT alone are generally less effective in the treatment of OCD than they are in the treatment of most other anxiety disorders. There has been a hope that combining these two treatments would improve outcomes. Furthermore, some of the potential problems with combined treatment for other anxiety disorders do not apply to OCD. For example, use of benzodiazepines and possible interference with CBT through a quick relief of anxiety symptoms are not relevant for OCD because these drugs are ineffective in OCD and are not used in its treatment.

In view of these considerations, it is not surprising that combining pharmacotherapy with ERP or CBT for OCD has apparently been a common practice. Although it appears less controversial, this approach to treatment has encountered problems very similar to those associated with combined treatments of panic disorder and reviewed in Chapter 2.

The first obstacle to the proper evaluation of combined treatments for OCD is the difficulty in ascertaining whether and to what extent various treatments have been combined. Although many studies have used both a medication and ERP or CBT, one treatment component, usually ERP or CBT, is often emphasized at the expense of the other (e.g., Abramowitz et al., 2003); this is not unlike a tendency to underreport medication use in treatment studies of panic disorder (see Chapter 2). Thus, some treatment studies of OCD misleadingly report that their results are a consequence of the use of one, not two, treatment modalities.

There are also divisions along the lines of allegiance to the therapists' primary professional identities (psychiatrists versus clinical psychologists) and therapeutic orientations (biological treatments versus psychological treatments). These divisions are not as deep in case of the more severe forms of OCD, for which it is easier to agree on the need for combined treatment. However, CBT therapists have generally been unenthusiastic about combined treatments, often citing evidence (see below) that combined treatments may not offer convincing advantages over ERP or CBT alone.

Finally, and perhaps most fundamentally, there is little evidence about the advantages and disadvantages of combined treatments for OCD over pharmacotherapy alone or psychological therapy alone. As a result, we do not have a clear answer to the key question of whether combined treatments for OCD achieve better results than either treatment alone, especially ERP or CBT. This situation obviously calls for more research.

Review of Research, Indications for Combined Treatments, and Sequence of Administering Treatments

Several studies have shown that adding ERP (Simpson et al., 1999, 2008) or CBT (Kampman et al., 2002; Tundo et al., 2007) to OCD patients who had a partial response or no response to pharmacotherapy produced significant treatment gains, suggesting that combination treatment might be superior to pharmacotherapy alone. Consistent with these findings, one placebo-controlled study found that a combination of clomipramine with ERP was superior to clomipramine alone (Foa et al., 2005).

When combined treatments for OCD were compared with ERP or CBT alone, the results were mixed. Marks et al. (1980, 1988) reported that clomipramine in combination with ERP was slightly and temporarily more efficacious than placebo plus ERP. In two studies, fluvoxamine combined with ERP also had some advantage over ERP alone (Cottraux et al., 1990; Hohagen et al., 1998), but in one of them, this advantage was lost at follow-up (Cottraux et al., 1990). Two studies with different designs reported that a combination of clomipramine (Foa et al., 2005) or fluvoxamine (van Balkom et al., 1998) with ERP was not superior to ERP alone.

The results of this research could be summarized to suggest that combined treatment for OCD is superior to pharmacotherapy alone, whereas it is either equally efficacious as ERP or CBT alone or only slightly and perhaps transiently superior to ERP or CBT alone. One study showed that the efficacy of CBT in OCD was not affected negatively by the previous administration of medication (O'Connor et al., 2006). Possible reasons for the lack of convincing advantage of combined treatment of OCD over ERP or CBT alone are similar to those discussed in Chapter 2.

Research findings also call into question the usefulness of combining treatments for OCD in routine clinical practice. Therefore, it is important to formulate possible indications for combined treatment. It appears that combined treatment is indicated for the more severe OCD (see Table 6–18) and for OCD co-occurring with depression (e.g., O'Connor et al., 2006). Combined treatment may also provide benefit to patients who have responded only partially to either pharmacotherapy alone or to ERP or CBT alone.

There is no established sequence of combining medications with ERP or CBT. Pharmacotherapy may be commenced for pragmatic reasons, that is, because it is more readily available and easier to administer than ERP or CBT. Also, the more severe OCD is, the more likely it is for treatment to begin with medication(s). Pharmacotherapy may then be augmented with ERP or CBT to improve patient's coping with obsessions and compulsions and decrease the risk of relapse after discontinuation of medication(s). Support is starting to emerge from controlled studies (e.g., Simpson et al., 2008) for the practice of augmenting pharmacotherapy with ERP in case of an insufficient response to pharmacotherapy alone.

If the treatment starts with ERP or CBT, the usual reasons for adding pharmacotherapy are a partial response to ERP or CBT and occurrence of depression. The sequencing of treatments is discussed in Chapter 2 in the context of panic disorder, and many of the sequencing issues also apply to OCD (see Table 2-31).

Studies investigating the efficacy of augmenting ERP with a fear extinction enhancer D-cycloserine (see Chapter 5) in OCD have reported conflicting results (Storch et al., 2007; Wilhelm et al., 2008). This combination strategy for OCD needs to be studied further.

OUTLOOK FOR THE FUTURE

There is a strong tendency to move OCD from the group of anxiety disorders to a new nosological group built around OCD. The advantages and disadvantages of this move, if the architects of the future classification systems decide to proceed with it, remain to be ascertained. Regardless of how OCD will be classified, further research is expected to advance our understanding of its psychopathology. It is not yet clear how best to address the heterogeneity of OCD. While conceptualizing OCD subtypes on the basis of the predominant clinical manifestations may not be optimal, alternative subtyping schemes need to be tested.

Despite progress made in understanding the pathogenesis of OCD, there is much to be learned about the pathophysiological and psychological mechanisms that bring about OCD. One way of moving forward is to study the neurobiological correlates of faulty information processing and psychological constructs such as underlying beliefs about and appraisals of OCD-relevant stimuli. Longitudinal studies could shed more light on the pathways leading from a predisposition to or a high risk for OCD to the actual occurrence of OCD. Factors relatively specific for OCD (e.g., involvement of the cortico-striatal-thalamic-cortical circuits, exaggerated appraisals of the importance of one's thoughts) require further study so that their role in the pathogenesis of OCD could be clarified.

Treatment results in OCD are generally unsatisfactory, and there is much room for improvement. The potential of the existing pharmacological agents may have been exhausted, and a possible breakthrough may occur through development of new drugs for OCD, based on a greater knowledge of its neurobiology. In the meantime, exploring novel ways of combining medications for OCD might improve the effectiveness of pharmacotherapy. Also, some drugs under investigation may improve currently used medications. For example, the "next generation" of SSRIs binding specifically to certain serotonin receptors may reduce side effects and other problems associated with traditional SSRIs.

With regard to psychological treatment, the techniques of behavior and cognitive therapy may need to be modified to increase patient motivation and compliance. Making these treatments more accessible is another priority. Adapting CBT to different clinical presentations of OCD, taking greater advantage of its most effective components, and improving treatment results in severe forms of OCD are additional challenging tasks. Finally, finding more successful ways of combining CBT with pharmacological treatment should receive full attention from clinicians and researchers.

7

Posttraumatic Stress Disorder

Posttraumatic stress disorder (PTSD) develops in predisposed individuals who have had a traumatic experience. There are many different ways in which PTSD presents itself, and only some of them (e.g., avoidance behavior, symptoms of hyperarousal) make it look like other anxiety disorders. Various manifestations of PTSD have led to its also being considered primarily a disorder of memory, a dissociative disorder, or a condition more closely related to depression. Given the presumed etiological link between a traumatic event and PTSD, there is a rare opportunity among psychiatric disorders for implementation of strategies that might prevent the development of PTSD. Most people recover after trauma, while many of those who do develop PTSD remit spontaneously. Still, a proportion of traumatized people develop a chronic form of PTSD—a condition that is often very difficult to treat.

KEY ISSUES

Posttraumatic stress disorder has been a controversial entity since its official introduction in the psychiatric classification in 1980. A number of issues have arisen, and many of them remain unresolved. Some of the key questions are listed below.

1. Is the concept of PTSD too heterogeneous?
2. Are there different types of PTSD or different disorders arising in the aftermath of trauma?
3. Has the concept of a traumatic event become too broad? Alternatively, can a greater variety of stressful events precipitate PTSD?
4. Is the occurrence of trauma necessary for the development of PTSD?
5. Are there any specific or unique features of PTSD, which would allow its differentiation from related disorders?

6. Has the concept of PTSD been overused or misused, especially in the context of compensation claims and litigation? Does PTSD reflect a "medicalization" of the normal human reactions and emotions in response to trauma?
7. What accounts for the fact that the majority of trauma victims recover spontaneously from early PTSD-like symptoms, whereas some go on to develop a chronic, severe, and debilitating PTSD? Has there been too much emphasis on vulnerability to developing post-trauma psychopathology and too little attention paid to factors such as resilience?
8. Why do we still have a difficulty understanding what combination of risk factors best predicts the development of PTSD?
9. Why have attempts at early intervention in the aftermath of trauma produced inconsistent results in terms of preventing full-blown PTSD?
10. How can the generally modest results of the treatment of chronic PTSD be improved? Should the current approach to treatment, which is largely "patchy" and symptom-oriented, be replaced by treatments (both pharmacological and psychological) that target some hypothetical, key feature or pathogenetic mechanism of PTSD?

CLINICAL FEATURES

Posttraumatic stress disorder is a very heterogeneous condition, and its clinical features may vary dramatically from one patient to another. The most common manifestations of PTSD are various ways through which the trauma is being reexperienced, avoidance of any cues that remind patients of the trauma, emotional numbing, difficulties in remembering all aspects of the trauma, various manifestations of hyperarousal, irritability, and negative expectations (Table 7–1). Some of these features may appear relatively quickly after the traumatic event whereas others develop later. A full clinical picture of PTSD is usually present several weeks or months after the trauma. With the more chronic course of PTSD, clinical presentation tends to be more complex, and PTSD is often complicated by depression, substance abuse, and/or personality changes, which lead to further impairment in various areas of functioning.

According to *DSM-IV-TR*, there are three main groups of symptoms and clinical manifestations of PTSD. These are symptoms of reexperiencing the trauma, avoidance and numbing of general responsiveness, and increased arousal. The description of PTSD cannot be complete without first revisiting what constitutes a traumatic event.

Table 7–1. Common Clinical Features of Posttraumatic Stress Disorder

---

Reexperiencing of the Traumatic Event

- Dreams and nightmares
- Intrusive and recurrent memories of the trauma
- Trauma-related perceptual experiences (e.g., flashbacks)

Ruminative Thinking (ruminations about trauma)

Avoidance of Various Reminders of the Trauma

Manifestations of Hyperarousal

- Hypervigilant behavior
- Insomnia
- Exaggerated startle response
- Difficulties with concentration

Irritability, Anger, and Impulsive Behavior

Restricted Range of Emotional Responsiveness (emotional numbing)

Manifestations Related to Depressive Features

- Loss of interests and anhedonia-like experiences
- Loss of purpose, meaning, and goals in life
- Guilt feelings

Social Withdrawal, Isolation

Various Dissociative Symptoms

Loss of Memory for Some Aspects of the Trauma

Various Somatic Symptoms, Somatization

Traumatic Event

In *DSM-IV-TR*, a trauma that may lead to PTSD has been defined as experiencing, witnessing, or being confronted with an event that involves actual or threatened death or serious injury to oneself or others (the actual event), with the person responding with intense fear, helplessness, or horror (response to the event). This conceptualization of the trauma is still very broad and encompasses very different experiences; it also means that traumas that precede PTSD do not include stressful events that are not (directly) life-threatening, such as loss of job or divorce. However, *DSM-IV-TR* considers as traumatic, and not only stressful, events such as finding out that someone close to the person has died suddenly, has had a serious injury, or has become ill with a life-threatening disease. This tendency to widen the concept of trauma may to some extent be related to a growing use of PTSD in litigation processes and has created some conceptual conundrums (see Diagnostic and Conceptual Issues, below).

Different traumas have different impacts not only because of the very nature of traumatic events but also because of the specific reactions of persons exposed to them and specific meanings attached to these events by different people (Figure 7–1). For example, traumatic events in which the life of a person was directly threatened are likely to be experienced differently from the person's witnessing someone's death. A sexual assault may be experienced as more traumatic than an armed robbery. A situation from which escape was possible or in which the person was able to fight for his or her life may be experienced less traumatically than a situation in which no escape and no fight were possible, and the person was completely helpless. Also, traumatic events that are recurrent and in which the person is unable to change his or her particular circumstances (for example, the experience of being a prisoner of war or of being sexually or physically abused as a child) are likely to be experienced differently from single, even severe, traumatic events.

Another aspect of traumatic events is the fact that most people do not expect such events to happen to them: people do not expect to be taken hostage, witness someone's suicide, or even have a traffic accident ("Disasters happen to others"). Because traumatic events are usually unexpected and unpredictable, they can elicit different feelings and be experienced in many different ways. While some people accept the trauma as a fact of life ("That was my fate"), others are angry and may feel as if they were unjustly punished ("Why did it happen to me? Surely, I did not deserve it"). Other victims are quick to point fingers and "know" who is guilty ("The accident wouldn't have happened if the driver hadn't driven too fast"). By their very nature, traumatic events suddenly and often brutally abolish the basic notions of civilized societies—that life proceeds in some orderly fashion, that it is largely predictable, and that it is governed by

Unexpected/unpredictable event involving possible or actual death or serious injury
(potential or real threat to one's own life or life of others)
↓
Reaction to the event:
(1) Intense fear
(2) Helplessness
(3) Horror
(4) Other emotions (e.g., shame, guilt)
↓
Appraisal of the meaning and/or consequences of the event
↓
Longer-lasting impact of the event
↓
Posttraumatic stress disorder

Figure 7–1. Characteristics of traumatic events and responses to these events that may lead to posttraumatic stress disorder (modified from *DSM-IV-TR*).

law and justice. Likewise, traumatic events may suddenly destroy any fantasy of personal invulnerability, thereby inflicting a deep narcissistic wound.

The *DSM-IV-TR* stipulation of emotional responses to traumatic events in the form of intense fear, sense of helplessness, and/or a feeling of horror (a complex state that combines fear, disgust, and/or disbelief) by no means represents all emotions elicited by such events. Some traumatized people feel an overwhelming shame or a sense of guilt, depending on the type of trauma, the nature of their involvement in the event (i.e., whether their lives were threatened or whether they witnessed an act of crime), and personality characteristics.

Reexperiencing the Traumatic Event

Intrusive and recurrent reexperiencing of the traumatic event is one of the most striking components of PTSD. Distressing dreams and nightmares involving a traumatic event are typical ways of reexperiencing the trauma. Many patients have intrusive and recurrent memories of the trauma. Others experience images or scenes of the trauma or some aspects of it, with an "as if real," visual quality of the experience (e.g., flashbacks). These phenomena are sometimes very difficult to distinguish from visual illusions and hallucinations. The perceptual component of reexperiencing the trauma may be very prominent, with one or more senses being involved. Thus, the patient can hear, see, and/or smell the perpetrator of the crime during an episode of reliving the assault.

Reexperiencing of the trauma is an involuntary phenomenon and it is almost always distressing or painful, with patients usually feeling that they have no control over it and that they are helpless. These experiences remind patients that they cannot escape the trauma or suggest to them that trauma is like an open, bleeding wound that will never heal.

Reexperiencing the trauma is usually brief but may recur very often. This may be precipitated by certain events, situations, or perceptual stimuli that patients associate with the particular traumatic situation. For example, a patient who survived a tram crash had very vivid and frightening images of the tram turning over every time she saw the tram or heard it approaching. At the same time, she felt "paralysis" in her legs, was short of breath, and her heart was racing, so that she also reexperienced the original trauma with a physiological response.

Avoidance Behavior

Patients with PTSD commonly resort to avoidance of certain situations, places, activities, or people because these remind them of the original trauma. The avoidance can be driven by a desire to minimize every possibility of reactivating a distressing memory of the trauma and reexperiencing it.

The patient who survived a tram crash avoided not only traveling on the tram but also stayed away from streets where trams were operating because the sight or sound of a tram might provoke unpleasant images of the accident.

The avoidance may provide PTSD patients with the badly needed sense that they are "in control," as if nothing bad could happen to them as long as they continued avoiding all potential dangers. This coping strategy often backfires and avoidance may become so prominent that it accounts for most impairment in PTSD. A typical example is that of a patient who became homebound because going out might remind her of a situation in which she was raped and because she no longer felt safe outside her house. The pattern of avoidance may be even more generalized in that it encompasses conversations about a traumatic event and any related internal mental activity (e.g., thinking about the trauma).

Hyperarousal Manifestations

Manifestations of hyperarousal in PTSD are related to patients' constant expectation of harm and to their consequent hypervigilance. These manifestations can become very severe and may dominate clinical presentation. Sometimes, hypervigilant behavior is so prominent that patients seem paranoid. They see danger everywhere, are constantly concerned about security, and often check whether all safety precautions have been taken. Symptoms of hyperarousal occur in different ways: through insomnia, exaggerated startle response, difficulties with concentration, and/or irritability.

Insomnia is a very common problem in PTSD. Sometimes it is related to distressing dreams and nightmares, and patients' overall sleep pattern is then quite disturbed. Insomnia may also be a consequence of tension, inability to relax, fear that "something bad" might happen, and the resultant need to be constantly alert. Insomnia may be particularly severe in patients whose trauma occurred at night or in darkness. It is not unusual for these patients to leave the lights or television on during the whole night.

Exaggerated startle response is another common manifestation of hyperarousal. Patients with PTSD seem hypersensitive to all sudden stimuli, particularly those that are auditory and cannot be seen—hence patients' occasionally extreme reaction to any sudden sound (e.g., a telephone ringing or someone knocking on the door).

Difficulties with concentration in PTSD may be selective. While patients seem to have no trouble concentrating on matters related to potential or real danger, their concentration may be poor when they attempt to focus on activities they perceive as distracting; focusing on the latter might lead to their being caught off guard. Difficulties with concentrating on simple activities such as reading a newspaper or watching television may make patients believe that their memory is not good, as they often have trouble remembering what they have read in the newspaper or seen on television.

Irritability, Anger, and Impulsive Behavior

Many patients with PTSD are irritable, have a "short fuse," and are prone to impulsive outbursts. These behaviors can sometimes be predicted, but they also occur without any obvious reason. The patients' apparent lack of control over their hostile impulses frightens them and may lead to feelings of remorse or guilt. Angry outbursts may be directed at anyone, including close friends and immediate family members. Such behaviors are difficult to understand, making it hard for others to empathize with patients' problems and contributing to their further social isolation and even rejection. As a result, patients may become even more prone to angry outbursts, thus creating a vicious cycle.

In addition to being related to general hyperarousal of PTSD patients, irritability may also be a consequence of other trauma-related feelings, thinking patterns, and experiences. For example, some patients feel almost entitled to be irritable and angry because the trauma gives them the "right" to have such feelings (e.g., "I won't be restrained after everything that I've gone through"). Other patients may be easily annoyed by what they perceive as a lack of understanding, lack of compassion, and lack of care. Irritability and anger may also be related to the sense of injustice for having been subjected to a traumatic experience, and, in such cases, patients may be preoccupied with the characteristic "Why me?" questions.

Changes in Emotional Responsiveness and Guilt Feelings

A common manifestation of PTSD is a change in emotional responsiveness, which may take many forms. For example, patients state that they have "lost all feelings" so that they are unable to feel happy, just as they cannot feel sad. Patients may report that they feel indifferent, "empty," "emotionally frozen," even toward their family members and friends. Sometimes it seems that their repertoire of emotional responsiveness has been reduced to fear and anger, both of which appear in response to a sense of danger associated with the trauma-related stimuli. This restricted range of emotional responsiveness is often referred to as "emotional numbing."

Emotional numbing may resemble depressive phenomena. Thus, patients who are emotionally numb often report that they have lost all interest in other people, events, or activities, and that there is nothing that could make them feel happy. A close relationship between emotional numbing and anhedonia has been observed, with both phenomena being crucially characterized by the loss of ability to experience positive feelings (e.g., Litz and Gray, 2002; Kashdan et al., 2006). Despite this overlap in phenomenology, emotional numbing has been considered relatively specific for PTSD and important for its development (e.g., Foa et al., 1995a; Litz and Gray, 2002; Ruscio et al., 2002; Breslau et al., 2005). Other common experiences related to emotional numbing are loss of purpose, meaning, and goals in life. Patients' typical statements are "Nothing seems important," "Everything is hopeless anyway," and "I see no future."

Guilt feelings are commonly seen among patients with PTSD. They may feel guilty mainly because they have survived horrific traumatic experiences whereas their fellow soldiers, other inmates, colleagues, travelers, family members, friends, or others have not ("survivor guilt"). In other situations, guilt feelings have a basis in reality, as some patients were directly responsible for someone's death or injury or failed to act responsibly and prevent a fatal accident. If guilt feelings are relentless, accompanied by vehement self-accusations, and way out of proportion to the patients' real responsibility for and involvement in a traumatic event, they suggest a strong depressive component. It is important to understand the nature and degree of guilt feelings, as they may be associated with suicidal tendencies.

Dissociative Symptoms and Memory Problems

Dissociative phenomena are often seen as part of the trauma response and they have been considered a key feature of acute stress disorder, a condition similar to PTSD, which develops very soon after a traumatic event (see Differential Diagnosis, below). Dissociative phenomena may occur as the traumatic event is still unfolding ("peritraumatic" dissociation) or immediately after the traumatic event. Dissociation can be conceptualized as a defense mechanism against the pain of the trauma so that some aspects of the traumatic experience are split off, pushed away, and then forgotten. Hence, loss of memory for some aspects of the traumatic experience is a common feature of PTSD. This inability to remember certain important aspects of the trauma is in striking contrast to a vivid and intrusive recollection of some other aspects of it (intrusive memories).

Dissociative mechanisms may separate memories for traumatic events (or memories for certain aspects of traumatic events) from feelings that accompanied these events. This separation can be manifested through patients' remembering the details of the trauma but forgetting how they felt at the time of the trauma. Sometimes patients seem emotionally detached or numb when they talk about their traumatic experience.

Dissociative phenomena also include a decreased awareness of one's surroundings and various depersonalization and derealization experiences. For example, patients may describe a sense of unreality and alienation with regard to how they appear to themselves or how they perceive some aspects of their surroundings. The feeling of unreality may extend to the trauma itself, so that patients may feel that the traumatic event never occurred. Others may feel that they have been permanently changed by the trauma and have trouble recognizing themselves, others, and their physical environment. Some patients describe various "out-of-body experiences" (e.g., watching their bodies from some distance).

There may also be a marked disturbance in the integration of the perception of time and space, particularly as it relates to the trauma. Thus, patients may exhibit a marked time distortion, and the traumatic event may seem longer to them (e.g., as if it were never ending). Sometimes they feel that the event occurred at a location different from the one where it really took place. Patients' description of the physical aspects of traumatic situation may be quite distorted.

The way in which dissociative symptoms are described in diagnostic manuals such as *DSM-IV-TR* has been criticized as vague, with many of these symptoms overlapping with each other or often being recorded in a manner inconsistent with the other elements of the clinical presentation (e.g., Bryant, 2007). It is also unclear what should be encompassed by dissociative experiences. For example, emotional numbing has been considered both a disorder of emotion and a dissociative phenomenon. The role of dissociative symptoms in the development of PTSD has been a subject of controversy (see Etiology and Pathogenesis, below).

Ruminative Thinking

Patients with PTSD often dwell on their trauma and its consequences in a way similar to ruminations of people with depression. That is, this thinking is somewhat intrusive (although not involuntary), recurrent, prolonged, fruitless, and does not contribute to solving problems and coping better. It has been demonstrated that ruminative thinking after trauma predicts PTSD (e.g., Ehlers et al., 1998; Murray et al., 2002; Kleim et al., 2007). Ruminations in PTSD have been found to trigger intrusive memories of the trauma and they have been associated with the unproductive "why" and "what if" type of questioning (Michael et al., 2007).

Somatic Symptoms

Somatic symptoms can sometimes be one of the leading features of PTSD, and PTSD patients generally report somatic symptoms very often (e.g., Shalev et al., 1990). This is seen particularly in patients who were injured during the traumatic event and who have certain physical consequences as a result of such injuries. A typical example of this is chronic pain.

Some PTSD patients complain of somatic symptoms (e.g., headache, various gastrointestinal problems) that do not have a clear organic basis; sometimes, patients are so preoccupied with these symptoms that they are diagnosed with a somatoform disorder. It appears that a response to trauma in the form of somatization is not at all rare. Certain somatoform symptoms, for example, pseudoneurological symptoms and symptoms associated with sexual functioning, may be particularly common among traumatized patients (Sack et al., 2007). As part of a response to trauma, somatization may change its forms over time. Whereas cardiovascular symptoms were prominent among soldiers in the American Civil War (hence the term "soldiers' heart"), tremor was a commonly observed symptom among German soldiers in the First World War. Extreme fatigue and exhaustion were reported among soldiers who participated in more recent wars.

Posttraumatic Stress Disorder in Patients With Different Types of Traumatic Experiences

Although the patterns of response to traumatic events are similar, regardless of the type of traumatic events, PTSD may have some specific features in patients who develop the condition after different types of traumatic events.

Posttraumatic Stress Disorder in Patients Who Participated in Military Combat (Combat-Related PTSD)

Posttraumatic stress disorder in these patients may have specific features related to the type of trauma and circumstances that led patients to find themselves in a combat situation. Social factors may play an important role in determining whether survivors of combat-related traumas develop PTSD. For example, participation in unpopular wars and being on the side that lost the war may increase the likelihood of developing PTSD. Under these circumstances, soldiers are not welcomed back as heroes; they are usually regarded as an unpleasant reminder of the loss, shame, and national humiliation and are rejected directly or indirectly by the society. Table 7–2 lists somewhat specific risk factors for developing combat-related PTSD (Kulka et al., 1990; King et al., 1999).

Table 7–2. Risk Factors that are Relatively Specific for Developing Combat-Related Posttraumatic Stress Disorder

- Involuntary participation in war—being drafted
- Participation in a war for which public support is lacking
- Discomforts of being in a combat zone, e.g., poor accommodation conditions, sleep deprivation, poor hygiene, inadequate food, exposure to unfavorable weather conditions
- Poor cohesiveness within the military unit, conflicts between members of the unit
- Prolonged and more direct threats to one's life
- Exposure to severe wounds and mutilated and/or dead bodies
- Being wounded in combat
- Participation in massacres or war crimes, or witnessing atrocities
- Absence of enthusiastic or supportive acceptance of soldiers after the war (lack of social support)

Features of combat-related PTSD do vary, but in this group of PTSD patients, social withdrawal, isolation, prominent guilt feelings, irritability, and aggressive outbursts seem to be more common. In addition, complications of PTSD such as alcoholism and drug abuse, depression, suicidal behavior, and impaired family, occupational, and social functioning are particularly frequent. If it becomes chronic, combat-related PTSD is very difficult to treat.

Posttraumatic Stress Disorder in Former Prisoners of War and Torture and Concentration Camp Survivors

Patients with PTSD who were detained as prisoners of war or were imprisoned in jails and concentration camps and tortured there because of belonging to a particular ethnic, religious, or political group have certain characteristics in common. This is because of the nature of the trauma to which these patients were subjected (Table 7–3).

After release from prison or liberation of a camp, many survivors have extremely strong guilt feelings. Not infrequently, suicide is the outcome of this guilt. These PTSD patients may have additional difficulties in adjusting to normal life circumstances. For example, they may have trouble accepting that they deserve basic human rights. Also, patients may find that the world to which they have returned has completely changed or that they no longer belong to it. In these situations, patients may have to leave their country and then subject themselves to another stress of adjusting to a foreign environment.

Posttraumatic Stress Disorder in Victims of Rape, Physical Assault, Armed Robbery, or Other Violent Crime

Patients with PTSD who are victims of rape, physical assault, armed robbery, shooting, abduction, terrorist attack, or other violent crime often become distrustful and suspicious, particularly toward people who in

Table 7–3. Characteristics of Traumatic Experience in Patients With Posttraumatic Stress Disorder Who Were Prisoners of War or Are Survivors of Torture and Concentration Camps

- Repetitive traumatization during detention or imprisonment
- Numerous or unlimited possibilities of being physically maltreated, starved, tortured, and/or subjected to ideological or religious conversion programs ("brainwashing")
- A possibility of being randomly selected for torture or execution
- Prominent sense of unpredictability and loss of control over one's life
- Marked feelings of helplessness
- Sharing the experience of detention or imprisonment with other detainees or prisoners may be marked by competition for survival (whether real or imagined), which fosters interpersonal mistrust, undermines the sense of solidarity, and makes it very difficult for the person to express how he or she feels

some way remind them of the perpetrators of the crime. These patients often present with intense fear of anything that reminds them of the location where the crime occurred or the person(s) who committed the crime. If this fear is accompanied by extensive avoidance, the clinical picture may be very similar to the one seen in phobias. The core issue for many of these patients is the loss of a sense of safety and the subsequent fear and expectation that they will be assaulted again. Therefore, various manifestations of hypervigilance and hyperarousal are a frequent component of their clinical presentation.

Posttraumatic stress disorder in victims of rape may be particularly severe because of the nature of rape and social attitudes toward rape and its victims. Rape is perhaps the most drastic way of violating one's physical integrity, leaving victims with a profoundly shattered sense of self-worth. As a result, the damage inflicted on self-image through rape can sometimes be irreparable. Rape may also have various symbolic meanings and corresponding consequences for its victims. Many of these pertain to the victims' sexuality and experience of intimacy, often leading to various types of sexual dysfunction and impairment of interpersonal functioning in general.

Society is often ambivalent in its attitude toward rape. Although rape is regarded as a crime punishable by law in most civilized countries, prejudice toward rape victims abounds. Among the latter are beliefs that victims of rape are somehow responsible for this crime, for example, by being "sexually provocative" or even by "seducing" the rapist. It does not come as a surprise, then, that rape victims often feel guilty of being raped, ashamed, "dirty," disgusted with themselves, overwhelmed by a sense of self-hatred, and in need of punishment. As a result, rape is still in many ways a taboo topic, with its victims often preferring to remain silent about it. The issues common to many victims of rape are summarized in Table 7–4.

Posttraumatic Stress Disorder in Victims of Traffic and Other Accidents

Patients who develop PTSD after road traffic accidents may present with a prominent phobia of driving or phobia of using certain vehicles. The functioning of these patients may be severely impaired if their job requires them to drive or use other means of transportation on a regular basis. In addition to features of PTSD, these patients may present with consequences of the injuries sustained during the accident, including pain. If permanent, as in case of the spinal cord injury or loss of a limb, such consequences may have an adverse impact on the course of PTSD.

The clinical picture and prognosis of PTSD in victims of traffic accidents may be further complicated if the accident has triggered litigation, from which the patient expects compensation—hence the formerly used term *compensation neurosis*. In these cases, some features of PTSD may seem exaggerated and patients are often labeled "attention-seeking" or "difficult." They can easily get angry and alienate their friends, families, or

Table 7–4. Common Issues Among Victims of Rape With Posttraumatic Stress Disorder

Changes in Perception of Self
- Shattered self-image
- Poor sense of self-worth and self-esteem

Emotional Responses to Rape
- Humiliation
- Shame
- Feeling guilty about rape

Behavioral Aspects
- Secrecy about rape
- Social withdrawal
- Marked safety concerns
- Extensive avoidance of places, situations, people, and other cues that remind victims of the rape

Other Changes
- Loss of interpersonal trust
- Fear of intimacy
- Sexual dysfunction

therapists and may appear unmotivated for treatment. Issues that are somewhat specific for road traffic accident victims with PTSD are summarized in Table 7–5.

Posttraumatic Stress Disorder in Victims of Natural Disasters

Natural disasters, such as earthquakes, floods, storms, forest fires, and volcano eruptions, usually happen suddenly, with little or no forewarning. They are often perceived as "acts of God," a stroke of misfortune, and events that are very difficult to predict or prevent. Disasters affect a large

Table 7–5. Issues Somewhat Specific for Victims of Road Traffic Accidents With Posttraumatic Stress Disorder

- Prominent phobia of driving or phobia of using certain vehicles
- Consequences of the injuries sustained during the accident, including pain
- Memory problems associated with posttraumatic stress disorder may be difficult to distinguish from memory problems caused by a head injury
- Guilt feelings may be prominent if someone died or was seriously injured in the accident
- Litigation or compensation issues

number of people at the same time and acute stress disorder is often seen among the survivors. The losses and suffering can be shared with other survivors, which facilitates the healing process and coming to terms with the consequences of the disaster. If PTSD develops, its prognosis is relatively good and may be crucially improved by effective relief efforts, massive social and psychological support, quick repair of the damage, and adequate compensation for the destroyed property and goods.

Varieties of Posttraumatic Stress Disorder

Partial Posttraumatic Stress Disorder

Some patients do not present with a full clinical picture of PTSD and do not meet criteria for a formal diagnosis of PTSD. In one community survey, this partial, subsyndromal, or diagnostically subthreshold form of PTSD was found in 3.4% of women and 0.3% of men (Stein MB et al., 1997b). A study in the primary care setting reported that 4.6% of trauma-exposed, mostly male veterans met criteria for current subthreshold PTSD (Grubaugh et al., 2005). Partial PTSD exhibits longitudinal stability, as it may be present for many months and years without transformation into full-blown PTSD, but also without spontaneous resolution (Carlier and Gersons, 1995). It may also represent a risk factor for delayed-onset PTSD (Carty et al., 2006). This form of PTSD may be associated with significant distress and functional impairment and it does *not* imply better response to treatment and better prognosis.

Complex Posttraumatic Stress Disorder

A form of PTSD with severe symptoms and permanent personality changes has been conceptualized under the terms *disorders of extreme stress not otherwise specified* (DESNOS) and *complex PTSD* (American Psychiatric Association, 1991; Herman, 1992, 1993; van der Kolk et al., 1996). In *ICD-10*, a similar condition was given a separate diagnostic designation and named "enduring personality change after catastrophic experience."

This form of PTSD is believed to be a consequence of prolonged exposure to severe and often multiple traumas (e.g., childhood abuse, torture, concentration camp experiences) and is characterized by lasting personality changes. They include profound disturbance in interpersonal relationships with estrangement from others, social withdrawal and isolation, pervasive mistrust, suspiciousness and hostility, changes in the experience of one's own identity, feeling of emptiness, and altered sense of meaning and purpose of life. Some patients with complex PTSD may also exhibit persistent irritability, outbursts of anger, and/or violent behavior. The concept of complex PTSD stands at the boundary of PTSD and personality disturbance and denotes effects of severe trauma and PTSD on personality. It has also generated an ongoing debate about the optimal ways of conceptualizing the relationship between severe trauma, PTSD, and trauma-related personality disorder (e.g., borderline personality disorder).

Posttraumatic Stress Disorder With Delayed Onset

A full syndrome of PTSD may sometimes develop many months or even years after a traumatic event. According to *DSM-IV-TR*, symptoms in PTSD with delayed onset emerge at least 6 months after the trauma. It appears that PTSD with delayed onset is relatively rare (e.g., Solomon et al., 1989a; Andrews et al., 2007). Patients who first present for treatment a long time after the occurrence of the traumatic event usually have long-standing but low-grade PTSD symptoms prior to seeking help, and many may have a partial, subthreshold form of PTSD (Carty et al., 2006). Delayed-onset PTSD may also occur as a consequence of "secondary traumatization" in patients who coped relatively well after the original trauma, and may be seen among patients who are seeking compensation.

Acute and Chronic Posttraumatic Stress Disorder

A distinction is made in *DSM-IV-TR* between acute (duration of less than 3 months) and chronic (duration of more than 3 months) PTSD. Acute and chronic PTSD are clinically indistinguishable, and the cut-off of 3 months appears arbitrary. If the distinction between acute and chronic PTSD is to be retained at all, it might be more meaningful to label as chronic those patients who have had symptoms for at least 6 months. Such a conceptualization of chronic PTSD might encompass a more homogenous group of patients and have clearer prognostic and treatment implications.

RELATIONSHIP BETWEEN POSTTRAUMATIC STRESS DISORDER AND OTHER DISORDERS

Patients with PTSD often have other mental disorders, and their clinical presentation may be colored by these co-occurring conditions. The overall lifetime psychiatric co-occurrence rate (at least one co-occurring mental disorder) in one epidemiological study was 79% for women and 88% for men (Kessler et al., 1995). Disorders that are most likely to co-occur with PTSD include depressive disorders (major depressive disorder and dysthymia), anxiety disorders, and alcohol and other substance abuse and dependence.

In view of the role of trauma in the etiology of disorders other than PTSD—for example, borderline personality disorder, various dissociative disorders, somatization disorder, and chronic "psychogenic" pain (pain disorder)—many patients present with various combinations of PTSD-like symptoms, features of borderline personality disorder, self-harming behavior, dissociative phenomena, medically unexplained somatic symptoms, and pain. These patients are often given different or multiple diagnostic labels at different times, depending on the mode of their pre-sentation. In many cases these labels represent different forms of expression of the single underlying, trauma-related psychopathology, and all these apparently different conditions may be considered to belong to a trauma-spectrum group of disorders. Some of these patients may also be described as having complex PTSD.

Posttraumatic Stress Disorder and Depressive Disorders

Major depressive disorder occurs in about one half of persons with PTSD in the community (Kessler et al., 1995). Dysthymia has also been commonly found in PTSD, for example, in one third of Vietnam veterans with PTSD (Kulka et al., 1990). The relationship between PTSD and depression is complex and important for several reasons (Table 7–6).

First, there is a substantial overlap in clinical manifestations, especially with regard to the symptoms of anhedonia, prominent guilt feelings, and suicidal behavior (see Clinical Features, above). The boundary between PTSD and depression may be difficult to draw, and PTSD is sometimes regarded as a variant of depression. Second, PTSD and depression may have a common genetic liability (Koenen et al., 2008a). Third, major depressive disorder may precede the onset of PTSD by many years; it may predispose to PTSD, complicate the course of PTSD, and appear in response to trauma at approximately the same time as PTSD. The occurrence of major depressive disorder after a traumatic event may be independent from the occurrence of PTSD and may represent a different, separate response to trauma (e.g., Shalev et al., 1998a; Erickson et al., 2001; Franklin

Table 7–6. Aspects of the Relationship Between Posttraumatic Stress Disorder and Depressive Disorders (Major Depressive Disorder, Dysthymia)

Frequent Co-occurrence

Significant Overlap in Clinical Manifestations

Common Genetic Liability

Temporal Relationships
- Major depressive disorder may precede the onset of PTSD by many years
- Major depressive disorder may predispose to PTSD
- Major depressive disorder may occur as a separate response to trauma, with or without PTSD
- Major depressive disorder may complicate the course of PTSD

Greater Severity of PTSD Symptoms, Greater Impairment and Disability

Increased Risk of Further Complications and Suicide

Negative Impact on the Treatment and Prognosis of PTSD

and Zimmerman, 2001), or the risk for developing both is shared (Breslau et al., 2000). Finally, the presence of depression in PTSD is associated with greater severity of PTSD symptoms, higher levels of impairment, and greater disability (e.g., Momartin et al., 2004); it also carries an increased risk of further complications and suicide, makes the treatment more difficult, and suggests a poorer prognosis.

Posttraumatic Stress Disorder and Anxiety Disorders

Anxiety disorders are found in approximately one third of individuals with PTSD in the community (Kessler et al., 1995). The rates with which various anxiety disorders co-occur with PTSD are similar in clinical samples. Most common among the anxiety disorders that co-occur with PTSD are generalized anxiety disorder, panic disorder, and phobias, with co-occurrence rates ranging between 25% and 40% (Kulka et al., 1990; McFarlane and Papay, 1992). In some studies, obsessive-compulsive disorder was also found to accompany PTSD more often than expected (Helzer et al., 1987; Breslau et al., 1991; McFarlane and Papay, 1992).

The co-occurrence of PTSD and anxiety disorders may be a consequence of their somewhat common developmental pathways (see Differential Diagnosis, below). The co-occurrence of PTSD and generalized anxiety disorder may reflect their shared clinical characteristics, such as hypervigilance, increased startle response, feelings of tension, restlessness, irritability, insomnia, and difficulties with concentration. The etiological, prognostic, and treatment implications of the co-occurrence of PTSD and anxiety disorders remain to be elucidated.

Posttraumatic Stress Disorder and Alcohol and Other Substance Abuse or Dependence

Chronic suffering of PTSD patients may lead to their seeking some symptom alleviation by means of alcohol or other psychotropic substances. Hence, alcohol or other substance use disorder is usually a complication of PTSD and is found in up to one half of men with PTSD and one third of women with PTSD (Kessler et al., 1995). The frequency of these disorders may be particularly high in certain PTSD patients: for example, lifetime prevalence of alcoholism in male Vietnam War veterans with PTSD was about 75% (Kulka et al., 1990).

Social factors, accessibility of alcohol and other drugs, and their specific effects determine the substance that may be abused. Alcohol and marijuana may be more likely to be abused because of their calming and relaxing effects, whereas stimulating drugs such as amphetamine seem to be avoided by patients with PTSD.

ASSESSMENT

Diagnostic and Conceptual Issues

The diagnosis of PTSD is based on the criteria spelled out in *DSM-IV-TR* and *ICD-10*. The diagnostic criteria in *DSM-IV-TR* are more detailed but also more complicated for routine use in clinical practice because of the need to memorize 17 symptoms grouped in three clusters (reexperiencing the trauma, avoidance and numbing of general responsiveness, and hyperarousal), with a minimum number of symptoms from each cluster required for making the diagnosis. An important aspect of the *DSM-IV-TR* conceptualization of PTSD is its definition of trauma that includes the event itself and response(s) to the event (see Clinical Features, above).

The cluster of symptoms of reexperiencing the trauma includes vivid memories and dreams of the traumatic event, experience of the trauma as if it were occurring in the present (e.g., through flashbacks), and distress and physiological reactivity on exposure to various reminders of the trauma. The cluster of symptoms of avoidance and numbing of general responsiveness includes attempts to avoid all activities, interpersonal interactions, people, and places that are associated with or remind one of the trauma, inability to recall certain aspects of the trauma, pervasively decreased interests, feeling of detachment or estrangement from others, restricted range of feelings, and a sense that there is little, if any, future. The cluster of symptoms of hyperarousal includes insomnia, irritability and outbursts of anger, difficulties with concentration, hypervigilance, and exaggerated startle response.

Unlike the *DSM-IV-TR* criteria, the *ICD-10* criteria for PTSD emphasize symptoms of reexperiencing of trauma as being most important, so that a diagnosis of PTSD can be made in the absence of avoidance behavior, numbing of general responsiveness, and symptoms of hyperarousal. Making a diagnosis of PTSD according to *ICD-10* is a matter of lower priority, as this diagnosis is justified if the criteria for diagnoses of major depressive disorder or another anxiety disorder have not been met. This approach to diagnostic conceptualization of PTSD may lead clinicians to overlook PTSD and underestimate its prevalence.

Although PTSD has received much attention by mental health professionals, nonprofessional organizations, and the media, there is a certain reluctance to use the diagnosis of PTSD. Traditional diagnostic labels, such as depression, anxiety, or some type of a "reactive state" are preferred by some, even when the clinical picture is consistent with the diagnosis of PTSD. Many of the reasons for this "avoidance" of PTSD are related to the controversies about this disorder (e.g., McHugh and Treisman, 2007; Rosen and Lilienfeld, 2008; Rosen et al., 2008), discussed below.

The first issue is that of an ever-expanding range of events considered to be traumatic. As already noted, *DSM-IV-TR* has allowed trauma to encompass instances in which a person has learned or heard about accidents, assaults, injuries, or other misfortunes befalling family members or close friends. This has resulted in a view that it is potentially traumatic to watch horrific events on television and film and that this could lead to PTSD (e.g., Eth, 2002; Pfefferbaum et al., 2002; Ahern et al., 2004). It has been calculated that this expansion of the definition of the trauma increased by 59% the total number of events considered traumatic (Breslau and Kessler, 2001).

Second, it appears that the clinical picture of PTSD is not necessarily related to or caused by the trauma preceding it. A full syndrome of PTSD has been reported in the absence of a traumatic event, for example, among people who experienced various non–life-threatening events (Helzer et al., 1987; Scott and Stradling, 1994; Olff et al., 2005) and people without any previous trauma (Gold et al., 2005; Mol et al., 2005), including those seeking treatment for depression (Bodkin et al., 2007). It has also been reported that pre-trauma vulnerability factors and lack of support after trauma contribute more to the post-trauma psychopathology than the magnitude of the trauma (Ozer et al., 2003). These findings raise doubts about a specific causal link between trauma and clinical features of PTSD and suggest that trauma may not be necessary for PTSD to develop.

Third, there is a question of the distinctiveness and uniqueness of clinical features of PTSD. It was found that the *DSM* criteria for PTSD might be met by a combination of symptoms of major depression and specific phobia (Spitzer et al., 2007), prompting some to call PTSD an "amalgam of other disorders" (Rosen et al., 2008). A substantial overlap between the clinical features of PTSD, depression, and a number of anxiety disorders contributes to a perception that PTSD is a nonspecific syndrome encountered among patients with various mood and anxiety disorders.

These considerations may account for apparently little agreement between clinicians about the diagnosis of PTSD, especially in routine clinical practice (Large and Nielssen, 2001; Nielssen and Large, 2008). Some authors have called for regular use of the structured or semistructured interviews in ordinary clinical settings to make sure PTSD is diagnosed reliably (Nielssen and Large, 2008).

Numerous factor analytic studies have attempted to ascertain whether there are specific symptoms in the structure of PTSD. The findings of these studies have been inconsistent, suggesting not only different numbers of factors or symptom clusters, but also labeling these factors differently. In addition, there have been different views as to which of these factors or symptom clusters might be specific for PTSD. As a result, the issue of the distinctiveness of PTSD features remains unresolved, casting a doubt on the validity of this psychopathological construct.

There are other ramifications of the concept of PTSD. Posttraumatic stress disorder has been criticized as a social and political construct because it legitimizes distress for certain social and political reasons and "medicalizes" normal trauma-related emotions and suffering (e.g., Summerfield, 2004). The social and political purposes of the concept of PTSD may to some extent explain its status as a "faddish" diagnosis. Some contemporary Western societies promote the notion that life is expected to be free of big disappointments and substantial distress. If something does go wrong and, for example, the person's marriage is dissolved or the person loses a job, the associated distress is transformed into a disorder. Hence, disorders modeled on PTSD have mushroomed since the introduction of the diagnosis of PTSD. They include "traumatic grief disorder" (Prigerson and Jacobs, 2001), "posttraumatic embitterment disorder" (Linden, 2003), "prolonged duress stress disorder" (Waddington et al., 2003), "posttraumatic relationship syndrome" (Vandervoort and Rokach, 2004), and potentially, many others.

Finally, misuse of the diagnosis of PTSD in compensation and litigation processes and the possibility of simulating PTSD cast a shadow over the concept of PTSD. The potential gain from simulating PTSD may make malingering of PTSD very attractive. It is disconcerting that rates of malingering among people considered to have PTSD may be as high as 50% (Resnick, 2003) and that lying about exposure to trauma appears to be common in patients with presumed PTSD (e.g., Frueh et al., 2005; Rosen and Taylor, 2007). Distancing PTSD from malingering will not be easy and requires significant changes in the societal attitudes toward stress and trauma as well as changes in the legal system that, unwittingly or not, rewards this psychiatric diagnosis.

In view of the aforementioned problems with the concept of PTSD, several changes have been proposed. They include either "tightening" the definition of a traumatic event (Spitzer et al., 2007) or omitting trauma both from the name of the disorder and from its diagnostic criteria (Nielssen and Large, 2008), omitting all the nonspecific symptoms of PTSD (e.g., difficulty concentrating, irritability, sleep disturbance, decreased interest) from the diagnostic criteria (Spitzer et al., 2007), and retaining only those features that appear to be relatively specific for PTSD, such as emotional numbing (Foa et al., 1995a). It has also been suggested that acute stress disorder should not be listed as a separate diagnosis because it lacks sufficient empirical support and does not perform well in its intended role as a predictor of the subsequent development of PTSD (Bryant, 2007).

Assessment Instruments

The gold standard for establishing the diagnosis of PTSD is the Clinician-Administered PTSD Scale (Blake et al., 1990). It is also used to assess the severity of PTSD and measure the changes that occur during treatment. This instrument is based on a structured clinical interview and should be administered only by experienced and trained clinicians. It is quite comprehensive but somewhat cumbersome and not suitable for routine clinical practice. The psychometric properties of this scale are excellent.

The Posttraumatic Diagnostic Scale (Foa, 1995) is a self-report instrument designed to assess the severity of PTSD and aid in making a diagnosis of PTSD. Because of its brevity, this instrument is relatively easy to administer and can be used as a tool for screening PTSD. It is also suitable for monitoring changes during treatment.

The Impact of Event Scale (Horowitz et al., 1979) is another self-report instrument that was originally constructed to measure the frequency of the symptoms of intrusion and avoidance associated with PTSD and other reactions to trauma and stress. The modified version (Weiss and Marmar, 1996) also assesses the frequency of hyperarousal symptoms. This instrument has been used for early detection of persons who are at high risk for developing PTSD.

Differential Diagnosis

It is erroneous to assume that PTSD-like symptoms that appear after trauma automatically imply that a person has developed PTSD. In terms of differential diagnosis of PTSD, the first step is to establish whether a traumatic event did occur and, if so, whether the symptoms appeared after the trauma. There are several conditions, mainly among the mood and anxiety disorders, that may be present before the trauma and are then exacerbated after the trauma, with or without additional PTSD-like symptoms or full-blown PTSD. Table 7–7 lists conditions that are likely to be considered in the differential diagnosis.

Table 7–7. Differential Diagnosis of Posttraumatic Stress Disorder

Trauma- and Stress-Related Disorders/Reactions
Acute stress disorder
Adjustment disorder
Acute psychotic reactions

Mood Disorders
Major depressive disorder
Dysthymia

Anxiety Disorders
Panic disorder
Agoraphobia
Generalized anxiety disorder
Specific phobia

Obsessive-compulsive disorder

Dissociative Disorders

Psychotic Disorder

Personality Disturbance (especially Borderline Personality Disorder)

Malingering

Acute Stress Disorder

As conceptualized by *DSM-IV-TR*, there are many similarities between PTSD and acute stress disorder (Table 7–8). The traumatic event that precedes both conditions is described in the same way, and the clinical picture is the same, except that acute stress disorder is also character-ized by prominent dissociative symptoms (derealization, depersonali-zation, dissociative amnesia, reduction in awareness of one's own surroundings and/or a sense of numbing, detachment, estrangement, or absence of emotional responsiveness). According to *DSM-IV-TR*, the symptoms of acute stress disorder appear and disappear within 4 weeks after the trauma, whereas the symptoms of PTSD last for at least 1 month. If the symptoms of acute stress disorder continue for more than 1 month, the diagnosis is changed to PTSD. The usefulness of the diagnosis of acute stress disorder and the status of acute stress disorder as a predictor of PTSD have been questioned (see Etiology and Pathogenesis, below).

Adjustment Disorder

In contrast to PTSD and acute stress disorder, the nature of a stressful event that precedes an adjustment disorder is less well defined (according to *DSM-IV-TR*). Such a stressor may be a traffic accident and witnessing the

Table 7–8. Similarities and Differences Between Posttraumatic Stress Disorder and Acute Stress Disorder (according to *DSM-IV-TR*)

Criteria	Acute Stress Disorder	Posttraumatic Stress Disorder
Traumatic event that precedes the disorder	Experiencing, witnessing, or being confronted with an event that involves actual or threatened death or serious injury to oneself or others, with the person responding with intense fear, helplessness, or horror	
Clinical features	1. Prominent dissociative symptoms essential for diagnosis	1. Prominent dissociative symptoms not essential for diagnosis
	2. Symptoms of reexperiencing the trauma, avoidance, numbing of general responsiveness, and hyperarousal	
Onset	Within 4 weeks of traumatic event	Any time after traumatic event
Duration	Minimum 2 days, maximum 4 weeks	Minimum 1 month, no maximum duration

death of a close family member, but also a marital conflict, problems at work, or failure to pass a school test. Usually, however, the event that precedes an adjustment disorder is less severe in terms of posing a direct danger to oneself or others.

Adjustment disorders are usually characterized by various symptoms of anxiety and depression and/or by disturbed behavior, and they rarely resemble acute stress disorder and PTSD. A diagnosis of adjustment disorder is one of exclusion and is warranted only in the absence of the full diagnostic criteria for PTSD, major depressive disorder, anxiety disorders, and other psychiatric conditions. In *DSM-IV-TR*, the symptoms of adjustment disorder persist for no more than 6 months after exposure to the stressor has ceased.

Major Depressive Disorder

Some trauma survivors develop both major depressive disorder and symptoms of PTSD. Ascertaining whether depression is present may be very difficult because of the significant overlap between the symptoms of these two conditions (see Clinical Features, and Relationship Between Posttraumatic Stress Disorder and Other Disorders, above). Symptoms such as loss of interest, diminished emotional reactivity, sleep disturbance, concentration difficulties, profound guilt feelings, and inability to imagine the future may be a consequence of both PTSD and major depression. Deciding whether these symptoms should be attributed to one or the other condition, or to both, requires a careful review of all aspects of clinical presentation. Although no symptom is entirely specific for a particular disorder, it is often assumed that symptoms of reexperiencing the trauma and emotional numbing are fairly specific for PTSD and that anhedonia is relatively specific for depression.

Dysthymia

Many patients with chronic PTSD have chronic and relatively low-grade depressive symptoms that are consistent with a pattern of dysthymia or with that of "double depression" (dysthymia plus major depressive disorder). Symptoms typical of dysthymia, such as poor self-esteem, feelings of hopelessness, chronic sleep disturbance, and poor concentration, are also frequently encountered in PTSD. As with major depression, the diagnostic attribution of these symptoms requires clinical judgment.

Anxiety Disorders

Panic attacks and symptoms of panic attacks sometimes occur for the first time in the context of the trauma or shortly thereafter, and it may seem that the trauma victim suffers from panic disorder rather than PTSD. In other cases, panic disorder is present before the onset of PTSD, with patients then exhibiting a genuine co-occurrence of panic disorder and PTSD. Panic attacks may also become incorporated into PTSD as part of the reaction to exposure to trauma reminders. As a result, symptoms of both conditions may be present at the same time and create diagnostic confusion. If panic attacks are only a part of panic disorder, they occur in a variety of settings and are not bound solely to the situations that remind patients of their traumatic experience.

In chronic PTSD, avoidance of various cues that remind patients of the trauma may become the most prominent component of clinical presentation, resembling specific phobia (e.g., a driving phobia) or agoraphobia (e.g., in case of the assault victims who become homebound). The distinction between phobic disorders and PTSD is based less on the presence of trauma (as the onset of both may be traced back to the specific traumatic event) and more on the reasons for avoidance behavior (which are not only associated with the reminders of the trauma in phobias) and presence of other PTSD symptoms.

Intrusive and recurrent reexperiencing of the trauma may sometimes resemble obsessions seen in obsessive-compulsive disorder. However, the latter are usually experienced as alien (ego-dystonic) and are generally not related to a traumatic event that the patient might have experienced.

Dissociative Disorders

Distinguishing various dissociative disorders (e.g., dissociative amnesia, depersonalization disorder, dissociative identity disorder) from PTSD may be difficult, particularly when their onset is preceded by the trauma, as is often the case. The absence of other characteristics of PTSD suggests a dissociative disorder.

Psychotic Reactions and Psychotic Disorders

The onset of psychosis sometimes occurs after a traumatic event. According to *DSM-IV-TR*, brief psychotic disorder with marked stressors (brief reactive psychosis) has a maximum duration of 1 month; if psychotic features persist for more than 1 month and have some characteristics of schizophrenia, a diagnosis of schizophreniform disorder should be considered. Acute psychotic features in the context of the trauma may also be related to bipolar affective disorder or be a part of delirium, substance-induced psychosis, or some other "organic" mental disorder.

Hallucinatory experiences (usually visual) as part of PTSD are always related to the trauma and constitute a way through which the trauma is reexperienced. They are short-lived and are often not true hallucinations. Persecutory delusions may occur in some patients with PTSD; if they are fleeting, not held firmly, and appear on the background of prominent hypervigilance, they can be considered a part of PTSD. In other cases, a psychotic illness may be present in addition to PTSD.

Personality Disturbance

The relationship between PTSD and personality disturbance is complex, as described in Clinical Features, and Relationship Between Posttraumatic Stress Disorder and Other Disorders (above). When a significant personality dysfunction co-occurs with PTSD, it is important to ascertain whether it preceded the traumatic event or developed as a complication of PTSD. There should be convincing evidence that personality disorder predated the traumatic event for the diagnosis of a personality disorder to be made. In many cases the personality disturbance manifestations seem to have begun at about the same time as PTSD or as a result of trauma (e.g., in borderline personality disorder). In these situations both diagnoses may be justified.

Malingering

Malingering should be taken into consideration in the differential diagnosis of PTSD if there is a litigation process, if criminal charges have been brought against the patient, or if political motives are implicated. The goals of malingering may be to receive financial compensation, elicit sympathy or public support, shift the blame to someone else, avoid punishment, and/or decrease the sentence. Malingering may be suspected in patients who seem to exaggerate their symptoms and distress and whose clinical presentation is inconsistent or very unusual, and who exhibit severe personality disturbance. It may be difficult to distinguish between PTSD and malingering, largely because the diagnosis of PTSD relies on patients' accounts of their symptoms and experiences, and it is not difficult to learn these from a variety of widely available sources. Guidelines for helping clinicians make this distinction have been developed (e.g., Resnick, 2003; Hall and Hall, 2006).

EPIDEMIOLOGY

Epidemiological considerations for PTSD are unique in that estimates of its frequency in the general population need to be made on the background of trauma exposure estimates. The likelihood with which people in the community are exposed to traumatic events varies substantially from one setting to another and from one country to another. There are also differences in the type of trauma to which different populations are likely to be exposed.

Trauma Exposure

Exposure rates to potentially traumatic events in the general adult population are high to extremely high, depending on the setting in which surveys took place and criteria for determining what constitutes a trauma (see Diagnostic and Conceptual Issues, above). In the National Comorbidity Survey, 61% of men and 51% of women from the representative sample of the U.S. population aged 15–54 reported being exposed to at least one traumatic event during their lives (Kessler et al., 1995). Exposure to multiple traumatic events was more frequent than exposure to a single event. The most common traumatic events were witnessing someone being injured or killed, being involved in a fire or natural disaster, and being involved in a life-threatening accident. Women were more likely to report rape, sexual assault or molestation, and abuse in childhood, whereas men more frequently reported being involved in a life-threatening accident, fire or other disaster and combat, physical assault, being threatened with a weapon, and being held captive.

Similar results were reported in one Australian epidemiological study, with the lifetime exposure rates to traumatic events for men being 65% and for women 50% (Creamer et al., 2001). In a study from Winnipeg, Canada, 81% of men and 74% of women experienced at least one traumatic event during their lifetime (Stein MB et al., 1997b), whereas in Detroit, the lifetime exposure rates to traumatic events were 97% for men and 87% for women (Breslau et al., 1998).

Exposure to traumatic events has been related to age and type of trauma. For example, the highest risk of violent trauma exposure in Detroit was recorded in adolescents and young adults (Breslau et al., 1998). Other studies have also found a frequent exposure to violent traumatic events in children and adolescents in the United States, with up to 47% of boys and 38% of girls reporting at least one such event (Boney-McCoy and Finkelhor, 1995; Schwab-Stone et al., 1995). Findings regarding trauma exposure rates in different ethnic groups in the United States have not been consistent, but these rates have been much higher among the urban and inner-city residents, regardless of ethnicity (e.g., Schwab-Stone et al., 1995). Children and adolescents seem to be at a particularly high risk of exposure to various forms of community violence in these usually impoverished, socioeconomically deprived, and crime-infested areas.

Exposure to traumatic experiences in various countries and populations depends on the particular social, economic, and political circumstances. Not surprisingly, trauma exposure rates have been exceedingly high among refugees and in some developing nations, countries with political and economic instability, societies with a high crime rate, and countries involved in recent armed conflicts or wars (e.g., Sack et al., 1994; de Jong et al., 2001).

When responses to traumatic events, as stipulated in the definition of trauma in *DSM-IV* (i.e., intense fear, helplessness, or horror), were taken into account, a vast majority of those exposed to traumatic events also endorsed such a response (Perkonigg and Wittchen, 1999; Breslau and Kessler, 2001; Norris et al., 2003). Of individuals exposed to traumatic events, females who also experienced intense fear, helplessness, or horror outnumbered males (80%–87% vs. 73%–74%; Perkonigg and Wittchen, 1999; Breslau and Kessler, 2001; Norris et al., 2003). The gender imbalance in terms of higher rates of exposure to traumatic events among males is largely offset by higher rates of relevant emotional responses to traumatic events in females, suggesting that there is little or no gender difference in exposure to trauma.

Epidemiological Findings for Posttraumatic Stress Disorder

The overall likelihood of developing PTSD over the lifetime after exposure to a traumatic event (conditional risk) was estimated to vary between 13% and 20.4% in women and between 6.2% and 8.2% in men (Kessler et al., 1995; Breslau et al., 1998). This likelihood differed substantially according to the type of trauma. The highest risk (45.9% for women and 65% for men) was found in victims of rape, followed by the risk in victims and survivors of combat and other crime (abuse and neglect in childhood, sexual molestation, physical assault) (Kessler et al., 1995; Breslau et al., 1998). The lifetime prevalence rates of PTSD among Vietnam War veterans were 30.9% in men and 26.9% in women (Kulka et al., 1990), but the more recent estimate of lifetime prevalence of PTSD in this population was lower, at 18.7% (Dohrenwend et al., 2006). The risk of developing PTSD was fairly low in survivors of natural disasters (3.8%) and victims of motor vehicle accidents (2.3%), while the lowest risk (0.2%) was recorded in persons who unexpectedly found a dead body (Breslau et al., 1998). The conditional risk for PTSD decreases with age and is higher in individuals whose trauma has occurred in childhood or early adolescence than in those whose trauma has occurred later in adolescence or adulthood (Kessler et al., 1995; Breslau et al., 1997).

Differences in the impact of various types of trauma and in the conditional risk for developing PTSD may to some extent be due to the ways in which the society responds to trauma. For example, the opportunities for recovering from rape are usually more limited than the opportunities for recovering from the consequences of a natural disaster.

The lifetime prevalence of PTSD in the general adult population in the United States was very low (1%) when using *DSM-III* criteria (Helzer et al., 1987). In the subsequent epidemiological studies, based on the *DSM-III-R* and *DSM-IV* criteria, estimates of the lifetime prevalence of PTSD in the general population in the United States were much higher, ranging from 6.8% (National Comorbidity Survey Replication; Kessler et al., 2005) to 9.2% (Breslau et al., 1991). There is some concern about these high prevalence rates because abuse of the diagnosis of PTSD by people who malinger or by those who are involved in litigation may artificially increase prevalence rates of PTSD (Rosen, 2004). No convincing differences in the prevalence rates of PTSD between various ethnic groups in the United States have been found (Kessler et al., 1995; Breslau et al., 1998).

Relatively few epidemiological studies of PTSD have been conducted outside of the United States and Canada. Not surprisingly, the lifetime prevalence rates of PTSD were very low in some countries (0.18% in Italy and 0.6% in Hong Kong; Faravelli et al., 1989; Chen et al., 1993) and high to extremely high in others (11.2% in Mexico and 37% in Algeria; de Jong et al., 2001; Norris et al., 2003). These differences mainly reflect different socioeconomic and political factors, particularly those that influence the likelihood of exposure to trauma and shape the societal response to trauma.

Epidemiological studies consistently show that more women than men suffer from PTSD. The lifetime prevalence of PTSD is about two times higher in women than in men in the United States (10.4%–11% vs. 5%–6%) (Breslau et al., 1991; Kessler et al., 1995). Studies in other countries found a similar preponderance of PTSD among women, except for Australia, where no gender difference was reported (Creamer et al., 2001), and Gaza, where there were more men with PTSD (de Jong et al., 2001). The reasons for generally higher prevalence rates of PTSD in women are not clear, especially since women are less likely to be exposed to traumatic events than men. As already noted, one possible explanation is women's apparently greater propensity to respond to trauma with intense fear, helplessness, or horror. Women are more likely than men to experience sexual assault and rape, which carry a particularly high risk for PTSD. Also, female victims of rape and other violent crime experience negative or stigmatizing social responses more often than male victims of the same crimes (e.g., Andrews et al., 2003).

The risk factors for developing PTSD are discussed in detail in Etiology and Pathogenesis (below). Table 7–9 summarizes main data about trauma exposure and epidemiology of PTSD.

Table 7–9. Epidemiological Data for Posttraumatic Stress Disorder

Prevalence rates of PTSD in the general population should be considered in conjunction with trauma exposure rates, as the latter vary significantly in different populations

Trauma Exposure Data

- Lifetime exposure rates to potentially traumatic events in the general adult population in the United States, Canada, and Australia: 61%–97% (men), 50%–87% (women)
- Children and adolescents in the United States are frequently exposed to violent traumatic events
- Exposure to multiple traumatic events is more frequent than exposure to a single traumatic event
- Findings regarding trauma exposure rates in different ethnic groups in the United States have not been consistent
- Trauma exposure rates are much higher among the urban and inner-city residents in the United States, regardless of ethnicity
- Trauma exposure rates tend to be extremely high among the refugees and in some developing countries, countries with political and economic instability, societies with a high crime rate, and countries involved in recent armed conflicts or wars
- Of individuals exposed to traumatic events in the United States, Germany, and Mexico, females who also experienced intense fear, helplessness, or horror outnumbered males (80%–87% vs. 73%–74%)

Table 7–9. (Continued)

Data for Posttraumatic Stress Disorder

- Overall likelihood of developing PTSD over lifetime after exposure to a traumatic event (conditional risk): 13%–20% (women), 6%–10% (men)
- Conditional risk for PTSD varies widely according to the type of trauma, with the highest risk being associated with rape, combat, and other crime (abuse and neglect in childhood, sexual molestation, physical assault)
- Conditional risk for PTSD decreases with age and is higher in individuals whose trauma has occurred in childhood or early adolescence than in those whose trauma has occurred later in adolescence or in adulthood
- Lifetime prevalence in the United States: 1% (*DSM-III* criteria, Epidemiologic Catchment Area Study), 9.2% (*DSM-III-R* criteria), 7.8% (*DSM-III-R* criteria, National Comorbidity Survey), 6.8% (*DSM-IV* criteria, National Comorbidity Survey Replication)
- No convincing differences in prevalence rates of PTSD between various ethnic groups in the United States have been found
- Lifetime prevalence in various countries, according to various diagnostic criteria: 0.18%–37%
- Lifetime prevalence is about 2 times higher in women than in men in most studies

COURSE AND PROGNOSIS

Although the course of PTSD (Table 7–10) varies from one patient to another, a remarkable finding about its course is the tendency to spontaneously diminish in intensity and disappear in a substantial number of patients. For example, the proportion of the trauma survivors with PTSD in one study was 39% 1 month after trauma, 17% 4 months after trauma, and 10% 1 year after trauma (Shalev et al., 1997; Freedman et al., 1999).

Table 7–10. Course of Posttraumatic Stress Disorder

A. Recovery

- Tendency to spontaneously diminish in intensity and disappear in a substantial number of patients within a few years of onset
- Recovery rates decrease sharply after PTSD has become chronic and, in particular, 1–2 years after onset
- Recovery rate 5 years after onset of PTSD: 18% (Zlotnick et al., 1999)

B. Fluctuating course (exacerbations and partial remissions)

C. Chronic, deteriorating course, often with various complications (depression, substance abuse or dependence, enduring personality change) and lasting impairment in most areas of functioning

Similarly, the prevalence of PTSD was 30.2% 1–3 months after a catastrophic earthquake, 26.9% 6–10 months after the earthquake, and 10.6% 18–20 months after the earthquake (Karamustafalioglu et al., 2006). Kessler et al. (1995) found a pattern of disappearance of symptoms within 1 year in the majority of people with PTSD, with rates of recovery decreasing sharply thereafter; the overall recovery rate was 60%. Similar rates of recovery (up to 66%) were reported by others (Blanchard et al., 1997; Shalev et al., 1997).

The main predictor of the course of PTSD is its duration: the longer the duration of PTSD, the lower the likelihood of recovery. One study has found that only 18% of patients recovered 5 years after the onset of PTSD (Zlotnick et al., 1999), while another reported that no recovery occurred after PTSD had lasted for 6 years (Kessler et al., 1995). A substantial number of chronic patients have a deteriorating course, with various complications (most commonly depression and/or substance abuse or dependence) and lasting impairments in most areas of functioning (marital/family, occupational, social). Some patients may exhibit an enduring personality change, as described in Varieties of Posttraumatic Stress Disorder (above).

Between the extremes of complete recovery and chronic, deteriorating course are PTSD patients with a course characterized by exacerbations and incomplete remissions. About one third of all patients with PTSD may have such a course. Exacerbations may be precipitated by exposure to reminders of the original trauma or by the occurrence of another traumatic event. Some patients may have a low tolerance for frustrating or stressful situations and experience difficulties in adjusting to any novelty or life change. They may react to these situations with anger or impulsive behavior, by further withdrawal, or by using alcohol, illicit drugs, or benzodiazepines. Some patients have persistent but relatively isolated symptoms of PTSD, such as nightmares and intrusive memories of the trauma. The clinical presentation of PTSD may also change over time.

Table 7–11 lists prognostic factors in PTSD. Poor prognosis of PTSD is generally predicted by early appearance and long duration of symptoms. Children and the elderly seem to have poorer prognosis. The prognosis of PTSD may also be linked with the type of trauma, with war-related traumas and physical and sexual assault generally being associated with poorer prognosis than traumas related to traffic accidents and natural disasters. Low levels of social support and unstable home and family situation also have a negative impact on the course and prognosis of PTSD. Additional factors that indicate poor prognosis of PTSD include female gender, childhood trauma, history of other anxiety and mood disorders, greater number of PTSD symptoms, more prominent numbing and hyperarousal symptoms, co-occurring medical conditions, and alcohol abuse (Breslau and Davis, 1992).

Table 7–11. Factors Indicating Poorer Prognosis of Posttraumatic Stress Disorder

Demographics
- Female gender
- Younger age (children)
- Older age (elderly)

Type of Trauma
- War-related traumas
- Traumas related to physical or sexual assault

PTSD Symptoms
- Early appearance of symptoms
- Long duration of symptoms
- Greater number of symptoms
- Prominent numbing and hyperarousal symptoms

Co-occurring Disorders
- Medical conditions
- Depression
- Alcohol and other substance abuse or dependence

Pre-trauma Factors
- History of childhood trauma
- History of anxiety and mood disorders

Social and Interpersonal Factors
- Low level of social support
- Unstable home and/or family situation
- Conflicts at home or workplace

With respect to impairment and negative impact on quality of life, PTSD has been found to be more severe than other anxiety disorders (e.g., Warshaw et al., 1993). Chronic PTSD may also be associated with poorer physical health in general, deleterious health habits (e.g., smoking), higher likelihood of cardiovascular, respiratory, gastrointestinal, and neurological disease, and greater use of health care services (e.g., Kulka et al., 1990; Kessler et al., 1995; Beckham et al., 1997).

ETIOLOGY AND PATHOGENESIS

There are several psychological and biological models of PTSD that account to a certain extent for its etiology and pathogenesis. These models are briefly presented after a review of our current understanding of the risk factors for developing PTSD.

RISK FACTORS FOR DEVELOPING POSTTRAUMATIC STRESS DISORDER

Despite reports of PTSD without a previous traumatic event (see Diagnostic and Conceptual Issues, above), PTSD has been conceptualized as a condition that does not occur in the absence of trauma. Of all mental disorders, PTSD is (controversially) rather unique in this regard. Even though a traumatic event is necessary for the development of PTSD, it is not sufficient. One study has reported that only a minority of trauma victims developed PTSD, despite 94% having PTSD symptoms 1 week after the trauma (Foa et al., 1991).

Epidemiological and clinical research into risk factors for developing PTSD has identified numerous factors that increase vulnerability to PTSD. It is possible that a combination of these factors, which may be unique for each individual, ultimately leads to PTSD. The risk factors are usually classified in accordance with their temporal relationship to the trauma. Some are present before the trauma (Table 7–12), others are related to the traumatic event itself (Table 7–12), and still a third group of risk factors includes those that manifest themselves in the period immediately after the trauma or many months and years following the trauma (Table 7–13).

In addition to understanding risk factors for developing PTSD, it is important to ascertain risk factors for exposure to trauma, because the latter risk may not be equally distributed. Men, extroverted persons, those with a history of childhood conduct problems and a family history of substance abuse, and persons with psychiatric disorders were found to be more likely to be exposed to trauma (Breslau et al., 1991). Some people, often those labeled as "risk takers," "not risk-aversive," or "accident-prone," and considered to be high on novelty-seeking and low on harm-avoidance dimensions of personality, may be more likely to be exposed to certain types of trauma. There has been little systematic and prospective research into this important area, with studies only starting to suggest that externalizing problems in childhood may increase risk of exposure to assaultive violence (Breslau et al., 2006) or to trauma in general (Koenen et al., 2007), whereas higher intelligence levels may decrease this risk (Breslau et al., 2006).

Risk factors for developing PTSD do not affect everyone in the same way and some appear to have a stronger predictive association with PTSD. In one meta-analysis of risk factors for PTSD, a lack of social support was found to have the strongest predictive power (Brewin et al., 2000). Some studies reported that negative social environment was a better predictor of PTSD than lack of support (Zoellner et al., 1999; Ullman and Filipas, 2001). Risk factors that pertain to the trauma itself and to the clinical features appearing in the period immediately after a traumatic event may be particularly important because their presence suggests that traumatized individuals should be recipients of early interventions for prevention of PTSD.

Table 7–12. Risk Factors for Developing Posttraumatic Stress Disorder that Are Present Before the Trauma and Related to the Trauma[a]

Risk Factors Present Before the Trauma

Demographic factors

- Female gender (Breslau and Davis, 1992; Kessler et al., 1995; Breslau et al., 1997, 1999)
- Lower socioeconomic status (Kessler et al., 1995; Koenen et al., 2007)

Family history

- Family history of mental disorders (Davidson et al., 1985; Kulka et al., 1990)
- Family or parental history of PTSD (Yehuda et al., 1998b), anxiety (Scrignar, 1984; Breslau et al., 1991), and antisocial behavior (Breslau and Davis, 1992)

Childhood-related and developmental factors

- Unstable family atmosphere (Kulka et al., 1990; Koenen et al., 2007)
- Disrupted parent-child attachments (Breslau et al., 1991)
- Early separation from parents (McFarlane, 1988; Breslau et al., 1991)
- Physical and sexual abuse in childhood (Bremner et al., 1993; Engel et al., 1993; Zaidi and Foy, 1994; Fontana et al., 1997)
- Chronic environmental adversity, chronic stress (Koenen et al., 2007)
- Presence of mental disorders during childhood or adolescence, e.g., enuresis (Gurvits et al., 1993) and anxiety disorders (Breslau et al., 2006)
- Behavioral disturbance during childhood, including externalizing tendencies and conduct disorder (Helzer et al., 1987; Kulka et al., 1990; Breslau et al., 2006; Koenen et al., 2007, 2008b)
- Interference with development of the central nervous system, neurological soft signs, lower intelligence (Macklin et al., 1998; Gurvits et al., 2000; Breslau et al., 2006; Koenen et al., 2007)

Psychopathology

- General psychological problems and psychiatric disorders (Helzer et al., 1987; McFarlane, 1989; Koenen et al., 2008b)
- Neuroticism, emotional immaturity (Kulka et al., 1990), negative self-appraisals (Bryant and Guthrie, 2007), high level of hostility combined with low level of self-efficacy (Heinrichs et al., 2005)
- Personality disorders (Ursano et al., 1999b), narcissistic vulnerability (Bachar et al., 2005)
- Past history of PTSD (Ursano et al., 1999b; Breslau et al., 2008)
- Depression and anxiety disorders (Scrignar, 1984; Breslau et al., 1991, 1997; Breslau and Davis, 1992; Kessler et al., 1995; Kleim et al., 2007)

Risk Factors Related to the Trauma

- Greater exposure to trauma (Shore et al., 1986; McFarlane, 1989)
- Greater severity of trauma (Foy et al., 1984; Winfield et al., 1990; Yehuda et al., 1998c)
- Type of trauma and meaning of the trauma for the person (traumatic experiences such as rape are more often associated with development of PTSD than other traumas)

[a] In some studies these risk factors also pertain to development of chronic posttraumatic stress disorder.

325

Table 7–13. Posttraumatic Stress Disorder Risk Factors That Appear After the Trauma

Clinical Factors

- Acute stress disorder (Bryant et al., 1998, 1999)
- Early development of PTSD-like symptoms (Koren et al., 1999; O'Donnell et al., 2007)
- Emotional numbing early after trauma (Feinstein and Dolan, 1991; Mayou et al., 1993; Shalev et al., 1996; Epstein et al., 1998)
- Prominent avoidance and other safety-seeking behaviors early after trauma (Bryant and Harvey, 1998; Ehlers et al., 1998; Dunmore et al., 2001; O'Donnell et al., 2007)
- Reexperiencing symptoms early after trauma (Creamer et al., 2004; O'Donnell et al., 2007)
- Symptoms of increased autonomic arousal early after trauma (Creamer et al., 2004; O'Donnell et al., 2007), including increased heart rate (Harvey and Bryant, 1998; Shalev et al., 1998b; Yehuda et al., 1998a; Brewin et al., 1999; Bryant et al., 2000, 2008a; Mellman et al., 2001) and increased respiration rate (Bryant et al., 2008a)
- Dissociative symptoms (Bremner et al., 1992; Koopman et al., 1994; Shalev et al., 1996; Ehlers et al., 1998; Ursano et al., 1999a; Holeva and Tarrier, 2001; Murray et al., 2002; Engelhard et al., 2003)
- Depressive symptoms (Shalev et al., 1998a; Freedman et al., 1999)
- Greater severity of symptoms in the immediate aftermath of the trauma (Denson et al., 2007)
- Serious physical consequences of the trauma, including severe injuries, chronic pain, and other health problems (Blanchard et al., 1997; Ehlers et al., 1998)
- Great difficulty in coping with and adjusting to everyday life situations and difficulty in solving problems in various situations (Solomon et al., 1989b, 1991)

Social and Environmental Factors

- Low levels of social and/or family support (King et al., 1998; Brewin et al., 2000)
- Unfavorable, stressful, or traumatic life events, not necessarily related to the original trauma (Blanchard et al., 1997; King et al., 1998; Brewin et al., 2000)
- Subsequent exposure to reactivating environmental factors (Kluznick et al., 1986; McFarlane, 1989)
- Being a refugee or being separated from family, relatives, and friends (Hunt and Gakenyi, 2005)

Biological Factors

- Lower cortisol levels shortly after trauma (McFarlane et al., 1997; Yehuda et al., 1998a)

Cognitive Factors

- Excessively negative appraisals of the trauma, its consequences, oneself, responses of other people to the trauma, and the future (Delahanty et al., 1997; Ehlers et al., 1998; Warda and Bryant, 1998a; Andrews et al., 2000; Smith and

Table 7–13. (Continued)

Bryant, 2000; Dunmore et al., 2001; Engelhard et al., 2002; Murray et al., 2002; Basoglu et al., 2005; Hagenaars et al., 2007; Kleim et al., 2007):

- Catastrophic appraisals of the traumatic event
- Negative appraisals of oneself
- Negative appraisals of symptoms of PTSD and other symptoms (e.g., negative appraisals of dissociative experiences)
- Negative appraisals of other people's attempts to offer support
- Exaggerated expectations of negative events in the future
- Attributions of responsibility for the trauma either to oneself (with subsequent feelings of shame or guilt) or to others
- Persistent, repetitive ruminations about the traumatic event

- "Mental defeat" (Kleim et al., 2007)
- Diminished sense of control over one's life and life events (Solomon et al., 1989b, 1991; Basoglu et al., 2005)
- Memory disturbances (Harvey et al., 1998; Warda and Bryant, 1998b; Guthrie and Bryant, 2000; Moulds and Bryant, 2002):

  - Difficulties in retrieving specific positive memories and positive personal information
  - Forgetting negative, trauma-related information and memories avoid, tendency to avoid

- Attribution of responsibility for one's own life to other people, one's environment, or circumstances beyond one's own control (Solomon et al., 1989b, 1991)

With respect to the trauma itself, there has been a suggestion that the more severe the trauma, the greater is the likelihood of developing PTSD (Foy et al., 1984; Winfield et al., 1990; Yehuda et al., 1998c). However, it is difficult to quantify and compare the severity of traumatic experiences because their nature is to a large extent subjective. Exposure to severe trauma repeatedly or continuously over time increases the risk of developing PTSD, and the greater the "amount" of trauma, the greater is the severity of PTSD, the so-called dose-effect relationship (e.g., Mollica et al., 1998).

The severity of symptoms occurring in the immediate aftermath of the assaultive traumatic events, regardless of the nature of the symptoms, was reported to be the most important predictor of PTSD in one study (Denson et al., 2007). The occurrence of certain symptoms during or shortly after trauma may increase the probability of the later development of PTSD. This appears to be the case with dissociative symptoms, depressive symptoms, and increased autonomic arousal, including elevated heart rate and respiration rate (Table 7–13).

There are at least two problems with claims that PTSD can be predicted on the basis of these early symptoms. First, certain early symptoms may not consistently predict PTSD. For example, peritraumatic dissociation has not uniformly been found to be a predictor of PTSD (e.g., Marshall and Schell, 2002; Creamer et al., 2004), and peritraumatic dissociation has been found to predict PTSD less well than persistent dissociation (dissociative symptoms continuing to be present for a longer time after the trauma) (Murray et al., 2002; Briere et al., 2005; Hagenaars et al., 2007). Second, while many early symptoms appear to be sensitive predictors of PTSD (because most PTSD patients have had some of these symptoms in the aftermath of the trauma; Freedman et al., 1999), they are nonspecific predictors, as the majority of traumatized individuals with these symptoms recover without developing PTSD. Therefore, the presence of the early symptoms *by itself* may be of little value for predicting PTSD.

The predictive value of acute stress disorder has also been scrutinized. Some research has found that acute stress disorder may be a poor predictor of the subsequent development of PTSD (Creamer et al., 2004). In trauma victims with acute stress disorder, there is a probability ranging widely from 30% (Staab et al., 1996) to 83% (Bryant and Harvey, 1998; Brewin et al., 1999) for later development of PTSD. Conversely, between 10% (Schnyder et al., 2001) and 72% (Harvey and Bryant, 2000) of patients with PTSD had acute stress disorder. Across the studies, it appears that a majority (70%–80%) of trauma victims with acute stress disorder go on to develop PTSD, whereas about one half of PTSD patients or even fewer (Bryant, 2007) do not have a history of acute stress disorder. These findings suggest that while the presence of acute stress disorder may have a high probability of leading to PTSD, the absence of acute stress disorder is by no means a guarantee that PTSD will not occur. Therefore, the pathway leading from traumatic event to PTSD may or may not involve acute stress disorder.

Using the knowledge of various risk factors for PTSD to introduce effective strategies for preventing PTSD remains a challenging task. We need to better understand how various risk and protective (resilience) factors interact to bring about PTSD or minimize the likelihood of its occurrence.

BIOLOGICAL MODELS

Table 7–14 lists findings of biological and neuroimaging studies that have been considered important for PTSD.

Genetic Factors

There may be a certain genetically based predisposition for the development of PTSD. This is suggested by findings that family history of psychopathology and psychiatric disorders in general increases the risk of

Table 7–14. Findings of Biological and Neuroimaging Studies That Have Been Considered Important, but Not Necessarily Specific for Posttraumatic Stress Disorder

Hypersensitivity of the Hypothalamic-Pituitary-Adrenal (HPA) Axis to Stress
- Abnormally low secretion of cortisol in response to stress, with subsequently decreased levels of cortisol
- Increased negative feedback regulation of cortisol
- Dysregulated mechanism of cortisol secretion

Decreased Hippocampal Volume on MRI Scans

PET Findings on Exposure to Stress or Reminders of the Trauma
- Excessive activation of limbic and perilimbic structures
- Activation of the visual cortex
- Decreased activity of the cortical areas involved in language expression

MRI, magnetic resonance imaging; PET, positron emission tomography.

developing PTSD (Davidson et al., 1985; Fontana and Rosenheck, 1994). Major depression and PTSD may share a common genetic risk, which could explain their frequent co-occurrence; according to this proposition, environmental influences determine whether a person develops one or the other of these disorders (Koenen et al., 2008a).

A study of male Vietnam veteran twins reported that a significant proportion of the variance in liability for 15 PTSD symptoms—between 13% and 34%, depending on the type of PTSD symptom clusters—was accounted for by genetic factors (True et al., 1993). The study did not find that premorbid environmental experiences shared by twins contributed to the development of PTSD symptoms.

Neuroendocrinology of Posttraumatic Stress Disorder

The neuroendocrinology of the normal response to stress involves the release of corticotropin-releasing hormone and arginine-vasopressin from the hypothalamus, which ultimately leads to the secretion of cortisol and catecholamines (mainly adrenaline) by the adrenal gland. As part of the hypothalamic-pituitary-adrenal (HPA) axis, cortisol in the blood then has a feedback effect on the hypothalamus and the pituitary gland, thereby controlling further release of hormones from these brain structures. Thus, with the diminution and disappearance of stress, the initially increased levels of cortisol normally decrease the secretion of corticotropin-releasing hormone and adrenocorticotropic hormone (ACTH), with the latter then bringing down cortisol levels to normal.

What happens with the HPA axis in PTSD? It has been hypothesized that the HPA axis in PTSD is hypersensitive to stress. This means decreased (rather than increased) plasma levels of cortisol (e.g., Mason et al., 1986; Yehuda et al.,

1990) and increased negative feedback regulation of cortisol via corticotropin-releasing hormone and ACTH. A low plasma cortisol level in the period immediately following the trauma has also been considered to suggest a higher likelihood of developing PTSD (e.g., McFarlane et al., 1997; Yehuda et al., 1998a).

Suggestions that lower levels of cortisol might be specific for PTSD have not been supported by other research (e.g., Liberzon et al., 1999; Young and Breslau, 2004; Fries et al., 2005). One systematic review and meta-analysis reported no differences in cortisol levels between people with and without PTSD and found low cortisol levels in studies conducted only in females with PTSD, in studies in which PTSD followed physical or sexual abuse, and in studies that measured cortisol levels in a certain way (Meewise et al., 2007). This indicates that neuroendocrinological abnormalities in PTSD may be more complex and that they may not characterize all people with PTSD.

Neuroanatomy and Pathophysiological Mechanisms

Neuroimaging Studies

Many magnetic resonance imaging studies have found a smaller hippo-campal volume in adults with chronic PTSD (Kitayama et al., 2005). This finding has been considered important for two reasons: (1) hippocampal atrophy may be caused by the stress-induced, persistently high levels of cortisol (Sapolsky, 1995) and (2) the hippocampus is believed to be crucially involved in memory processes, so that reduced hippocampal volume might account for memory disturbances that are often prominent in PTSD. Research has not supported these propositions unequivocally. As already noted, many PTSD patients have decreased, not increased, levels of cortisol. While a long-term treatment of PTSD with paroxetine was found to increase hippocampal volume and improve hippocampus-based verbal declarative memory (Vermetten et al., 2003), one study failed to find a correlation between memory impairment in PTSD and hippocampal volume (Lindauer et al., 2006). In addition, some studies could not replicate the finding of a smaller hippocampal volume in PTSD patients (e.g., Golier et al., 2005), and others also found a reduced hippocampal volume in patients with depression (e.g., Bremner et al., 2000b). Therefore, it does not seem that decreased hippo-campal volume represents a specific neurobiological correlate of PTSD.

Several positron emission tomography studies used PTSD symptom provocation paradigms (e.g., visualizing or viewing traumatic scenes, recalling or listening to the accounts of one's own traumatic experiences). These studies did not produce consistent findings about regional cerebral blood flow changes in PTSD patients, but some preliminary conclusions may be made on the basis of these findings. It appears that in response to traumatic stimuli, there may be a decreased activity of the inferior frontal cortex (Rauch et al., 1996; Shin et al., 1999), Broca's area (Shin et al., 1997), middle temporal cortex (Rauch et al., 1996), medial prefrontal cortex, hippocampus, and visual association cortex (Bremner et al., 1999). Under the same circumstances, there was increased activity of the limbic, paralimbic, and visual cortex (Rauch et al., 1996), anterior cingulate, amygdala (Shin et al., 1997), orbitofrontal cortex, and anterior temporal pole (Shin et al., 1999). These findings suggest that PTSD may be characterized by an excessive but nonspecific response of the limbic and perilimbic structures to the trauma, in conjunction with an activation of the visual cortex and decreased response of parts of the cortex that are pivotal for language expression. In clinical terms, this may help account for nonverbal visual reexperiencing of the trauma along with hyperarousal, which is so common in PTSD.

Neurotransmitter Systems

Noradrenaline Many patients with PTSD exhibit hyperarousal as a consequence of centrally increased noradrenergic stimulation and involvement of the locus coeruleus. This is similar to the changes in the noradrenaline system that may be present in panic disorder. Another similarity with panic disorder comes from the results of studies using yohimbine, which increases noradrenergic function as an α_2 adrenergic antagonist. When yohimbine was administered to PTSD patients, a significant proportion experienced panic attacks, flashbacks, intrusive recollection of the trauma, and emotional numbing (Southwick et al., 1993, 1997). Also, noradrenergic suppressors (clonidine, propranolol) alleviate symptoms of autonomic hyperactivity (e.g., increased heart rate and blood pressure) and intrusive reexperiencing of the trauma (Kolb et al., 1984).

The potential role of noradrenaline and adrenaline in PTSD is underscored by their involvement in the normal response to stress. It has been suggested that in PTSD there may be a hyperresponsiveness of noradrenaline and adrenaline to stress (e.g., McFall et al., 1990). However, studies in which the levels of adrenaline and/or noradrenaline were measured in blood and urine of PTSD patients produced conflicting results.

Serotonin Several findings support the role of the serotonin system in the pathogenesis of PTSD. For example, the administration of *m*-chlorophenylpiperazine (an agonist at some serotonin receptors and antagonist at other serotonin receptors) to PTSD patients induced panic attacks and intensified symptoms of PTSD (Southwick et al., 1997). Serotonergic activity may be affected by stress, for example, by corticotropin-releasing hormone, which is a part of the HPA axis (Kirby et al., 2000). Increased irritability, anger, impulsivity, and aggressive and suicidal behavior, which are often encountered in PTSD patients, have been associated with decreased functioning of the serotonin system (Evenden, 1999; Mann, 1999). The efficacy of selective serotonin reuptake inhibitors in the treatment of PTSD may also suggest a role of serotonin in the pathogenesis of PTSD.

Kindling

Kindling was originally proposed as an explanation for epilepsy but has also been invoked to account for some features of PTSD. In epilepsy, kindling involves sensitization of the neurons to repeatedly administered, subthreshold electrical stimuli so that they eventually start firing spontaneously and produce seizures, without any external stimulation (Goddard et al., 1969). In PTSD, the limbic structures become kindled, that is, sensitized to the trauma-related stimuli as a result of exposure, so that even in the absence of these stimuli and absence of stress, limbic structures demonstrate an exaggerated response, with abrupt changes in mood, anger, and impulsive and aggressive behavior. Kindling in PTSD may involve an excessive noradrenergic stimulation of the amygdala from the locus coeruleus (Post et al., 1997). This theory may explain the efficacy of some anticonvulsants in the treatment of PTSD manifestations such as mood instability and impulsive outbursts.

PSYCHOLOGICAL MODELS

Psychological models of PTSD have grappled with more or less success to explain a condition with complex disturbances in the realms of emotion (e.g., fear, anger), cognition (e.g., memory, attention, interpretations, beliefs about trauma, oneself, and the world), and behavior (e.g., avoidance, impulsivity). A review of the most prominent psychological models is presented below.

Behavioral Model

This model proposes that fear in PTSD is a consequence of classical conditioning, as a learned response to a wide variety of the initially neutral stimuli that become associated with the traumatic event (Keane et al., 1985). Any aspect of the traumatic situation or experience may acquire the ability to elicit fear through stimulus generalization and higher order conditioning. People with PTSD become very sensitive to these trauma-associated stimuli or reminders of the trauma and react with high levels of anxiety. Analogous to the role of avoidance in phobias, PTSD is maintained through avoidance of trauma-related stimuli because such avoidance "protects" against fear. Although the behavioral model is somewhat simplistic, it has been useful as an explanation for the seemingly inextinguishable fear of the wide variety of trauma-related stimuli and for the role of avoidance in perpetuating PTSD.

Theory of Shattered Assumptions and Beliefs

This theory highlights the impact of the trauma on PTSD patients' basic, preexisting assumptions and beliefs (e.g., Horowitz, 1986; Janoff-Bulman, 1992). Since the traumatic event is unpredictable and brutal, it shatters assumptions and beliefs that people may have about adherence to rules and law, safety, justice, fairness, reciprocity in interactions with others, and meaningfulness. The traumatic event turns upside down the person's whole assumptive world in which structure, order, stability, hope, and predictability play important roles. According to this model, PTSD reflects poor adjustment to the trauma, with the traumatized person failing to come to terms with post-trauma reality that is so incongruous with pre-trauma assumptions and beliefs.

Horowitz's Model of Alternate Reprocessing and Avoidance

This theory (Horowitz, 1976, 1986), based on psychodynamic ideas, postulates that PTSD is characterized by alternating attempts to reprocess (work through) and avoid trauma-related information. As a result, PTSD patients oscillate between unpleasant, painful, and frightening "compulsive repetition" of the trauma (e.g., through intrusive memories and flashbacks) and the temporarily comforting avoidance of all reminders of the trauma or even denial of the trauma. Trauma-related information remains active and fails to be adequately reprocessed and integrated with pre-trauma experience.

Cognitively Based Models

Cognitively based models emphasize specific assumptions, beliefs, appraisals, and faulty information processing in the pathogenesis of PTSD. These models attempt to account for traumatic (or emotional) memories as the most characteristic feature of PTSD. That is, they explicitly or implicitly conceptualize PTSD as largely being based on the failure of the traumatic memories to be adequately processed so that they appear intrusively and repeatedly and are accompanied by overwhelming, negative emotions.

Information-Processing Theories

The basic tenet of the information-processing theories is that PTSD results from faulty or incomplete cognitive and emotional processing of the trauma-related experience. The origin of these theories can be found in Lang's (1979) theory of emotional imagery. In the context of PTSD, traumatic or emotional memory is conceptualized as a network that connects the following:

- Information about the physical (perceptual) aspects of the traumatic situation
- Information about the person's reaction (emotional and physiological) to the situation
- Information about the personal meaning of the situation

Although any of these components of the network can activate traumatic memory, it is usually activated by stimuli that remind the person of the physical aspects of the traumatic situation. For example, exposure to the

sights or sounds reminiscent of the traumatic situation automatically activates the original emotional and physiological reactions to the trauma. These
reactions lead to an appraisal of the situation as currently threatening, with
the consequent urge to escape. The memory is strengthened by its link with
the sympathetic nervous system, so that every time the person experiences
autonomic arousal, the memory of the trauma reawakens.

Lang's theory served as the basis for the "network model" of PTSD (Foa
et al., 1989). There are several important components of this model:

1. Traumatic memory is conceived of as a network in which concepts
   of safety and danger play a salient role. Various stimuli associated
   with the notions of danger and lack of safety activate traumatic
   memory in PTSD.
2. There is a lowered threshold for the activation of the traumatic
   memory in PTSD and memory of the trauma is easily accessed.
3. It is difficult for PTSD patients to habituate to trauma-related
   stimuli because of their tendency to avoid such stimuli.

Emotional Processing Theory

The emotional processing theory brings together several aspects of the
work of Foa and associates, including components of the network model
(Foa and Kozak, 1986; Foa et al., 1989; Foa and Riggs, 1993; Foa and
Rothbaum, 1998). In its original form, this theory postulated a memory-
fear structure in PTSD, which consists of neuronal networks that participate
in selective emotional processing of trauma-related fear stimuli. This structure is maintained by avoidance, beliefs about constant external threat,
perception of oneself as weak and inadequate, and appraisal of PTSD
symptoms as a sign of personal failure.

In an updated version of the theory, it is proposed that cognitive rigidity
makes selective emotional processing of the trauma more likely. The cognitive
rigidity pertains to inflexible pre-trauma attitudes and views about oneself
(especially one's own competence) and/or the surrounding world (in terms of
it being safe or dangerous). If these are excessively optimistic, the expectations
and assumptions will be contradicted by the trauma; if they are excessively
negative, the expectations and assumptions will be confirmed by the trauma.

The emotional processing theory has served as the basis for a successful
treatment approach to PTSD, which uses both exposure and modification of
the hypothesized memory-fear structure (see Psychological Treatment,
below). The latter entails adoption of positive, corrective information that is
incompatible with the pathological memory-fear structure (Foa and
Rothbaum, 1998).

Dual Representation Theory

The dual representation theory of PTSD (Brewin et al., 1996) proposes that
traumatic experience is represented in two different memory systems. One

system is called "verbally accessible memory." Within this system, the trauma clearly belongs to the past and memory of the trauma has been well integrated with other aspects of the personality, allowing deliberate and easy retrieval of the trauma-related information and verbal expression of this information. The other system is "situationally accessible memory," which is activated involuntarily (usually in the form of flashbacks and intrusive memories) by the situations that remind the person of the trauma. Within situationally accessible memory, the trauma is experienced as if it were occurring in the present. The memory of the trauma is represented on a perceptual level (containing sights, sounds, and/or smells) and is associated with "raw," unprocessed emotions (as they were experienced at the time of the trauma) and physiological responses to the trauma (with various symptoms of hyperarousal).

According to this theory, PTSD may result from an imbalance between the two memory systems. That is, verbally accessible memory of the trauma cannot neutralize situationally accessible memory, with the latter being easily activated by numerous, unpredictable, and uncontrollable reminders of the trauma and enjoying a retrieval advantage. Therefore, when the memory of the trauma is retrieved, it is automatically experienced as if the trauma were occurring in the present, along with perceptual, emotional, and physiological components of the traumatic experience.

The treatment of PTSD is seen as a modification of the highly distressing trauma memories within situationally accessible memory so that the relatively benign trauma representations are created during exposure and cognitive restructuring. The trauma-related information contained in situationally accessible memory is thereby reprocessed, followed by its transfer to the verbally accessible memory because it can be better represented there. Trauma reminders will then retrieve reprocessed, trauma-related information from verbally accessible memory only. Ultimately, the dissociated, automatic, uncontrollable, distressing, and largely nonverbal and incommunicable memories of the trauma are replaced by fully integrated, well-controlled, verbally expressible, and communicable memories of the trauma.

Comprehensive Cognitive Model

This model (Ehlers and Clark, 2000) suggests that trauma victims who go on to develop PTSD appraise the traumatic experience and its consequences in a way that generates a sense of constant, unpredictable, and generalized threat. Such an appraisal of the trauma is made more likely by the presence of "mental defeat" (Ehlers et al., 2000). This refers to a state of mind of traumatized individuals at the time of the event, which is characterized by a sense of helplessness, loss of all control and autonomy, and readiness to give up and surrender. This experience leads to specific appraisals of oneself as weak and unable to cope and protect against omnipresent danger. Many other factors related to negative pre-trauma experiences and certain personality characteristics also contribute to a negative appraisal of oneself, one's own future, and the surrounding world. A combination of mental defeat, ruminations, and pre-trauma anxiety or depression has been found to be the most reliable predictor of PTSD (Kleim et al., 2007).

The model postulates that there are several specific memory disturbances in PTSD and that memory of the trauma is poorly integrated, poorly elaborated, and poorly contextualized. This is manifested clinically through fragmented memories of the trauma, difficulties in intentional recall of certain aspects of the trauma, and misplacing of traumatic memories as if the trauma were occurring in the present. A strong associative memory accounts for the firm link between memories of the trauma and certain cues or triggers and explains a quick, unexpected reactivation of traumatic memories by various stimuli and a disturbing lack of control over such memories.

Many behavioral and cognitive factors and processes maintain PTSD. Behavioral factors include various attempts to avoid trauma reminders and thereby prevent a return of the trauma memories, safety behaviors designed to minimize trauma-related threat, and use of alcohol and drugs to suppress discomfort or anxiety. The cognitive processes that maintain PTSD include persistent, maladaptive ruminations about various aspects of the trauma and its consequences and selective attention to trauma-related threat cues.

The comprehensive cognitive model has received some empirical support (e.g., Fairbrother and Rachman, 2006), but its various components need further testing and validation. The model serves as the basis for cognitive therapy of PTSD, which has shown efficacy in several studies (Gillespie et al., 2002; Ehlers et al., 2003, 2005).

Psychodynamic Approaches

There are several psychodynamic contributions to our understanding of PTSD. Freud speculated that "traumatic neurosis," a conceptual forerunner of PTSD, develops through "repetition compulsion"; patients keep on reliving the trauma to obtain a greater sense of control over trauma, but failing to do so leads to neurosis.

Krystal (1988) proposed that the essence of PTSD is in the patients' inability to use trauma-related emotions as signals that would activate adequate defense mechanisms against painful recollections of the trauma. Instead, patients experience trauma-related emotions as a warning that the trauma will recur and resort to somatization or use alcohol or other substances in an attempt to alleviate discomfort, avoid painful emotions, and prevent recurrence of the trauma. This may explain a relatively high frequency of psychosomatic conditions, alexithymia, and substance abuse among trauma survivors and patients with PTSD.

The psychodynamic approach to PTSD also takes into account the defense mechanisms used by PTSD patients. The purpose of these mechanisms is to alleviate the consequences of the trauma and avoid painful trauma-related feelings. Patients with PTSD often use immature defense mechanisms, such as denial and projection: they may deny their own feelings or project anger and guilt feelings onto others. Traumatized individuals sometimes defend themselves against the feeling of helplessness through anger, revenge fantasies, or relentless pursuit of compensation.

All psychodynamic approaches to PTSD emphasize importance of the personal meaning of the trauma. Understanding of this meaning is considered crucial for treatment and is related to patient's personality characteristics.

TREATMENT

Many people with PTSD seek professional help only reluctantly and relatively late, after a full clinical picture has emerged. There are several reasons for this. Some people feel ashamed or embarrassed about their traumatic experience; others feel that seeking treatment is a sign of weakness, poor coping, or lack of resilience; there are also people with chronic PTSD who harbor beliefs that they do not have a real disorder and expect their symptoms to go away with the passage of time. This ambivalent and sometimes quite negative attitude toward treatment can affect the treatment process adversely. Some mental health professionals, on their part, are reluctant to treat PTSD patients; this may be due to factors such as discomfort about having to address very unpleasant and painful issues in the course of treatment, lack of readiness to work with patients who are often very difficult to treat, or unwillingness to be drawn into a PTSD-related litigation process.

It is being increasingly recognized that the timing of therapeutic intervention in PTSD is critical and that the best results may be achieved by secondary prevention. In other words, if traumatic events cannot be prevented, perhaps pathological reactions to such events can. Hence the expectation from early treatment to prevent development of the disabling features of PTSD and its complications and improve prognosis of PTSD.

The issues in early treatment of PTSD revolve around two questions. First, who should be treated? All victims of the trauma or only those who appear to be at risk for developing PTSD? Second, how should the early treatment be conducted? Through specific psychological interventions, pharmacotherapy, or some combination of psychological and pharmacological treatment?

Considering the findings that most trauma victims recover without any treatment, it appears reasonable to institute early treatment in individuals who are more likely to develop PTSD. A large body of research has revealed numerous risk factors for PTSD (see Etiology and Pathogenesis, above), but most of them are not specific for PTSD and are therefore of limited value for identification of at-risk individuals who should be offered early treatment. Clinicians are often left with their own judgment as to which combination of risk factors might be predictive of PTSD. As for the most appropriate early treatment approach, there is an increasing knowledge about psychological strategies that might be useful in this phase but little information on effective pharmacotherapy.

A full-blown PTSD presents with different combinations of symptoms. It is unknown whether a single, underlying mechanism leads to different manifestations of PTSD, and current treatments can only target "surface" clinical features, for example, flashbacks, avoidance, or hyperarousal. Considering clinical heterogeneity of PTSD, no treatment approach is likely to be applicable to all patients. It follows that when making a decision about treatment of PTSD, one should take into account specific characteristics of each patient's clinical presentation and personality.

Various treatments are often combined in clinical practice. The severity of PTSD can serve only as a rough guide to the selection of treatment: in mild forms of PTSD, psychological treatments alone may be preferred, whereas in the more severe forms, a combination of psychological and pharmacological treatments is usually used (Ballenger et al., 2000). Only a few studies have compared the efficacy of pharmacological and psychological treatment in PTSD. There is some indication that over short-term treatment, pharmacotherapy (paroxetine) may be as efficacious as cognitive-behavioral therapy (CBT) (Frommberger et al., 2004) or that pharmacotherapy (fluoxetine) may not fare as well as eye movement desensitization and reprocessing (EMDR) (van der Kolk et al., 2007). In the long run, CBT and EMDR tend to produce better outcomes than pharmacotherapy (Frommberger et al., 2004; van der Kolk et al., 2007).

Once the full clinical picture of PTSD has emerged, it may not be realistic to expect all of its features to completely and permanently disappear with treatment. In an effort to avoid unrealistic expectations and disappointment, it is important to set realistic goals of treatment (Table 7–15).

Table 7–15. Goals of Treatment in Posttraumatic Stress Disorder

- Alleviation of symptoms and behavioral disturbances
- Alleviation of the manifestations of any co-occurring conditions
- Better understanding of the trauma, its meanings, implications, and consequences, with sensible incorporation of the traumatic experience and traumatic memories into one's identity
- Increased resilience to stress
- Improvement in functioning
- Minimization of disability
- Prevention of complications

PHARMACOLOGICAL TREATMENT

Aspects of pharmacotherapy that are specific for PTSD are presented in Table 7–16. The precise role of pharmacotherapy in the treatment of PTSD remains to be elaborated. While there is evidence that some medications are efficacious, the magnitude of their effects is not impressive. The response to pharmacotherapy is achieved in just over one half of patients, and many responders still have significant symptoms. A remission (almost complete disappearance of all symptoms, with return to normal functioning) with pharmacotherapy occurs less often, perhaps in one fifth to one quarter of PTSD patients (although in one study, the remission rate achieved after 6 months of pharmacological treatment was 50.9% [Davidson et al., 2006a]). Therefore, there is much room for improvement when using pharmacological treatment for PTSD and a role for psychological therapy to maximize the benefits of pharmacotherapy.

Different symptoms with which PTSD patients present may have different neurobiological underpinnings, with different patterns of response to pharmacological agents. For this reason, it may be very difficult to find a medication that would be equally effective for all the major symptoms of PTSD or for many different combinations of these symptoms. This may

Table 7–16. Aspects of Pharmacotherapy that Are Relatively Specific for Posttraumatic Stress Disorder

- Use of pharmacotherapy for secondary prevention of PTSD (i.e., medications administered early in the aftermath of trauma may prevent full-blown PTSD)
- Rates of response and remission are generally lower in PTSD than in other anxiety disorders, except for obsessive-compulsive disorder
- More classes of medications are used for PTSD than for other anxiety disorders
- Simultaneous use of two or more medications is more frequently seen in PTSD than in other anxiety disorders (with the possible exception of obsessive-compulsive disorder)
- Antidepressants are considered the treatment of choice, but other medications are often combined with antidepressants, sometimes from the very beginning of treatment
- When a combination of medications is used for PTSD, antidepressants are an essential component of any pharmacotherapy "package"
- Choice of medications other than antidepressants may be based, at least in part, on predominant type of symptoms
- When selective serotonin reuptake inhibitors are used, their propensity to cause or worsen insomnia and to initially cause or worsen agitation may have significant practical implications
- Benzodiazepines have a very limited role in treatment
- Boundary between routine treatment and treatment resistance in PTSD is often blurred

help explain why the simultaneous use of two or more medications is more frequently seen in PTSD than in other anxiety disorders (with the possible exception of obsessive-compulsive disorder).

Pharmacological treatment in PTSD is used with the goals of significantly decreasing the most prominent and disabling symptoms and improving functioning. Pharmacotherapy may also be used for treatment of co-occurring psychiatric disorders and prevention of complications. The efficacy of medications in reaching these goals varies dramatically from one patient to another. Main indications for pharmacological treatment of PTSD include its greater severity, presence of symptoms that may be likely to respond to pharmacotherapy (e.g., sleep disturbance, restlessness, impulsivity), and co-occurrence of psychiatric conditions such as depression.

An early pharmacological treatment should target symptoms that appear within several weeks of the traumatic event and are both predictive of the later development of PTSD and responsive to pharmacotherapy. These include depressive manifestations and symptoms of autonomic hyperarousal (e.g., increased heart rate). One recommendation is to start treatment of PTSD symptoms with an antidepressant about 3 weeks after the traumatic event if the acute response to trauma has not subsided by that time, and in particular, if depressive symptoms are prominent (Ballenger et al., 2000). In addition, an early, short-term use of medications that decrease autonomic arousal, such as clonidine and propranolol, may be beneficial (e.g., Taylor and Cahill, 2002; Vaiva et al., 2003). These medications can be administered in conjunction with or instead of muscle relaxation that also aims to alleviate symptoms of hyperarousal. An early use of benzodiazepines was not found to prevent development of the full-blown PTSD (Gelpin et al., 1996).

Certain medications may work better for some symptoms of PTSD than for others, but it is still unclear to what extent medications can be combined to complement each other's effects and how best to use them in combination. Because of the heterogeneity of the clinical picture, it is not surprising that several quite different classes of medications have been used in PTSD (Table 7–17). The choice of medication, *apart from antidepressants*, may depend to some extent on the predominant symptomatology of the PTSD patient (Table 7–18), but we do not have specific pharmacological treatments for specific clusters of PTSD symptoms.

Antidepressants are considered to be the most important pharmacological agents for PTSD. They are used to treat PTSD both because they have direct and specific effects on a wide range of PTSD symptoms and because they are effective in treating the commonly co-occurring depression and anxiety disorders. If not used alone, antidepressants are an essential component of any pharmacotherapy "package" for PTSD. Several classes of antidepressants have been found to be useful in PTSD, but the evidence of efficacy is strongest for selective serotonin reuptake inhibitors (SSRIs) and venlafaxine (in its extended-release [XR] formulation), a serotonin and

Table 7–17. Classes of Medications Used in Treatment of Posttraumatic Stress Disorder

Antidepressants

Selective serotonin reuptake inhibitors
Venlafaxine extended-release (serotonin and noradrenaline reuptake inhibitor)
Tricyclic antidepressants
Mirtazapine (noradrenergic and specific serotonergic antidepressant)
Classical monoamine oxidase inhibitors

Second-Generation Antipsychotics

Risperidone, olanzapine, quetiapine

Anticonvulsants/Mood Stabilizers

Lamotrigine, carbamazepine, valproate, gabapentin, tiagabine, topiramate, lithium

α_1-*adrenergic Antagonist*
Prazosin

Benzodiazepines

Non-benzodiazepine Hypnotics
Zolpidem, zopiclone, eszopiclone, zaleplon

Noradrenergic Suppressors
Clonidine, propranolol

Buspirone (azapirone anxiolytic)

---

noradrenaline reuptake inhibitor. Consequently, these medications represent first- and second-line pharmacotherapy for PTSD (Table 7–19). Tricyclic antidepressants (TCAs), mirtazapine, a noradrenergic and specific serotonergic antidepressant, and phenelzine, a classical and irreversible monoamine oxidase inhibitor (MAOI), have also been efficacious in the treatment of PTSD, but with less evidence. Major tolerability and other problems with TCAs and phenelzine make them less suitable for treatment.

Several other medications—second-generation antipsychotics, anticonvulsants/mood stabilizers, prazosin, a centrally active α_1-adrenergic antagonist, and benzodiazepines—have demonstrated some efficacy for PTSD, whether used alone or, more commonly, in conjunction with an antidepressant. Their role in the treatment of PTSD has not been defined precisely because they can be used as an alternative monotherapy, along with an antidepressant from the very beginning of treatment, and/or for treatment-resistant PTSD, when they are usually added to an antidepressant. In the text below, these medications (listed in Table 7–21) are referred to as alternative and/or adjunctive pharmacotherapy for PTSD.

Table 7–18. Aspects of Patients' Clinical Presentation That May Guide the Choice of Medication in Posttraumatic Stress Disorder, Apart From Antidepressants

Predominant Symptomatology	Choice of Medication
Recurrent, intrusive reexperiencing of the trauma	Second-generation antipsychotics
Quasi-hallucinatory experiences (e.g., flashbacks)	Second-generation antipsychotics
Psychotic symptoms (e.g., hallucinations, delusions)	Second-generation antipsychotics
Irritability, outbursts of anger, impulsive, aggressive behavior (behavioral disturbance)	Anticonvulsants/mood stabilizers(?) Second-generation antipsychotics(?)
Nightmares	Prazosin
Sleep disturbance, insomnia	Prazosin Non-benzodiazepine hypnotics Benzodiazepines(?)
Autonomic hyperactivity and hyperarousal	Clonidine Propranolol Benzodiazepines(?)

Table 7–19. Choice of Medication in Treatment of Posttraumatic Stress Disorder

Rank	Medication
First-line	SSRIs (especially fluoxetine, sertraline, and paroxetine)
Second-line	Venlafaxine extended-release (XR)
Third-line	TCAs (amitriptyline, imipramine)
Fourth-line	Mirtazapine
Fifth-line	Phenelzine

SSRI, selective serotonin reuptake inhibitor; TCA, tricyclic antidepressant.

Antidepressants in Treatment of Posttraumatic Stress Disorder

Selective Serotonin Reuptake Inhibitors

Owing to their broad efficacy and relatively good tolerability, SSRIs have become the first-line pharmacotherapy for PTSD. The efficacy in PTSD in controlled trials has been established for fluoxetine (van der Kolk et al., 1994, 2007; Connor et al., 1999; Meltzer-Brody et al., 2000; Martenyi et al., 2002a), sertraline (Brady et al., 2000; Davidson et al., 2001a; Zohar et al., 2002; Stein DJ et al., 2006), and paroxetine (Marshall et al., 2001; Tucker et al., 2001). There is also some evidence of efficacy for citalopram (Seedat et al., 2000; Tucker et al., 2003) and fluvoxamine (Marmar et al., 1996; Davidson et al., 1998; Escalona et al., 2002), but it comes from open-label studies and one small, controlled trial. Response rates to SSRIs in most of the controlled trials varied between 50% and 60%, with fairly high placebo response rates. In a number of trials, the difference between response rate to an SSRI and to a placebo was barely significant, and some studies failed to distinguish between the effects of SSRIs and those of placebo in certain groups of PTSD patients (e.g., veterans with combat-related PTSD).

There are conflicting findings with regard to the type of PTSD symptoms that may be most responsive to SSRIs. It appears that SSRIs are efficacious in treating various symptom clusters of PTSD but not to the same extent, and that pattern of response varies from one patient to another. Therefore, SSRIs do not seem to be more suitable for any particular type or cluster of PTSD symptoms, and their choice is not necessarily suggested by the presence of specific PTSD symptoms. A study of the effects of sertraline on PTSD symptoms found an early decrease (after 1 week of treatment) in irritability and anger and a more pronounced impact on the psychological than on the somatic symptoms of PTSD (Davidson et al., 2002).

Some improvement in the symptoms of PTSD usually occurs after 2–4 weeks of treatment, but full response can be expected only after a patient has been on a therapeutic dose for 4–6 weeks. Therefore, a trial of an SSRI should last for at least 6 weeks, although an adequate trial requires about 12 weeks of treatment.

Several studies have suggested that SSRIs may be more useful for PTSD related to civilian trauma than for PTSD associated with combat trauma (van der Kolk et al., 1994; Connor et al., 1999; Hertzberg et al., 2000; Davidson et al., 2001a; Zohar et al., 2002). Other studies have reported efficacy of fluvox-amine in combat-related PTSD (e.g., Marmar et al., 1996; Escalona et al., 2002). Posttraumatic stress disorder associated with war-related traumas, and especially with combat experiences, tends to have more severe features and to be more resistant to treatment. It does not come as a surprise, therefore, that SSRIs seem to underperform in the treatment of this type of PTSD. One clinical situation in which SSRIs may be useful is when PTSD co-occurs with alcohol-related problems (Brady et al., 1995).

Side effects of SSRIs and other issues associated with their use are described in Chapter 2. The main specific drawback of SSRIs in the treatment of PTSD is their propensity to cause or worsen insomnia, which, along with recurrent dreams of the trauma, nightmares, and other sleep disturbances, is often a prominent feature of PTSD. Selective serotonin reuptake inhibitors are not necessarily implicated in sleep disturbances, but it is very important to discuss with patients their possible association with insomnia before commencing treatment. Patients with sleep disturbance should be encouraged to follow the principles of sleep hygiene; if that is not sufficient to improve sleep, hypnotic medications can be combined with SSRIs. Non-benzodiazepine hypnotics (e.g., zolpidem, zopiclone, eszopiclone, and zaleplon) should be given preference over benzodiazepines, and if possible, they should be used on a short-term or as-needed (prn) basis. Treatment with hypnotics need not begin immediately; it is recommended that hypnotic medication be commenced after the patient has had at least four consecutive nights of disturbed sleep (Ballenger et al., 2000).

The other relatively specific feature of treatment of PTSD with SSRIs is the propensity of these medications to worsen anxiety and cause agitation in some patients during initial treatment. This effect is similar to that seen in patients with panic disorder treated with SSRIs (see Chapter 2), and may be more frequently encountered when fluoxetine or sertraline is used. As a result, it is prudent to initiate treatment with an SSRI in the same way as in panic disorder—at a very low dose, which is usually one quarter to one half of the dose used to treat depression. Depending on the side effects and treatment response, the dose of an SSRI is then gradually and very carefully increased to a level that is often above its dose usually used in the treatment of depression. The range of effective doses of SSRIs and other antidepressants for PTSD tends to be quite wide (Table 7–20).

Table 7–20. Doses of Antidepressants Usually Used in Treatment of Posttraumatic Stress Disorder

Medication	Dose Range
Selective serotonin reuptake inhibitors	
Fluoxetine	20–60 mg/day
Sertraline	50–200 mg/day
Paroxetine	20–60 mg/day
Citalopram	20–60 mg/day
Fluvoxamine	100–300 mg/day
Venlafaxine extended-release	75–300 mg/day
Tricyclic antidepressants	
Amitriptyline	75–250 mg/day
Imipramine	75–250 mg/day
Mirtazapine	30–60 mg/day
Classical monoamine oxidase inhibitors	
Phenelzine	45–90 mg/day

Venlafaxine Extended Release

One controlled trial has established the efficacy of venlafaxine extended release (venlafaxine XR) in the treatment of PTSD (Davidson et al., 2006b). Interestingly, that study compared venlafaxine XR with sertraline and placebo, and found that only venlafaxine XR, but not sertraline, was superior to placebo. Venlafaxine XR may be particularly useful for PTSD patients who have a severe, co-occurring depression, and where dual action of this drug may be advantageous. Many of the issues regarding the treatment of PTSD with SSRIs also pertain to venlafaxine XR. Side effects of venlafaxine XR and other matters surrounding its use are discussed in more detail in Chapter 2.

Tricyclic Antidepressants

Of the TCAs, the efficacy for PTSD was demonstrated in controlled trials of amitriptyline (Davidson et al., 1990) and imipramine (Kosten et al., 1991). These trials were conducted in patients with combat-related PTSD, and improvements were not impressive. Unlike SSRIs, TCAs do not interfere with sleep and may be useful in the treatment of patients with severe sleep disturbance, restlessness, and agitation. However, this advantage may come at a cost of excessive sedation. The tolerability of TCAs and their toxicity in overdose makes them less desirable as a treatment option (see Chapter 2).

Mirtazapine

Mirtazapine was found to be efficacious in one small placebo-controlled study, where the response rate was over 60% (Davidson et al., 2003). Like TCAs, the specific advantage of this drug is that it does not interfere with sleep and that it may be used to treat PTSD patients with severe insomnia; its main side effects are sedation and weight gain.

Phenelzine

Phenelzine, a classical and irreversible MAOI, has demonstrated efficacy for PTSD in one placebo-controlled comparison study with imipramine (Kosten et al., 1991). In another comparison trial with imipramine, there was no difference in overall efficacy, but phenelzine appeared to be superior in terms of alleviating symptoms of intrusive reexperiencing of the trauma (Frank et al., 1988). Because of the side effects, special dietary requirements and numerous interactions with other drugs (see Chapter 4), phenelzine is reserved for PTSD patients who have not responded to other antidepressants. It may be very difficult and potentially dangerous to use phenelzine whenever compliance with its proper use is in doubt; this is particularly relevant for PTSD patients who lack behavioral control and are prone to act impulsively.

Alternative and/or Adjunctive Pharmacotherapy for Posttraumatic Stress Disorder

Second-Generation Antipsychotics

Second-generation antipsychotics (risperidone, olanzapine, quetiapine) are increasingly used in the treatment of PTSD, regardless of the presence of psychotic symptoms. They are administered either as monotherapy or, more frequently, in combination with an antidepressant. The rationale for this practice is second-generation antipsychotics' anxiolytic, antidepressant, and mood-stabilizing properties (Hamner and Robert, 2005), although there is some evidence that these agents also have specific effects on some PTSD symptoms. Second-generation antipsychotics also have serotonergic and noradrenergic effects, which is of relevance for PTSD because mechanisms involving the corresponding neurotransmitter systems have been implicated in its development (see Etiology and Pathogenesis, above).

The evidence of efficacy of second-generation antipsychotics for PTSD has been somewhat mixed. In controlled studies, monotherapy with olanzapine was not superior to placebo (Butterfield et al., 2001), whereas monotherapy with risperidone showed a significantly better result (Padala et al., 2006). When used as an add-on to antidepressant therapy for PTSD in controlled trials, both risperidone (Hamner et al., 2003a; Monnelly et al., 2003; Reich et al., 2004; Bartzokis et al., 2005) and olanzapine (Stein MB et al., 2002b) have shown efficacy. One controlled trial in which risperidone was added to sertraline did not show an unequivocal advantage of this combination (Rothbaum et al., 2008). No placebo-controlled study of quetiapine in PTSD has been published yet, but open-label trials have reported favorable results of its use as monotherapy (Kozaric-Kovacic and Pivac, 2007) and adjunctive therapy (Hamner et al., 2003b) in PTSD. The doses of second-generation antipsychotics that may be useful in PTSD may be generally lower than those used in the treatment of schizophrenia and bipolar disorder (e.g., risperidone, 0.5–3 mg/day).

Second-generation antipsychotics seem to be commonly prescribed to PTSD patients with behavioral disturbances (e.g., Monnelly et al., 2003), but evidence-based justification for this practice is sparse. These medications are clearly indicated in the presence of psychotic symptoms, which may be more common in combat-related PTSD (Hamner et al., 1999; Kozaric-Kovacic and Borovecki, 2005). Several studies in which adjunctive risperidone and olanzapine demonstrated efficacy, were conducted in patients with combat-related PTSD (Stein MB et al., 2002b; Hamner et al., 2003a; Monnelly et al., 2003; Bartzokis et al., 2005); these patients are often difficult to treat and may benefit from adjunctive second-generation antipsychotics. One meta-analysis has found that adjunctive treatment with risperidone may have beneficial effects on the cluster of intrusion symptoms of PTSD, which include flashbacks and various quasi-hallucinatory experiences (Pae et al., 2008).

Potential side effects of second-generation antipsychotic drugs include extrapyramidal symptoms, sexual dysfunction, and metabolic complications such as weight gain, diabetes, and hyperlipidemias. These adverse events need to be weighed carefully against the possible benefits of these drugs.

Anticonvulsants and Mood Stabilizers

Anticonvulsants and mood stabilizers have usually been considered as adjunctive treatment for PTSD patients, particularly for those with prominent irritability, outbursts of anger, and impulsive, aggressive behavior. The rationale for using anticonvulsants and mood stabilizers may be found in the conceptualization of PTSD as a disorder of affective instability, based on the kindling phenomenon (see Etiology and Pathogenesis, above). Many case reports, case series, and open-label studies involving carbamazepine, valproate, lamotrigine, gabapentin, tiagabine, topiramate, and lithium have suggested potential benefits of these drugs. However, a few controlled trials (e.g., with valproate as monotherapy for male military veterans with PTSD, [Davis et al., 2008] and with tiagabine as monotherapy for a mixed group of PTSD patients [Davidson et al., 2007]) did not show efficacy in PTSD. Only one small controlled study reported that lamotrigine was more efficacious than placebo as monotherapy for PTSD (Hertzberg et al., 1999). A lack of efficacy of some anticonvulsants and mood stabilizers as monotherapy for PTSD in controlled studies does not preclude their use as adjunctive treatment.

Prazosin

Several case series and open-label trials have shown that prazosin, a centrally active α_1-adrenergic antagonist, has a specific effect on nightmares in patients with PTSD. In a small controlled trial, combat-related PTSD patients treated with prazosin (either as adjunctive therapy or monotherapy) showed a significant decrease in nightmares and improvement in other sleep disturbances and other features of PTSD (Raskind et al., 2003). Hypotension, tachycardia, and dizziness are the main side effects of prazosin. Its therapeutic dose is 4–9 mg/day, but some patients may need a higher dose. When prazosin is ceased, it is common for nightmares to return.

Benzodiazepines

In the only controlled study with a benzodiazepine in PTSD, alprazolam decreased anxiety levels but had no effect on the specific symptoms of PTSD (Braun et al., 1990). There is some support for the short-term or as-needed (prn) use of benzodiazepines in the treatment of symptoms of hyperarousal in PTSD patients (e.g., Shalev and Rogel-Fuchs, 1992). Benzodiazepines could also be used for short-term treatment of insomnia, but other medications are preferable.

Long-term treatment of PTSD with benzodiazepines is not recommended, particularly in patients who have poor impulse control. Benzodiazepines may make it more likely for these patients to exhibit aggression. In addition, PTSD patients seem to have more difficulty than patients with other anxiety

disorders with the discontinuation of benzodiazepines and with benzodiazepine withdrawal symptoms (Risse et al., 1990). Benzodiazepines should
also be avoided in patients who abuse alcohol or other substances. For all
these reasons, the role of benzodiazepines in the treatment of PTSD is very
limited. If they have to be used at all, that should be for clear symptom targets
(e.g., insomnia, autonomic hyperarousal), in conjunction with antidepressants or other drugs, and for a very brief period.

Long-Term Pharmacological Treatment of Posttraumatic Stress Disorder

There are no data on long-term treatment of PTSD with medications other
than antidepressants. Therefore, it is unknown whether and to what extent
these medications, when efficacious in acute treatment, maintain their
efficacy in the course of long-term treatment of PTSD.

Several antidepressants have demonstrated efficacy in controlled, long-
term and/or relapse prevention studies in PTSD over periods of up to 28
weeks. These include fluoxetine (Martenyi et al., 2002b; Davidson et al.,
2005; Martenyi and Soldatenkova, 2006), sertraline (Davidson et al., 2001b),
and venlafaxine XR (Davidson et al., 2006a). In one long-term, open-label
study, patients who previously responded to sertraline in a 12-week placebo-controlled study, maintained their improvement over an additional 24
weeks of treatment; some PTSD patients who did not respond to sertraline
during initial treatment subsequently became responders (Londborg et al.,
2001). The latter finding suggests that some patients need to be treated with
an SSRI longer (more than 12 weeks) to respond.

The optimal duration of pharmacological treatment of PTSD is
unknown. For most cases of chronic PTSD, it is recommended that pharmacotherapy with an antidepressant be continued for at least 1 year after a
satisfactory response to acute treatment has been achieved (Ballenger et al.,
2000). In clinical practice, this recommendation often translates to an even
longer treatment. The dose administered during that time should probably
be the same as the dose that produced the initial response.

As with other anxiety disorders, there is a risk of relapse upon discontinuation of pharmacotherapy. Therefore, if the medication is to be ceased, it
is imperative that its dose be gradually and carefully reduced (e.g., by not
more than 25% every 2–3 months). Psychological treatment techniques may
be combined with pharmacotherapy to decrease the risk of relapse.

Pharmacotherapy of Treatment-Resistant Posttraumatic Stress Disorder

Although not precisely established, it is reasonable to postulate that an
adequate pharmacological trial for chronic PTSD consists of a minimum
of 12 weeks of treatment with an antidepressant at the highest

recommended dose or the highest dose tolerated by the patient. In case of intolerable side effects, an adequate pharmacological trial is shorter.

Treatment resistance in PTSD has not been well defined. Theoretically, a patient is not treatment resistant if he or she has not had a trial with all classes of antidepressants that have been found to be efficacious for PTSD. In practice, many clinicians consider treatment resistance to be present if the patient has not responded to two antidepressants, usually one or two SSRIs, or an SSRI and venlafaxine XR. It should be emphasized, however, that PTSD patients who do not respond to SSRIs and venlafaxine should be treated with other antidepressants that have shown efficacy in PTSD, unless use of the latter might be hazardous on medical grounds.

A sharp distinction between routine pharmacotherapy of PTSD and management of treatment-resistant PTSD cannot be made in clinical practice. As an illustration of this, some patients commence treatment with an antidepressant and another medication from the very beginning, as if they were already treatment resistant. A decision as to whether a patient will be administered only an antidepressant at that time or an antidepressant with another drug will likely depend on the clinician's assessment of the antidepressant's ability to target most of the symptoms that the individual patient presents with. Thus, if some symptoms, such as insomnia and nightmares, are particularly prominent, and TCAs or mirtazapine cannot be used, a medication targeting these symptoms (e.g., prazosin or a non-benzodiazepine hypnotic) may be administered with an SSRI or venlafaxine XR from the onset of treatment.

A "true" treatment resistance probably begins after the patient has completely failed trials with several antidepressants, alone or in combination with other drugs. What options are then available to clinicians?

Besides initiating psychological treatment or intensifying it if the patient has already been engaged in psychological therapy, it is reasonable to administer medications that have not been used up to that point (Table 7–21). The choice of medication and decision about using one or more medications again depend on the circumstances of the individual patient, his or her clinical presentation, and nature of the medications under consideration. In practical terms, this means either combining an antidepressant with one of the alternative and/or adjunctive medication options for PTSD or using the latter alone. Alternative medications can also be combined, for example, a second-generation antipsychotic plus an anticonvulsant/mood stabilizer. In addition, several other medications, for which there is very little, inconsistent, or questionable evidence of efficacy can be used. These include noradrenergic suppressors clonidine and propranolol, and buspirone, an azapirone that acts as a partial agonist on serotonin 1_A receptors.

Clonidine, which is an α_2 adrenergic agonist, and propranolol, a β-adrenergic blocker, may be used to counteract autonomic hyperactivity and decrease autonomic hyperarousal. There is some evidence that clonidine may also decrease hypervigilance, alleviate various symptoms of reexperiencing trauma, and improve sleep and impulse control (Kolb et al., 1984). Clonidine may cause hypotension, and tolerance seems to develop to its therapeutic effects during long-term administration.

If there has been partial response to one of the antidepressants used alone or to an antidepressant in combination with another drug, various augmentation strategies could be considered. The choice of an augmenting agent is usually guided by the symptoms and behaviors that are still prominent, despite pharmacotherapy (Table 7–21). Thus, patients with severe outbursts of anger and impulse control problems can be administered a second-generation antipsychotic or an anticonvulsant/mood stabilizer, whereas patients with autonomic hyperarousal symptoms may respond to clonidine, propranolol, or even a benzodiazepine. In case of

Table 7–21.Alternative and/or Adjunctive Pharmacotherapy Options and Pharmacological Options for Treatment-Resistant Posttraumatic Stress Disorder

Alternative and/or adjunctive pharmacotherapy options (used alone or in combination with first-, second-, third-, or fourth-line antidepressants)

- Second-generation antipsychotics (risperidone, olanzapine, quetiapine)
- Anticonvulsants and mood stabilizers (carbamazepine, valproate, lamotrigine, gabapentin, tiagabine, topiramate, lithium)
- Prazosin
- Benzodiazepines (caution when using them; combination treatment preferred over monotherapy)

Lack of response to first-, second-, third-, and fourth-line antidepressants, used alone or in combination with other medications

- Medications (from the list of alternative and/or adjunctive pharmacotherapy options for PTSD) that have not been used previously, administered alone or in combination with antidepressants
- Combinations of alternative and/or adjunctive pharmacotherapy options for PTSD
- Symptom-driven augmentation with noradrenergic suppressors (clonidine, propranolol)
- Augmentation with buspirone

Partial response to a first-, second-, third-, or fourth-line antidepressant, used alone or in combination with another medication

Augmentation strategies (usually symptom-driven)

- With second-generation antipsychotics (risperidone, olanzapine, quetiapine)
- With anticonvulsants and mood stabilizers (carbamazepine, valproate, lamotrigine, gabapentin, tiagabine, topiramate, lithium)
- With prazosin
- With noradrenergic suppressors (clonidine, propranolol)
- With buspirone
- With non-benzodiazepine hypnotics (zolpidem, zopiclone, eszopiclone, zaleplon)
- With benzodiazepines

severe insomnia, a hypnotic medication can be added; augmentation with prazosin may be reasonable in the presence of frequent nightmares. There are no clear guidelines as to how and when to combine these and other medications, and physicians and psychiatrists have to rely on their clinical judgment when making these decisions.

PSYCHOLOGICAL TREATMENT

General Issues in Psychological Treatment of Posttraumatic Stress Disorder

Regardless of the type of psychological treatment used for PTSD, the nature of the therapeutic relationship is likely to play a major role in affecting the outcome. This is a consequence of the specific needs and characteristics of PTSD patients. Above all, they need to feel safe in a therapeutic setting, probably more so than other patients. The sense of safety should be fostered by the therapist in multiple ways, some of which are listed below.

- The therapist should communicate an unconditional acceptance of patients.
- The therapist should convey a nonjudgmental attitude, which helps create an atmosphere in which patients feel free to express their feelings and attitudes (without negative consequences to follow).
- The therapist needs to be sensitive about issues that are important to patients, compassionate about their plight, and able to empathize.
- The therapist should pay particular attention to aspects of the patients' traumatic experience that they feel ashamed of, or guilty, embarrassed, angry, or desperate about. These aspects should be neither avoided nor emphasized too much.
- The therapist should promote a positive attitude toward the future while demonstrating to patients that he or she is fully aware of and understands their past traumatic experience and its impact.

Patients with PTSD who have become mistrustful through a traumatic experience or its consequences can have their sense of trust restored only within a safe therapeutic environment. Other issues that often need to be addressed in the course of psychotherapy include effects of the trauma on patients' sense of self-worth and their perception of other people and life in general, and their own future in particular.

Phase-Based Approach to Psychological Treatment of Posttraumatic Stress Disorder

The period shortly after the trauma has occurred seems ideal for using psychological interventions to prevent PTSD or alleviate PTSD-like symptoms. While the use of early psychological interventions in trauma victims is generally not disputable, there are some unresolved issues. Thus, which interventions should be used, for which trauma victims, at what time after a traumatic event, and for how long? Only those trauma victims who are at risk for developing PTSD may need psychological intervention. Therefore, the main tasks following a traumatic event are identification of victims who are at risk for developing PTSD (see Tables 7–12 and 7–13) and offering specific psychological intervention to them. Early psychological interventions involve psychological debriefing and CBT.

After full-blown PTSD has developed, well-established psychological treatments can be used. They include several types of CBT, EMDR, group therapy, and psychodynamic psychotherapy. Of these, trauma-focused therapies (individually delivered CBT and EMDR) have been most efficacious (e.g., Bisson et al., 2007).

Early Psychological Interventions

Psychological Debriefing Psychological debriefing (Mitchell, 1983; Dyregrov, 1989) was the first intervention developed specifically for use during the first several days after a traumatic event. It was designed for both group and individual format but has increasingly been used as an individual intervention. Psychological debriefing is usually administered in a single session that takes about 2 hours. It is provided to all victims of the trauma (and even more broadly, to relatives of the victims, military personnel, emergency care workers, and others who may be in contact with the victims), regardless of the degree of their distress and presence of any symptoms of acute stress disorder.

Psychological debriefing provides victims with support and reassurance, information about normal and abnormal responses to trauma, and the opportunity to go over the event in full detail, express their feelings and thoughts associated with the event, and learn basic skills for coping with the impact of the trauma. In addition, personal meaning(s) of the trauma may be explored. The goals of psychological debriefing include promotion of normal emotional and cognitive processing of the trauma, symptom alleviation, empowerment of the victims to deal effectively with trauma-related consequences, and prevention of PTSD.

Despite the appeal of psychological debriefing as simple, based on common sense, pragmatic, and intuitively useful for alleviating acute distress and preventing PTSD, long-term efficacy studies of single-session psychological debriefing have not produced encouraging results. Two systematic reviews and one meta-analysis failed to demonstrate superiority of psychological debriefing over the absence of any intervention (Rose and Bisson, 1998; Van Emmerick et al., 2002; Rose et al., 2003). Two studies showed that the outcome following psychological debriefing was even worse (Bisson et al., 1997; Mayou et al., 2000). These studies have been criticized on methodological grounds and as not being representative of psychological debriefing as it is carried out in the real world (Deahl, 2003). One study did not find any particular advantage of group debriefing over the lack of any intervention, but it did not show that group debriefing was detrimental (Devilly and Annab, 2008). The usefulness of psychological debriefing has been debated, with some arguing that it is a "waste of time" (Wessely, 2003) and others emphasizing that it is unethical "not to do anything" in the aftermath of trauma (Deahl, 2003).

Resolution of this controversy does not appear to be in either complete rejection of psychological debriefing nor in its endorsement for routine use after traumatic events. Psychological debriefing is often perceived by its recipients to have short-term benefits and play an important educational role (Deahl, 2003). The way in which this intervention is administered may determine whether or not it works. Proponents of psychological debriefing emphasize that this is not meant to be a one-off, stand-alone intervention, but merely the initial one, and usually as a part of a treatment package (Mitchell and Everly, 1995; Deahl, 2003).

Psychological debriefing should not be mandatory and should preferably not be conducted by people who are strangers to the victims (Wessely, 2003). Anyone contemplating to use psychological debriefing should be mindful of potential reasons for its lack of efficacy:

- Inadvertent re-traumatization through imaginal exposure to the trauma-related material too soon after the traumatic event (Rose et al., 2003)
- Emergence of the sense of shame that cannot be adequately addressed during a single session of debriefing (Rose et al., 2003)
- Interference with the natural process of healing through medicalization of the trauma-related distress (Rose et al., 2003; Wessely, 2003)
- Erroneous assumptions that it is *always* salubrious for trauma victims to "open up," express their feelings, and give an account of what happened (Rose et al., 2003; Wessely, 2003).

Early Cognitive-Behavioral Therapy

There are several reports of CBT used early after a traumatic event and in patients with acute stress disorder (Foa et al., 1995b; Bryant et al., 1998, 1999, 2003, 2008b; Gidron et al., 2001). In contrast to psychological debriefing, which is administered to all trauma victims, early CBT has been used mainly in victims at high risk for developing PTSD, including those with acute stress disorder. The technical aspects of administering this version of CBT and its efficacy have received most attention.

Patients with early symptoms of PTSD who commenced treatment 2 weeks after a traumatic event and received a four-session CBT package had a better post-treatment outcome than patients without any structured treatment (Foa et al., 1995b). At follow-up, however, these differences in efficacy disappeared, suggesting that CBT might be useful in accelerating recovery of trauma victims with PTSD symptoms.

Studies by Bryant et al. (1998, 1999, 2003, 2008b) were conducted in patients with acute stress disorder during the first month after a traumatic event. The version of CBT used in these studies relied mainly on exposure therapy and was similar to the standard CBT for PTSD, except that it was condensed, lasting 5 instead of the usual 12–16 sessions. Earlier studies (Bryant et al., 1998, 1999, 2003) demonstrated that this version of CBT was superior to "supportive counseling," and that this difference in favor of CBT was maintained at 4-year follow-up. The comparison treatment modality, supportive counseling, specifically excluded components of CBT (exposure, cognitive restructuring, and anxiety management techniques) and consisted of psychoeducation, training in problem-solving skills, and support. Therefore, the superiority of CBT could be attributed to its specific ingredients. These studies also reported a higher dropout rate among patients treated with CBT, suggesting that use of CBT early after a traumatic event may not be suitable for some traumatized patients, perhaps because of its intensity and temporal proximity to a traumatic event.

In the subsequent, controlled study, five sessions of exposure-based therapy were compared with five sessions of cognitive restructuring and lack of any treatment in patients with acute stress disorder (Bryant et al., 2008b). Exposure-based therapy was superior in terms of greater symptom reduction, decreased likelihood of developing PTSD, and increased rates of remission. This led to a conclusion that exposure-based therapy is efficacious as an early intervention for trauma victims at high risk for developing PTSD.

Psychological Treatments for Chronic Posttraumatic Stress Disorder

Cognitive-Behavioral Therapy

There are several components of a typical CBT package for PTSD. They include psychoeducation, exposure, cognitive restructuring, and anxiety management techniques. In various versions of CBT these components are used in different proportions, and different techniques are used within each component of CBT.

Psychoeducation This is carried out at the very beginning of treatment. Patients are informed about normal and pathological responses to trauma and nature of CBT. The main goals of psychoeducation are to dispel misconceptions about PTSD by providing appropriate information and agree on treatment goals through collaborative negotiation.

Exposure This is usually considered to be the main ingredient of CBT for PTSD. The general principles of exposure therapy are the same as those for treatment of agoraphobia and other phobias (see Chapters 2 and 5). They are based on constructing hierarchies of the feared situations and stimuli to which patients are gradually being exposed, from the least fear- or

Table 7–22. Aspects of Cognitive-Behavioral Therapy That Are Relatively Specific for Posttraumatic Stress Disorder

Exposure

- Prolonged imaginal exposure is used
- In vivo exposure usually follows imaginal exposure
- Gradual exposure is preferable to flooding
- Patients should be fully emotionally engaged during exposure
- Greater flexibility may be needed to devise situations and stimuli that patients are exposed to
- Some improvement achieved during in-session, therapist-assisted exposure should generally precede self-exposure

Cognitive Restructuring

Identifying, challenging, and modifying the specific trauma-related appraisals, such as

- Feeling responsible or blaming oneself for the occurrence of trauma
- Perceiving oneself as too weak
- Negative appraisal of one's own coping abilities
- Perceiving symptoms of PTSD (especially reexperiencing of the trauma) as personal defeat
- Negative (mistrustful, hostile) attitude toward others, often because of their perceived failure to be supportive or offer help

---

discomfort-eliciting situation or stimulus to the strongest fear- or discomfort-eliciting situation or stimulus. There are several aspects of exposure that are relatively specific for PTSD (Table 7–22).

Most exposure-based programs for PTSD include prolonged imaginal exposure. This technique requires that patients vividly imagine the traumatic situation for prolonged periods of time—preferably for 1–2 hours every day, both in sessions and as homework exercises. When imaginal exposure occurs in sessions, the therapist can assist with the exposure by requesting that patients provide a detailed account of their traumatic experience. To enhance this process, patients need to be emotionally engaged, which can be achieved by asking them to speak in the present tense and in the first person, while including in their accounts a detailed description of their emotional responses to the trauma (e.g., feelings of fear, helplessness, despair, disgust, shame, or loss of control). Patients' accounts should also include trauma-related sensory cues (e.g., sounds, sights, or smells); these can subsequently be used to enhance exposure and reliving of the trauma. For example, an audiotape with a sound of a helicopter can be played to patients with combat-related PTSD.

In vivo exposure usually follows imaginal exposure and involves exposure to situations and stimuli that remind patients of the trauma or activate traumatic memories. In vivo exposure in PTSD is conducted in a way similar to in vivo exposure in agoraphobia (see Chapter 2).

As in other anxiety disorders, exposure is beneficial in treating PTSD because it promotes habituation to patients' fears and a sense of self-mastery. In addition, there may be specific benefits of exposure in treating PTSD as it allows patients to relive their traumatic experience in a controlled manner. It then becomes possible for patients to reappraise the trauma, adopt relevant corrective information (e.g., about threat and safety), and reprocess corresponding emotional reactions. Ultimately, successful exposure treatment leads to a reconstruction of the trauma within the patients' memory system. This reconstruction encompasses both cognitive and emotional levels, without any component of the traumatic experience being split off.

Some patients are unable to complete a full exposure program because it is too unpleasant and painful. This is understandable because exposure requires patients to face and fully re-create a traumatic event that they are desperately trying to push aside. To minimize the risk of dropout, the therapist should carefully explain to patients the rationale and goals of exposure and be attentive to any signs that they are becoming overwhelmed by the experience of reliving the trauma.

There have been attempts to enhance adherence to exposure-based therapy, minimize the risk of dropping out, improve its delivery, and make it more accessible. Thus, virtual reality exposure therapy has been found to be useful in the treatment of PTSD and recommended for patients who are unable to fully engage in standard exposure therapy (e.g., Difede et al., 2007). Internet-based, self-management, and therapist-assisted CBT was shown to be efficacious in one controlled trial (Litz et al., 2007).

Cognitive Restructuring Cognitive techniques for PTSD (Table 7–22) involve identifying and challenging specific appraisals and beliefs pertaining to patients, their future, the traumatic event, other people, and the world in general. In a broad sense, the goal of cognitive approaches is for patients to "normalize" the traumatic experience through reappraisal of the trauma and its consequences and change in their meaning. A more balanced appraisal and understanding of the trauma would then ensue. Patients need to come to terms with traumatic experience and incorporate it into their lives so that they do not have to try to forget it, deny it, or be afraid or ashamed of it.

There are several types of cognitive distortions that are relatively specific for PTSD and, if present, should be addressed in the course of CBT. For example, patients may hold themselves responsible or guilty for the occurrence of a traumatic event despite a lack of any indicator that they were indeed responsible or guilty. Some patients have a particularly distorted view of others and the world, which is permeated with mistrust, suspiciousness, and hostility. Such a view is often based on exaggerated appraisals of danger that need to be modified during treatment. Any beliefs that the trauma has permanently damaged the person and prevented some accomplishments also need to be addressed.

Anxiety Management Techniques These techniques are often used as part of the CBT package, with the goals of alleviating tension, anxiety, and hyper-arousal symptoms. They may also assist PTSD patients in their struggle to regain some control over their symptoms and may help them engage with anxiety-provoking CBT procedures, particularly exposure.

Anxiety management techniques often involve use of muscle relaxation and breathing retraining in a way similar to their use in other anxiety disorders. "Stress inoculation training," originally proposed by Meichenbaum (1975), includes psychoeducation, role-playing, modeling, some cognitive restructuring, and "thought stopping" and "self-instruc-tion" (or "self-talk"). The latter entails attempts to suppress intrusive, trauma-related thoughts. However, these attempts often do not work and may even intensify intrusive thoughts (e.g., Harvey and Bryant, 1998; Rassin et al., 2000). Therefore, the original stress inoculation training is now used less often or, when used, it is substantially modified.

Efficacy of Cognitive-Behavioral Therapy Cognitive-behavioral therapy has been used in PTSD associated with different types of trauma, which has required adaptations of some of its techniques. For example, frequent themes in the course of treatment of sexual assault victims are guilt, shame, secrecy about the trauma, safety, trust, power, self-esteem, inti-macy, and avoidance (Table 7–4). When treating PTSD related to sexual assault, CBT is often modified to address these themes adequately, usually through a greater emphasis on cognitive approaches. Issues of pain, injury, litigation, and persistent, disabling avoidance of trauma-related reminders are common during the treatment of motor vehicle accident survivors with PTSD (Table 7–5), which calls for these issues to be attended to during CBT.

In victims of assault and violent crime, CBT has been efficacious. Foa et al. (1991, 1999) found prolonged exposure (over 9 sessions) among female victims of sexual and nonsexual assault to be superior to stress inoculation training and supportive counseling, whereas stress inoculation training was more efficacious than supportive counseling. When exposure plus specific cognitive interventions (in "cognitive processing therapy") was compared with prolonged exposure alone (both conducted over 13 ses-sions) in the treatment of female victims of sexual assault, the two treat-ments were approximately equally efficacious; however, patients who were treated with specific cognitive techniques improved more on measures of guilt (Resick et al., 2002).

Cognitive-behavioral therapy has also been successfully used in treat-ment of PTSD related to motor vehicle accidents. Studies have shown that 8–12 sessions of CBT are superior to supportive psychotherapy and no treatment in survivors of road traffic accidents with PTSD (Fecteau and Nicki, 1999; Blanchard et al., 2003). At 1- and 2-year follow-up, CBT gen-erally continued to show superiority over supportive psychotherapy, but there was little improvement from the end of treatment to the 2-year follow-up (Blanchard et al., 2004).

The results of CBT for war veterans with PTSD have been less encouraging. Possible reasons include greater severity of PTSD in many of these patients, presence of complications (alcohol or other substance abuse, enduring personality changes, depression), and the fact that many patients commenced CBT years after traumatic events. Nevertheless, several studies suggest that CBT may be beneficial to this group of patients (e.g., Cooper and Clum, 1989; Keane et al., 1989; Glynn et al., 1999). Cognitive-behavioral therapy for combat-related PTSD may need to last longer (14–20 sessions instead of 8–12) than CBT for PTSD related to other types of trauma. The outcome of CBT in these patients may crucially depend on how exposure is conducted (i.e., what proportion of exposure is imaginal and in vivo, whether exposure is gradual enough, and how traumatic memories elicited by exposure and the accompanying feelings are dealt with).

The efficacy of a standard course of prolonged, imaginal exposure alone was compared to that of cognitive restructuring alone in two large studies involving PTSD patients with various types of traumas (Marks et al., 1998; Tarrier et al., 1999). There were no significant differences between the outcomes of the two treatments, suggesting that exposure does not have to be an ingredient of CBT in the treatment of *all* PTSD patients.

The efficacy of cognitive therapy based on the comprehensive cognitive model of PTSD (Ehlers and Clark, 2000) has been tested in several studies. In one of these, cognitive therapy was used to treat PTSD in survivors of a terrorist attack and produced substantial improvement after an average of eight sessions (Gillespie et al., 2002). In two randomized controlled trials, cognitive therapy demonstrated a similarly good outcome, with a very low dropout rate and maintenance of treatment gains at 6-month follow-up (Ehlers et al., 2003, 2005). It should be noted that this form of cognitive therapy also uses both imaginal and in vivo exposure. The emphasis, however, is on reappraisal of the trauma-related material elicited through exposure and on the elimination of avoidance, other safety behaviors, and maladaptive cognitive strategies that play a crucial role in maintaining PTSD.

Eye Movement Desensitization and Reprocessing

Eye movement desensitization and reprocessing combines behavioral and cognitive techniques with eye movements (Shapiro, 1995). Patients are required to focus on trauma-related stimuli and memories (in a way similar to imaginal exposure), while simultaneously tracking the therapist's finger as it moves quickly across their visual field. This procedure is repeated and accompanied by cognitive techniques aimed at changing dysfunctional assumptions and beliefs about the trauma.

This technique has generated some controversy, largely because the role of eye movements is poorly understood. Numerous studies have examined the efficacy of EMDR. It appears that EMDR is more efficacious than fluoxetine (van der Kolk et al., 2007) and nonspecific psychological interventions (e.g., supportive listening), relaxation, and stress management (Carlson et al., 1998; Bisson et al., 2007). When EMDR was compared to CBT, it was found to be somewhat less efficacious (Devilly and Spence, 1999; Taylor et al., 2003), but two subsequent meta-analyses found no difference in efficacy (Seidler and Wagner, 2006; Bisson et al., 2007). While some research suggests that initial treatment gains with EMDR may not be maintained over time (e.g., Macklin et al., 2000), other studies have reported that EMDR produces a lasting improvement (e.g., van der Kolk et al., 2007). It is important to ascertain which PTSD patients might benefit the most from EMDR, as there has been some question about the suitability and efficacy of EMDR for combat-related PTSD (e.g., Feske, 1998).

Group Therapy

It is not clear whether group therapy for PTSD is useful and how it should optimally be conducted. A group format may allow its members to share their experiences and support each other. It may also facilitate exposure to traumatic stimuli through encouragement from group members and observation of other patients' exposure during the group sessions. Some PTSD patients feel that only people who have undergone similar traumatic experiences can understand them and are therefore keen to join groups composed of other PTSD patients. Others feel too embarrassed to talk about their trauma and their symptoms in front of others and look for safety within a therapeutic relationship with their therapist. The anger and hostility of some PTSD patients are destructive to the group processes. Therefore, patients' suitability for group therapy should be assessed on a case-by-case basis.

The efficacy of group therapy for PTSD has not been well established, although there are many reports of its successful use within different theoretical frameworks, in a variety of contexts, and for victims of various traumas. One study in adult female victims of childhood sexual abuse found a significant decrease in PTSD symptoms following "affect management" in the course of CBT-based group therapy (Zlotnick et al., 1997). In another study, the outcome of CBT-based group therapy of Vietnam veterans with PTSD was not better than that of supportive group therapy (Schnurr et al., 2003). One meta-analysis reported a greater improvement in PTSD symptoms with group CBT than with "usual care" and no treatment (Bisson et al., 2007).

Psychodynamic Psychotherapy

Psychodynamic psychotherapy may be suitable only for a subset of patients with PTSD. It may be indicated for patients who are motivated to explore their traumatic experiences and whose goal is not merely to have these experiences "under control." It should not be used if patients have disruptive emotional dysregulation, poor impulse control, or a significant substance use problem. The goal of psychodynamic psychotherapy is a healing reconstruction of traumatic experiences by means of transference. The therapeutic process focuses on the meaning of the trauma for PTSD sufferers and may include reliving of the traumatic event and emotional catharsis.

Patients' transferrential reactions may be vehement, as they direct much of their frustration and anger to the therapist. The outcome of psychodynamic psychotherapy may then depend on the therapist's response and on his or her countertransference. The therapist must be careful not to succumb to feelings of helplessness that may permeate the relationship with the patient. Also, the therapist should be attentive to issues of mistrust and expectation of rejection, which PTSD patients often bring into the therapeutic situation. Some patients test the therapeutic relationship by challenging the therapist's authority or by insisting that the therapist is unable to understand them. In these situations, the therapist should not hurry to offer "proofs" of competence, availability, and compassion. In other instances, the therapist must not plunge to "rescue" the patient and should be vigilant about his or her omnipotence fantasies.

COMBINED TREATMENTS

Combining pharmacotherapy with psychological treatments, especially CBT, for chronic PTSD seems reasonable because either treatment alone often produces a partial improvement or is effective only for some symptoms. This has created an expectation that combining pharmacotherapy and CBT would improve outcome. While combined treatments are apparently used frequently in clinical practice, their efficacy in PTSD has hardly been tested. There have been no large-scale comparisons of the efficacy of combined pharmacotherapy and CBT to that of either treatment alone. Many of the issues regarding combined treatment for panic disorder discussed in Chapter 2 also apply to the combined treatment for PTSD.

As with other anxiety disorders, a combination of pharmacotherapy and CBT in PTSD may produce better results than pharmacotherapy alone. This is suggested by the finding of a pilot study that treatment with a 10-session CBT and sertraline was superior to treatment with sertraline alone in PTSD patients who had not responded to previous pharmacotherapy (Otto et al., 2003).

The issue of whether combined treatment of PTSD produces better results than CBT alone is controversial. Many CBT therapists are opposed to combined treatment because its advantage over CBT alone has often been doubtful in studies of other anxiety disorders (see Chapters 2 and 6). In practical terms, it would be important to know whether and to what extent the use of medications (especially antidepressants) might interfere with prolonged exposure and other more specific CBT techniques for PTSD.

In the absence of research findings for PTSD, clinicians may rely on considerations for other anxiety disorders regarding indications for combined treatment and the sequence of combining pharmacotherapy and CBT (see Chapter 2). Thus, combined treatments may be useful in treating patients with severe forms of PTSD, those whose illness has been complicated by depression or other mental disorders, and patients who have had only a limited response to pharmacotherapy alone or CBT alone. Patients treated originally or primarily with pharmacotherapy may benefit from augmentation with CBT to decrease the likelihood of relapse after stopping the medication(s). It is uncertain whether pharmacotherapy may facilitate exposure therapy for PTSD, but adding a medication seems reasonable when patients have great difficulty engaging in exposure therapy.

OUTLOOK FOR THE FUTURE

The concept of PTSD has been seriously challenged. The way in which this challenge is responded to will ultimately determine the fate of PTSD so that its validity is confirmed or it becomes just another chapter in the history of psychiatry. Considering only the vast intellectual and financial resources invested into PTSD-inspired research, the latter outcome seems unlikely. Additional resources are now needed to disentangle some of the key conundrums surrounding PTSD. These include better understanding of the interactions between vulnerability to PTSD and trauma, elucidation of the mechanisms that lead to various clinical presentations of PTSD, identification of its unique features, conceptualization of any subtypes of PTSD, and clarification of what may be specific for PTSD at the neurobiological level and with regard to psychological mechanisms. All this will play a major role in the process of validating the concept of PTSD. Once this is achieved, PTSD will have a greater chance of becoming a "respectable" diagnosis, provided also that society does not foster its unjustified use and abuse.

As with numerous other illnesses in psychiatry and medicine, we cannot wait for the outcome of conceptual debates and for the discoveries that would allow us to understand better why and how PTSD develops. Posttraumatic stress disorder is an important public health problem and a pragmatic approach is essential; much of it should revolve around endeavors to identify more precisely trauma victims who are at high risk of developing PTSD, and then treat them early whenever possible.

Research into risk factors for developing PTSD has enhanced only to some extent our understanding of the trajectory from trauma to PTSD. One way of advancing in this area is to improve research methodology, for example, by studying risk factors prospectively, while controlling for confounding variables, and taking into account the ways in which various risk factors are interrelated. The other strategy would be to shift the focus and study resilience in the face of adversity and trauma. Both of these approaches would converge to provide a clearer picture of the pathways leading from trauma to PTSD, related syndromes, and other forms of psychopathology.

Perhaps the most puzzling aspect of PTSD is the fact that most trauma victims do not develop PTSD and of those who do, the majority recovers spontaneously. Better understanding of this phenomenon might help devise more effective treatments insofar as the natural healing processes can be used both to intervene early in the aftermath of trauma and to treat chronic PTSD. Treatment results will also improve to the extent that the target of treatment is shifted from symptoms or "surface" manifestations of PTSD to the underlying (pathophysiological and psychological) mechanisms and meanings of the trauma and its consequences. This is likely to reduce polypharmacy and decrease a tendency to assess treatment outcomes mainly through reductions in symptoms.

REFERENCES

Abel JL, Borkovec TD. 1995. Generalizability of DSM-III-R generalized anxiety disorders to proposed DSM-IV criteria and cross-validation of proposed changes. Journal of Anxiety Disorders, 9: 303–315.

Abelson JL, Curtis GC, Sagher O, et al. 2005. Deep brain stimulation for refractory obsessive-compulsive disorder. Biological Psychiatry, 57: 510–516.

Abraham K. 1921/1942. Contributions to the theory of the anal character. In Selected Papers of Karl Abraham, M.D. London: Hogarth Press, pp. 370–392.

Abramowitz J, Franklin ME, Foa EB. 2002. Empirical status of cognitive behavioral therapy for obsessive-compulsive disorder. Romanian Journal of Cognitive Behavioral Therapy, 2: 89–104.

Abramowitz J, Moore K, Carmin C, et al. 2001. Acute onset of obsessive- compulsive disorder in males following childbirth. Psychosomatics, 42: 429–431.

Abramowitz JS. 1996. Variants of exposure and response prevention in the treatment of obsessive-compulsive disorder: A meta-analysis. Behavior Therapy, 27: 583–600.

Abramowitz JS. 1997. Effectiveness of psychological and pharmacological treatments for obsessive-compulsive disorder: A quantitative review. Journal of Consulting and Clinical Psychology, 65: 44–52.

Abramowitz JS, Deacon BJ. 2005. The OC spectrum: A closer look at the arguments and the data. In Abramowitz JS, Houts AC, editors: Concepts and Controversies in Obsessive-Compulsive Disorder. New York: Springer, pp. 141–149.

Abramowitz JS, Franklin ME, Schwartz SA, et al. 2003. Symptom presentation and outcome of cognitive behavioral therapy for obsessive-compulsive disorder. Journal of Consulting and Clinical Psychology, 71: 1049– 1057.

Abramowitz JS, Franklin ME, Street GP, et al. 2000. Effects of comorbid depression on response to treatment for obsessive-compulsive disorder. Behavior Therapy, 31: 517–528.

Abramowitz JS, Wheaton MG, Storch EA. 2008. The status of hoarding as a symptom of obsessive-compulsive disorder. Behaviour Research and Therapy, 46: 1026–1033.

Abrams K, Rassovsky Y, Kushner MG. 2006. Evidence for respiratory and non-respiratory subtypes in panic disorder. Depression and Anxiety, 23: 474–481.

Ackerman DL, Greenland S. 2002. Multivariate meta-analysis of controlled drug studies for obsessive-compulsive disorder. Journal of Clinical Psychopharmacology, 22: 309–317.

Ackerman DL, Greenland S, Bystritsky A. 1998. Clinical characteristics of response to fluoxetine treatment of obsessive-compulsive disorder. Journal of Clinical Psychopharmacology, 18: 185–192.

Ackerman DL, Greenland S, Bystritsky A, et al. 1994. Predictors of treatment response in obsessive-compulsive disorder: Multivariate analyses from a multi-center trial of clomipramine. Journal of Clinical Psychopharmacology, 14: 247–254.

Aderka IM. 2009. Factors affecting treatment efficacy in social phobia: The use of video feedback and individual vs. group formats. Journal of Anxiety Disorders, 23: 12–17.

Adler CM, Craske MG, Kirshenbaum S, et al. 1989. "Fear of panic": An investigation of its role in panic occurrence, phobic avoidance, and treatment outcome. Behaviour Research and Therapy, 27: 391–396.

Adler CM, McDonough-Ryan P, Sax KW. 2000. fMRI of neuronal activation with symptom provocation in unmedicated patients with obsessive compulsive disorder. Journal of Psychiatric Research, 34: 317–324.

Agras WS, Chapin HM, Oliveau DC. 1972. The natural history of phobias: Course and prognosis. Archives of General Psychiatry, 26: 315–317.

Agras WS, Sylvester D, Oliveau D. 1969. The epidemiology of common fears and phobias. Comprehensive Psychiatry, 10: 151–156.

Ahern J, Galea S, Resnick H, et al. 2004. Television images and probable posttraumatic stress disorder after September 11: The role of background characteristics, event exposures, and peri-event panic. Journal of Nervous and Mental Disease, 192: 217–226.

Akiskal HS. 1998. Toward a definition of generalized anxiety disorder as an anxious temperament type. Acta Psychiatrica Scandinavica, 98 (Suppl. 393): 66–73.

Alarcon RD, Libb JW, Spitler D. 1993. A predictive study of obsessive-compulsive disorder response to clomipramine. Journal of Clinical Psychopharmacology, 13: 210–213.

Albert U, Aguglia E, Maina G, et al. 2002. Venlafaxine versus clomipramine in the treatment of obsessive-compulsive disorder: A preliminary single-blind, 12-week, controlled study. Journal of Clinical Psychiatry, 63: 1004–1009.

Aliyev NA, Aliyev ZN. 2008. Valproate (depakine-chrono) in the acute treatment of outpatients with generalized anxiety disorder without psychiatric comorbidity: Randomized, double-blind, placebo-controlled study. European Psychiatry, 23: 109–114.

Allen AJ, Leonard HL, Swedo SE. 1995. Case study: A new infection-triggered autoimmune subtype of pediatric OCD and Tourette's syndrome. Journal of the American Academy of Child and Adolescent Psychiatry, 34: 307–311.

Allgulander C. 1999. Paroxetine in social phobia: A randomized placebo-controlled study. Acta Psychiatrica Scandinavica, 100: 193–198.

Allgulander C, Dahl AA, Austin C, et al. 2004a. Efficacy of sertraline in a 12-week trial for generalized anxiety disorder. American Journal of Psychiatry, 161: 1642–1649.

Allgulander C, Florea I, Huusom AKT. 2006. Prevention of relapse in generalized anxiety disorder by escitalopram treatment. International Journal of Neuropsychopharmacology, 9: 495–505.

Allgulander C, Hackett D, Salinas E. 2001. Venlafaxine extended release (ER) in the treatment of generalised anxiety disorder: Twenty-four week placebo-controlled dose-ranging study. British Journal of Psychiatry, 179: 15–22.

Allgulander C, Lavori PW. 1991. Excess mortality among 3302 patients with "pure" anxiety neurosis. Archives of General Psychiatry, 48: 599–602.

Allgulander C, Mangano R, Zhang J, et al. 2004b. Efficacy of venlafaxine ER in patients with social anxiety disorder: A double-blind, placebo-controlled, parallel-group comparison with paroxetine. Human Psychopharmacology, 19: 387–396.

Allgulander C, Nutt D, Detke M, et al. 2008. A non-inferiority comparison of duloxetine and venlafaxine in the treatment of adult patients with generalized anxiety disorder. Journal of Psychopharmacology, 22: 417–425.

Alnaes R, Torgersen S. 1988. The relationship between DSM-III symptom disorders (axis I) and personality disorders (axis II) in an outpatient population. Acta Psychiatrica Scandinavica, 78: 485–492.

Alonso P, Menchon JM, Pifarre J, et al. 2001a. Long-term follow-up and predictors of clinical outcome in obsessive-compulsive patients treated with serotonin reuptake inhibitors and behavioral therapy. Journal of Clinical Psychiatry, 62: 535–540.

Alonso P, Pujol J, Cardoner N, et al. 2001b. Right prefrontal repetitive transcranial magnetic stimulation in obsessive-compulsive disorder: A double-blind, placebo-controlled study. American Journal of Psychiatry, 158: 1143–1145.

American Psychiatric Association. 1980. Diagnostic and Statistical Manual of Mental Disorders, 3rd Edition (DSM-III). Washington, DC: American Psychiatric Association.

American Psychiatric Association. 1987. Diagnostic and Statistical Manual of Mental Disorders, 3rd Edition Revised (DSM-III-R). Washington, DC: American Psychiatric Association.

American Psychiatric Association. 1991. DSM-IV Draft Criteria. Washington, DC: American Psychiatric Association.

American Psychiatric Association. 1994. Diagnostic and Statistical Manual of Mental Disorders, 4th Edition (DSM-IV). Washington, DC: American Psychiatric Association.

American Psychiatric Association. 1998. Practice guidelines for the treatment of patients with panic disorder. American Journal of Psychiatry, 155 (May Supplement): 1–34.

American Psychiatric Association. 2000. Diagnostic and Statistical Manual of Mental Disorders, 4th Edition, Text Revision (DSM-IV-TR). Washington, DC: American Psychiatric Association.

Amering M, Bankier B, Berger P, et al. 1999. Panic disorder and cigarette smoking behavior. Comprehensive Psychiatry, 40: 35–38.

Amering M, Katschnig H, Berger P, et al. 1997. Embarrassment about the first panic attack predicts agoraphobia in panic disorder patients. Behaviour Research and Therapy, 35: 517–521.

Amies PL, Gelder MG, Shaw PM. 1983. Social phobia: A comparative clinical study. British Journal of Psychiatry, 142: 174–179.

Amir N, Foa EB, Coles ME. 1998. Negative interpretation bias in social phobia. Behaviour Research and Therapy, 36: 945–957.

Amir N, Foa EB, Coles ME. 2000. Implicit memory bias for threat-relevant information in individuals with generalized social phobia. Journal of Abnormal Psychology, 109: 713–720.

Amir N, Klumpp H, Elias J, et al. 2005. Increased activation of the anterior cingulate cortex during processing of disgust faces in individuals with social phobia. Biological Psychiatry, 57: 975–981.

Ananth J, Pecknold JC, Van Den Steen N, et al. 1981. Double-blind comparative study of clomipramine and amitriptyline in obsessive neurosis. Progress in Neuropsychopharmacology and Biological Psychiatry, 5: 257–262.

Andersch S, Hetta J. 2003. A 15-year follow-up study of patients with panic disorder. European Psychiatry, 18: 401–408.

Andrade L, Eaton WW, Chilcoat H. 1994. Lifetime comorbidity of panic attacks and major depression in a population-based study: Symptom profiles. British Journal of Psychiatry, 165: 363–369.

Andrews B, Brewin CR, Philpott R, et al. 2007. Delayed-onset posttraumatic stress disorder: A systematic review of the evidence. American Journal of Psychiatry, 164: 1319–1326.

Andrews B, Brewin CR, Rose S. 2003. Gender, social support, and PTSD in victims of violent crime. Journal of Traumatic Stress, 16: 421–427.

Andrews B, Brewin CR, Rose S, et al. 2000. Predicting PTSD in victims of violent crime: The role of shame, anger and blame. Journal of Abnormal Psychology, 109: 69–73.

Andrews G, Stewart G, Allen R, et al. 1990. The genetics of six neurotic disorders: A twin study. Journal of Affective Disorders, 19: 23–29.

Angst J, Gamma A, Baldwin DS. 2009. The generalized anxiety spectrum: Prevalence, onset, course and outcome. European Archives of Psychiatry and Clinical Neurosciences, 259: 37–45.

Anholt GE, Kempe P, de Haan E, et al. 2008. Cognitive versus behavior therapy: Processes of change in the treatment of obsessive-compulsive disorder. Psychotherapy and Psychosomatics, 77: 38–42.

Antony MM, Roth D, Swinson RP, et al. 1998. Illness intrusiveness in individuals with panic disorder, obsessive-compulsive disorder, or social phobia. Journal of Nervous and Mental Disease, 186: 311–315.

Arch JJ, Craske MG. 2007. Implications of naturalistic use of pharmacotherapy in CBT treatment for panic disorder. Behaviour Research and Therapy, 45: 1435–1447.

Arntz A. 2003. Cognitive therapy versus applied relaxation as treatment of generalized anxiety disorder. Behaviour Research and Therapy, 41: 633–646.

Aronson TA, Logue CM. 1987. On the longitudinal course of panic disorder: Developmental history and predictors of phobic complications. Comprehensive Psychiatry, 28: 344–355.

Arrindell WA, Emmelkamp PMG. 1986. Marital adjustment, intimacy and needs in female agoraphobics and their partners: A controlled study. British Journal of Psychiatry, 149: 592–602.

Arrindell WA, Emmelkamp PMG, Monsma A, et al. 1983. The role of perceived parental rearing practices in the aetiology of phobic disorders: A controlled study. British Journal of Psychiatry, 143: 183–187.

Asakura S, Tajima O, Koyama T. 2007. Fluvoxamine treatment of generalized social anxiety disorder in Japan: A randomized double-blind, placebo-controlled study. International Journal of Neuropsychopharmacology, 10: 263–274.

Aston-Jones G, Foote SL, Bloom FE. 1984. Anatomy and physiology of locus coeruleus neurons: Functional implications. In Ziegler M, Lake CR, editors: Norepinephrine (Frontiers of Clinical Neuroscience), Volume 2. Baltimore: Williams & Wilkins, pp. 92–116.

Austin LS, Lydiard RB, Ballenger JC, et al. 1991. Dopamine blocking activity of clomipramine in patients with obsessive-compulsive disorder. Biological Psychiatry, 30: 225–232.

Bachar E, Hadar H, Shalev AY. 2005. Narcissistic vulnerability and the development of PTSD: A prospective study. Journal of Nervous and Mental Disease, 193: 762–765.

Baer L. 1994. Factor analysis of symptom subtypes of obsessive-compulsive disorder and their relation to personality and tic disorders. Journal of Clinical Psychiatry, 55 (Suppl. 3): 18–23.

Baer L, Jenike MA, Black DW, et al. 1992. Effect of axis II diagnoses on treatment outcome with clomipramine in 55 patients with obsessive-compulsive disorder. Archives of General Psychiatry, 49: 862–866.

Baer L, Jenike MA, Ricciardi JN, et al. 1990. Standardized assessment of personality disorders in obsessive-compulsive disorder. Archives of General Psychiatry, 47: 826–830.

Baer L, Rauch SL, Ballantine HT, et al. 1995. Cingulotomy for intractable obsessive-compulsive disorder: Prospective long-term follow-up of 18 patients. Archives of General Psychiatry, 52: 384–392.

Baetz M, Bowen R. 1998. Efficacy of divalproex sodium in patients with panic disorder and mood instability who have not responded to conventional therapy. Canadian Journal of Psychiatry, 43: 73–77.

Bajwa WK, Asnis GM, Sanderson WC, et al. 1992. High cholesterol levels in patients with panic disorder. American Journal of Psychiatry, 149: 376–378.

Bakker A, Spinhoven P, van Balkom AJLM, et al. 2002a. Relevance of assessment of cognitions during panic attacks in the treatment of panic disorder. Psychotherapy and Psychosomatics, 71: 158–161.

Bakker A, van Balkom AJLM, Spinhoven P. 2002b. SSRIs vs. TCAs in the treatment of panic disorder: A meta-analysis. Acta Psychiatrica Scandinavica, 106: 163–167.

Baldwin D, Bobes J, Stein DJ, et al. 1999. Paroxetine in the treatment of social phobia: Randomized, double-blind, placebo-controlled study. British Journal of Psychiatry, 175: 120–126.

Baldwin DS, Huusom AKT, Maehlum E. 2006. Escitalopram and paroxetine in the treatment of generalised anxiety disorder: Randomised, placebo-controlled, double-blind study. British Journal of Psychiatry 189: 264–272.

Ball SG, Kuhn A, Wall D, et al. 2005. Selective serotonin reuptake inhibitor treatment for generalized anxiety disorder: A double-blind, prospective comparison between paroxetine and sertraline. Journal of Clinical Psychiatry, 66: 94–99.

Ball SG, Otto MW, Pollack MH, et al. 1994. Predicting prospective episodes of depression in patients with panic disorder: A longitudinal study. Journal of Consulting and Clinical Psychology, 62: 359–365.

Ballenger JC, Burrows GD, DuPont RL, et al. 1988. Alprazolam in panic disorder and agoraphobia: Results from a multicenter trial: I. Efficacy in short-term treatment. Archives of General Psychiatry, 45: 413–422.

Ballenger JC, Davidson JRT, Lecrubier Y, et al. 2000. Consensus statement on post-traumatic stress disorder from the International Consensus Group on Depression and Anxiety. Journal of Clinical Psychiatry, 61 (Suppl. 5): 60–66.

Ballenger JC, Lydiard RB. 1997. Panic disorder: Results of a patient survey. Human Psychopharmacology, 12: S27–S33.

Ballenger JC, Wheadon DE, Steiner M, et al. 1998. Double-blind, fixed-dose, placebo-controlled study of paroxetine in the treatment of panic disorder. American Journal of Psychiatry, 155: 36–42.

Bandelow B. 1995. Assessing the efficacy of treatment for panic disorder and agoraphobia. II. The Panic and Agoraphobia Scale. International Clinical Psychopharmacology, 10: 73–81.

Bandelow B. 1999. Panic and Agoraphobia Scale (PAS). Seattle: Hogrefe & Huber Publishers.

Bandelow B, Behnke K, Lenoir S, et al. 2004. Sertraline versus paroxetine in the treatment of panic disorder: An acute, double-blind noninferiority comparison. Journal of Clinical Psychiatry, 65: 405–413.

Bandelow B, Bobes J, Ahokas A, et al. 2007. Results from a phase III study of once-daily extended release quetiapine fumarate (quetiapine XR) monotherapy in patients with generalised anxiety disorder. International Journal of Psychiatry in Clinical Practice, 11: 314–315.

Barger SD, Sydeman SJ. 2005. Does generalized anxiety disorder predict coronary heart disease risk factors independently of major depressive disorder? Journal of Affective Disorders, 88: 87–91.

Barlow DH. 1988. Anxiety and Its Disorders: The Nature and Treatment of Anxiety and Panic. New York: Guilford Press.

Barlow DH, Blanchard RB, Vermilyea JB, et al. 1986. Generalized anxiety and generalized anxiety disorder: Description and reconceptualization. American Journal of Psychiatry, 143: 40–44.

Barlow DH, Craske MG, Cerny JA, et al. 1989. Behavioral treatment of panic disorder. Behavior Therapy, 20: 261–282.

Barlow DH, Gorman JM, Shear MK, et al. 2000. Cognitive-behavioral therapy, imipramine, or their combination for panic disorder: A randomized controlled trial. Journal of the American Medical Association, 283: 2529–2536.

Barlow DH, Rapee RM, Brown TA. 1992. Behavioral treatment of generalized anxiety disorder. Behavior Therapy, 23: 551–570.

Barsky AJ, Delamater BA, Clancy SA, et al. 1996. Somatized psychiatric disorder presenting as palpitations. Archives of Internal Medicine, 156: 1102–1108.

Bartzokis G, Lu PH, Turner J, et al. 2005. Adjunctive risperidone in the treatment of chronic combat-related posttraumatic stress disorder. Biological Psychiatry, 57: 474–479.

Basoglu M, Lax T, Kasvikis Y, et al. 1988. Predictors of improvement in obsessive-compulsive disorder. Journal of Anxiety Disorders, 2: 299–317.

Basoglu M, Livanou M, Crnobaric C, et al. 2005. Psychiatric and cognitive effects of war in former Yugoslavia: Association of lack of redress for trauma and post-traumatic stress reactions. Journal of the American Medical Association, 294: 580–590.

Basoglu M, Marks IM, Kilic K, et al. 1994. Alprazolam and exposure for panic disorder with agoraphobia: Attribution of improvement to medication predicts subsequent relapse. British Journal of Psychiatry, 164: 652–659.

Baxter LR, Phelps ME, Mazziotta JC, et al. 1987. Local cerebral glucose metabolic rates in obsessive-compulsive disorder: A comparison with rates in unipolar depression and in normal controls. Archives of General Psychiatry, 44: 211–218.

Baxter LR, Schwartz JM, Bergman KS, et al. 1992. Caudate glucose metabolic rate changes with both drug and behavior therapy for obsessive-compulsive disorder. Archives of General Psychiatry, 49: 681–689.

Beck AT, Emery G, Greenberg RI. 1985. Anxiety Disorders and Phobias: A Cognitive Perspective. New York: Basic Books.

Beck AT, Epstein N, Brown G, et al. 1988. An inventory for measuring clinical anxiety: Psychometric properties. Journal of Consulting and Clinical Psychology, 56: 893–897.

Becker ES, Goodwin R, Hölting C, et al. 2003. Content of worry in the community: What do people with generalized anxiety disorder or other disorders worry about? Journal of Nervous and Mental Disease, 191: 688–691.

Becker ES, Rinck M, Türke V, et al. 2007. Epidemiology of specific phobia subtypes: Findings from the Dresden Mental Health Study. European Psychiatry, 22: 69–74.

Beckham J, Kirby AC, Feldman ME, et al. 1997. Prevalence and correlates of heavy smoking in Vietnam veterans with chronic posttraumatic stress disorder. Addictive Behaviors, 22: 637–647.

Beesdo K, Bittner A, Pine DS, et al. 2007. Incidence of social anxiety disorder and the consistent risk for secondary depression in the first three decades of life. Archives of General Psychiatry, 64: 903–912.

Beidel DC, Turner SM. 1999. The natural course of shyness and related syndromes. In Schmidt LA, Schulkin JS, editors: Extreme Fear, Shyness, and Social Phobia: Origins, Biological Mechanisms, and Clinical Outcomes. New York: Oxford University Press, pp. 203–223.

Beitman BD, Basha I, Flaker G, et al. 1987. Non-fearful panic disorder: Panic attacks without fear. Behaviour Research and Therapy, 25: 487–492.

Beitman BD, Thomas AM, Kushner MG. 1992. Panic disorder in the families of patients with normal coronary arteries and non-fearful panic disorder. Behaviour Research and Therapy, 30: 403–406.

Benedetti A, Perugi G, Toni C, et al. 1997. Hypochondriasis and illness phobia in panic-agoraphobic patients. Comprehensive Psychiatry, 38: 124–131.

Berle D, Starcevic V. 2005. Thought-action fusion: Review of the literature and future directions. Clinical Psychology Review, 25: 263–284.

Berle D, Starcevic V, Hannan A, et al. 2008. Cognitive factors in panic disorder, agoraphobic avoidance and agoraphobia. Behaviour Research and Therapy, 46: 282–291.

Bernstein DA, Borkovec TD. 1973. Progressive Relaxation Training. Champaign, IL: Research Press.

Biber B, Alkin T. 1999. Panic disorder subtypes: Differential response to CO_2 challenge. American Journal of Psychiatry, 156: 739–744.

Biederman J, Petty CR, Hirshfeld-Becker DR, et al. 2007. Developmental trajectories of anxiety disorders in offspring at high risk for panic disorder and major depression. Psychiatry Research, 153: 245–252.

Bielski RJ, Bose A, Chang C-C. 2005. A double-blind comparison of escitalopram and paroxetine in the long-term treatment of generalized anxiety disorder. Annals of Clinical Psychiatry, 17: 65–69.

Bienvenu OJ, Nestadt G, Eaton WW. 1998. Characterizing generalized anxiety: Temporal and symptomatic thresholds. Journal of Nervous and Mental Disease, 186: 51–56.

Bienvenu OJ, Samuels JF, Riddle MA, et al. 2000. The relationship of obsessive–compulsive disorder to possible spectrum disorders: Results from a family study. Biological Psychiatry, 48: 287–293.

Bijl R, Ravelli A, van Zessen G. 1998. Prevalence of psychiatric disorder in the general population: Results of the Netherlands Mental Health Survey and Incidence Study (NEMESIS). Social Psychiatry and Psychiatric Epidemiology, 33: 587–595.

Biondi M, Picardi A. 2003. Increased probability of remaining in remission from panic disorder with agoraphobia after drug treatment in patients who received concurrent cognitive-behavioural therapy: A follow-up study. Psychotherapy and Psychosomatics, 72: 34–42.

Birbaumer N, Grodd W, Diedrich O, et al. 1998. fMRI reveals amygdala activation to human faces in social phobics. Neuroreport, 9: 1223–1226.

Bisserbe JC, Lane RM, Flament MF. 1997. A double-blind comparison of sertraline and clomipramine in outpatients with obsessive-compulsive disorder. European Psychiatry, 12: 82–93.

Bisson JI, Ehlers A, Matthews R, et al. 2007. Psychological treatments for chronic post-traumatic stress disorder: Systematic review and meta-analysis. British Journal of Psychiatry, 190: 97–104.

Bisson JI, Jenkins PL, Alexander J, et al. 1997. Randomised controlled trial of psychological debriefing for victims of acute burn trauma. British Journal of Psychiatry, 171: 78–81.

Black A. 1974. The natural history of obsessional neurosis. In Beech HR, editor: Obsessional States. London: Methuen Press, pp. 1–23.

Black DW, Monahan P, Gable J, et al. 1998. Hoarding and treatment response in 38 non-depressed subjects with obsessive-compulsive disorder. Journal of Clinical Psychiatry, 59: 420–425.

Black DW, Wesner R, Bowers W, et al. 1993. A comparison of fluvoxamine, cognitive therapy, and placebo in the treatment of panic disorder. Archives of General Psychiatry, 50: 44–50.

Blair K, Geraci M, Devido J, et al. 2008b. Neural response to self- and other referential praise and criticism in generalized social phobia. Archives of General Psychiatry, 65: 1176–1184.

Blair K, Shaywitz J, Smith BW, et al. 2008a. Response to emotional expressions in generalized social phobia and generalized anxiety disorder: Evidence for separate disorders. American Journal of Psychiatry, 165: 1193–1202.

Blake DD, Weathers FW, Nagy LN, et al. 1990. A clinician rating scale for assessing current and lifetime PTSD: The CAPS-1. Behavior Therapist, 18: 187–188.

Blanchard EB, Hickling EJ, Devineni T, et al. 2003. A controlled evaluation of cognitive behavioral therapy for posttraumatic stress in motor vehicle accident survivors. Behaviour Research and Therapy, 41: 79–96.

Blanchard EB, Hickling EJ, Forneris CA, et al. 1997. Prediction of remission of acute posttraumatic stress disorder in motor vehicle accident victims. Journal of Traumatic Stress, 10: 215–234.

Blanchard EB, Hickling EJ, Malta LS, et al. 2004. One- and two-year prospective follow-up of cognitive behavior therapy or supportive psychotherapy. Behaviour Research and Therapy, 42: 745–759.

Bland RC, Newman SC, Orn H. 1988. Age of onset of psychiatric disorders. Acta Psychiatrica Scandinavica, 77 (Suppl. 338): 43–49.

Blashfield R, Noyes R, Reich J, et al. 1994. Personality disorder traits in generalized anxiety and panic disorder patients. Comprehensive Psychiatry, 35: 329–334.

Blaya C, Seganfredo AC, Dornelles M, et al. 2007. The efficacy of milnacipran in panic disorder: An open trial. International Clinical Psychopharmacology, 22: 153–158.

Blazer DG, Hughes D, George LK, et al. 1991. Generalized anxiety disorder. In Robins LN, Regier DA, editors: Psychiatric Disorders in America: The Epidemiologic Catchment Area Study. New York: Free Press, pp. 180–203.

Bloch MH, Landeros-Weisenberger A, Kelmendi B, et al. 2006. A systematic review: Antipsychotic augmentation with treatment refractory obsessive-compulsive disorder. Molecular Psychiatry, 11: 622–632.

Blomhoff S, Haug TT, Hellström K, et al. 2001. Randomised controlled general practice trial of sertraline, exposure therapy and combined treatment in generalised social phobia. British Journal of Psychiatry, 179: 23–30.

Bodkin JA, Pope HG, Detke MJ, et al. 2007. Is PTSD caused by traumatic stress? Journal of Anxiety Disorders, 21: 176–182.

Boersma K, Den Hengst S, Dekker J, et al. 1976. Exposure and response prevention in the natural environment: A comparison with obsessive-compulsive patients. Behaviour Research and Therapy, 14: 19–24.

Bogetto F, Bellino S, Vaschetto P, et al. 2000. Olanzapine augmentation in fluvoxamine-refractory obsessive-compulsive disorder: A 12-week open trial. Psychiatry Research, 96: 91–98.

Boney-McCoy S, Finkelhor D. 1995. Psychosocial sequelae of violent victimization in a national youth sample. Journal of Consulting and Clinical Psychology, 63: 726–736.

Book SW, Thomas SE, Randall PK, et al. 2008. Paroxetine reduces social anxiety in individuals with a co-occurring alcohol use disorder. Journal of Anxiety Disorders, 22: 310–318.

Booth R, Rachman S. 1992. The reduction of claustrophobia – I. Behaviour Research and Therapy, 30: 207–221.

Borkovec TD, Costello E. 1993. Efficacy of applied relaxation and cognitive-behavioral therapy in the treatment of generalized anxiety disorder. Journal of Consulting and Clinical Psychology, 61: 611–619.

Borkovec TD, Inz J. 1990. The nature of worry in generalized anxiety disorder: A predominance of thought activity. Behaviour Research and Therapy, 28: 153–158.

Borkovec TD, Ray WJ, Stoeber J. 1998. Worry: A cognitive phenomenon intimately linked to affective, physiological, and interpersonal behavioral processes. Cognitive Therapy and Research, 22: 561–576.

Borkovec TD, Shadick RN, Hopkins M. 1991. The nature of normal and pathological worry. In Rapee RM, Barlow DH, editors: Chronic Anxiety: Generalized Anxiety Disorder and Mixed Anxiety-Depression. New York: Guilford Press, pp. 29–51.

Boschen MJ. 2008. Paruresis (psychogenic inhibition of micturition): Cognitive behavioral formulation and treatment. Depression and Anxiety, 25: 903–912.

Bose A, Korotzer A, Gommoll C, et al. 2008. Randomized placebo-controlled trial of escitalopram and venlafaxine XR in the treatment of generalized anxiety disorder. Depression and Anxiety, 25: 854–861.

Bourdon KH, Boyd JH, Rae DS, et al. 1988. Gender differences in phobias: Results of the ECA community survey. Journal of Anxiety Disorders, 2: 227–241.

Bourdon KH, Rae DS, Locke BZ, et al. 1992. Estimating the prevalence of mental disorders in US adults from the Epidemiologic Catchment Area Study. Public Health Reports, 107: 663–668.

Bourque P, Ladouceur R. 1980. An investigation of various performance-based treatments with acrophobics. Behaviour Research and Therapy, 18: 161–170.

Bowen RC, Offord DR, Boyle MH. 1990. The prevalence of overanxious disorder and separation anxiety disorder: Results from the Ontario Child Health Study. Journal of the American Academy of Child and Adolescent Psychiatry, 29: 753–758.

Bowlby J. 1973. Separation: Anxiety and Anger, Vol. 2. New York: Basic Books.

Boyd JH, Rae DS, Thompson JW, et al. 1990. Social phobia: Prevalence and risk factors. Social Psychiatry and Psychiatric Epidemiology, 25: 314–323.

Boyer WF, Feighner JP. 1993. A placebo-controlled double-blind multicenter trial of two doses of ipsapirone versus diazepam in generalized anxiety disorder. International Clinical Psychopharmacology, 8: 173–176.

Brady K, Pearlstein T, Asnis GM, et al. 2000. Efficacy and safety of sertraline treatment of posttraumatic stress disorder: A randomized controlled trial. Journal of the American Medical Association, 283: 1837–1844.

Brady KT, Sonne SC, Roberts JM. 1995. Sertraline treatment of comorbid posttraumatic stress disorder and alcohol dependence. Journal of Clinical Psychiatry, 56: 502–505.

Brantigan CO, Brantigan TA, Joseph N. 1982. Effect of beta blockade and beta stimulation on stage fright. American Journal of Medicine, 72: 88–94.

Brantley PJ, Mehan DJ, Ames SC, et al. 1999. Minor stressors and generalized anxiety disorder among low-income patients attending primary care clinics. Journal of Nervous and Mental Disease, 187: 435–440.

Braun P, Greenberg D, Dasberg H, et al. 1990. Core symptoms of posttraumatic stress disorder unimproved by alprazolam treatment. Journal of Clinical Psychiatry, 51: 236–238.

Brawman-Mintzer O, Lydiard RB. 1996. Generalized anxiety disorder: Issues in epidemiology. Journal of Clinical Psychiatry, 57 (Suppl. 7): 3–8.

Brawman-Mintzer O, Lydiard RB. 1997. Biological basis of generalized anxiety disorder. Journal of Clinical Psychiatry, 58 (Suppl. 3): 16–25.

Brawman-Mintzer O, Lydiard RB, Crawford MM, et al. 1994. Somatic symptoms in generalized anxiety disorder with and without comorbid psychiatric disorders. American Journal of Psychiatry, 151: 930–932.

Brawman-Mintzer O, Lydiard RB, Emmanuel N, et al. 1993. Psychiatric comorbidity in patients with generalized anxiety disorder. American Journal of Psychiatry, 150: 1216–1218.

Brawman-Mintzer O, Knapp RG, Nietert PJ. 2005. Adjunctive risperidone in generalized anxiety disorder: A double-blind, placebo-controlled study. Journal of Clinical Psychiatry, 66: 1321–1325.

Brawman-Mintzer O, Knapp RG, Rynn M, et al. 2006. Sertraline treatment for generalized anxiety disorder: A randomized, double-blind, placebo-controlled study. Journal of Clinical Psychiatry, 67: 874–881.

Breier A, Charney DS, Heninger GR. 1984. Major depression in patients with agoraphobia and panic disorder. Archives of General Psychiatry, 41: 1129–1135.

Breier A, Charney DS, Heninger GR. 1986. Agoraphobia with panic attacks: Development, diagnostic stability, and course of illness. Archives of General Psychiatry, 43: 1029–1036.

Breiter HC, Rauch SL, Kwong KK, et al. 1996. Functional magnetic resonance imaging of symptom provocation in obsessive-compulsive disorder. Archives of General Psychiatry, 53: 595–606.

Bremner JD, Innis RB, White T, et al. 2000a. SPECT [I-123]iomazenil measurement of the benzodiazepine receptor in panic disorder. Biological Psychiatry, 47: 96–106.

Bremner JD, Narayan M, Anderson ER, et al. 2000b. Hippocampal volume reduction in major depression. American Journal of Psychiatry, 157: 115–118.

Bremner JD, Narayan M, Staib LH, et al. 1999. Neural correlates of memories of childhood sexual abuse in women with and without posttraumatic stress disorder. American Journal of Psychiatry, 156: 1787–1795.

Bremner JD, Southwick SM, Brett E, et al. 1992. Dissociation and posttraumatic stress disorder in Vietnam combat veterans. American Journal of Psychiatry, 149: 328–332.

Bremner JD, Southwick SM, Johnson DR, et al. 1993. Childhood physical abuse and combat-related posttraumatic stress disorder in Vietnam veterans. American Journal of Psychiatry, 150: 235–239.

Breslau N, Chilcoat HD, Kessler RC, et al. 1999. Vulnerability to assaultive violence: Further specification of the sex difference in post-traumatic stress disorder. Psychological Medicine, 29: 813–821.

Breslau N, Davis GC. 1992. Posttraumatic stress disorder in an urban population of young adults: Risk factors for chronicity. American Journal of Psychiatry, 149: 671–675.

Breslau N, Davis GC, Andreski P, et al. 1991. Traumatic events and posttraumatic stress disorder in an urban population of young adults. Archives of General Psychiatry, 48: 216–222.

Breslau N, Davis GC, Andreski P, et al. 1997. Sex differences in posttraumatic stress disorder. Archives of General Psychiatry, 54: 1044–1048.

Breslau N, Davis GC, Peterson EL, et al. 2000. A second look at comorbidity in victims of trauma: The posttraumatic stress disorder–major depression connection. Biological Psychiatry, 48: 902–909.

Breslau N, Kessler RC. 2001. The stressor criterion in DSM-IV posttraumatic stress disorder: An empirical investigation. Biological Psychiatry, 50: 699–704.

Breslau N, Kessler RC, Chilcoat HD, et al. 1998. Trauma and posttraumatic stress disorder in the community: The 1996 Detroit Area Survey of Trauma. Archives of General Psychiatry, 55: 626–632.

Breslau N, Klein D. 1999. Smoking and panic attacks. Archives of General Psychiatry, 56: 1141–1147.

Breslau N, Lucia VC, Alvarado GF. 2006. Intelligence and other predisposing factors in exposure to trauma and posttraumatic stress disorder: A follow-up study at age 17 years. Archives of General Psychiatry, 63: 1238–1245.

Breslau N, Peterson EL, Schultz LR. 2008. A second look at prior trauma and the posttraumatic stress disorder effects of subsequent trauma: A prospective epidemiological study. Archives of General Psychiatry, 65: 431–437.

Breslau N, Reboussin BA, Anthony JC, et al. 2005. The structure of posttraumatic stress disorder: Latent class analysis in 2 community samples. Archives of General Psychiatry, 62: 1343–1351.

Brewin CR, Andrews B, Rose S, et al. 1999. Acute stress disorder and posttraumatic stress disorder in victims of violent crime. American Journal of Psychiatry, 156: 360–365.

Brewin CR, Andrews B, Valentine JD. 2000. Meta-analysis of risk factors for post-traumatic stress disorder in trauma-exposed adults. Journal of Consulting and Clinical Psychology, 68: 748–766.

Brewin CR, Dalgleish T, Joseph S. 1996. A dual representation theory of post trau-matic stress disorder. Psychological Review, 103: 670–686.

Briere J, Scott C, Weathers F. 2005. Peritraumatic and persistent dissociation in the presumed etiology of PTSD. American Journal of Psychiatry, 162: 2295–2301.

Briggs A, Stretch D, Brandon S. 1993. Subtyping of panic disorder by symptom profile. British Journal of Psychiatry, 163: 201–209.

Bringager CB, Dammen T, Friis A. 2004. Nonfearful panic disorder in chest pain patients. Psychosomatics, 45: 69–79.

Brooks RB, Baltazar PL, Munjack DJ. 1989. Co-occurrence of personality disorders with panic disorder, social phobia, and generalized anxiety disorder: A review of the literature. Journal of Anxiety Disorders, 3: 259–285.

Brown EJ, Heimberg RG, Juster HR. 1995. Social phobia subtype and avoidant personality disorder: Effect on severity of social phobia, impairment, and out-come of cognitive-behavioral treatment. Behavior Therapy, 26: 467–486.

Brown M, Smits JA, Powers MB, et al. 2003. Differential sensitivity of the three ASI factors in predicting panic disorder patients' subjective and behavioral response to hyperventilation challenge. Journal of Anxiety Disorders, 17: 583–591.

Brown TA. 1997. The nature of generalized anxiety disorder and pathological worry: Current evidence and conceptual models. Canadian Journal of Psychiatry, 42: 817–825.

Brown TA, Barlow DH, Liebowitz MR. 1994. The empirical basis of generalized anxiety disorder. American Journal of Psychiatry, 151: 1272–1280.

Brown TA, Chorpita BF, Barlow DH. 1998. Structural relationships among dimen-sions of the DSM-IV anxiety and mood disorders and dimensions of negative affect, positive affect, and autonomic arousal. Journal of Abnormal Psychology, 107: 179–192.

Brown TA, DiNardo PA, Lehman CL, et al. 2001. Reliability of DSM-IV anxiety and mood disorders: Implications for classification of emotional disorders. Journal of Abnormal Psychology, 110: 49–58.

Brown TA, Marten PA, Barlow DH. 1995. Discriminant validity of the symptoms constituting the DSM-III-R and DSM-IV associated symptom criterion of gen-eralized anxiety disorder. Journal of Anxiety Disorders, 9: 317–328.

Brown TA, O'Leary TA, Barlow DH. 1993. Generalized anxiety disorder. In Barlow DH, editor: Clinical Handbook of Psychological Disorders, 2nd Edition. New York: Guilford Press, pp. 137–188.

Bruce SE, Machan JT, Dyck I, et al. 2001. Infrequency of "pure" GAD: Impact of psychiatric comorbidity on clinical course. Depression and Anxiety, 14: 219–225.

Bruce SE, Vasile RG, Goisman RM, et al. 2003. Are benzodiazepines still the medica-tion of choice for patients with panic disorder with or without agoraphobia? American Journal of Psychiatry, 160: 1432–1438.

Bryant RA. 2007. Does dissociation further our understanding of PTSD? Journal of Anxiety Disorders, 21: 183–191.

Bryant RA, Creamer M, O'Donnell M, et al. 2008a. A multisite study of initial respiration rate and heart rate as predictors of posttraumatic stress disorder. Journal of Clinical Psychiatry, 69: 1694–1701.

Bryant RA, Guthrie RM. 2007. Maladaptive self-appraisals before trauma exposure predict posttraumatic stress disorder. Journal of Consulting and Clinical Psychology, 75: 812–815.

Bryant RA, Harvey AG. 1998. Relationship of acute stress disorder and posttraumatic stress disorder following mild traumatic brain injury. American Journal of Psychiatry, 155: 625–629.

Bryant RA, Harvey AG, Dang ST, et al. 1998. Treatment of acute stress disorder: A comparison of cognitive-behavioral therapy and supportive counseling. Journal of Consulting and Clinical Psychology, 66: 862–866.

Bryant RA, Harvey AG, Guthrie RM, et al. 2000. A prospective study of psychophysiological arousal, acute stress disorder and posttraumatic stress disorder. Journal of Abnormal Psychology, 109: 341–344.

Bryant RA, Mastrodomenico J, Felmingham KL, et al. 2008b. Treatment of acute stress disorder: A randomized controlled trial. Archives of General Psychiatry, 65: 659–667.

Bryant RA, Moulds ML, Nixon RVD. 2003. Cognitive behaviour therapy of acute stress disorder: A four-year follow-up. Behaviour Research and Therapy, 41: 489–494.

Bryant RA, Sackville T, Dang ST, et al. 1999. Treating acute stress disorder: An evaluation of cognitive behavior therapy and supportive counseling techniques. American Journal of Psychiatry, 156: 1780–1786.

Buchanan AW, Meng KS, Marks IM. 1996. What predicts improvement and compliance during the behavioral treatment of obsessive compulsive disorder? Anxiety, 2: 22–27.

Buckner JD, Schmidt NB, Lang AR, et al. 2008. Specificity of social anxiety disorder as a risk factor for alcohol and cannabis dependence. Journal of Psychiatric Research, 42: 230–239.

Buckner JD, Timpano KR, Zvolensky MJ, et al. 2008. Implications of comorbid alcohol dependence among individuals with social anxiety disorder. Depression and Anxiety, 25: 1028–1037.

Buglass D, Clarke J, Henderson A, et al. 1977. A study of agoraphobic housewives. Psychological Medicine, 7: 73–86.

Buhr K, Dugas MJ. 2006. Investigating the construct validity of intolerance of uncertainty and its unique relationship with worry. Journal of Anxiety Disorders, 20: 222–236.

Burke KC, Burke JD, Rae DS, et al. 1991. Comparing age at onset of major depression and other psychiatric disorders by birth cohorts in five U.S. community populations. Archives of General Psychiatry, 48: 789–795.

Burns LE, Thorpe GL, Cavallaro LA. 1986. Agoraphobia eight years after behavioral treatment: A follow-up study with interview, self-report, and behavioral data. Behavior Therapy, 17: 580–591.

Butler G, Cullington A, Munby M, et al. 1984. Exposure and anxiety management in the treatment of social phobia. Journal of Consulting and Clinical Psychology, 52: 642–650.

Butler G, Fennell M, Robson P, et al. 1991. A comparison of behavior therapy and cognitive-behavior therapy in the treatment of generalized anxiety disorder. Journal of Consulting and Clinical Psychology, 59: 167–175.

Butler G, Mathews A. 1983. Cognitive processes in anxiety. Advances in Behaviour Research and Therapy, 5: 51–62.

Butler G, Wells A. 1995. Cognitive-behavioral treatments: Clinical applications. In Heimberg RG, Liebowitz MR, Hope DA, Schneier FR, editors: Social Phobia: Diagnosis, Assessment, and Treatment. New York: Guilford Press, pp. 310–333.

Butterfield MI, Becker ME, Connor KM, et al. 2001. Olanzapine in the treatment of post-traumatic stress disorder: A pilot study. International Clinical Psychopharmacology, 16: 197–203.

Bystritsky A, Ackerman DL, Rosen RM, et al. 2004. Augmentation of serotonin reuptake inhibitors in refractory obsessive-compulsive disorder using adjunctive olanzapine: A placebo-controlled trial. Journal of Clinical Psychiatry, 65: 565–568.

Bystritsky A, Pontillo D, Powers M, et al. 2001. Functional MRI changes during panic anticipation and imagery exposure. Neuroreport, 12: 3953–3957.

Candilis PJ, McLean RY, Otto MW, et al. 1999. Quality of life in patients with panic disorder. Journal of Nervous and Mental Disease, 187: 429–434.

Canino GJ, Bird HR, Shrout PE, et al. 1987. The prevalence of specific psychiatric disorders in Puerto Rico. Archives of General Psychiatry, 44: 727–735.

Carlier IV, Gersons BPR. 1995. Partial posttraumatic stress disorder (PTSD): The issue of psychological scars and the occurrence of PTSD symptoms. Journal of Nervous and Mental Disease, 183: 107–109.

Carlson JG, Chemtob CM, Rusnak K, et al. 1998. Eye movement desensitization and reprocessing (EMDR) treatment for combat-related posttraumatic stress disorder. Journal of Traumatic Stress, 11: 3–24.

Carpenter LL, Leon Z, Yasmin S, et al. 1999. Clinical experience with mirtazapine in the treatment of panic disorder. Annals of Clinical Psychiatry, 11: 81–86.

Carrigan M, Randall C. 2003. Self-medication in social phobia: A review of the alcohol literature. Addictive Behaviors, 28: 269–284.

Carty J, O'Donnell ML, Creamer M. 2006. Delayed-onset PTSD: A prospective study of injury survivors. Journal of Affective Disorders, 90: 257–261.

Casacalenda N, Boulenger JP. 1998. Pharmacologic treatments effective in both generalized anxiety disorder and major depressive disorder: Clinical and theoretical implications. Canadian Journal of Psychiatry, 43: 722–730.

Cassano GB, Petracca A, Perugi G. 1988. Clomipramine for panic disorder: I. The first 10 weeks of a long-term comparison with imipramine. Journal of Affective Disorders, 14: 123–127.

Castle DJ, Deale A, Marks IM, et al. 1994. Obsessive-compulsive disorder: Prediction of outcome from behavioral psychotherapy. Acta Psychiatrica Scandinavica, 89: 393–398.

Catapano F, Perris F, Masella M, et al. 2006. Obsessive-compulsive disorder: A 3-year prospective follow-up study of patients treated with serotonin reuptake inhibitors. OCD follow-up study. Journal of Psychiatric Research, 40: 502–510.

Chambers J, Yeragani VK, Keshavan MS. 1986. Phobias in India and the United Kingdom: A trans-cultural study. Acta Psychiatrica Scandinavica, 74: 388–391.

Chambless DL, Caputo GC, Bright P, et al. 1984. Assessment of fear in agoraphobics: The Body Sensations Questionnaire and the Agoraphobic Cognitions Questionnaire. Journal of Consulting and Clinical Psychology, 52: 1090–1097.

Chambless DL, Caputo GC, Jasin SE, et al. 1985. The Mobility Inventory for Agoraphobia. Behaviour Research and Therapy, 23: 35–44.

Chambless DL, Fydrich T, Rodebaugh TL. 2008. Generalized social phobia and avoidant personality disorder: Meaningful distinction or useless duplication? Depression and Anxiety, 25: 8–19.

Chambless DL, Mason J. 1986. Sex, sex role stereotyping, and agoraphobia. Behaviour Research and Therapy, 24: 231–235.

Chambless DL, Renneberg B, Goldstein A, et al. 1992. MCMI-diagnosed personality disorders among agoraphobic outpatients: Prevalence and relationship to severity and treatment outcome. Journal of Anxiety Disorders, 6: 193–211.

Charney DS, Heninger GR. 1986. Abnormal regulation of noradrenergic function in panic disorders: Effects of clonidine in healthy subjects and patients with agoraphobia and panic disorder. Archives of General Psychiatry, 43: 1042–1054.

Charney DS, Heninger GR, Breier A. 1984. Noradrenergic function in panic anxiety: Effects of yohimbine in healthy subjects and patients with agoraphobia and panic disorder Archives of General Psychiatry, 41: 751–763.

Chartier MJ, Hazen AL, Stein MB. 1998. Lifetime patterns of social phobia: A retrospective study of the course of social phobia in a nonclinical population. Depression and Anxiety, 7: 113–121.

Chavira DA, Stein MB, Malcarne VL. 2002. Scrutinizing the relationship between shyness and social phobia. Journal of Anxiety Disorders, 16: 585–598.

Chelminski I, Zimmerman M. 2003. Pathological worry in depressed and anxious patients. Journal of Anxiety Disorders, 17: 533–546.

Chen CN, Wong J, Lee N, et al. 1993. The Shatin Community Mental Health Survey in Hong Kong. Archives of General Psychiatry, 50: 125–133.

Chen YP, Ehlers A, Clark DM, et al. 2002. Patients with generalized social phobia direct their attention away from faces. Behaviour Research and Therapy, 40: 677–687.

Chen YW, Dilsaver SC. 1995. Comorbidity of panic disorder in bipolar illness: Evidence from the Epidemiologic Catchment Area survey. American Journal of Psychiatry, 152: 280–282.

Chignon JM, Lepine JP, Ades J. 1993. Panic disorder in cardiac outpatients. American Journal of Psychiatry, 150: 780–785.

Chouinard G, Goodman W, Greist J, et al. 1990. Results of a double-blind placebo-controlled trial of a new serotonin uptake inhibitor, sertraline, in the treatment of obsessive-compulsive disorder. Psychopharmacology Bulletin, 26: 279–284.

Christensen H, Hadzi-Pavlovic D, Andrews G, et al. 1987. Behavior therapy and tricyclic medication in the treatment of obsessive-compulsive disorder: A quantitative review. Journal of Consulting and Clinical Psychology, 55: 701–711.

Clark DA. 2005. Lumping versus splitting: A commentary on subtyping in OCD. Behavior Therapy, 36: 401–404.

Clark DA, Steer RA, Beck AT. 1994. Common and specific dimensions of self-reported anxiety and depression: Implications for the cognitive and tripartite models. Journal of Abnormal Psychology, 103: 645–654.

Clark DM. 1986. A cognitive approach to panic. Behaviour Research and Therapy, 24: 461–470.

Clark DM. 1988. A cognitive model of panic attacks. In Rachman S, Maser JD, editors: Panic: Psychological Perspectives. Hillsdale, NJ: Erlbaum, pp. 71–89.

Clark DM, Beck AT. 1988. Cognitive approaches. In Last CG, Hersen M, editors: Handbook of Anxiety Disorders. New York: Pergamon Press, pp. 362–385.

Clark DM, Ehlers A, McManus F, et al. 2003. Cognitive therapy versus fluoxetine in generalized social phobia: A randomized placebo-controlled trial. Journal of Consulting and Clinical Psychology, 71: 1058–1067.

Clark DM, Salkovskis PM, Hackmann A, et al. 1994. A comparison of cognitive therapy, applied relaxation and imipramine in the treatment of panic disorder. British Journal of Psychiatry, 164: 759–769.

Clark DM, Wells A. 1995. A cognitive model of social phobia. In Heimberg R, Liebowitz M, Hope DA, Schneier FR, editors: Social Phobia: Diagnosis, Assessment and Treatment. New York: Guilford Press, pp. 69–93.

Clark LA, Watson D. 1991. Tripartite model of anxiety and depression: Psychometric evidence and taxonomic implications. Journal of Abnormal Psychology, 100: 316–336.

Clarvit SR, Schneier FR, Liebowitz MR. 1996. The offensive subtype of Taijin-kyofu-sho in New York City: The phenomenology and treatment of a social anxiety disorder. Journal of Clinical Psychiatry, 57: 523–527.

Clayton IC, Richards JC, Edwards CJ. 1999. Selective attention in obsessive-compulsive disorder. Journal of Abnormal Psychology, 108: 171–175.

Cloitre M, Shear MK. 1995. Psychodynamic perspectives. In Stein MB, editor: Social Phobia: Clinical and Research Perspectives. Washington, DC: American Psychiatric Press, pp. 163–187.

Clomipramine Collaborative Study Group. 1991. Clomipramine in the treatment of patients with obsessive-compulsive disorder. Archives of General Psychiatry, 48: 730–738.

Clum GA, Knowles SL. 1991. Why do some people with panic disorders become avoidant? A review. Clinical Psychology Review, 11: 295–313.

Coles ME, Frost RO, Heimberg RG, et al. 2003. "Not just right experiences": Perfectionism, obsessive-compulsive features and general psychopathology. Behaviour Research and Therapy, 41: 681–700.

Connor KM, Sutherland SM, Tupler LA, et al. 1999. Fluoxetine in post-traumatic stress disorder. Randomised, double-blind study. British Journal of Psychiatry, 175: 17–22.

Cooper NA, Clum GA. 1989. Imaginal flooding as a supplementary treatment for PTSD in combat veterans: A controlled study. Behavior Therapy, 20: 381–391.

Cooper PJ, Eke M. 1999. Childhood shyness and maternal social phobia: A community study. British Journal of Psychiatry, 174: 439–443.

Cordioli AV, Heldt E, Bochi DB, et al. 2003. Cognitive-behavioral group therapy in obsessive-compulsive disorder: A randomized clinical trial. Psychotherapy and Psychosomatics, 72: 211–216.

Coryell W, Noyes R, Clancy J. 1982. Excess mortality in panic disorder: A comparison with primary unipolar depression. Archives of General Psychiatry, 39: 701–703.

Coryell W, Noyes R, House JD. 1986. Mortality among outpatients with anxiety disorders. American Journal of Psychiatry, 143: 508–510.

Cottraux J, Messy P, Marks IM, et al. 1993. Predictive factors in the treatment of obsessive-compulsive disorders with fluvoxamine and/or behaviour therapy. Behavioural Psychotherapy, 21: 45–50.

Cottraux J, Mollard E, Bouvard M, et al. 1990. A controlled study of fluvoxamine and exposure in obsessive-compulsive disorder. International Clinical Psychopharmacology, 5: 17–30.

Cowley DS, Arana GW. 1990. The diagnostic utility of lactate sensitivity in panic disorder. Archives of General Psychiatry, 47: 277–284.

Cowley DS, Dager SR, McClellan J, et al. 1988. Response to lactate infusion in generalized anxiety disorder. Biological Psychiatry, 24: 409–414.

Cowley DS, Ha EH, Roy-Byrne PP. 1997. Determinants of pharmacologic treatment failure in panic disorder. Journal of Clinical Psychiatry, 58: 555–561.

Cox BJ, Direnfeld DM, Swinson RP, et al. 1994a. Suicidal ideation and suicide attempts in panic disorder and social phobia. American Journal of Psychiatry, 151: 882–887.

Cox BJ, Endler NS, Swinson RP, et al. 1992. Situations and specific coping strategies associated with clinical and nonclinical panic attacks. Behaviour Research and Therapy, 30: 67–69.

Cox BJ, Fuentes K, Borger SC, et al. 2001. Psychopathological correlates of anxiety sensitivity: Evidence from clinical interviews and self-report measures. Journal of Anxiety Disorders, 15: 317–332.

Cox BJ, Swinson RP, Endler NS, et al. 1994b. The symptom structure of panic attacks. Comprehensive Psychiatry, 35: 349–353.

Craske MG. 1996. An integrated approach to panic disorder. Bulletin of the Menninger Clinic, 60 (Suppl.): A87–A104.

Craske MG, Barlow DH, O'Leary TA. 1992. Mastery of Your Anxiety and Worry. Albany, NY: Graywind.

Craske MG, Brown TA, Barlow DH. 1991. Behavioral treatment of panic disorder: A two-year follow-up. Behavior Therapy, 22: 289–304.

Craske MG, Golinelli D, Stein MB, et al. 2005. Does the addition of cognitive-behavioral therapy improve panic disorder treatment outcome relative to medication alone in the primary-care setting? Psychological Medicine, 35: 1645–1654.

Craske MG, Lang AJ, Mystkowski JL, et al. 2002. Does nocturnal panic represent a more severe form of panic disorder? Journal of Nervous and Mental Disease, 190: 611–618.

Craske MG, Mohlman J, Yi J, et al. 1995. Treatment of claustrophobia and snake/ spider phobias: Fear of arousal and fear of context. Behaviour Research and Therapy, 33: 197–203.

Craske MG, Rapee RM, Barlow DH. 1988. The significance of panic-expectancy for individual patterns of avoidance. Behavior Therapy, 19: 577–592.

Craske MG, Rapee RM, Jackel L, et al. 1989. Qualitative dimensions of worry in DSM-III-R generalized anxiety disorder subjects and nonanxious controls. Behaviour Research and Therapy, 27: 397–402.

Craske MG, Sipsas A. 1992. Animal phobias vs. claustrophobias: Exteroceptive vs. interoceptive cues. Behaviour Research and Therapy, 30: 569–581.

Creamer M, Burgess P, McFarlane AC. 2001. Post-traumatic stress disorder: Findings from the Australian National Survey of Mental Health and Well-Being. Psychological Medicine, 31: 1237–1247.

Creamer M, O'Donnell MJ, Pattison P. 2004. The relationship between acute stress disorder and posttraumatic stress disorder in severely injured trauma survivors. Behaviour Research and Therapy, 42: 315–328.

Crino RD. 1999. Obsessive-compulsive spectrum disorders. Current Opinion in Psychiatry, 12: 151–155.

Crits-Christoph PC, Connolly MB, Azarian K, et al. 1996. An open trial of brief supportive-expressive psychotherapy in the treatment of generalized anxiety disorder. Psychotherapy, 33: 418–430.

Cross-National Collaborative Panic Study, Second Phase Investigators. 1992. Drug treatment of panic disorder: Comparative efficacy of alprazolam, imipramine, and placebo. British Journal of Psychiatry, 160: 191–202.

Crowe RR, Noyes R, Pauls DL, et al. 1983. A family study of panic disorder. Archives of General Psychiatry, 40: 1065–1069.

Curtis GC, Magee WJ, Eaton WW, et al. 1998. Specific fears and phobias: Epidemiology and classification. British Journal of Psychiatry, 173: 212–217.

Darcis T, Ferreri M, Natens J, et al. 1995. A multicentre double-blind, placebo-controlled study investigating the anxiolytic efficacy of hydroxyzine in patients with generalized anxiety. Human Psychopharmacology, 10: 181–187.

Davey GCL, Levy S. 1998. Catastrophic worrying: Personal inadequacy and a perseverative iterative style as features of the catastrophizing process. Journal of Abnormal Psychology, 107: 576–586.

Davey GCL, McDonald AS, Hirisave U, et al. 1998. A cross-cultural study of animal fears. Behaviour Research and Therapy, 36: 735–750.

Davidson J, Baldwin D, Stein DJ, et al. 2006a. Treatment of posttraumatic stress disorder with venlafaxine extended release: A 6-month randomized controlled trial. Archives of General Psychiatry, 63: 1158–1165.

Davidson J, Kudler H, Smith R, et al. 1990. Treatment of posttraumatic stress disorder with amitriptyline and placebo. Archives of General Psychiatry, 47: 259–266.

Davidson J, Pearlstein T, Londborg P, et al. 2001b. Efficacy of sertraline in preventing relapse of posttraumatic stress disorder: Results of a 28-week double-blind, placebo-controlled study. American Journal of Psychiatry, 158: 1974–1981.

Davidson J, Rothbaum BO, Tucker P, et al. 2006b. Venlafaxine extended release in posttraumatic stress disorder: A sertraline- and placebo-controlled study. Journal of Clinical Psychopharmacology, 26: 259–267.

Davidson J, Swartz M, Storck M, et al. 1985. A diagnostic and family study of posttraumatic stress disorder. American Journal of Psychiatry, 142: 90–93.

Davidson J, Yaryura-Tobias J, DuPont R, et al. 2004c. Fluvoxamine-controlled release formulation for the treatment of generalized social anxiety disorder. Journal of Clinical Psychopharmacology, 24: 118–125.

Davidson JR, Bose A, Korotzer A, et al. 2004a. Escitalopram in the treatment of generalized anxiety disorder: Double-blind, placebo controlled, flexible-dose study. Depression and Anxiety, 19: 234–240.

Davidson JR, Brady K, Mellman TA, et al. 2007. The efficacy and tolerability of tiagabine in adult patients with post-traumatic stress disorder. Journal of Clinical Psychopharmacology, 27: 85–88.

Davidson JR, Connor KM, Hertzberg MA, et al. 2005. Maintenance therapy with fluoxetine in posttraumatic stress disorder: A placebo-controlled discontinuation study. Journal of Clinical Psychopharmacology, 25: 166–169.

Davidson JR, Foa EB, Huppert JD, et al. 2004b. Fluoxetine, comprehensive cognitive behavioral therapy, and placebo in generalized social phobia. Archives of General Psychiatry, 61: 1005–1013.

Davidson JR, Landerman LR, Farfel GM, et al. 2002. Characterizing the effects of sertraline in post-traumatic stress disorder. Psychological Medicine, 32: 661–670.

Davidson JR, Weisler RH, Butterfield MI, et al. 2003. Mirtazapine vs. placebo in posttraumatic stress disorder: A pilot trial. Biological Psychiatry, 53: 188–191.

Davidson JR, Weisler RH, Malik M, et al. 1998. Fluvoxamine in civilians with posttraumatic stress disorder. Journal of Clinical Psychopharmacology, 18: 93–95.

Davidson JRT, DuPont RL, Hedges D, et al. 1999. Efficacy, safety and tolerability of venlafaxine extended release and buspirone in outpatients with generalized anxiety disorder. Journal of Clinical Psychiatry, 60: 528–535.

Davidson JRT, Hughes DL, George LK, et al. 1993a. The epidemiology of social phobia: Findings from the Duke Epidemiological Catchment Area Study. Psychological Medicine, 23: 709–718.

Davidson JRT, Petts N, Richichi E, et al. 1993b. Treatment of social phobia with clonazepam and placebo. Journal of Clinical Psychopharmacology, 13: 423–428.

Davidson JRT, Rothbaum BO, van der Kolk BA, et al. 2001a. Multicenter, double-blind comparison of sertraline and placebo in the treatment of posttraumatic stress disorder. Archives of General Psychiatry, 58: 485–492.

Davies SJ, Ghahramani P, Jackson PR, et al. 1999. Association of panic disorder and panic attacks with hypertension. American Journal of Medicine, 107: 310–316.

Davis LL, Davidson JR, Ward LC, et al. 2008. Divalproex in the treatment of posttraumatic stress disorder: A randomized, double-blind, placebo-controlled trial in a veteran population. Journal of Clinical Psychopharmacology, 28: 84–88.

Deahl M. 2003. In debate: Psychological debriefing is a waste of time. Against. British Journal of Psychiatry, 183: 13–14.

de Araujo LA, Ito LM, Marks IM. 1996. Early compliance and other factors predicting outcome of exposure for obsessive-compulsive disorder. British Journal of Psychiatry, 169: 747–752.

DeBellis MD, Casey BJ, Dahl RE, et al. 2000. A pilot study of amygdala volumes in pediatric generalized anxiety disorder. Biological Psychiatry, 48: 51–57.

de Beurs E, van Balkom AJ, Lange A, et al. 1995. Treatment of panic disorder with agoraphobia: Comparison of fluvoxamine, placebo, and psychological panic management combined with exposure and of exposure in vivo alone. American Journal of Psychiatry, 152: 683–691.

Degonda M, Angst J. 1993. The Zurich Study, XX: Social phobia and agoraphobia. European Archives of Psychiatry and Clinical Neuroscience, 243: 95–102.

de Haan HE, van Oppen P, van Balkom AJLM, et al. 1997. Prediction of outcome and early vs. late improvement in OCD patients treated with cognitive behavior therapy and pharmacotherapy. Acta Psychiatrica Scandinavica, 96: 354–361.

de Jong JT, Komproe IH, Van Ommeren M, et al. 2001. Lifetime events and posttraumatic stress disorder in 4 postconflict settings. Journal of the American Medical Association, 286: 555–562.

De Jongh A, Muris P, Ter Horst G, et al. 1995. One-session cognitive treatment of dental phobia: Preparing dental phobics for treatment by restructuring negative cognitions. Behaviour Research and Therapy, 33: 947–954.

Delahanty DL, Herberman HB, Craig KJ, et al. 1997. Acute and chronic distress and posttraumatic stress disorder as a function of responsibility for serious motor vehicle accidents. Journal of Consulting and Clinical Psychology, 65: 560–567.

Delahanty DL, Raimonde AJ, Spoonster E. 2000. Initial posttraumatic urinary cortisol levels predict subsequent PTSD symptoms in motor vehicle accident victims. Biological Psychiatry, 48: 940–947.

Delle Chiaie R, Pancheri P, Casacchia M, et al. 1995. Assessment of the efficacy of buspirone in patients affected by generalized anxiety disorder, shifting to buspirone from prior treatment with lorazepam: A placebo-controlled, double-blind study. Journal of Clinical Psychopharmacology, 15: 12–19.

Demal U, Gerhardt L, Mayrhofer A, et al. 1993. Obsessive compulsive disorder and depression. Psychopathology, 26: 145–150.

DeMartinis N, Rynn M, Rickels K, et al. 2000. Prior benzodiazepine use and buspirone response in the treatment of generalized anxiety disorder. Journal of Clinical Psychiatry, 61: 91–94.

Demartino R, Mollica RF, Wilk V. 1995. Monoamine oxidase inhibitors in posttraumatic stress disorder. Journal of Nervous and Mental Disease, 183: 510–515.

den Boer JA, Westenberg HGM, Kamerbeek WDJ. 1987. Effect of serotonin uptake inhibitors in anxiety disorders: A double-blind comparison of clomipramine and fluvoxamine. International Clinical Psychopharmacology, 2: 21–32.

Denson TF, Marshall GN, Schell TL, et al. 2007. Predictors of posttraumatic distress 1 year after exposure to community violence: The importance of acute symptom severity. Journal of Consulting and Clinical Psychology, 75: 683–692.

Denys D, Burger H, van Megen H, et al. 2003a. A score for predicting response to pharmacotherapy in obsessive-compulsive disorder. International Clinical Psychopharmacology, 18: 315–322.

Denys D, de Geus F, van Megen HJGM, et al. 2004c. A double-blind, randomized, placebo-controlled trial of quetiapine addition in patients with obsessive-compulsive disorder refractory to serotonin reuptake inhibitors. Journal of Clinical Psychiatry, 65: 1040–1048.

Denys D, Fineberg N, Carey PD, et al. 2007. Quetiapine addition in obsessive-compulsive disorder: Is treatment outcome affected by type and dose of serotonin reuptake inhibitors? Biological Psychiatry, 61: 412–414.

Denys D, van der Wee N, van Megen HJGM, et al. 2003b. A double blind comparison of venlafaxine and paroxetine in obsessive-compulsive disorder. Journal of Clinical Psychopharmacology, 23: 568–575.

Denys D, van Megen HJGM, van der Wee N, et al. 2004b. A double-blind switch study of paroxetine and venlafaxine in obsessive-compulsive disorder. Journal of Clinical Psychiatry, 65: 37–43.

Denys D, Zohar J, Westenberg HGM. 2004a. The role of dopamine in obsessive-compulsive disorder: Preclinical and clinical evidence. Journal of Clinical Psychiatry, 65 (Suppl. 14): 11–17.

de Ruiter C, Rijken H, Garssen B, et al. 1989. Comorbidity among the anxiety disorders. Journal of Anxiety Disorders, 3: 57–68.

DeVeaugh-Geiss J, Katz R, Landau P, et al. 1990. Clinical predictors of treatment response in obsessive-compulsive disorder: Exploratory analyses from multicenter trials of clomipramine. Psychopharmacology Bulletin, 26: 54–59.

Devilly GJ, Annab R. 2008. A randomised controlled trial of group debriefing. Journal of Behavior Therapy and Experimental Psychiatry, 39: 42–56.

Devilly GJ, Spence SH. 1999. The relative efficacy and treatment distress of EMDR and a cognitive-behavior trauma treatment protocol in the amelioration of posttraumatic stress disorder. Journal of Anxiety Disorders, 13: 131–157.

DeWit DJ, Ogborne A, Offord DR, et al. 1999. Antecedents of the risk of recovery from DSM-III social phobia. Psychological Medicine, 29: 569–582.

Diaferia G, Sciuto G, Perna G, et al. 1993. DSM-III-R personality disorders in panic disorder. Journal of Anxiety Disorders, 7: 153–161.

Diamond DB. 1985. Panic attacks, hypochondriasis, and agoraphobia: A self-psychology formulation. American Journal of Psychotherapy, 39: 114–125.

Diamond DB. 1987. Psychotherapeutic approaches to the treatment of panic attacks, hypochondriasis and agoraphobia. British Journal of Medical Psychology, 60: 79–84.

Difede J, Cukor J, Jayasinghe N, et al. 2007. Virtual reality exposure therapy for the treatment of posttraumatic stress disorder following September 11, 2001. Journal of Clinical Psychiatry, 68: 1639–1647.

DiNardo PA, Guzy LT, Jenkins JA, et al. 1988. Etiology and maintenance of dog fears. Behaviour Research and Therapy, 26: 241–244.

Dohrenwend BP, Turner JB, Turse N, et al. 2006. The psychological risks of Vietnam for U.S. veterans: A revisit with new data and methods. Science, 313: 979–982.

Dougherty DD, Baer L, Cosgrove GR, et al. 2002. Prospective long-term follow-up of 44 patients who received cingulotomy for treatment-refractory obsessive-compulsive disorder. American Journal of Psychiatry, 159: 269–275.

Dreessen L, Arntz A, Luttels C, et al. 1994. Personality disorders do not influence the results of cognitive behavior therapies for anxiety disorders. Comprehensive Psychiatry, 35: 265–274.

Dreessen L, Hoekstra R, Arntz A. 1997. Personality disorders do not influence the results of cognitive and behavior therapy for obsessive compulsive disorder. Journal of Anxiety Disorders, 11: 503–521.

Dugas MJ, Freeston MH, Ladouceur R, et al. 1998a. Worry themes in primary GAD, secondary GAD, and other anxiety disorders. Journal of Anxiety Disorders, 12: 253–261.

Dugas MJ, Gagnon F, Ladouceur R, et al. 1998b. Generalized anxiety disorder: A preliminary test of a conceptual model. Behaviour Research and Therapy, 36: 215–226.

Dugas MJ, Ladouceur R, Leger E, et al. 2003. Group cognitive-behavioral therapy for generalized anxiety disorder: Treatment outcome and long-term follow-up. Journal of Consulting and Clinical Psychology, 71: 821–825.

Dunmore E, Clark DM, Ehlers A. 2001. A prospective investigation of the role of cognitive factors in persistent posttraumatic stress disorder (PTSD) after physical or sexual assault. Behaviour Research and Therapy, 39: 1063–1084.

Durham RC, Murphy T, Allan T, et al. 1994. Cognitive therapy, analytic psychotherapy and anxiety management training for generalised anxiety disorder. British Journal of Psychiatry, 165: 315–323.

Dyregrov A. 1989. Caring for helpers in disaster situations: Psychological debriefing. Disaster Management, 2: 25–30.

Eaton WW, Dryman A, Weissman MM. 1991. Panic and phobias. In Robins LN, Regier DA, editors: Psychiatric Disorders in America: The Epidemiologic Catchment Area Study. New York: Free Press, pp. 155–179.

Eaton WW, Kessler RC, Wittchen HU, et al. 1994. Panic and panic disorder in the United States. American Journal of Psychiatry, 151: 413–420.

Echeburua E, De Corral P, Bajos EG, et al. 1993. Interactions between self-exposure and alprazolam in the treatment of agoraphobia without current panic: An exploratory study. Behavioural and Cognitive Psychotherapy 21: 219–238.

Eddy KT, Dutra L, Bradley R, et al. 2004. A multidimensional meta-analysis of psychotherapy and pharmacotherapy for obsessive-compulsive disorder. Clinical Psychology Review, 24: 1011–1030.

Ehlers A, Clark DM. 2000. A cognitive model of posttraumatic stress disorder. Behaviour Research and Therapy, 38: 319–345.

Ehlers A, Clark DM, Hackmann A, et al. 2003. A randomized controlled trial of cognitive therapy, a self-help booklet, and repeated assessments as early interventions for posttraumatic stress disorder. Archives of General Psychiatry, 60: 1024–1032.

Ehlers A, Clark DM, Hackmann A, et al. 2005. Cognitive therapy for post-traumatic stress disorder: Development and evaluation. Behaviour Research and Therapy, 43: 413–431.

Ehlers A, Hofmann SG, Herda CA, et al. 1994. Clinical characteristics of driving phobia. Journal of Anxiety Disorders, 8: 323–339.

Ehlers A, Maercker A, Boos A. 2000. Posttraumatic stress disorder following political imprisonment: The role of mental defeat, alienation, and perceived permanent change. Journal of Abnormal Psychology, 109: 45–55.

Ehlers A, Mayou RA, Bryant RA. 1998. Psychological predictors of chronic PTSD after motor vehicle accidents. Journal of Abnormal Psychology, 107: 508–519.

Eisen JL, Beer DA, Pato MT, et al. 1997. Obsessive-compulsive disorder in patients with schizophrenia or schizoaffective disorder. American Journal of Psychiatry, 154: 271–273.

Eisen JL, Coles ME, Shea TT, et al. 2006. Clarifying the convergence between obsessive-compulsive personality disorder criteria and obsessive-compulsive disorder. Journal of Personality Disorders, 20: 294–305.

Eisen JL, Phillips KA, Baer L, et al. 1998. The Brown Assessment of Beliefs Scale: Reliability and validity. American Journal of Psychiatry, 155: 102–108.

Eisen JL, Rasmussen SA. 1993. Obsessive-compulsive disorder with psychotic features. Journal of Clinical Psychiatry, 54: 373–379.

Eisen JL, Rasmussen SA, Phillips KA, et al. 2001. Insight and treatment outcome in obsessive-compulsive disorder. Comprehensive Psychiatry, 42: 494–497.

Elie R, Lamontagne Y. 1984. Alprazolam and diazepam in the treatment of generalized anxiety. Journal of Clinical Psychopharmacology, 4: 125–129.

Emmelkamp P, Krijn M, Hulsbosch AM, et al. 2002. Virtual reality treatment versus exposure in vivo: A comparative evaluation in acrophobia. Behaviour Research and Therapy, 40: 509–516.

Emmelkamp PM, Beens H. 1991. Cognitive therapy with obsessive-compulsive disorder: A comparative evaluation. Behaviour Research and Therapy, 29: 293–300.

Emmelkamp PMG, Gerlsma C. 1994. Marital functioning and the anxiety disorders. Behavior Therapy, 25: 407–429.

Emmelkamp PMG, van den Heuvell C, van Linden RM, et al. 1989. Home-based treatment of obsessive-compulsive patients: Intersession interval and therapist involvement. Behaviour Research and Therapy, 27: 89–93.

Engel CC, Engel AL, Campbell SJ, et al. 1993. Posttraumatic stress disorder symptoms and precombat sexual and physical abuse in Desert Storm veterans. Journal of Nervous and Mental Disease, 181: 683–688.

Engelhard IM, van den Hout MA, Arntz A. 2002. A longitudinal study of "intrusion-based reasoning" and posttraumatic stress disorder after exposure to a train disaster. Behaviour Research and Therapy, 40: 1415–1425.

Engelhard IM, van den Hout MA, Kindt M, et al. 2003. Peritraumatic dissociation and posttraumatic stress after pregnancy loss: A prospective study. Behaviour Research and Therapy, 41; 67–78.

Epstein RS, Fullerton CS, Ursano RJ. 1998. Posttraumatic stress disorder following an air disaster: A prospective study. American Journal of Psychiatry, 155: 934–938.

Erickson DJ, Wolfe J, King DW, et al. 2001. Posttraumatic stress disorder and depression symptomatology in a sample of Gulf War veterans: A prospective analysis. Journal of Consulting and Clinical Psychology, 69: 41–49.

Erzegovesi S, Cavallini MC, Cavedini P, et al. 2001. Clinical predictors of drug response in obsessive-compulsive disorder. Journal of Clinical Psychopharmacology, 21: 488–492.

Erzegovesi S, Guglielmo E, Siliprandi F, et al. 2005. Low-dose risperidone augmentation of fluvoxamine treatment in obsessive-compulsive disorder: A double-blind, placebo-controlled study. European Neuropsychopharmacology, 15: 69–74.

Escalona R, Canive JM, Calais LA, et al. 2002. Fluvoxamine treatment in veterans with combat-related post-traumatic stress disorder. Depression and Anxiety, 15: 29–33.

Esler M, Alvarenga M, Lambert G, et al. 2004. Cardiac sympathetic nerve biology and brain monoamine turnover in panic disorder. Annals of the New York Academy of Sciences, 1018: 505–514.

Eth S. 2002. Television viewing as a risk factor. Psychiatry, 65: 301–303.

Evans KC, Wright CI, Wedig MM, et al. 2008. A functional MRI study of amygdala responses to angry schematic faces in social anxiety disorder. Depression and Anxiety, 25: 496–505.

Evenden J. 1999. Impulsivity: A discussion of clinical and experimental findings. Journal of Psychopharmacology, 13: 180–192.

Fahy TJ, O'Rourke DO, Bropky J, et al. 1992. The Galway study of panic disorder. I. Clomipramine and lofepramine in DSM-III-R panic disorder: A placebo-controlled trial. Journal of Affective Disorders, 25: 63–76.

Fairbrother N, Rachman S. 2006. PTSD in victims of sexual assault: Test of a major component of the Ehlers-Clark theory. Journal of Behavior Therapy and Experimental Psychiatry, 37: 74–93.

Fallon BA, Liebowitz MR, Campeas R, et al. 1998. Intravenous clomipramine for obsessive-compulsive disorder refractory to oral clomipramine: A placebo-controlled study. Archives of General Psychiatry, 55: 918–924.

Faravelli C, Cosci F, Rotella F, et al. 2008. Agoraphobia between panic and phobias: Clinical epidemiology from the Sesto Fiorentino Study. Comprehensive Psychiatry, 49: 283–287.

Faravelli C, Degl'Innocenti BG, Giardinelli L. 1989. Epidemiology of anxiety disorders in Florence. Acta Psychiatrica Scandinavica, 79: 308–312.

Faravelli C, Pallanti S. 1989. Recent life events and panic disorder. American Journal of Psychiatry, 146: 622–626.

Faravelli C, Panichi C, Pallanti S, et al. 1991. Perception of early parenting in panic and agoraphobia. Acta Psychiatrica Scandinavica, 84: 6–8.

Faravelli C, Paterniti S, Scarpato MA. 1995. A 5-year prospective, naturalistic follow-up study of panic disorder. Comprehensive Psychiatry, 36: 271–277.

Faravelli C, Webb T, Ambonetti A, et al. 1985. Prevalence of traumatic early life events in 31 agoraphobic patients with panic attacks. American Journal of Psychiatry, 142: 1493–1494.

Fava GA, Grandi S, Canestrari R. 1988. Prodromal symptoms in panic disorder with agoraphobia. American Journal of Psychiatry, 145: 1564–1567.

Fava GA, Grandi S, Rafanelli C, et al. 1992. Prodromal symptoms in panic disorder with agoraphobia: A replication study. Journal of Affective Disorders, 25: 85–88.

Fava GA, Grandi S, Saviotti FM, et al. 1990. Hypochondriasis with panic attacks. Psychosomatics, 31: 351–353.

Fava GA, Zielezny M, Savron G, et al. 1995. Long-term effects of behavioural treatment for panic disorder with agoraphobia. British Journal of Psychiatry, 166: 87–92.

Fecteau G, Nicki R. 1999. Cognitive behavioural treatment of posttraumatic stress disorder after motor vehicle accident. Behavioural and Cognitive Psychotherapy, 27: 201–215.

Feighner JP, Merideth CH, Hendrickson GA. 1982. A double-blind comparison of buspirone and diazepam in outpatients with generalized anxiety disorder. Journal of Clinical Psychiatry, 43: 103–108.

Feinstein A, Dolan R. 1991. Predictors of post-traumatic stress disorder following physical trauma: An examination of the stressor criterion. Psychological Medicine, 21: 85–91.

Feinstein SB, Fallon BA, Petkova E, et al. 2003. Item-by-item factor analysis of the Yale-Brown Obsessive Compulsive Scale Symptom Checklist. Journal of Neuropsychiatry and Clinical Neurosciences, 15: 187–193.

Feltner D, Wittchen H-U, Kavoussi R, et al. 2008. Long-term efficacy of pregabalin in generalized anxiety disorder. International Clinical Psychopharmacology, 23: 18–28.

Feltner DE, Crockatt JG, Dubovsky SJ, et al. 2003. A randomized, double-blind, placebo-controlled, fixed-dose, multicenter study of pregabalin in patients with generalized anxiety disorder. Journal of Clinical Psychopharmacology, 23: 240–249.

Fenichel O. 1945. The Psychoanalytic Theory of Neurosis. New York: W.W. Norton.

Fenigstein F, Scheier MF, Buss AK. 1975. Public and private self-consciousness: Assessment and theory. Journal of Consulting and Clinical Psychology, 43: 522–527.

Fenton WS, McGlashan TH. 1986. The prognostic significance of obsessive-compulsive symptoms in schizophrenia. American Journal of Psychiatry, 143: 437–441.

Ferguson JM, Khan A, Mangano R, et al. 2007. Relapse prevention of panic disorder in adult outpatient responders to treatment with venlafaxine extended release. Journal of Clinical Psychiatry, 68: 58–68.

Feske U. 1998. Eye movement desensitization and reprocessing treatment for posttraumatic stress disorder. Clinical Psychology: Science and Practice, 5: 171–181.

Feske U, Chambless DL. 1995. Cognitive-behavioral versus exposure only treatment for social phobia: A meta-analysis. Behavior Therapy, 26: 695–720.

Fifer SK, Mathias SD, Patrick DL, et al. 1994. Untreated anxiety among adult primary care patients in a health maintenance organization. Archives of General Psychiatry, 51: 740–750.

Fineberg N, Hughes A, Gale T, et al. 2005. Group cognitive-behaviour therapy in obsessive-compulsive disorder (OCD): A controlled study. International Journal of Psychiatry in Clinical Practice, 9: 257–263.

Fineberg NA, O'Doherty C, Rajagopal S, et al. 2003. How common is obsessive-compulsive disorder in a dermatology outpatient clinic? Journal of Clinical Psychiatry, 64: 152–155.

Fineberg NA, Stein DJ, Premkumar P, et al. 2006. Adjunctive quetiapine for serotonin reuptake inhibitor-resistant obsessive-compulsive disorder: A meta-analysis of randomized controlled treatment trials. International Clinical Psychopharmacology, 21: 337–343.

Fineberg NA, Tonnoir B, Lemming O, et al. 2007. Escitalopram prevents relapse of obsessive-compulsive disorder. European Neuropsychopharmacology, 17: 430–439.

Fishbein M, Middlestadt SE, Ottati V, et al. 1988. Medical problems among ICSOM musicians: Overview of a national survey. Medical Problems of Performing Artists, 3: 1–8.

Fisher PL, Durham RC. 1999. Recovery rates in generalized anxiety disorder following psychological therapy: An analysis of clinically significant change in the STAI-T across outcome studies since 1990. Psychological Medicine, 29: 1425–1434.

Fisher PL, Wells A. 2005. How effective are cognitive and behavioural treatments for obsessive-compulsive disorder? A clinical significance analysis. Behaviour Research and Therapy, 43: 1543–1558.

Flament MF, Whitaker A, Rapoport JL, et al. 1988. Obsessive compulsive disorder in adolescence: An epidemiological study. Journal of the American Academy of Child and Adolescent Psychiatry, 27: 764–771.

Fleet R, Lespérance F, Arsenault A, et al. 2005. Myocardial perfusion study of panic attacks in patients with coronary artery disease. American Journal of Cardiology, 96: 1064–1068.

Fleet RP, Dupuis G, Marchand A, et al. 1996. Panic disorder in emergency department chest pain patients: Prevalence, comorbidity, suicidal ideation, and physician recognition. American Journal of Medicine, 101: 371–380.

Fleet RP, Lavoie K, Beitman BD. 2000a. Is panic disorder associated with coronary artery disease? A critical review of the literature. Journal of Psychosomatic Research, 48: 347–356.

Fleet RP, Martel J-P, Lavoie KL, et al. 2000b. Non-fearful panic disorder: A variant of panic in medical patients? Psychosomatics, 41: 311–320.

Fleming B, Faulk A. 1989. Discriminating factors in panic disorder with and without agoraphobia. Journal of Anxiety Disorders, 3: 209–219.

Foa EB. 1979. Failure in treating obsessive compulsives. Behaviour Research and Therapy, 17: 169–179.

Foa EB. 1995. Posttraumatic Diagnostic Scale Manual. Minneapolis: National Computer Systems.

Foa EB, Dancu CV, Hembree EA, et al. 1999. A comparison of exposure therapy, stress inoculation training, and their combination for reducing posttraumatic stress disorder in female assault victims. Journal of Consulting and Clinical Psychology, 67: 194–200.

Foa EB, Goldstein A. 1978. Continuous exposure and complete response prevention of obsessive-compulsive disorder. Behavior Therapy, 9: 821–829.

Foa EB, Grayson JB, Steketee G, et al. 1983. Success and failure in behavioral treatment of obsessive compulsives. Journal of Consulting and Clinical Psychology, 51: 287–297.

Foa EB, Hearst-Ikeda D, Perry KJ. 1995b. Evaluation of a brief cognitive-behavioral program for the prevention of chronic PTSD in recent assault victims. Journal of Consulting and Clinical Psychology, 63: 948–955.

Foa EB, Kozak MJ. 1986. Emotional processing of fear: Exposure to corrective information. Psychological Bulletin, 99: 20–35.

Foa EB, Kozak MJ. 1995. DSM-IV field trial: Obsessive-compulsive disorder. American Journal of Psychiatry, 152: 90–96.

Foa EB, Kozak MJ. 1996. Psychological treatment for obsessive-compulsive disorder. In Mavissakalian MR, Prien RF, editors: Long-Term Treatments of Anxiety Disorders. Washington, DC: American Psychiatric Press, pp. 285–309.

Foa EB, Liebowitz MR, Kozak MJ, et al. 2005. Randomized, placebo-controlled trial of exposure and ritual prevention, clomipramine, and their combination in the treatment of obsessive-compulsive disorder. American Journal of Psychiatry, 162: 151–161.

Foa EB, Riggs DS. 1993. Post-traumatic stress disorder in rape victims. In Oldham J, Riba MB, Tasman A, editors: American Psychiatric Press Review of Psychiatry, Volume 12. Washington, DC: American Psychiatric Press, pp. 273–303.

Foa EB, Riggs DS, Gershuny BS. 1995a. Arousal, numbing, and intrusion: Symptom structure of PTSD following assault. American Journal of Psychiatry, 152: 116–120.

Foa EB, Rothbaum BO. 1998. BKT Treating the Trauma of Rape: Cognitive-Behavioral Therapy for PTSD. New York: Guilford Press.

Foa EB, Rothbaum BO, Riggs DS, et al. 1991. Treatment of posttraumatic stress disorder in rape victims: A comparison between cognitive-behavioral procedures and counseling. Journal of Consulting and Clinical Psychology, 59: 715–723.

Foa EB, Steketee GS, Grayson JB. 1981. Success and failure in treating obsessive-compulsives. Biological Psychiatry, 5: 1099–1102.

Foa EB, Steketee GS, Grayson JB, et al. 1984. Deliberate exposure and blocking of obsessive-compulsive rituals: Immediate and long-term effects. Behavior Therapy, 15: 450–472.

Foa EB, Steketee GS, Ozarow BJ. 1985. Behavior therapy with obsessive compulsives: From theory to treatment. In Mavissakalian M, Turner SM, Michelsen L, editors: Obsessive Compulsive Disorder: Psychological and Pharmacological Treatments. New York: Plenum Press, pp. 49–129.

Foa EB, Steketee G, Rothbaum BO. 1989. Behavioral/cognitive conceptualization of post-traumatic stress disorder. Behavior Therapy, 20: 155–176.

Fodor IG. 1974. The phobic syndrome in women: Implications for treatment. In Franks V, Burtle V, editors: Women in Therapy. New York: Brunner/Mazel, pp. 132–168.

Fontana A, Rosenheck R. 1994. Posttraumatic stress disorder among Vietnam theater veterans: A causal model of etiology in a community sample. Journal of Nervous and Mental Disease, 182: 677–684.

Fontana A, Schwartz LS, Rosenheck R. 1997. Posttraumatic stress disorder among female Vietnam veterans: A causal model of etiology. American Journal of Public Health, 87: 169–175.

Foy DW, Sipprelle RC, Rueger DB, et al. 1984. Etiology of posttraumatic stress disorder in Vietnam veterans. Journal of Consulting and Clinical Psychology, 40: 1323–1328.

Frances A, Dunn P. 1975. The attachment-autonomy conflict in agoraphobia. International Journal of Psychoanalysis, 56: 435–439.

Frank E, Cyranowski JM, Rucci P, et al. 2002. Clinical significance of lifetime panic spectrum symptoms in the treatment of patients with bipolar I disorder. Archives of General Psychiatry, 59: 905–911.

Frank JB, Kosten TR, Giller EL, et al. 1988. A randomized clinical trial of phenelzine and imipramine for posttraumatic stress disorder. American Journal of Psychiatry, 145: 1289–1291.

Franklin CL, Zimmerman M. 2001. Posttraumatic stress disorder and major depressive disorder: Investigating the role of overlapping symptoms in diagnostic comorbidity. Journal of Nervous and Mental Disease, 189: 548–551.

Franklin JA. 1987. The changing nature of agoraphobic fears. British Journal of Clinical Psychology, 26: 127–133.

Franklin ME, Abramowitz JS, Kozak MJ, et al. 2000. Effectiveness of exposure and ritual prevention for obsessive-compulsive disorder: Randomized compared with nonrandomized samples. Journal of Consulting and Clinical Psychology, 68: 594–602.

Fredrikson M, Annas P, Fischer H, et al. 1996. Gender and age differences in the prevalence of specific fears and phobias. Behaviour Research and Therapy, 34: 33–39.

Freedman SA, Peri T, Brandes D, et al. 1999. Predictors of chronic PTSD – A prospective study. British Journal of Psychiatry, 174: 353–359.

Freeman CPL, Trimble MR, Deakin JFW, et al. 1994. Fluvoxamine versus clomipramine in the treatment of obsessive compulsive disorder: A multicenter, randomized, double-blind, parallel group comparison. Journal of Clinical Psychiatry, 55: 301–305.

Freeman D, Gittins M, Pugh K, et al. 2008. What makes one person paranoid and another person anxious? The differential prediction of social anxiety and persecutory ideation in an experimental situation. Psychological Medicine, 38: 1121–1132.

Freeston MH, Ladouceur R, Gagnon F, et al. 1997. Cognitive-behavioral treatment of obsessive thoughts: A controlled study. Journal of Consulting and Clinical Psychology, 65: 405–413.

Freeston MH, Rhéaume JL, Dugas MJ, et al. 1994. Why do people worry? Personality and Individual Differences, 17: 791–802.

Freeston MH, Rhéaume J, Ladouceur R. 1996. Correcting faulty appraisals of obsessional thoughts. Behaviour Research and Therapy, 34: 433–446.

Fresco DM, Mennin DS, Heimberg RG, et al. 2003. Using the Penn State Worry Questionnaire to identify individuals with generalized anxiety disorder: A receiver operating characteristic analysis. Journal of Behavior Therapy and Experimental Psychiatry, 34: 283–291.

Freud S. 1908/1959. Character and anal erotism. In Strachey J, editor: The Standard Edition of the Complete Psychological Works of Sigmund Freud, Vol. 9. London: Hogarth Press, pp. 167–175.

Freud S. 1909/1955a. Analysis of a phobia in a five-year-old boy. In Strachey J, editor: The Standard Edition of the Complete Psychological Works of Sigmund Freud, Vol. 10. London: Hogarth Press, pp. 3–149.

Freud S. 1909/1955b. Notes upon a case of obsessional neurosis. In Strachey J, editor: The Standard Edition of the Complete Psychological Works of Sigmund Freud, Vol. 10. London: Hogarth Press, pp. 151–318.

Freud S. 1913/1958. The disposition to obsessional neurosis. In Strachey J, editor: The Standard Edition of the Complete Psychological Works of Sigmund Freud, Vol. 12. London: Hogarth Press, pp. 317–326.

Freud S. 1926/1959. Inhibitions, symptoms and anxiety. In Strachey J, editor: The Standard Edition of the Complete Psychological Works of Sigmund Freud, Vol. 20. London: Hogarth Press, pp. 77–175.

Fries E, Hesse J, Hellhammer J, et al. 2005. A new view of hypocortisolism. Psychoneuroendocrinology, 30: 1010–1016.

Frommberger U, Stieglitz R-D, Nyberg E, et al. 2004. Comparison between paroxetine and behaviour therapy in patients with posttraumatic stress disorder (PTSD): A pilot study. International Journal of Psychiatry in Clinical Practice, 8: 19–23.

Frost RO, Krause MS, Steketee G. 1996. Hoarding and obsessive-compulsive symptoms. Behavior Modification, 20: 116–132.

Frost RO, Steketee G, Williams LF, et al. 2000. Mood, personality disorder symptoms and disability in obsessive-compulsive hoarders: A comparison with clinical and nonclinical controls. Behaviour Research and Therapy, 38: 1071–1081.

Frueh BC, Elhai JD, Grubaugh AL, et al. 2005. Documented combat exposure of US veterans seeking treatment for combat-related post-traumatic stress disorder. British Journal of Psychiatry, 186: 467–472.

Furer P, Walker JR, Chartier MJ, et al. 1997. Hypochondriacal concerns and somatization in panic disorder. Depression and Anxiety, 6: 78–85.

Furmark T, Appel L, Michelgard A, et al. 2005. Cerebral blood flow changes after treatment of social phobia with the neurokinin-1 antagonist GR205171, citalopram, or placebo. Biological Psychiatry, 58: 132–142.

Furmark T, Tillfors M, Marteinsdottir I, et al. 2002. Common changes in cerebral blood flow in patients with social phobia treated with citalopram or cognitive-behavioral therapy. Archives of General Psychiatry, 59: 425–433.

Furmark T, Tillfors M, Stattin H, et al. 2000. Social phobia subtypes in the general population revealed by cluster analysis. Psychological Medicine, 30: 1335–1344.

Furukawa TA, Watanabe N, Churchill R. 2006. Psychotherapy plus antidepressant for panic disorder with or without agoraphobia: Systematic review. British Journal of Psychiatry, 188: 305–312.

Fyer AJ, Mannuzza S, Chapman TF, et al. 1993. A direct interview family study of social phobia. Archives of General Psychiatry, 50: 286–293.

Fyer AJ, Mannuzza S, Chapman TF, et al. 1995. Specificity in familial aggregation of phobic disorders. Archives of General Psychiatry, 52: 564–573.

Fyer AJ, Mannuzza S, Gallops MS, et al. 1990. Familial transmission of simple phobias and fears. Archives of General Psychiatry, 47: 252–256.

Gabbard GO. 1992. Psychodynamics of panic disorder and social phobia. Bulletin of the Menninger Clinic, 56 (Suppl. A): A3–A13.

Garvey MJ, Cook B, Noyes R. 1988. The occurrence of a prodrome of generalized anxiety in panic disorder. Comprehensive Psychiatry, 29: 445–449.

Gelenberg AJ, Lydiard RB, Rudolph RL, et al. 2000. Efficacy of venlafaxine extended-release capsules in nondepressed outpatients with generalized anxiety disorder: A 6-month randomized controlled trial. Journal of the American Medical Association, 283: 3082–3088.

Gelernter CS, Uhde TW, Cimbolic P, et al. 1991. Cognitive-behavioral and pharmacological treatments of social phobia: A controlled study. Archives of General Psychiatry, 48: 938–945.

Gelpin E, Bonne O, Peri T, et al. 1996. Treatment of recent trauma survivors with benzodiazepines: A prospective study. Journal of Clinical Psychiatry, 57: 390–394.

Gentil V, Lotufoo-Neto F, Andrade L, et al. 1993. Clomipramine, a better reference drug for panic/agoraphobia. I. Effectiveness comparison with imipramine. Journal of Psychopharmacology, 7: 316–324.

Germine M, Goddard AW, Woods SW, et al. 1992. Anger and anxiety responses to *m*-chlorophenylpiperazine in generalized anxiety disorder. Biological Psychiatry, 32: 457–461.

Gidron Y, Gal R, Freedman S, et al. 2001. Translating research findings to PTSD prevention: Results of a randomized controlled trial. Journal of Traumatic Stress, 14: 773–780.

Giedd JN, Rapoport JL, Garvey MA, et al. 2000. MRI assessment of children with obsessive-compulsive disorder or tics associated with streptococcal infection. American Journal of Psychiatry, 157: 281–283.

Gilbert AR, Moore GJ, Keshavan MS, et al. 2000. Decrease in thalamic volumes of pediatric patients with obsessive-compulsive disorder who are taking paroxetine. Archives of General Psychiatry, 57: 449–456.

Gillespie K, Duffy M, Hackmann A, et al. 2002. Community based cognitive therapy in the treatment of post-traumatic stress disorder following the Omagh bomb. Behaviour Research and Therapy, 40: 345–357.

Gittelman R, Klein DF. 1984. Relationship between separation anxiety and agoraphobic disorders. Psychopathology, 17 (Suppl. 1): 56–65.

Gladstone GL, Parker GB, Mitchell PB, et al. 2005. A Brief Measure of Worry Severity (BMWS): Personality and clinical correlates of severe worriers. Journal of Anxiety Disorders, 19: 877–892.

Glynn SM, Eth S, Randolph ET, et al. 1999. A test of behavioral family therapy to augment exposure for combat-related posttraumatic stress disorder. Journal of Consulting and Clinical Psychology, 67: 243–251.

Goddard AW, Brouette T, Almai A, et al. 2001a. Early coadministration of clonazepam with sertraline for panic disorder. Archives of General Psychiatry, 58: 681–686.

Goddard AW, Mason GF, Almai A, et al. 2001b. Reductions in occipital cortex GABA levels in panic disorder detected with ^{1}H-magnetic resonance spectroscopy. Archives of General Psychiatry, 58: 556–561.

Goddard GV, McIntyre DC, Leech CK. 1969. A permanent change in brain function resulting from daily electrical stimulation. Experimental Neurology, 25: 295–330.

Goisman RM, Warshaw MG, Steketee GS, et al. 1995. DSM-IV and the disappearance of agoraphobia without a history of panic disorder: New data on a controversial diagnosis. American Journal of Psychiatry, 152: 1438–1443.

Gold SD, Marx BP, Soler-Baillo JM, et al. 2005. Is life stress more traumatic than traumatic stress? Journal of Anxiety Disorders, 19: 687–698.

Goldberg DP, Lecrubier Y. 1995. Form and frequency of mental disorders across centres. In Ustun TB, Sartorius N, editors: Mental Illness in General Health Care: An International Study. New York: Wiley, pp. 323–334.

Goldstein AJ, Chambless DL. 1978. A reanalysis of agoraphobia. Behavior Therapy, 9: 47–59.

Goldstein RB, Weissman MM, Adams PB, et al. 1994. Psychiatric disorders in relatives of probands with panic disorder and/or major depression. Archives of General Psychiatry, 51: 383–394.

Goldstein RB, Wickramaratne PJ, Horwath E, et al. 1997. Familial aggregation and phenomenology of 'early'-onset (at or before age 20 years) panic disorder. Archives of General Psychiatry, 54: 271–278.

Golier JA, Yehuda R, De Santi S, et al. 2005. Absence of hippocampal volume differences in survivors of the Nazi Holocaust with and without posttraumatic stress disorder. Biological Psychiatry, 139: 53–64.

Goodman WK, Bose A, Wang Q. 2005. Treatment of generalized anxiety disorder with escitalopram: Pooled results from double-blind, placebo-controlled trials. Journal of Affective Disorders, 87: 161–167.

Goodman WK, Kozak MJ, Liebowitz M, et al. 1996. Treatment of obsessive-compulsive disorder with fluvoxamine: A multicentre, double-blind, placebo-controlled trial. International Clinical Psychopharmacology, 11: 21–29.

Goodman WK, McDougle CJ, Price LH, et al. 1990a. Beyond the serotonin hypothesis: A role for dopamine in some forms of obsessive compulsive disorder? Journal of Clinical Psychiatry, 51 (Suppl. 8): 36–43.

Goodman WK, Price LH, Delgado PL, et al. 1990b. Specificity of serotonin reuptake inhibitors in the treatment of obsessive-compulsive disorder: Comparison of fluvoxamine and desipramine. Archives of General Psychiatry, 47: 577–585.

Goodman WK, Price LH, Rasmussen SA, et al. 1989a. The Yale-Brown Obsessive Compulsive Scale: I. Development, use, and reliability. Archives of General Psychiatry, 46: 1006–1011.

Goodman WK, Price LH, Rasmussen SA, et al. 1989b. Efficacy of fluvoxamine in obsessive-compulsive disorder: A double-blind comparison with placebo. Archives of General Psychiatry, 46: 36–44.

Goodwin DW, Guze SB, Robbins E. 1969. Follow-up studies in obsessional neurosis. Archives of General Psychiatry, 20: 182–187.

Goossens L, Sunaert S, Spellmeyer G, et al. 2007. Amygdala hyperfunction in phobic fear normalizes after exposure. Biological Psychiatry, 62: 1119–1125.

Gorman JM, Askanazi J, Liebowitz MR, et al. 1984. Response to hyperventilation in a group of patients with panic disorder. American Journal of Psychiatry, 141: 857–861.

Gorman JM, Fyer MR, Goetz R, et al. 1988. Ventilatory physiology of patients with panic disorder. Archives of General Psychiatry, 45: 31–39.

Gorman JM, Kent JM, Sullivan GM, et al. 2000. Neuroanatomical hypothesis of panic disorder, revised. American Journal of Psychiatry, 157: 493–505.

Gorman JM, Liebowitz MR, Fyer AJ, et al. 1989. A neuroanatomical hypothesis for panic disorder. American Journal of Psychiatry, 146: 148–161.

Gorman JM, Papp LA. 1990. Respiratory physiology of panic. In Ballenger JC, editor: Neurobiology of Panic Disorder. New York: Wiley-Liss, pp. 187–203.

Gorman JM, Sloan RP. 2000. Heart rate variability in depressive and anxiety disorders. American Heart Journal, 140 (Suppl. 4): 77–83.

Grant BF, Hasin DS, Blanco C, et al. 2005b. The epidemiology of social anxiety disorder in the United States: Results from the National Epidemiologic Survey on Alcohol and Related Conditions. Journal of Clinical Psychiatry, 66: 1351–1361.

Grant BF, Hasin DS, Stinson FS, et al. 2005a. Prevalence, correlates, co-morbidity, and comparative disability of DSM-IV generalized anxiety disorder in the USA: Results from the National Epidemiologic Survey on Alcohol and Related Conditions. Psychological Medicine, 35: 1747–1759.

Green MA, Curtis GC. 1988. Personality disorders in panic patients: Response to termination of antipanic medication. Journal of Personality Disorders, 2: 303–314.

Greenberg BD, Malone DA, Friehs GM, et al. 2006. Three-year outcomes in deep brain stimulation for highly resistant obsessive-compulsive disorder. Neuropsychopharmacology, 31: 2384–2393.

Greenberg PE, Sisitsky T, Kessler RC, et al. 1999. The economic burden of anxiety disorders in the 1990s. Journal of Clinical Psychiatry, 60: 427–435.

Gregory AM, Caspi A, Moffitt TE, et al. 2007. Juvenile mental health histories of adults with anxiety disorders. American Journal of Psychiatry, 164: 301–308.

Greist J, Chouinard G, DuBoff E, et al. 1995a. Double-blind parallel comparison of three dosages of sertraline and placebo in outpatients with obsessive-compulsive disorder. Archives of General Psychiatry, 52: 289–295.

Greist JH. 1994. Behavior therapy for obsessive-compulsive disorder. Journal of Clinical Psychiatry, 55 (Suppl.): 60–68.

Greist JH, Jefferson JW, Kobak KA, et al. 1995c. Efficacy and tolerability of serotonin transport inhibitors in obsessive-compulsive disorder: A meta-analysis. Archives of General Psychiatry, 52: 53–60.

Greist JH, Jefferson JW, Kobak KA, et al. 1995b. A 1 year double-blind placebo-controlled fixed dose study of sertraline in the treatment of obsessive-compulsive disorder. International Clinical Psychopharmacology, 10: 57–65.

Grubaugh AL, Magruder KM, Waldrop AE, et al. 2005. Subthreshold PTSD in primary care: Prevalence, psychiatric disorders, healthcare use, and functional status. Journal of Nervous and Mental Disease, 193: 658–664.

Grunhaus L, Pande AC, Brown MB, et al. 1994. Clinical characteristics of patients with concurrent major depressive disorder and panic disorder. American Journal of Psychiatry, 151: 541–546.

Guastella AJ, Dadds MR, Lovibond PF, et al. 2007. A randomized controlled trial of the effect of D-cycloserine on exposure therapy for spider fear. Journal of Psychiatric Research, 41: 466–471.

Guastella AJ, Richardson R, Lovibond PF, et al. 2008. A randomized controlled trial of D-cycloserine enhancement of exposure therapy for social anxiety disorder. Biological Psychiatry, 63: 544–549.

Gurvits TV, Gilbertson MW, Lasko NB, et al. 2000. Neurologic soft signs in chronic posttraumatic stress disorder. Archives of General Psychiatry, 57: 181–186.

Gurvits TV, Lasko NB, Schachter SC, et al. 1993. Neurological status of Vietnam veterans with chronic posttraumatic stress disorder. Journal of Neuropsychiatry and Clinical Neurosciences, 150: 183–188.

Guthrie R, Bryant RA. 2000. Attempting suppression of traumatic memories over extended periods in acute stress disorder. Behaviour Research and Therapy, 38: 899–907.

Hackmann A, Surawy C, Clark DM. 1998. Seeing yourself through others' eyes: A study of spontaneously occurring images in social phobia. Behavioural and Cognitive Psychotherapy, 26: 3–12.

Hafner RJ. 1977. The husbands of agoraphobic women and their influence on treatment outcome. British Journal of Psychiatry, 131: 289–294.

Hagenaars MA, van Minnen A, Hoogduin KAL. 2007. Peritraumatic psychological and somatoform dissociation in predicting PTSD symptoms: A prospective study. Journal of Nervous and Mental Disease, 195: 952–954.

Hall RCW, Hall RCW. 2006. Malingering of PTSD: Forensic and diagnostic considerations, characteristics of malingerers and clinical presentations. General Hospital Psychiatry, 28: 525–535.

Hallam RS. 1978. Agoraphobia: A critical review of the concept. British Journal of Psychiatry, 133: 314–319.

Hallam RS, Hafner J. 1978. Fears of phobic patients: Factor analyses of self-report data. Behaviour Research and Therapy, 16: 1–6.

Hamilton M. 1959. The assessment of anxiety states by rating. British Journal of Medical Psychology, 32: 50–55.

Hamner MB, Deitsch SE, Brodrick PS, et al. 2003b. Quetiapine treatment in patients with posttraumatic stress disorder: An open trial of adjunctive therapy. Journal of Clinical Psychopharmacology, 23: 15–20.

Hamner MB, Faldowski RA, Ulmer HG, et al. 2003a. Adjunctive risperidone treatment in post-traumatic stress disorder: A preliminary controlled trial of effects on comorbid psychotic symptoms. International Clinical Psychopharmacology, 18: 1–8.

Hamner MB, Frueh B, Ulmer H, et al. 1999. Psychotic features and illness severity in combat veterans with chronic posttraumatic stress disorder. Biological Psychiatry, 45: 846–852.

Hamner MB, Robert S. 2005. Emerging roles for atypical antipsychotics in chronic post-traumatic stress disorder. Expert Review of Neurotherapeutics, 5: 267–275.

Hartford J, Kornstein S, Liebowitz M, et al. 2007. Duloxetine as an SNRI treatment for generalized anxiety disorder: Results from a placebo- and active-controlled trial. International Clinical Psychopharmacology, 22: 167–174.

Hartley LR, Ungapen S, Davie I, et al. 1983. The effect of beta adrenergic blocking drugs on speakers' performance and memory. British Journal of Psychiatry, 142: 512–517.

Harvey AG, Bryant RA. 1998. The effect of attempted thought suppression in acute stress disorder. Behaviour Research and Therapy, 36: 583–590.

Harvey AG, Bryant RA. 2000. Two-year prospective evaluation of the relationship between acute stress disorder and posttraumatic stress disorder following mild traumatic brain injury. American Journal of Psychiatry, 157: 626–628.

Harvey AG, Bryant RA, Dang S. 1998. Autobiographical memory in acute stress disorder. Journal of Consulting and Clinical Psychology, 66: 500–506.

Hasler G, Nugent AC, Carlson PJ, et al. 2008. Altered cerebral γ-aminobutyric acid type A-benzodiazepine receptor binding in panic disorder determined by [^{11}C]flumazenil positron emission tomography. Archives of General Psychiatry, 65: 1166–1175.

Haug TT, Blomhoff S, Hellstrom K, et al. 2003. Exposure therapy and sertraline in social phobia: 1-year follow-up of a randomised controlled trial. British Journal of Psychiatry, 182: 312–318.

Heimberg RG, Dodge CS, Hope DA, et al. 1990a. Cognitive-behavioral treatment of social phobia: Comparison to a credible placebo control. Cognitive Therapy and Research, 14: 1–23.

Heimberg RG, Hope DA, Dodge CS, et al. 1990b. DSM-III-R subtypes of social phobia: Comparison of generalized social phobics and public speaking phobics. Journal of Nervous and Mental Disease, 178: 172– 179.

Heimberg RG, Liebowitz MR, Hope DA, et al. 1998. Cognitive-behavioral group therapy versus phenelzine in social phobia: 12-week outcome. Archives of General Psychiatry, 55: 1133–1141.

Heimberg RG, Salzman DG, Holt CS, et al. 1993. Cognitive-behavioral group treatment for social phobia: Effectiveness at five-year follow-up. Cognitive Therapy and Research, 17: 325–339.

Heinrichs M, Wagner D, Schoch W, et al. 2005. Predicting posttraumatic stress symptoms from pretraumatic risk factors: A 2-year prospective follow-up study in firefighters. American Journal of Psychiatry, 162: 2276–2282.

Heiser NA, Turner SM, Beidel DC. 2003. Shyness: Relationship to social phobia and other psychiatric disorders. Behaviour Research and Therapy, 41: 209–221.

Hellström K, Öst L-G. 1995. One-session therapist-directed exposure vs. two forms of manual-directed self-exposure in the treatment of spider phobia. Behaviour Research and Therapy, 33: 959–965.

Helzer JE, Robins LN, McEvoy L. 1987. Post-traumatic stress disorder in the general population: Findings of the Epidemiologic Catchment Area survey. New England Journal of Medicine, 317: 1630–1634.

Hemmings SMJ, Stein DJ. 2006. The current status of association studies in obsessive-compulsive disorder. Psychiatric Clinics of North America, 29: 411–444.

Herbert JD, Gaudiano BA, Rheingold AA, et al. 2005. Social skills training augments the effectiveness of cognitive behavioral group therapy for social anxiety disorder. Behavior Therapy, 36: 125–138.

Herbert JD, Hope DA, Bellack AS. 1992. Validity of the distinction between generalized social phobia and avoidant personality disorder. Journal of Abnormal Psychology, 101: 332–339.

Herman JL. 1992. Trauma and Recovery. New York: Basic Books.

Herman JL. 1993. Sequelae of prolonged and repeated trauma: Evidence for a complex posttraumatic syndrome (DESNOS). In Davidson JRT, Foa EB, editors: Posttraumatic Stress Disorder: DSM-IV and Beyond. Washington, DC: American Psychiatric Press, pp. 213–228.

Hermann A, Schafer A, Walter B, et al. 2007. Diminished medial prefrontal cortex activity in blood-injection-injury phobia. Biological Psychiatry, 75: 124–130.

Hertzberg MA, Butterfield MI, Feldman ME, et al. 1999. A preliminary study of lamotrigine for the treatment of posttraumatic stress disorder. Biological Psychiatry, 45: 1226–1229.

Hertzberg MA, Feldman ME, Beckham JC. 2000. Lack of efficacy for fluoxetine in PTSD: A placebo-controlled trial in combat veterans. Annals of Clinical Psychiatry, 12: 101–105.

Hettema JM, Prescott CA, Kendler KS. 2003. The effects of anxiety, substance use and conduct disorders on risk of major depressive disorder. Psychological Medicine, 33: 1423–1432.

Hiller W, Leibbrand R, Rief W, et al. 2005. Differentiating hypochondriasis from panic disorder. Journal of Anxiety Disorders, 19: 29–49.

Himle JA, McPhee K, Cameron OG, et al. 1989. Simple phobia: Evidence for heterogeneity. Psychiatry Research, 28: 25–30.

Hirschmann S, Dannon PN, Iancu I, et al. 2000. Pindolol augmentation in patients with treatment-resistant panic disorder: A double-blind, placebo-controlled trial. Journal of Clinical Psychopharmacology, 20: 556–559.

Hodgson RJ, Rachman S. 1977. Obsessional compulsive complaints. Behaviour Research and Therapy, 15: 389–395.

Hoehn-Saric R, Hazlett RL, McLeod DR. 1993a. Generalized anxiety disorder with early and late onset of anxiety symptoms. Comprehensive Psychiatry, 34: 291–298.

Hoehn-Saric R, McLeod D. 1985. Generalized anxiety disorder. Psychiatric Clinics of North America, 8: 73–88.

Hoehn-Saric R, McLeod DR, Hipsley PA. 1993b. Effect of fluvoxamine on panic disorder. Journal of Clinical Psychopharmacology, 13: 321–326.

Hoehn-Saric R, McLeod DR, Zimmerli WD. 1988. Differential effects of alprazolam and imipramine in generalized anxiety disorder: Somatic versus psychic symptoms. Journal of Clinical Psychiatry, 49: 293–301.

Hoehn-Saric R, McLeod DR, Zimmerli WD. 1989. Somatic manifestations in women with generalized anxiety disorder: Psychophysiological responses to psychological stress. Archives of General Psychiatry, 46: 1113–1119.

Hoehn-Saric R, Merchant AF, Keyser ML, et al. 1981. Effects of clonidine on anxiety disorders. Archives of General Psychiatry, 38: 1278–1282.

Hoehn-Saric R, Ninan P, Black DW, et al. 2000. Multicenter, double-blind comparison of sertraline and desipramine for concurrent obsessive-compulsive and major depressive disorders. Archives of General Psychiatry, 57: 76–82.

Hoffart A, Martinsen E. 1993. The effects of personality disorders and anxious-depressive comorbidity on outcome of patients with unipolar depression and with panic disorder and agoraphobia. Journal of Personality Disorders, 7: 304–311.

Hofmann SG. 2004. Cognitive mediation of treatment change in social phobia. Journal of Consulting and Clinical Psychology, 72: 392–399.

Hofmann SG. 2008. Cognitive processes during fear acquisition and extinction in animals and humans: Implications for exposure therapy of anxiety disorders. Clinical Psychology Review, 28: 200–211.

Hofmann SG, Lehman CL, Barlow DH. 1997. How specific are specific phobias? Journal of Behavior Therapy and Experimental Psychiatry, 28: 233–240.

Hofmann SG, Meuret AE, Smits JAJ, et al. 2006. Augmentation of exposure therapy with D-cycloserine for social anxiety disorder. Archives of General Psychiatry, 63: 298–304.

Hofmann SG, Moscovitch DA, Kim H-J, et al. 2004. Changes in self-perception during treatment of social phobia. Journal of Consulting and Clinical Psychology, 72: 588–596.

Hoge EA, Tamrakar SM, Christian KM, et al. 2006. Cross-cultural differences in somatic presentation in patients with generalized anxiety disorder. Journal of Nervous and Mental Disease, 194: 962–966.

Hohagen F, Winkelmann G, Rasche-Rauchle H, et al. 1998. Combination of behaviour therapy with fluvoxamine in comparison with behaviour therapy and placebo: Results of a multicentre study. British Journal of Psychiatry (Suppl. 35), 173: 71–78.

Holeva V, Tarrier N. 2001. Personality and peritraumatic dissociation in the prediction of PTSD in victims of road traffic accidents. Journal of Psychosomatic Research, 51: 687–692.

Hollander E. 1993. Obsessive-Compulsive Related Disorders. Washington, DC: American Psychiatric Press.

Hollander E, Allen A, Steiner M, et al. 2003b. Acute and long-term treatment and prevention of relapse of obsessive-compulsive disorder with paroxetine. Journal of Clinical Psychiatry, 64: 1113–1121.

Hollander E, Benzaquen S. 1997. The obsessive-compulsive spectrum disorders. International Review of Psychiatry, 9: 99–109.

Hollander E, Bienstock CA, Koran LM, et al. 2002. Refractory obsessive-compulsive disorder: State-of-the-art treatment. Journal of Clinical Psychiatry, 63 (Suppl. 6): 20–29.

Hollander E, Braun A, Simeon D. 2008. Should OCD leave the anxiety disorders in DSM-V? The case for obsessive compulsive-related disorders. Depression and Anxiety, 25: 317–329.

Hollander E, Koran LM, Goodman WK, et al. 2003a. A double-blind, placebo-controlled study of the efficacy and safety of controlled-release fluvoxamine in patients with obsessive-compulsive disorder. Journal of Clinical Psychiatry, 64: 640–647.

Hollander E, Kwon J, Stein D, et al. 1996. Obsessive-compulsive and spectrum disorders: Overview and quality of life issues. Journal of Clinical Psychiatry, 57 (Suppl. 8): 3–6.

Hollander E, Rossi NB, Sood E, et al. 2003c. Risperidone augmentation in treatment-resistant obsessive-compulsive disorder: A double-blind, placebo-controlled study. International Journal of Neuropsychopharmacology, 6: 397–401.

Hollander E, Wong CM. 1995. Obsessive-compulsive spectrum disorders. Journal of Clinical Psychiatry, 56 (Suppl. 4): 3–6.

Hollander E, Wong CM. 1998. Psychosocial functions and economic costs of obsessive compulsive disorder. CNS Spectrums, 3 (Suppl. 1): 48–58.

Hollifield M, Thompson PM, Ruiz JE, et al. 2005. Potential effectiveness and safety of olanzapine in refractory panic disorder. Depression and Anxiety, 21: 33–40.

Holt CS, Heimberg RG, Hope DA. 1992. Avoidant personality disorder and the generalized subtype of social phobia. Journal of Abnormal Psychology, 101: 318–325.

Hope DA, Heimberg RG. 1988. Public and private self-consciousness and social phobia. Journal of Personality Assessment, 52: 626–639.

Hope DA, Heimberg RG, Klein JF. 1990. Social anxiety and the recall of interpersonal information. Journal of Cognitive Psychotherapy, 4: 185–195.

Hornig CD, McNally RJ. 1995. Panic disorder and suicide attempt: A reanalysis of data from the Epidemiologic Catchment Area study. British Journal of Psychiatry, 167: 76–79.

Horowitz MJ. 1976. Stress Response Syndromes. New York: Aronson.

Horowitz MJ. 1986. Stress Response Syndromes, 2nd Edition. Northvale, NJ: Jason Aronson.

Horowitz MJ, Wilner N, Alvarez W. 1979. Impact of Event Scale: A measure of subjective distress. Psychosomatic Medicine, 41: 209–218.

Horwath E, Lish JD, Johnson J, et al. 1993. Agoraphobia without panic: Clinical reappraisal of an epidemiological finding. American Journal of Psychiatry, 150: 1496–1501.

Hoyer J, Becker ES, Roth WT. 2001. Characteristics of worry in GAD patients, social phobics, and controls. Depression and Anxiety, 13: 89–96.

Hubbard J, Realmuto GM, Northwood AK, et al. 1995. Comorbidity of psychiatric diagnoses with posttraumatic stress disorder in survivors of childhood trauma. Journal of the American Academy of Child and Adolescent Psychiatry, 34: 1167–1173.

Hunt C, Issakidis C, Andrews G. 2002. DSM-IV generalized anxiety disorder in the Australian National Survey of Mental Health and Well-being. Psychological Medicine, 32: 649–659.

Hunt N, Gakenyi M. 2005. Comparing refugees and nonrefugees: The Bosnian experience. Journal of Anxiety Disorders, 19: 717–723.

Hwu HG, Yeh EK, Chang LY. 1989. Prevalence of psychiatric disorders in Taiwan defined by the Chinese Diagnostic Interview Schedule. Acta Psychiatrica Scandinavica, 79: 136–147.

IMCTGMSP. 1997. The International Multicenter Clinical Trial Group on Moclobemide in Social Phobia. Moclobemide in social phobia: A double-blind, placebo-controlled clinical study. European Archives of Psychiatry and Clinical Neuroscience, 247: 71–80.

Ingram IM. 1961. The obsessional personality and obsessional illness. American Journal of Psychiatry, 117: 1016–1019.

Insel TR. 1992. Toward a neuroanatomy of obsessive-compulsive disorder. Archives of General Psychiatry, 49: 739–744.

Insel TR, Akiskal HS. 1986. Obsessive-compulsive disorder with psychotic features: A phenomenological analysis. American Journal of Psychiatry, 143: 1527–1533.

Insel TR, Murphy DL, Cohen RM, et al. 1983. Obsessive-compulsive disorder: A double-blind trial of clomipramine and clorgyline. Archives of General Psychiatry, 40: 605–612.

Jacob RG, Furman JM, Durrant JD, et al. 1996. Panic, agoraphobia, and vestibular dysfunction. American Journal of Psychiatry, 153: 503–512.

Jacobson E. 1938. Progressive Relaxation. Chicago: University of Chicago Press.

Jacobson NS, Wilson L, Tupper C. 1988. The clinical significance of treatment gains resulting from exposure-based interventions for agoraphobia: A re-analysis of outcome data. Behavior Therapy, 19: 539–554.

Jaisoorya TS, Reddy YCJ, Srinath S. 2003. The relationship of obsessive-compulsive disorder to putative spectrum disorders: Results from an Indian study. Comprehensive Psychiatry, 44: 317–323.

James IA, Blackburn IM. 1995. Cognitive therapy with obsessive-compulsive disorder. British Journal of Psychiatry, 166: 444–450.

Janoff-Bulman R. 1992. Shattered Assumptions: Towards a New Psychology of Trauma. New York: Free Press.

Jansson L, Jerremalm A, Öst L-G. 1986. Follow-up of agoraphobic patients treated with exposure in vivo or applied relaxation. British Journal of Psychiatry, 149: 486–490.

Jansson L, Öst L-G. 1982. Behavioral treatments for agoraphobia: An evaluative review. Clinical Psychology Review, 2: 311–336.

Jenike MA. 1998. Neurosurgical treatment of obsessive-compulsive disorder. British Journal of Psychiatry, 173 (Suppl. 35): 79–90.

Jenike MA, Baer L, Ballantine T, et al. 1991. Cingulotomy for refractory obsessive-compulsive disorder: A long-term follow-up of 33 patients. Archives of General Psychiatry, 48: 548–555.

Jenike MA, Baer L, Minichiello WE, et al. 1986. Concomitant obsessive-compulsive disorder and schizotypal personality disorder. American Journal of Psychiatry, 143: 530–532.

Jenike MA, Baer L, Minichiello WE, et al. 1997. Placebo-controlled trial of fluoxetine and phenelzine for obsessive-compulsive disorder. American Journal of Psychiatry, 154: 1261–1264.

Jensen HH, Poulsen JC. 1982. Amnestic effects of diazepam: "Drug dependence" explained by state dependent learning. Scandinavian Journal of Psychology, 23: 107–111.

Jiang W, Glassman A, Krishnan R, et al. 2005. Depression and ischemic heart disease. American Heart Journal, 150: 54–78.

Johnson J, Weissman MM, Klerman GL. 1990. Panic disorder, comorbidity, and suicide attempts. Archives of General Psychiatry, 47: 805–808.

Johnston DG, Troyer IE, Whitsett SF. 1988. Clomipramine treatment of agoraphobic women: An 8-week controlled trial. Archives of General Psychiatry, 45: 453–459.

Jones MK, Menzies RG. 1998. Danger ideation reduction therapy (DIRT) for obsessive-compulsive washers: A controlled trial. Behaviour Research and Therapy, 36: 959–970.

Joormann J, Stöber J. 1999. Somatic symptoms of generalized anxiety disorder from the DSM-IV: Associations with pathological worry and depression symptoms in a nonclinical sample. Journal of Anxiety Disorders, 13: 491–503.

Juster HR, Heimberg RG. 1995. Social phobia: Longitudinal course and long-term outcome of cognitive-behavioral treatment. Psychiatric Clinics of North America, 18: 821–842.

Kagan J, Reznick JS, Clarke C, et al. 1984. Behavioral inhibition to the unfamiliar. Child Development, 55: 2212–2225.

Kagan J, Reznick JS, Snidman N. 1987. The physiology and psychology of behavioral inhibition in children. Child Development, 58: 1459–1473.

Kagan J, Reznick JS, Snidman N. 1988. Biological basis of childhood shyness. Science, 240: 167–171.

Kahn RJ, McNair DM, Lipman RS, et al. 1986. Imipramine and chlordiazepoxide in depressive and anxiety disorders: II. Efficacy in anxious outpatients. Archives of General Psychiatry, 43: 79–85.

Kampman M, Keijsers GPJ, Hoogduin CAL, et al. 2002. Addition of cognitive-behaviour therapy for obsessive-compulsive disorder patients non- responding to fluoxetine. Acta Psychiatrica Scandinavica, 106: 314–319.

Karamustafalioglu OK, Zohar J, Güveli M, et al. 2006. Natural course of posttraumatic stress disorder: A 20-month prospective study of Turkish earthquake survivors. Journal of Clinical Psychiatry, 67: 882–889.

Karasu TB. 1994. A developmental metatheory of psychopathology. American Journal of Psychotherapy, 48: 581–599.

Karno M, Golding JM, Sorenson SB, et al. 1988. The epidemiology of obsessive-compulsive disorder in five US communities. Archives of General Psychiatry, 45: 1094–1099.

Kasahara T. 2005. Taijin-Kyofu and Social Anxiety Disorder. Tokyo: Kongo publishing.

Kashdan TB, Elhai JD, Frueh C. 2006. Anhedonia and emotional numbing in combat veterans with PTSD. Behaviour Research and Therapy, 44: 457–467.

Kasper S, Stein DJ, Loft H, et al. 2005. Escitalopram in the treatment of social anxiety disorder: Randomised, placebo-controlled, flexible-dosage study. British Journal of Psychiatry, 186: 222–226.

Katerndahl DA. 1990. Infrequent and limited-symptom panic attacks. Journal of Nervous and Mental Disease, 178: 313–317.

Katerndahl DA. 1993. Panic and prolapse: Meta-analysis. Journal of Nervous and Mental Disease, 181: 539–544.

Katerndahl DA, Realini JP. 1993. Lifetime prevalence of panic states. American Journal of Psychiatry, 150: 246–249.

Katon W. 1990. Chest pain, cardiac disease and panic disorder. Journal of Clinical Psychiatry, 51: 27–30.

Katon W. 1996. Panic disorder: Relationship to high medical utilization, unexplained physical symptoms, and medical costs. Journal of Clinical Psychiatry, 57 (Suppl. 10): 11–18.

Katon W, Vitaliano PP, Russo J, et al. 1986. Panic disorder: Epidemiology in primary care. Journal of Family Practice, 23: 233–239.

Katschnig H, Amering M, Stolk JM, et al. 1995. Long-term follow-up after a drug trial for panic disorder. British Journal of Psychiatry, 167: 487–494.

Katz RJ, DeVeaugh-Geiss J, Landau P. 1990. Clomipramine in obsessive-compulsive disorder. Biological Psychiatry, 28: 401–414.

Katzelnick DJ, Kobak KA, Greist JH, et al. 1995. Sertraline for social phobia: A double-blind, placebo-controlled crossover study. American Journal of Psychiatry, 152: 1368–1371.

Kawachi I, Golditz GA, Ascherio A, et al. 1994. Prospective study of phobic anxiety and risk of coronary heart disease in men. Circulation, 89: 1992–1997.

Kawachi I, Sparrow D, Vokonas PS, et al. 1995. Decreased heart rate variability in men with phobic anxiety: Data from the Normative Aging Study. American Journal of Cardiology, 75: 882–885.

Keane TM, Fairbank JA, Caddell JM, et al. 1989. Implosive (flooding) therapy reduced symptoms of PTSD in Vietnam combat veterans. Behavior Therapy, 20: 245–260.

Keane TM, Zimering RT, Caddell RT. 1985. A behavioral formulation of PTSD in Vietnam veterans. Behavior Therapist, 8: 9–12.

Keijsers GPJ, Hoogduin CAL, Schaap CPDR. 1994. Predictors of treatment outcome in the behavioural treatment of obsessive-compulsive disorder. British Journal of Psychiatry, 165: 781–786.

Kelly CB, Cooper SJ. 1998. Differences in variability in plasma noradrenaline between depressive and anxiety disorders. Journal of Psychopharmacology, 12: 161–167.

Kendler KS. 1996. Major depression and generalised anxiety disorder: Same genes, (partly) different environments—revisited. British Journal of Psychiatry, 168 (Suppl. 30): 68–75.

Kendler KS, Gardner CO, Gatz M, et al. 2007. The sources of co-morbidity between major depression and generalized anxiety disorder in a Swedish national twin sample. Psychological Medicine, 37: 453–462.

Kendler KS, Karkowski LM, Prescott CA. 1999. Fears and phobias: Reliability and heritability. Psychological Medicine, 29: 539–553.

Kendler KS, Neale MC, Kessler RC, et al. 1992a. Generalized anxiety disorder in women: A population-based twin study. Archives of General Psychiatry, 49: 267–272.

Kendler KS, Neale MC, Kessler RC, et al. 1992b. Major depression and generalized anxiety disorder: Same genes, (partly) different environments? Archives of General Psychiatry, 49: 716–722.

Kendler KS, Neale MC, Kessler RC, et al. 1992c. The genetic epidemiology of phobias in women: The interrelationship of agoraphobia, social phobia, situational phobia, and simple phobia. Archives of General Psychiatry, 49: 273–281.

Kendler KS, Neale MC, Kessler RC, et al. 1993. Panic disorder in women: A population-based twin study. Psychological Medicine, 23: 397–406.

Kennedy BL, Schwab JJ. 1997. Utilization of medical specialists by anxiety disorder patients. Psychosomatics, 38: 109–112.

Kent G, Gibbons R. 1987. Self-efficacy and the control of anxious cognitions. Journal of Behavior Therapy and Experimental Psychiatry, 18: 33–40.

Kessler RC, Berglund P, Demler O, et al. 2005. Lifetime prevalence and age-of-onset distributions of DSM-IV disorders in the National Comorbidity Survey Replication. Archives of General Psychiatry, 62: 593–602.

Kessler RC, Chiu WT, Jin R, et al. 2006. The epidemiology of panic attacks, panic disorder, and agoraphobia in the National Comorbidity Survey Replication. Archives of General Psychiatry, 63: 415–424.

Kessler RC, Crum RM, Warner LA, et al. 1997a. Lifetime co-occurrence of DSM-III-R alcohol abuse and dependence with other psychiatric disorders in the National Comorbidity Survey. Archives of General Psychiatry, 54: 313–321.

Kessler RC, DuPont RL, Berglund P, et al. 1999a. Impairment in pure and comorbid generalized anxiety disorder and major depression at 12 months in two national surveys. American Journal of Psychiatry, 156: 1915–1923.

Kessler RC, Gruber M, Hettema JM, et al. 2008. Co-morbid major depression and generalized anxiety disorders in the National Comorbidity Survey follow-up. Psychological Medicine, 38: 365–374.

Kessler RC, Keller MB, Wittchen H-U. 2001. The epidemiology of generalized anxiety disorder. Psychiatric Clinics of North America, 24: 19–40.

Kessler RC, McGonagle KA, Zhao S, et al. 1994. Lifetime and 12-month prevalence of DSM-III-R psychiatric disorders in the United States: Results from the National Comorbidity Survey. Archives of General Psychiatry, 51: 8–19.

Kessler RC, McGonagle KA, Zhao S, et al. 1997b. Differences in the use of psychiatric outpatient services between the US and Ontario. New England Journal of Medicine, 336: 551–557.

Kessler RC, Sonnega A, Bromet E, et al. 1995. Posttraumatic stress disorder in the National Comorbidity Survey. Archives of General Psychiatry, 52: 1048–1060.

Kessler RC, Stang P, Wittchen HU, et al. 1999b. Lifetime co-morbidities between social phobia and mood disorders in the US National Comorbidity Survey. Psychological Medicine, 29: 555–567.

Kessler RC, Stein MB, Berglund P. 1998. Social phobia subtypes in the National Comorbidity Survey. American Journal of Psychiatry, 155: 613–619.

Khantzian E. 1985. The self-medication hypothesis of addictive disorders: Focus on heroin and cocaine dependence. American Journal of Psychiatry, 142: 1259–1264.

Kimble CE, Zehr HD. 1982. Self-consciousness, information load, self-presentation, and memory in a social situation. Journal of Social Psychology, 118: 39–46.

King DW, King LA, Foy DW, et al. 1999. Posttraumatic stress disorder in a national sample of female and male Vietnam veterans: Risk factors, war-zone stressors, and resilience-recovery variables. Journal of Abnormal Psychology, 108: 164–170.

King LA, King DW, Fairbank JA. 1998. Resilience-recovery factors in post-traumatic stress disorder among female and male Vietnam veterans: Hardiness, postwar social support, and additional stressful life events. Journal of Personality and Social Psychology: Personality Processes and Individual Differences, 74: 420–434.

Kinoshita Y, Chen J, Rapee RM, et al. 2008. Cross-cultural study of conviction subtype Taijin Kyofu: Proposal and reliability of Nagoya-Osaka diagnostic criteria for social anxiety disorder. Journal of Nervous and Mental Disease, 196: 307–313.

Kirby L, Rice K, Valentino R. 2000. Effects of corticotropin-releasing factor on neuronal activity in the serotonergic dorsal raphe nucleus. Neuropsychopharmacology, 22: 148–162.

Kitayama N, Vaccarino V, Kutner M, et al. 2005. Magnetic resonance imaging (MRI) measurement of hippocampal volume in posttraumatic stress disorder: A meta-analysis. Journal of Affective Disorders, 88: 79–86.

Kleim B, Ehlers A, Glucksman E. 2007. Early predictors of chronic post-traumatic stress disorder in assault survivors. Psychological Medicine, 37: 1457–1467.

Klein DF. 1981. Anxiety reconceptualized. In Klein DF, Rabkin JG, editors: Anxiety: New Research and Changing Concepts. New York: Raven Press, pp. 235–264.

Klein DF. 1993. False suffocation alarms, spontaneous panics, and related conditions: An integrative hypothesis. Archives of General Psychiatry, 50: 306–317.

Klein DF, Klein HM. 1989. The definition and psychopharmacology of spontaneous panic and phobia. In Tyrer P, editor: Psychopharmacology of Anxiety. New York: Oxford University Press, pp. 135–162.

Kleiner L, Marshall WL. 1987. The role of interpersonal problems in the development of agoraphobia with panic attacks. Journal of Anxiety Disorders, 1: 313–323.

Klerman GL, Weissman MM, Ouellette R, et al. 1991. Panic attacks in the community: Social morbidity and health care utilization. Journal of the American Medical Association, 265: 742–746.

Klosko JS, Barlow DH, Tassinari R, et al. 1990. A comparison of alprazolam and behavior therapy in the treatment of panic disorder. Journal of Consulting and Clinical Psychology, 58: 77–84.

Kluznick JC, Speed N, Van Valkenburg C, et al. 1986. Forty-year follow-up of United States prisoners of war. American Journal of Psychiatry, 143: 1443–1446.

Kobak KA, Greist JH, Jefferson JW, et al. 1998. Behavioral versus pharmacological treatments of obsessive-compulsive disorder: A meta-analysis. Psychopharmacology (Berlin), 136: 205–216.

Kobak KA, Greist JH, Jefferson JW, et al. 2002. Fluoxetine in social phobia: A double-blind, placebo-controlled pilot study. Journal of Clinical Psychopharmacology, 22: 257–262.

Koenen KC, Fu QJ, Ertel K, et al. 2008a. Common genetic liability to major depression and posttraumatic stress disorder in men. Journal of Affective Disorders, 105: 109–115.

Koenen KC, Moffitt TE, Caspi A, et al. 2008b. The developmental mental-disorder histories of adults with posttraumatic stress disorder: A prospective longitudinal birth cohort study. Journal of Abnormal Psychology, 117: 460–466.

Koenen KC, Moffitt TE, Poulton R, et al. 2007. Early childhood factors associated with the development of post-traumatic stress disorder: Results from a longitudinal birth cohort. Psychological Medicine, 37: 181–192.

Kohut H. 1971. The Analysis of the Self. New York: International Universities Press.

Kohut H. 1977. The Restoration of the Self. New York: International Universities Press.

Kolb LC, Burris BC, Griffiths S. 1984. Propranolol and clonidine in treatment of the chronic post-traumatic stress disorder of war. In van der Kolk BA, editor: Post-Traumatic Stress Disorder: Psychological and Biological Sequelae. Washington, DC: American Psychiatric Press, pp. 97–105.

Koopman C, Classen C, Spiegel D. 1994. Predictors of posttraumatic stress symptoms among survivors of the Oakland/Berkeley, California firestorm. American Journal of Psychiatry, 151: 888–894.

Koponen H, Allgulander C, Erickson J, et al. 2007. Efficacy of duloxetine for the treatment of generalized anxiety disorder: Implications for primary care physicians. Primary Care Companion to Journal of Clinical Psychiatry, 9: 100–107.

Koran LM, Gamel NN, Choung HW, et al. 2005. Mirtazapine for obsessive-compulsive disorder: An open trial followed by double-blind discontinuation. Journal of Clinical Psychiatry, 66: 515–520.

Koran LM, Hackett E, Rubin A, et al. 2002. Efficacy of sertraline in the long-term treatment of obsessive-compulsive disorder. American Journal of Psychiatry, 159: 88–95.

Koran LM, McElroy SL, Davidson JRT, et al. 1996. Fluvoxamine versus clomipramine for obsessive-compulsive disorder: A double-blind comparison. Journal of Clinical Psychopharmacology, 16: 121–129.

Koran LM, Sallee FR, Pallanti S. 1997. Rapid benefit of intravenous pulse loading of clomipramine in obsessive-compulsive disorder. American Journal of Psychiatry, 154: 396–401.

Koren D, Arnon I, Klein E. 1999. Acute stress response and posttraumatic stress disorder in traffic accident victims: A one-year prospective, follow-up study. American Journal of Psychiatry, 156: 367–373.

Kosten TR, Frank JB, Dan E, et al. 1991. Pharmacotherapy for posttraumatic stress disorder using phenelzine or imipramine. Journal of Nervous and Mental Disease, 179: 366–370.

Kozak MJ, Foa EB. 1994. Obsessions, overvalued ideas, and delusions in obsessive-compulsive disorder. Behaviour Research and Therapy, 32: 343–353.

Kozaric-Kovacic D, Borovecki A. 2005. Prevalence of psychotic comorbidity in combat-related post-traumatic stress disorder. Military Medicine, 170: 223–226.

Kozaric-Kovacic D, Pivac N. 2007. Quetiapine treatment in an open trial in combat-related post-traumatic stress disorder with psychotic features. International Journal of Neuropsychopharmacology, 10: 253–261.

Kringlen E. 1965. Obsessional neurotics: A long term follow-up. British Journal of Psychiatry, 111: 709–722.

Kristensen AS, Mortensen EL, Mors O. 2008. Social phobia with sudden onset – Post-panic social phobia? Journal of Anxiety Disorders, 22: 684–692.

Kronig MH, Apter J, Asnis G, et al. 1999. Placebo-controlled, multicenter study of sertraline treatment for obsessive-compulsive disorder. Journal of Clinical Psychopharmacology, 19: 172–176.

Krueger RF. 1999. The structure of common mental disorders. Archives of General Psychiatry, 56: 921–926.

Krystal H. 1988. Integration and Self-Healing: Affect, Trauma, Alexithymia. Hillsdale, NJ: Analytic Press.

Krystal JH, Niehoff-Deutsch DN, Charney DS. 1996. The biological basis of panic disorder. Journal of Clinical Psychiatry, 57: 23–31.

Kulka RA, Schlenger WE, Fairbank JA, et al. 1990. Trauma and the Vietnam War Generation: Report of Findings from the National Vietnam Veterans Readjustment Study. New York: Brunner/Mazel.

Kushner MG, Beitman BD. 1990. Panic attacks without fear: An overview. Behaviour Research and Therapy, 28: 469–479.

Labbate LA, Pollack MH, Otto MW, et al. 1994. Sleep panic attacks: An association with childhood anxiety and adult psychopathology. Biological Psychiatry, 36: 57–60.

Lader M, Scotto JC. 1998. A multicentre double-blind comparison of hydroxyzine, buspirone and placebo in patients with generalized anxiety disorder. Psychopharmacology, 139: 402–406.

Lader M, Stender K, Burger V, et al. 2004. Efficacy and tolerability of escitalopram in 12- and 24-week treatment of social anxiety disorder: Randomised, double-blind, placebo-controlled, fixed-dose study. Depression and Anxiety, 19: 241–248.

Ladouceur R, Blais F, Freeston MH, et al. 1998. Problem solving and problem orientation in generalized anxiety disorder. Journal of Anxiety Disorders, 12: 139–152.

Ladouceur R, Dugas MJ, Freeston MH, et al. 2000. Efficacy of a cognitive-behavioral treatment for generalized anxiety disorder: Evaluation in a controlled clinical trial. Journal of Clinical and Consulting Psychology, 68: 957–964.

Ladouceur R, Freeston MH, Dugas MJ. 1993. L'intolérance à l'incertitude et les raisons pour s'inquiéter dans le trouble d'anxiété généralisée. Presented at the Annual Convention of the Quebec Society for Research in Psychology, Quebec City, Quebec, Canada.

Ladouceur R, Talbot F, Dugas MJ. 1997. Behavioral expressions of intolerance of uncertainty in worry: Experimental findings. Behavior Modification, 21: 355–371.

Lampe L, Slade T, Issakidis C, et al. 2003. Social phobia in the Australian National Survey of Mental Health and Well-Being (NSMHWB). Psychological Medicine, 33: 637–646.

Lane C. 2008. Shyness: How Normal Behavior Became a Sickness. New Haven, CT: Yale University Press.

Lang PJ. 1979. A bio-informational theory of emotional imagery. Journal of Psychophysiology, 16: 495–512.

Lange A, van Dyck R. 1992. The function of agoraphobia in the marital relationship. Acta Psychiatrica Scandinavica, 85: 89–93.

Langlois F, Freeston MH, Ladouceur R. 2000. Differences and similarities between obsessive intrusive thoughts and worry in a non-clinical population: Study 2. Behaviour Research and Therapy, 38: 175–189.

Large M, Nielssen O. 2001. An audit of medico-legal reports prepared for claims of psychiatric injury following motor vehicle accidents. Australian and New Zealand Journal of Psychiatry, 35: 535–540.

Lavoie KL, Fleet RP, Laurin C, et al. 2004. Heart rate variability in coronary artery disease patients with and without panic disorder. Psychiatry Research, 128: 289–299.

Leckman JF, Walker DE, Cohen DJ. 1993. Premonitory urges in Tourette's syndrome. American Journal of Psychiatry, 150: 98–102.

Leckman JF, Walker DE, Goodman WK, et al., 1994. "Just right" perceptions associated with compulsive behavior in Tourette's syndrome. American Journal of Psychiatry, 151: 675–680.

Lecrubier Y. 1998. Comorbidity in social anxiety disorder: Impact on disease burden and management. Journal of Clinical Psychiatry, 59: 33–37.

Lecrubier Y, Bakker A, Judge R. 1997. A comparison of paroxetine, clomipramine, and placebo in the treatment of panic disorder. Acta Psychiatrica Scandinavica, 95: 145–152.

Lecrubier Y, Judge R. 1997. Long-term evaluation of paroxetine, clomipramine and placebo in panic disorder. Acta Psychiatrica Scandinavica, 95: 153–160.

Lecrubier Y, Weiller E. 1997. Comorbidities in social phobia. International Clinical Psychopharmacology, 12 (Suppl. 6): 17–21.

Lecrubier Y, Wittchen H-U, Faravelli C, et al. 2000. A European perspective on social anxiety disorder. European Psychiatry, 15: 5–16.

Lee CK, Kwak YS, Yamamoto J, et al. 1990. Psychiatric epidemiology in Korea. Part I: Gender and age differences in Seoul. Journal of Nervous and Mental Disease, 178: 242–246.

Lelliott P, Marks I, McNamee G, et al. 1989. Onset of panic disorder with agoraphobia: Toward an integrated model. Archives of General Psychiatry, 46: 1000–1004.

Lelliott PT, Noshirvani HF, Basoglu M, et al. 1988. Obsessive-compulsive beliefs and treatment outcome. Psychological Medicine, 18: 697–702.

Lenane MC, Swedo SE, Leonardo H, et al. 1990. Psychiatric disorders in first degree relatives of children and adolescents with obsessive compulsive disorder. Journal of the American Academy of Child and Adolescent Psychiatry, 29: 407–412.

Leon AC, Porter AL, Weissman MM. 1995. The social costs of anxiety disorders. British Journal of Psychiatry, 166 (Suppl. 27): 19–22.

Leon CA, Leon A. 1990. Panic disorder and parental bonding. Psychiatric Annals, 20: 503–508.

Leonard HL, Swedo SE. 2001. Paediatric autoimmune neuropsychiatric disorders associated with streptococcal infection (PANDAS). International Journal of Neuropsychopharmacology, 4: 191–198.

Leonard HL, Swedo SE, Lenane MC, et al. 1991. A double-blind desipramine substitution during long-term clomipramine treatment in children and adolescents with obsessive-compulsive disorder. Archives of General Psychiatry, 48: 922–927.

Leonard HL, Swedo SE, Lenane MC, et al. 1993. A 2- to 7-year follow-up study of 54 obsessive-compulsive children and adolescents. Archives of General Psychiatry, 50: 429–439.

Leonard HL, Swedo SE, Rapoport JL, et al. 1989. Treatment of obsessive-compulsive disorder with clomipramine and desipramine in children and adolescents: A double-blind crossover comparison. Archives of General Psychiatry, 46: 1088–1092.

Lepine JP, Chignon JM, Teherani M. 1993. Suicide attempts in patients with panic disorder. Archives of General Psychiatry, 50: 144–149.

Lepine JP, Lellouch J. 1994. Classification and epidemiology of anxiety disorders. In Darcourt G, Mendlewicz J, Racagni G, Brunello N, editors: Current Therapeutic Approaches to Panic and Other Anxiety Disorders. Basel: Karger, pp. 1–14.

Lepola U, Bergtholdt B, Lambert JS, et al. 2004. Controlled-release paroxetine in the treatment of patients with social anxiety disorder. Journal of Clinical Psychiatry, 65: 222–229.

Lepola UM, Wade AG, Leinonen EV, et al. 1998. A controlled, prospective, 1-year trial of citalopram in the treatment of panic disorder. Journal of Clinical Psychiatry, 59: 528–534.

Lesch KP, Wiesmann M, Hoh A, et al. 1992. 5-HT1A receptor-effector system responsivity in panic disorder. Psychopharmacology, 106: 111–117.

Lesser IM, Rubin RT, Pecknold JC, et al. 1988. Secondary depression in panic disorder and agoraphobia: I. Frequency, severity, and response to treatment. Archives of General Psychiatry, 45: 437–443.

Levy S, Guttman L. 1976. Worry, fear, and concern differentiated. Israel Annals of Psychiatry and Related Disciplines, 14: 211–228.

Liberzon I, Abelson JL, Flagel SB, et al. 1999. Neuroendocrine and psychophysiologic responses in PTSD: A symptom provocation study. Neuropsychopharmacology, 21: 40–50.

Lieb R, Wittchen H-U, Hoefler M, et al. 2000. Parental psychopathology, parenting styles, and the risk of social phobia in offspring: A prospective-longitudinal community study. Archives of General Psychiatry, 57: 859–866.

Liebowitz MR. 1987. Social phobia. Modern Problems in Pharmacopsychiatry, 22: 141–173.

Liebowitz MR, Campeas R, Hollander E. 1987. Possible dopamine dysregulation in social phobia and atypical depression. Psychiatry Research, 22: 89–90.

Liebowitz MR, DeMartinis NA, Weihs K, et al. 2003. Efficacy of sertraline in severe generalized social phobia: Results of a double-blind, placebo-controlled study. Journal of Clinical Psychiatry, 64: 785–792.

Liebowitz MR, Gelenberg AJ, Munjack D. 2005a. Venlafaxine extended release vs. placebo and paroxetine in social anxiety disorder. Archives of General Psychiatry, 62: 190–198.

Liebowitz MR, Gorman JM, Fyer AJ, et al. 1985. Lactate provocation of panic attacks: II. Biochemical and physiological findings. Archives of General Psychiatry, 42: 709–719.

Liebowitz MR, Heimberg RG, Fresco DM, et al. 2000. Social phobia or social anxiety disorder: What's in a name? Archives of General Psychiatry, 57: 191–192.

Liebowitz MR, Heimberg RG, Schneier FR, et al. 1999. Cognitive-behavioral group therapy versus phenelzine in social phobia: Long-term outcome. Depression and Anxiety, 10: 89–98.

Liebowitz MR, Mangano RM, Bradwejn J, et al. 2005b. A randomized controlled trial of venlafaxine extended release in generalized social anxiety disorder. Journal of Clinical Psychiatry, 66: 238–247.

Liebowitz MR, Quitkin FM, Stewart JW, et al. 1988. Antidepressant specificity in atypical depression. Archives of General Psychiatry, 45: 129–137.

Liebowitz MR, Schneier F, Campeas R, et al. 1992. Phenelzine vs. atenolol in social phobia: A placebo-controlled comparison. Archives of General Psychiatry, 49: 290–300.

Liebowitz MR, Stein MB, Tancer M, et al. 2002. A randomized, double-blind, fixed-dose comparison of paroxetine and placebo in the treatment of generalized social anxiety disorder. Journal of Clinical Psychiatry 63: 66–74.

Lindauer RJL, Olff M, van Meijel EPM, et al. 2006. Cortisol, learning, memory, and attention in relation to smaller hippocampal volume in police officers with posttraumatic stress disorder. Biological Psychiatry, 59: 171–177.

Lindemann CG, Zitrin CM, Klein DF. 1984. Thyroid dysfunction in phobic patients. Psychosomatics, 25: 603–606.

Linden M. 2003. Posttraumatic embitterment disorder. Psychotherapy and Psychosomatics, 72: 195–202.

Lindsay M, Crino R, Andrews G. 1997. Controlled trial of exposure and response prevention in obsessive-compulsive disorder. British Journal of Psychiatry, 171: 135–139.

Lipsitz, JD, Barlow DH, Mannuzza S, et al. 2002. Clinical features of four DSM-IV-specific phobia subtypes. Journal of Nervous and Mental Disease, 190: 471–478.

Lister RG. 1985. The amnesic action of benzodiazepines in man. Neuroscience and Biobehavioral Reviews, 9: 87–94.

Litz BT, Engel CC, Bryant RA, et al. 2007. A randomized, controlled proof-of-concept trial of an Internet-based, therapist-assisted self-management treatment for posttraumatic stress disorder. American Journal of Psychiatry, 164: 1676–1683.

Litz BT, Gray MJ. 2002. Emotional numbing in posttraumatic stress disorder: Current and future research directions. Australian and New Zealand Journal of Psychiatry, 36: 198–204.

Llorca PM, Spadone C, Sol O, et al. 2002. Efficacy and safety of hydroxyzine in the treatment of generalized anxiety disorder: A 3-month double-blind study. Journal of Clinical Psychiatry, 63: 1020–1027.

Loerch B, Graf-Morgenstern M, Hautzinger M, et al. 1999. Randomised placebo-controlled trial of moclobemide, cognitive-behavioural therapy and their combination in panic disorder with agoraphobia. British Journal of Psychiatry, 174: 205–212.

Logue MB, Thomas AM, Barbee JG, et al. 1993. Generalized anxiety disorder patients seek evaluation for cardiological symptoms at the same frequency as patients with panic disorder. Journal of Psychiatric Research, 27: 55–59.

Londborg PD, Hegel MT, Goldstein S, et al. 2001. Sertraline treatment of posttraumatic stress disorder: Results of 24 weeks of open-label continuation treatment. Journal of Clinical Psychiatry, 62: 325–331.

Londborg PD, Wolkow R, Smith WT. 1998. Sertraline in the treatment of panic disorder: A multi-site, double-blind, placebo-controlled, fixed-dose investigation. British Journal of Psychiatry, 173: 54–60.

Lopez-Ibor JJ Jr, Saiz J, Cottraux J, et al. 1996. Double-blind comparison of fluoxetine versus clomipramine in the treatment of obsessive-compulsive disorder. European Neuropsychopharmacology, 6: 111–118.

Lteif GN, Mavissakalian MR. 1995. Life events and panic disorder/agoraphobia. Comprehensive Psychiatry, 36: 118–122.

Lucock MP, Salkovskis PM. 1988. Cognitive factors in social anxiety and its treatment. Behaviour Research and Therapy, 26: 297–302.

Lydiard RB, Ballenger JC, Rickels K. 1997. A double-blind evaluation of the safety and efficacy of abecarnil, alprazolam, and placebo in outpatients with generalized anxiety disorder. Journal of Clinical Psychiatry, 58: 11–18.

Lydiard RB, Greenwald S, Weissman MM, et al. 1994. Panic disorder and gastrointestinal symptoms: Findings from the National Institute of Mental Health Epidemiologic Catchment Area project. American Journal of Psychiatry, 151: 64–70.

Macdonald PA, Antony MM, Macleod CM, et al. 1997. Memory and confidence in memory judgments among individuals with obsessive compulsive disorder and non-clinical controls. Behaviour Research and Therapy, 35: 497–505.

Mackinnon D, Xu J, McMahon F, et al. 1997. Panic disorder with familial bipolar disorder. Biological Psychiatry, 42: 90–95.

Macklin ML, Metzger LJ, Lasko NB, et al. 2000. Five-year follow-up study of eye movement desensitization and reprocessing therapy for combat-related posttraumatic stress disorder. Comprehensive Psychiatry, 41: 24–27.

Macklin ML, Metzger LJ, Litz BT, et al. 1998. Lower precombat intelligence is a risk factor for posttraumatic stress disorder. Journal of Consulting and Clinical Psychology, 66: 323–326.

MacLeod C, Mathews A, Tata P. 1986. Attentional bias in emotional disorders. Journal of Abnormal Psychology, 95: 15–20.

Magee WJ, Eaton WW, Wittchen H-U, et al. 1996. Agoraphobia, simple phobia, and social phobia in the National Comorbidity Survey. Archives of General Psychiatry, 53: 159–168.

Maier W, Gaensicke M, Freyberger HJ, et al. 2000. Generalized anxiety disorder (ICD-10) in primary care from a cross-cultural perspective: A valid diagnostic entity? Acta Psychiatrica Scandinavica, 101: 29–36.

Maier W, Minges J, Lichtermann D. 1995. The familial relationship between panic disorder and unipolar depression. Journal of Psychiatric Research, 29: 375–388.

Maina G, Pessina E, Albert U, et al. 2008. 8-week, single-blind, randomized trial comparing risperidone versus olanzapine augmentation of serotonin reuptake inhibitors in treatment-resistant obsessive-compulsive disorder. European Neuropsychopharmacology, 18: 364–372.

Malizia AL, Cunningham VJ, Bell CJ, et al. 1998. Decreased brain GABA$_A$-benzodiazepine receptor binding in panic disorder: Preliminary results from a quantitative PET study. Archives of General Psychiatry, 55: 715–720.

Maller RG, Reiss S. 1992. Anxiety sensitivity in 1984 and panic attacks in 1987. Journal of Anxiety Disorders, 6: 241–247.

Mallet L, Polosan M, Jaafari N, et al. 2008. Subthalamic nucleus stimulation in severe obsessive-compulsive disorder. New England Journal of Medicine, 359: 2121–2134.

Mancuso DM, Townsend MH, Mercante DE. 1993. Long-term follow-up of generalized anxiety disorder. Comprehensive Psychiatry, 34: 441–446.

Mann JJ. 1999. Role of the serotonergic system in the pathogenesis of major depression and suicidal behavior. Neuropsychopharmacology, 21: 99S–105S.

Mannuzza S, Schneier FR, Chapman TF, et al. 1995. Generalized social phobia: Reliability and validity. Archives of General Psychiatry, 52: 230–237.

Mansell W, Clark DM. 1999. How do I appear to others? Social anxiety and processing of the observable self. Behaviour Research and Therapy, 37: 419–434.

Mantovani A, Lisanby SH, Pieraccini F, et al. 2006. Repetitive transcranial magnetic stimulation (rTMS) in the treatment of obsessive-compulsive disorder (OCD) and Tourette's syndrome (TS). International Journal of Neuropsychopharmacology, 9: 95–100.

Marazziti D, Dell'Osso L, Di Nasso E, et al. 2002. Insight in obsessive-compulsive disorder: A study of an Italian sample. European Psychiatry, 17: 407–410.

Marcaurelle R, Belanger C, Marchand A. 2003. Marital relationship and the treatment of panic disorder with agoraphobia: A critical review. Clinical Psychology Review, 23: 247–276.

Margraf J, Barlow DH, Clark DM. et al. 1993. Psychological treatment of panic: Work in progress in outcome, active ingredients, and follow-up. Behaviour Research and Therapy, 31: 1–8.

Margraf J, Ehlers A, Roth WT. 1986. Sodium lactate infusions and panic attacks: A review and critique. Psychosomatic Medicine, 48: 23–51.

Margraf J, Ehlers A, Roth WT. 1988. Mitral valve prolapse and panic disorder: A review of their relationship. Psychosomatic Medicine, 50: 93–113.

Markowitz JS, Weissman MM, Ouellette R, et al. 1989. Quality of life in panic disorder. Archives of General Psychiatry, 46: 984–992.

Marks IM. 1988. Blood-injury phobia: A review. American Journal of Psychiatry, 145: 1207–1213.

Marks IM, Boulogouris JC, Marcet P. 1971. Flooding versus desensitization in the treatment of phobic patients: A cross-over study. British Journal of Psychiatry, 119: 353–375.

Marks IM, Gray S, Cohen D, et al. 1983. Imipramine and brief therapist-aided exposure in agoraphobics having self-exposure homework. Archives of General Psychiatry, 40: 153–162.

Marks IM, Hodgson R, Rachman S. 1975. Treatment of chronic obsessive-compulsive neurosis by in vivo exposure: A 2-year follow-up and issues in treatment. British Journal of Psychiatry, 127: 349–364.

Marks IM, Lelliott P, Basoglu M, et al. 1988. Clomipramine, self-exposure and therapist-aided exposure for obsessive compulsive rituals. British Journal of Psychiatry, 152: 522–534.

Marks IM, Lovell K, Noshirvani H, et al. 1998. Treatment of posttraumatic stress disorder by exposure and/or cognitive restructuring: A controlled study. Archives of General Psychiatry, 55: 317–325.

Marks IM, Mathews AM. 1979. Brief standard self-rating scale for phobic patients. Behaviour Research and Therapy, 17: 263–267.

Marks IM, Stern RS, Mawson D, et al. 1980. Clomipramine and exposure for obsessive-compulsive rituals. British Journal of Psychiatry, 136: 1–25.

Marks IM, Swinson RP, Basoglu M, et al. 1993. Alprazolam and exposure alone and combined in panic disorder with agoraphobia: A controlled study in London and Toronto. British Journal of Psychiatry, 162: 776–787.

Marmar CR, Schoenfeld F, Weiss DS, et al. 1996. Open trial of fluvoxamine treatment for combat-related posttraumatic stress disorder. Journal of Clinical Psychiatry, 57 (Suppl. 8): 66–72.

Maron E, Nikopensius T, Koks S, et al. 2005. Association study of 90 candidate gene polymorphisms in panic disorder. Psychiatric Genetics, 15: 17–24.

Marshall GN, Schell TL. 2002. Reappraising the link between peritraumatic dissociation and PTSD symptom severity: Evidence from a longitudinal study of community violence survivors. Journal of Abnormal Psychology, 111: 626–636.

Marshall RD, Beebe KL, Oldham M, et al. 2001. Efficacy and safety of paroxetine treatment for chronic PTSD: A fixed–dose, placebo–controlled study. American Journal of Psychiatry, 158: 1982–1988.

Marten PA, Brown TA, Barlow DH, et al. 1993. Evaluation of the ratings comprising the associated symptom criterion of DSM-III-R generalized anxiety disorder. Journal of Nervous and Mental Disease, 181: 676–682.

Martenyi F, Brown EB, Zhang H, et al. 2002b. Fluoxetine v. placebo in prevention of relapse in post-traumatic stress disorder. British Journal of Psychiatry, 181: 315–320.

Martenyi F, Brown EB, Zhang H, et al. 2002a. Fluoxetine versus placebo in posttraumatic stress disorder. Journal of Clinical Psychiatry, 63: 199–206.

Martenyi F, Soldatenkova V. 2006. Fluoxetine in the acute treatment and relapse prevention of combat-related post-traumatic stress disorder: Analysis of the veteran group of a placebo-controlled, randomized clinical trial. European Neuropsychopharmacology, 16: 340–349.

Martin JLR, Sainz-Pardo M, Furukawa TA, et al. 2007. Benzodiazepines in generalized anxiety disorder: Heterogeneity of outcomes based on a systematic review and meta-analysis of clinical trials. Journal of Psychopharmacology, 21: 774–782.

Marzillier JS, Lambert C, Kellett J. 1976. A controlled evaluation of systematic desensitization and social skills training for socially inadequate psychiatric patients. Behaviour Research and Therapy, 14: 225–238.

Mason JW, Giller EL, Kosten TR, et al. 1986. Urinary free-cortisol levels in posttraumatic stress disorder patients. Journal of Nervous and Mental Disease, 174: 145–149.

Massion AO, Dyck IR, Shea MT, et al. 2002. Personality disorders and time to remission in generalized anxiety disorder, social phobia, and panic disorder. Archives of General Psychiatry, 59: 434–440.

Massion AO, Warshaw MG, Keller MB. 1993. Quality of life and psychiatric morbidity in panic disorder and generalized anxiety disorder. American Journal of Psychiatry, 150: 600–607.

Mataix-Cols D, Marks IM, Greist JH, et al. 2002b. Obsessive-compulsive symptom dimensions as predictors of compliance with and response to behaviour therapy: Results from a controlled trial. Psychotherapy and Psychosomatics, 71: 255–262.

Mataix-Cols D, Pertusa A, Leckman JF. 2007. Issues for DSM-V: How should obsessive-compulsive and related disorders be classified? American Journal of Psychiatry, 164: 1313–1314.

Mataix-Cols D, Rauch SL, Baer L, et al. 2002a. Symptom stability in adult obsessive-compulsive disorder: Data from a naturalistic two-year follow-up study. American Journal of Psychiatry, 159: 263–268.

Mataix-Cols D, Rauch SL, Manzo PA, et al. 1999. Use of factor-analyzed symptom dimensions to predict outcome with serotonin reuptake inhibitors and placebo in the treatment of obsessive-compulsive disorder. American Journal of Psychiatry, 156: 1409–1416.

Mathews A, Mogg K, May J, et al. 1989. Implicit and explicit memory bias in anxiety. Journal of Abnormal Psychology, 98: 236–240.

Mattick RP, Peters L. 1988. Treatment of severe social phobia: Effects of guided exposure with and without cognitive restructuring. Journal of Consulting and Clinical Psychology, 56: 251–260.

Mattick RP, Peters L, Clarke JC. 1989. Exposure and cognitive restructuring for social phobia: A controlled study. Behavior Therapy, 20: 3–23.

Mavissakalian M. 1988. The relationship between panic, phobic and anticipatory anxiety in agoraphobia. Behaviour Research and Therapy, 26: 235–240.

Mavissakalian M, Hamman MS. 1987. DSM-III personality disorders in agoraphobia: II. Changes with treatment. Comprehensive Psychiatry, 28: 356–361.

Mavissakalian M, Hamman MS, Haidar SA, et al. 1993. DSM-III personality disorders in generalized anxiety, panic/agoraphobia, and obsessive-compulsive disorders. Comprehensive Psychiatry, 34: 243–248.

Mavissakalian M, Michelson L. 1986a. Two-year follow-up of exposure and imipramine treatment of agoraphobia. American Journal of Psychiatry 143: 1106–1112.

Mavissakalian M, Michelson L. 1986b. Agoraphobia: Relative and combined effectiveness of therapist-assisted in vivo exposure and imipramine. Journal of Clinical Psychiatry, 47: 117–122.

Mavissakalian M, Perel JM. 1989. Imipramine dose-response relationship in panic disorder with agoraphobia: Preliminary findings. Archives of General Psychiatry, 46: 127–131.

Mavissakalian M, Perel JM. 1992. Protective effects of imipramine maintenance treatment in panic disorder with agoraphobia. American Journal of Psychiatry, 149: 1053–1057.

Mavissakalian M, Perel JM. 1995. Imipramine treatment of panic disorder with agoraphobia: Dose ranging and plasma level-response relationships. American Journal of Psychiatry, 152: 673–682.

Mavissakalian MR, Guo S. 2004. Early detection of relapse in panic disorder. Acta Psychiatrica Scandinavica, 110: 393–399.

Mavissakalian MR, Perel JM. 2002. Duration of imipramine therapy and relapse in panic disorder with agoraphobia. Journal of Clinical Psychopharmacology, 22: 294–299.

Mayerovitch JI, du Fort GG, Kakuma R, et al. 2003. Treatment seeking for obsessive-compulsive disorder: Role of obsessive-compulsive disorder symptoms and comorbid psychiatric diagnoses. Comprehensive Psychiatry, 44: 162–168.

Mayou R, Bryant B, Duthie R. 1993. Psychiatric consequences of road traffic accidents. British Medical Journal, 307: 647–651.

Mayou R, Ehlers A, Hobbs M. 2000. Psychological debriefing for road traffic accident victims: Three year follow-up of a randomised controlled trial. British Journal of Psychiatry, 176: 589–593.

McClure EB, Monk CS, Nelson EE, et al. 2007. Abnormal attention modulation of fear circuit function in pediatric generalized anxiety disorder. Archives of General Psychiatry, 64: 97–106.

McDougle CJ, Epperson CN, Pelton GH, et al. 2000. A double-blind, placebo-controlled study of risperidone addition in serotonin reuptake inhibitor-refractory obsessive-compulsive disorder. Archives of General Psychiatry, 57: 794–801.

McDougle CJ, Goodman WK, Leckman JF, et al. 1994. Haloperidol addition in fluvoxamine-refractory obsessive-compulsive disorder: A double-blind, placebo-controlled study in patients with and without tics. Archives of General Psychiatry, 51: 302–308.

McDougle CJ, Goodman WK, Price LH, et al. 1990. Neuroleptic addition in fluvoxamine-refractory obsessive-compulsive disorder. American Journal of Psychiatry, 147: 652–654.

McElroy SL, Altshuler LL, Suppes T, et al. 2001. Axis I psychiatric comorbidity and its relationship to historical illness variables in 288 patients with bipolar disorder. American Journal of Psychiatry, 158: 420–426.

McEwan KL, Devins GM. 1983. Is increased arousal in social anxiety noticed by others? Journal of Abnormal Psychology, 92: 417–421.

McFall M, Murburg M, Ko G, et al. 1990. Autonomic response to stress in Vietnam combat veterans with post-traumatic stress disorder. Biological Psychiatry, 27: 1165–1175.

McFarlane AC. 1988. The longitudinal course of posttraumatic morbidity: The range of outcomes and their predictors. Journal of Nervous and Mental Disease, 176: 30–39.

McFarlane AC. 1989. The etiology of post-traumatic morbidity: Predisposing, precipitating and perpetuating factors. British Journal of Psychiatry, 154: 221–228.

McFarlane AC, Atchison M, Yehuda R. 1997. The acute stress response following motor vehicle accidents and its relation to PTSD. Annals of the New York Academy of Sciences, 821: 437–441.

McFarlane AC, Papay P. 1992. Multiple diagnoses in posttraumatic stress disorder in the victims of a natural disaster. Journal of Nervous and Mental Disease, 180: 498–504.

McGee R, Feehan M, Williams S, et al. 1990. DSM-III disorders in a large sample of adolescents. Journal of the American Academy of Child and Adolescent Psychiatry, 29: 611–619.

McHugh PR, Treisman G. 2007. PTSD: A Problematic diagnostic category. Journal of Anxiety Disorders, 21: 211–222.

McHugh RK, Otto MW, Barlow DH, et al. 2007. Cost-efficacy of individual and combined treatments for panic disorder. Journal of Clinical Psychiatry, 68: 1038–1044.

McKay D. 1997. A maintenance program for obsessive-compulsive disorder using exposure with response prevention: 2-year follow-up. Behaviour Research and Therapy, 35: 367–369.

McKay D, Abramowitz JS, Taylor S. 2008. Discussion: The obsessive-compulsive spectrum. In Abramowitz JS, McKay D, Taylor S, editors: Obsessive-Compulsive Disorder: Subtypes and Spectrum Conditions. New York: Elsevier, pp. 287–300.

McKay D, Neziroglu F, Todaro J, et al. 1996. Changes in personality disorders following behavior therapy for obsessive-compulsive disorder. Journal of Anxiety Disorders, 10: 47–57.

McLean PD, Whittal ML, Söchting I, et al. 2001. Cognitive versus behavior therapy in the group treatment of obsessive-compulsive disorder. Journal of Consulting and Clinical Psychology, 69: 205–214.

McLeod JD. 1994. Anxiety disorders and marital quality. Journal of Abnormal Psychology, 103: 767–776.

McNally RJ. 1987. Preparedness and phobias: A review. Psychological Bulletin, 101: 283–303.

McNally RJ. 2002. Disgust has arrived. Journal of Anxiety Disorders, 16: 561–566.

McNally RJ, Lorenz M. 1987. Anxiety sensitivity in agoraphobics. Journal of Behavior Therapy and Experimental Psychiatry, 18: 3–11.

McPherson FM, Brougham L, McLaren S. 1980. Maintenance of improvement in agoraphobic patients treated by behavioural methods: A four-year follow-up. Behaviour Research and Therapy, 18: 150–152.

Meewisse M-L, Reitsma JB, de Vries G-J, et al. 2007. Cortisol and post-traumatic stress disorder in adults: Systematic review and meta-analysis. British Journal of Psychiatry, 191: 387–392.

Meibach RC, Dunner D, Wilson LG, et al. 1987. Comparative efficacy of propranolol, chlordiazepoxide, and placebo in the treatment of anxiety: A double-blind trial. Journal of Clinical Psychiatry, 48: 355–358.

Meichenbaum D. 1975. Self-instructional methods. In Kanfer FH, Goldstein AP, editors: Helping People Change. New York: Pergamon Press, pp. 357–391.

Mellings TMB, Alden LE. 2000. Cognitive processes in social anxiety: The effects of self-focus, rumination and anticipatory processing. Behaviour Research and Therapy, 38: 243–257.

Mellman TA, David D, Bustamante V, et al. 2001. Predictors of post-traumatic stress disorder following severe injury. Depression and Anxiety, 14: 226–231.

Meltzer-Brody S, Connor KM, Churchill E, et al. 2000. Symptom-specific effects of fluoxetine in post-traumatic stress disorder. International Clinical Psychopharmacology, 15: 227–231.

Mendels J, Krajewski TF, Huffer V, et al. 1986. Effective short-term treatment of generalized anxiety with trifluoperazine. Journal of Clinical Psychiatry, 47: 170–174.

Mendlewicz J, Papadimitriou G, Wilmotte J. 1993. Family study of panic disorder: Comparison with generalized anxiety disorder, major depression, and normal subjects. Psychiatric Genetics, 3: 73–78.

Mennin DS, Heimberg RG, Jack MS. 2000. Comorbid generalized anxiety disorder in primary social phobia: Symptom severity, functional impairment, and treatment response. Journal of Anxiety Disorders, 14: 325–343.

Menzies RG, Clarke JC. 1993a. The etiology of childhood water phobia. Behaviour Research and Therapy, 31: 499–501.

Menzies RG, Clarke JC. 1993b. The etiology of fear of heights and its relationship to severity and individual response patterns. Behaviour Research and Therapy, 31: 355–365.

Menzies RG, Clarke JC. 1995. The etiology of phobias: A nonassociative account. Clinical Psychology Review, 15: 23–48.

Mersch PPA. 1995. The treatment of social phobia: The differential effectiveness of exposure in vivo and an integration of exposure in vivo, rational emotive therapy and social skills training. Behaviour Research and Therapy, 33: 259–269.

Mersch PPA, Emmelkamp PMG, Bögel SM, et al. 1989. Social phobia: Individual response patterns and the effects of behavioral and cognitive interventions. Behaviour Research and Therapy, 27: 421–434.

Mersch PPA, Emmelkamp PMG, Lips C. 1991. Social phobia: Individual response patterns and the long-term effects of behavioral and cognitive interventions: A follow-up study. Behaviour Research and Therapy, 29: 357–362.

Meyer TJ, Miller RL, Metzger R, et al. 1990. Development and validation of the Penn State Worry Questionnaire. Behaviour Research and Therapy, 28: 487–495.

Michael T, Halligan SL, Clark DM, et al. 2007. Rumination in posttraumatic stress disorder. Depression and Anxiety, 24: 307–317.

Michelson D, Allgulander C, Dantendorfer K, et al. 2001. Efficacy of usual antidepressant dosing regimens of fluoxetine in panic disorder: Randomised, placebo-controlled trial. British Journal of Psychiatry, 179: 514–518.

Michelson D, Lydiard RB, Pollack MH, et al. 1998. Outcome assessment and clinical improvement in panic disorder: Evidence from a randomized controlled trial of fluoxetine and placebo. American Journal of Psychiatry, 155: 1570–1577.

Michelson D, Pollack M, Lydiard RB. 1999. Continuing treatment of panic disorder after acute response: Randomised, placebo-controlled trial with fluoxetine. British Journal of Psychiatry, 172: 213–218.

Mick MA, Telch MJ. 1998. Social anxiety and history of behavioral inhibition in young adults. Journal of Anxiety Disorders, 12: 1–20.

Miguel EC, Coffey BJ, Baer L, et al. 1995. Phenomenology of intentional repetitive behaviors in obsessive-compulsive disorder and Tourette's disorder. Journal of Clinical Psychiatry, 56: 246–255.

Miguel EC, do Rosario-Campos MC, da Silva Prado H, et al. 2000. Sensory phenomena in obsessive-compulsive disorder and Tourette's disorder. Journal of Clinical Psychiatry, 61: 150–156.

Mikkelson EJ, Deltor J, Cohen DJ. 1981. School avoidance and social phobia triggered by haloperidol in patients with Tourette's syndrome. American Journal of Psychiatry, 138: 1572–1576.

Milanfranchi A, Ravagli S, Lensi P, et al. 1997. A double-blind study of fluvoxamine and clomipramine in the treatment of obsessive-compulsive disorder. International Clinical Psychopharmacology, 12: 131–136.

Miller ML. 1953. On street fear. International Journal of Psychoanalysis, 34: 232–252.

Milrod B, Busch F, Cooper A, et al. 1997. Manual of Panic-Focused Psychodynamic Psychotherapy. Washington, DC: American Psychiatric Press.

Milrod B, Leon AC, Busch F, et al. 2007a. A randomized controlled clinical trial of psychoanalytic psychotherapy for panic disorder. American Journal of Psychiatry, 164: 265–272.

Milrod BL, Leon AC, Barber JP, et al. 2007b. Do comorbid personality disorders moderate panic-focused psychotherapy? An exploratory examination of the American Psychiatric Association Practice Guidelines. Journal of Clinical Psychiatry, 68: 885–891.

Mineka S, Watson D, Clark LA. 1998. Comorbidity of anxiety and unipolar mood disorders. Annual Review of Psychology, 49: 377–412.

Minichiello WE, Baer L, Jenike MA. 1987. Schizotypal personality disorder: A poor prognostic indicator for behavior therapy in the treatment of obsessive-compulsive disorder. Journal of Anxiety Disorders, 1: 273–276.

Miranda R, Fontes M, Marroquín B. 2008. Cognitive content-specificity I future expectancies: Role of hopelessness and intolerance of uncertainty in depression and GAD symptoms. Behaviour Research and Therapy, 46: 1151–1159.

Mitchell JT. 1983. When disaster strikes ... the critical incident stress debriefing process. Journal of Emergency Medical Services, 8: 36–39.

Mitchell JT, Everly GS. 1995. Critical Incident Stress Debriefing: An Operation Manual for the Prevention of Traumatic Stress among Emergency Services and Disaster Workers. Elliott City, MD: Chevron Publishing.

Mitte K. 2005. A meta-analysis of the efficacy of psycho- and pharmacotherapy in panic disorder with and without agoraphobia. Journal of Affective Disorders, 88: 27–45.

Mitte K, Noack P, Steil R, et al. 2005. A meta-analytic review of the efficacy of drug treatment in generalized anxiety disorder. Journal of Clinical Psychopharmacology, 25: 141–150.

Modigh K, Westberg P, Eriksson E. 1992. Superiority of clomipramine over imipramine in the treatment of panic disorder: A placebo-controlled trial. Journal of Clinical Psychopharmacology, 12: 251–261.

Moffitt TE, Caspi A, Harrington H, et al. 2007b. Generalized anxiety disorder and depression: Childhood risk factors in a birth cohort followed to age 32. Psychological Medicine, 37: 441–452.

Moffitt TE, Harrington H, Caspi A, et al. 2007a. Depression and generalized anxiety disorder: Cumulative and sequential comorbidity in a birth cohort followed prospectively to age 32 years. Archives of General Psychiatry, 64: 651–660.

Mogg K, Bradley BP, Miller T, et al. 1994. Interpretation of homophones related to threat: Anxiety or response bias effects? Cognitive Therapy and Research, 18: 461–477.

Mohlman J, de Jesus M, Gorenstein EE, et al. 2004. Distinguishing generalized anxiety disorder, panic disorder, and mixed anxiety states in older treatment-seeking adults. Journal of Anxiety Disorders, 18: 275–290.

Mol SSL, Arntz A, Metsemakers JFM, et al. 2005. Symptoms of post-traumatic stress disorder after non-traumatic events: Evidence from an open population study. British Journal of Psychiatry, 186: 494–499.

Mollica RF, Mcinnes K, Pham T, et al. 1998. The dose-effect relationships between torture and psychiatric symptoms in Vietnamese ex-political detainees and a comparison group. Journal of Nervous and Mental Disease, 186: 543–553.

Momartin S, Silove D, Manicavasagar V, et al. 2004. Comorbdity of PTSD and depression: Associations with trauma exposure, symptom severity and functional impairment in Bosnian refugees resettled in Australia. Journal of Affective Disorders, 80: 231–238.

Monk CS, Nelson EE, McClure EB, et al. 2006. Ventrolateral prefrontal cortex activation and attentional bias in response to angry faces in adolescents with generalized anxiety disorder. American Journal of Psychiatry, 163: 1091–1097.

Monk CS, Telzer EH, Mogg K, et al. 2008. Amygdala and ventrolateral prefrontal cortex activation to masked angry faces in children and adolescents with generalized anxiety disorder. Archives of General Psychiatry, 65: 568–576.

Monnelly EP, Ciraulo DA, Knapp C, et al. 2003. Low-dose risperidone as adjunctive therapy for irritable aggression in posttraumatic stress disorder. Journal of Clinical Psychopharmacology, 23: 193–196.

Montgomery SA, Kasper S, Stein DJ, et al. 2001. Citalopram 20 mg, 40 mg and 60 mg are all effective and well tolerated compared with placebo in obsessive-compulsive disorder. International Clinical Psychopharmacology, 16: 75–86.

Montgomery SA, Mahe V, Haudiquet V, et al. 2002. Effectiveness of venlafaxine, extended release formulation, in short-term and long-term treatment of generalized anxiety disorder: Results of a survival analysis. Journal of Clinical Psychopharmacology, 21: 561–567.

Montgomery SA, McIntyre A, Osterheider M, et al. 1993. A double-blind, placebo-controlled study of fluoxetine in patients with DSM-III-R obsessive-compulsive disorder. European Neuropsychopharmacology, 3: 143–152.

Montgomery SA, Nil R, Durr-Pal N, et al. 2005. A 24-week randomized, double-blind, placebo-controlled study of escitalopram for the prevention of generalized social anxiety disorder. Journal of Clinical Psychiatry, 66: 1270–1278.

Montgomery SA, Tobias K, Zornberg GL, et al. 2006. Efficacy and safety of pregabalin in the treatment of generalized anxiety disorder: A 6-week, multicenter, randomized, double-blind, placebo-controlled comparison of pregabalin and venlafaxine. Journal of Clinical Psychiatry, 67: 771–782.

Morgenstern J, Langenbucher J, Labouvie E, et al. 1997. The comorbidity of alcoholism and personality disorders in a clinical population: Prevalence rates and relation to alcohol typology. Journal of Abnormal Psychology, 106: 74–84.

Morissette SB, Spiegel DA, Barlow DH. 2008. Combining exposure and pharmacotherapy in the treatment of social anxiety disorder: A preliminary study of state dependent learning. Journal of Psychopathology and Behavioral Assessment, 30: 211–219.

Moritz S, Fricke S, Jacobsen D, et al. 2004. Positive schizotypal symptoms predict treatment outcome in obsessive-compulsive disorder. Behaviour Research and Therapy, 42: 217–227.

Moulds ML, Bryant RA. 2002. Directed forgetting in acute stress disorder. Journal of Abnormal Psychology, 111: 175–179.

Mowrer O. 1960. Learning Theory and Behavior. New York: Wiley.

Muehlbacher M, Nickel MK, Nickel C, et al. 2005. Mirtazapine treatment of social phobia in women: A randomized, double-blind, placebo-controlled study. Journal of Clinical Psychopharmacology, 25: 580–583.

Mulkens S, de Jong PJ, Dobbelaar A, et al. 1999. Fear of blushing: Fearful preoccupation irrespective of facial coloration. Behaviour Research and Therapy, 37: 1119–1128.

Mullaney JA, Trippett CJ. 1979. Alcohol dependence and phobias: Clinical description and relevance. British Journal of Psychiatry, 135: 565–573.

Muller JE, Koen L, Stein DJ. 2004. The spectrum of social anxiety disorders. In Bandelow B, Stein DJ, editors: Social Anxiety Disorder. New York: Marcel Dekker, pp. 19–34.

Munby J, Johnston DW. 1980. Agoraphobia: The long-term follow-up of behavioral treatment. British Journal of Psychiatry, 137: 418–427.

Mundo E, Mainia G, Uslenghi C. 2000. Multicentre, double-blind comparison of fluvoxamine and clomipramine in the treatment of obsessive-compulsive disorder. International Clinical Psychopharmacology, 15: 69–76.

Murray J, Ehlers A, Mayou RA. 2002. Dissociation and post-traumatic stress disorder: Two prospective studies of road traffic accident survivors. British Journal of Psychiatry, 180: 363–368.

Nagy LM, Krystal JH, Woods SW, et al. 1989. Clinical and medication outcome after short-term alprazolam and behavioral group treatment in panic disorder: 2.5 year naturalistic follow-up study. Archives of General Psychiatry, 46: 993–999.

Nakatani E, Nakagawa A, Nakao T, et al. 2005. A randomized controlled trial of Japanese patients with obsessive-compulsive disorder – Effectiveness of behavior therapy and fluvoxamine. Psychotherapy and Psychosomatics, 74: 269–276.

Nardi AE, Nascimento I, Valença AM, et al. 2003. Respiratory panic disorder subtype: Acute and long-term response to nortriptyline, a noradrenergic tricyclic antidepressant. Psychiatry Research, 120: 283–293.

Nardi AE, Valença AM, Nascimento I, et al. 2005. A three-year follow-up study of patients with the respiratory subtype of panic disorder after treatment with clonazepam. Psychiatry Research, 137: 61–70.

Narrow WE, Rae DS, Robins LN, et al. 2002. Revised prevalence estimates of mental disorders in the United States: Using a clinical significance criterion to reconcile 2 surveys' estimates. Archives of General Psychiatry, 59: 115–123.

Nash JR, Sargent PA, Rabiner EA, et al. 2008. Serotonin 5-HT$_{1A}$ receptor binding in people with panic disorder: Positron emission tomography study. British Journal of Psychiatry, 193: 229–234.

National Institute for Clinical Excellence. 2004. The Management of Panic Disorder and Generalised Anxiety Disorder in Primary and Secondary Care. London: National Collaborating Centre for Mental Health.

Neftel KA, Adler RH, Kappell K, et al. 1982. Stage fright in musicians: A model illustrating the effect of beta-blockers. Psychosomatic Medicine, 44: 461–469.

Nelson EC, Grant JD, Bucholz KK, et al. 2000. Social phobia in a population-based female adolescent twin sample: Co-morbidity and associated suicide-related symptoms. Psychological Medicine, 30: 797–804.

Nemiah JC. 1988. Psychoneurotic disorders. In Nicholi AM, editor: The New Harvard Guide to Psychiatry. Cambridge, MA: Belknap Press of Harvard University Press, pp. 234–258.

Nestadt G, Samuels J, Riddle M, et al. 2000. A family study of obsessive-compulsive disorder. Archives of General Psychiatry, 57: 358–363.

Newman MG, Hofmann SG, Trabert W, et al. 1994. Does behavioral treatment of social phobia lead to cognitive changes? Behavior Therapy, 25: 503–517.

Neziroglu F, Anemone R, Yaryura-Tobias JA. 1992. Onset of obsessive-compulsive disorder in pregnancy. American Journal of Psychiatry, 149: 947–950.

Neziroglu F, McKay D, Yaryura-Tobias JA, et al. 1999. The Overvalued Ideas Scale: Development, reliability and validity in obsessive-compulsive disorder. Behaviour Research and Therapy, 37: 881–902.

Nicolini H, Bakish D, Duenas H, et al. 2009. Improvement of psychic and somatic symptoms in adult patients with generalized anxiety disorder: Examination from a duloxetine, venlafaxine extended-release and placebo-controlled trial. Psychological Medicine, 39: 267–276.

Nielssen O, Large M. 2008. Post-traumatic stress disorder's future (letter). British Journal of Psychiatry, 192: 394.

Nimatoudis I, Zissis NP, Kogeorgos J, et al. 2004. Remission rates with venlafaxine extended release in Greek outpatients with generalized anxiety disorder: A double-blind, randomized, placebo controlled study. International Clinical Psychopharmacology, 19: 331–336.

Ninan PT, Koran LM, Kiev A, et al. 2006. High-dose sertraline strategy for nonresponders to acute treatment for obsessive-compulsive disorder: A multicenter double-blind trial. Journal of Clinical Psychiatry, 67: 15–22.

Nisita C, Petracca A, Akiskal HS, et al. 1990. Delimitation of generalized anxiety disorder: Clinical comparisons with panic and major depressive disorders. Comprehensive Psychiatry, 31: 409–415.

Norris FH, Murphy AD, Baker CK, et al. 2003. Epidemiology of trauma and post-traumatic stress disorder in Mexico. Journal of Abnormal Psychology, 112: 646–656.

Norton GR, Dorward J, Cox BJ. 1986. Factors associated with panic attacks in nonclinical subjects. Behavior Therapy, 17: 239–252.

Noyes R. 1999. The relationship of hypochondriasis to anxiety disorders. General Hospital Psychiatry, 21: 8–17.

Noyes R, Clancy J, Garvey MJ, et al. 1987a. Is agoraphobia a variant of panic disorder or a separate illness? Journal of Anxiety Disorders, 1: 3–13.

Noyes R, Clancy J, Woodman C, et al. 1993. Environmental factors related to the outcome of panic disorder: A seven-year follow-up study. Journal of Nervous and Mental Disease, 181: 529–538.

Noyes R, Clarkson C, Crowe RR, et al. 1987b. A family study of generalized anxiety disorder. American Journal of Psychiatry, 144: 1019–1024.

Noyes R, Crowe RR, Harris EL, et al. 1986. Relationship between panic disorder and agoraphobia: A family study. Archives of General Psychiatry, 43: 227–232.

Noyes R, Garvey MJ, Cook B. 1991. Controlled discontinuation of benzodiazepine treatment for patients with panic disorder. American Journal of Psychiatry, 148: 517–523.

Noyes R, Moroz G, Davidson JTR, et al. 1997. Moclobemide in social phobia: A controlled dose-response trial. Journal of Clinical Psychopharmacology, 17: 247–254.

Nutt D, Argyropoulos S, Hood S, et al. 2006. Generalized anxiety disorder: A comorbid disease. European Neuropsychopharmacology, 16 (Suppl. 2): S109–S118.

Nutt DJ, Glue P, Lawson C, et al. 1990. Flumazenil provocation of panic attacks: Evidence for altered benzodiazepine receptor sensitivity in panic disorder. Archives of General Psychiatry, 47: 917–925.

Nuttin BJ, Gabriels LA, Cosyns PR, et al. 2003. Long-term electrical capsular stimulation in patients with obsessive-compulsive disorder. Neurosurgery, 52: 1263–1272.

Oakley-Browne MA, Joyce PR, Wells E, et al. 1989. Christchurch Psychiatric Epidemiology Study, Part II: Six month and other period prevalences of specific psychiatric disorders. Australian and New Zealand Journal of Psychiatry, 23: 327–340.

O'Connor KP, Aardema F, Robillard S, et al. 2006. Cognitive behaviour therapy and medication in the treatment of obsessive-compulsive disorder. Acta Psychiatrica Scandinavica, 113: 408–419.

O'Donnell ML, Elliott P, Lau W, et al. 2007. PTSD symptom trajectories: From early to chronic response. Behaviour Research and Therapy, 45: 601–606.

Obsessive Compulsive Cognitions Working Group. 1997. Cognitive assessment of obsessive-compulsive disorder. Behaviour Research and Therapy, 35: 667–681.

Oehrberg S, Christiansen PE, Behnke K, et al. 1995. Paroxetine in the treatment of panic disorder: A randomised, double-blind, placebo-controlled study. British Journal of Psychiatry, 167: 374–379.

Oei TP, Llamas M, Evans L. 1997. Does concurrent drug intake affect the long-term outcome of group cognitive behaviour therapy in panic disorder with or without agoraphobia? Behaviour Research and Therapy, 35: 851–857.

Öhman A. 1986. Face the beast and fear the face: Animal and social fears as prototypes for evolutionary analyses of emotion. Psychophysiology, 23: 123–145.

Olatunji BO, Smits JAJ, Connolly K, et al. 2007. Examination of the decline in fear and disgust during exposure to threat-relevant stimuli in blood-injection-injury phobia. Journal of Anxiety Disorders, 21: 445–455.

Olff M, Koeter MWJ, Van Haaften EH, et al. 2005. Impact of a foot and mouth disease crisis on post-traumatic stress symptoms in farmers. British Journal of Psychiatry, 186: 165–166.

Olfson M, Fireman B, Weissman MM, et al. 1997. Mental disorders and disability among patients in primary care practice. American Journal of Psychiatry, 154: 1734–1740.

Olfson M, Kessler RC, Berglund PA, et al. 1998. Psychiatric disorder onset and first treatment contact in the United States and Ontario. American Journal of Psychiatry, 155: 1415–1422.

O'Neill GW. 1985. Is worry a valuable concept? Behaviour Research and Therapy, 23: 479–480.

Onur E, Alkin T, Tural Ü. 2007. Panic disorder subtypes: Further clinical differences. Depression and Anxiety, 24: 479–486.

O'Rourke D, Fahy TJ, Brophy J, et al. 1996. The Galway Study of Panic Disorder: III. Outcome at 5 to 6 years. British Journal of Psychiatry, 168: 462–469.

Orsillo SM, Lilienfeld SO, Heimberg RG. 1994. Social phobia and response to challenge procedures: Examining the interaction between anxiety sensitivity and trait anxiety. Journal of Anxiety Disorders, 8: 247–258.

Öst L-G. 1987a. Applied relaxation: Description of a coping technique and review of controlled studies. Behaviour Research and Therapy, 25: 397–409.

Öst L-G. 1987b. Age of onset in different phobias, Journal of Abnormal Psychology, 96: 223–229.

Öst L-G. 1988. Applied relaxation vs. progressive relaxation in the treatment of panic disorder. Behaviour Research and Therapy, 26: 13–22.

Öst L-G. 1989. One-session treatment for specific phobias. Behaviour Research and Therapy, 27: 1–7.

Öst L-G. 1996. One-session group treatment of spider phobia. Behaviour Research and Therapy, 34: 707–715.

Öst L-G, Breitholtz E. 2000. Applied relaxation vs. cognitive therapy in the treatment of generalized anxiety disorder. Behaviour Research and Therapy, 38: 777–790.

Öst L-G, Hugdahl K. 1981. Acquisition of phobias and anxiety response patterns in clinical patients. Behaviour Research and Therapy, 19: 439–447.

Öst L-G, Sterner U. 1987. Applied tension: A specific behavioural method for treatment of blood phobia. Behaviour Research and Therapy, 25: 25–29.

O'Sullivan G, Noshirvani H, Marks I, et al. 1991. Six year follow-up after exposure and clomipramine therapy for obsessive compulsive disorder. Journal of Clinical Psychiatry, 52: 150–155.

Otto MW, Hinton D, Korbly NB, et al. 2003. Treatment of pharmacotherapy-refractory posttraumatic stress disorder among Cambodian refugees: A pilot study of combination treatment with cognitive-behavior therapy vs sertraline alone. Behaviour Research and Therapy, 41: 1271–1276.

Otto MW, Pollack MH, Fava M, et al. 1995. Elevated Anxiety Sensitivity Index scores in patients with major depression: Correlates and changes with antidepressant treatment. Journal of Anxiety Disorders, 9: 117–123.

Otto MW, Pollack MH, Gould RA, et al. 2000. A comparison of the efficacy of clonazepam and cognitive-behavioral group therapy for the treatment of social phobia. Journal of Anxiety Disorders, 14: 345–358.

Otto MW, Pollack MH, Sabatino SA. 1996. Maintenance of remission following cognitive behavior therapy for panic disorder: Possible deleterious effects of concurrent medication treatment. Behavior Therapy, 27: 473–482.

Otto MW, Pollack MH, Sachs GS, et al. 1992. Alcohol dependence in panic disorder patients. Journal of Psychiatric Research, 26: 29–38.

Otto MW, Pollack MH, Sachs GS, et al. 1993. Discontinuation of benzodiazepine treatment: Efficacy of cognitive-behavioral therapy for patients with panic disorder. American Journal of Psychiatry, 150: 1485–1490.

Otto MW, Tuby KS, Gould RA, et al. 2001. An effect-size analysis of the relative efficacy and tolerability of serotonin selective reuptake inhibitors for panic disorder. American Journal of Psychiatry, 158: 1989–1992.

Ozer EJ, Best SR, Lipsey TL, et al. 2003. Predictors of posttraumatic stress disorder and symptoms in adults: A meta-analysis. Psychological Bulletin, 129: 52–73.

Padala PR, Madison J, Monnahan M, et al. 2006. Risperidone monotherapy for posttraumatic stress disorder related to sexual assault and domestic abuse in women. International Clinical Psychopharmacology, 21: 275–280.

Pae C-U, Lim H-K, Peindl K, et al. 2008. The atypical antipsychotics olanzapine and risperidone in the treatment of posttraumatic stress disorder: A meta-analysis of randomized, double-blind, placebo-controlled clinical trials. International Clinical Psychopharmacology, 23: 1–8.

Page AC. 1994. Blood-injury phobia. Clinical Psychology Review, 14: 443–461.

Page AC, Bennett K, Carter O, et al. 1997. The Blood-Injection Symptom Scale (BISS): Assessing a structure of phobic symptoms elicited by blood and injections. Behaviour Research and Therapy, 35: 457–464.

Pande AC, Crockatt JG, Feltner DE, et al. 2003. Pregabalin in generalized anxiety disorder: A placebo-controlled trial. American Journal of Psychiatry, 160: 533–540.

Pande AC, Davidson JRT, Jefferson JW, et al. 1999. Treatment of social phobia with gabapentin: A placebo-controlled study. Journal of Clinical Psychopharmacology, 19: 341–348.

Pande AC, Feltner DE, Jefferson JW, et al. 2004. Efficacy of the novel anxiolytic pregabalin in social anxiety disorder: A placebo-controlled, multicenter study. Journal of Clinical Psychopharmacology, 24: 141–149.

Pande AC, Pollack MH, Crockatt J, et al. 2000. Placebo-controlled study of gabapentin treatment of panic disorder. Journal of Clinical Psychopharmacology, 20: 467–471.

Papadimitriou GN, Kerkhofs M, Kempenaers C, et al. 1988. EEG sleep studies in patients with generalized anxiety disorder. Psychiatry Research, 26: 183–190.

Papp LA, Klein DF, Gorman JM. 1993. Carbon dioxide hypersensitivity, hyperventilation, and panic disorder. American Journal of Psychiatry, 150: 1149–1157.

Pato MT, Zohar-Kadouch R, Zohar J, et al. 1988. Return of symptoms after discontinuation of clomipramine in patients with obsessive-compulsive disorder. American Journal of Psychiatry, 145: 1521–1525.

Pauls DL, Alsobrook JP, Goodman W, et al. 1995. A family study of obsessive-compulsive disorder. American Journal of Psychiatry, 152: 76–84.

Perani D, Colombo C, Bressi S, et al. 1995. [18F]FDG PET study in obsessive-compulsive disorder: A clinical/metabolic correlation study after treatment. British Journal of Psychiatry, 166: 244–250.

Perkonigg A, Wittchen H-U. 1999. Prevalence and comorbidity of traumatic events and posttraumatic stress disorder in adolescents and young adults. In Maercker A, Solomon Z, Schützwohl M, editors: Post-Traumatic Stress Disorder: A Lifespan Developmental Perspective. Seattle: Hogrefe & Huber Publishers, pp. 113–133.

Perna G, Bussi R, Allevi L, et al. 1999. Sensitivity to 35% carbon dioxide in patients with generalized anxiety disorder. Journal of Clinical Psychiatry, 60: 379–384.

Perse TL, Greist JH, Jefferson JW, et al. 1987. Fluvoxamine treatment of obsessive-compulsive disorder. American Journal of Psychiatry, 144: 1543–1548.

Pertusa A, Fullana MA, Singh S, et al. 2008. Compulsive hoarding: OCD symptom, distinct clinical syndrome, or both? American Journal of Psychiatry, 165: 1289–1298.

Pfefferbaum B, Pfefferbaum RL, North CS, et al. 2002. Does television viewing satisfy criteria for exposure to posttraumatic stress disorder? Psychiatry, 65: 306–309.

Phan KL, Fitzgerald DA, Nathan PJ, et al. 2006. Association between amygdala hyperactivity to harsh faces and severity of social anxiety in generalized social phobia. Biological Psychiatry, 59: 424–429.

Piccinelli M, Pini S, Bellantuono C, et al. 1995. Efficacy of drug treatment in obsessive-compulsive disorder: A meta-analytic review. British Journal of Psychiatry, 166: 424–443.

Pigott TA, Pato MT, Bernstein SE, et al. 1990. Controlled comparisons of clomipramine and fluoxetine in the treatment of obsessive-compulsive disorder: Behavioral and biological results. Archives of General Psychiatry, 47: 926–932.

Pilkonis PA, Zimbardo PG. 1979. The personal and social dynamics of shyness. In Izard CE, Editor: Emotions in Personality and Psychopathology. New York: Plenum.

Pini S, Cassano GB, Simonini E, et al. 1997. Prevalence of anxiety disorder comorbidity in bipolar depression, unipolar depression and dysthymia. Journal of Affective Disorders, 42: 145–153.

Pini S, Dell'Osso L, Mastrocinque C, et al. 1999. Axis I comorbidity in bipolar disorder with psychotic features. British Journal of Psychiatry, 175: 467–471.

Plehn K, Peterson RA. 2002. Anxiety sensitivity as a predictor of the development of panic symptoms, panic attacks, and panic disorder: A prospective study. Journal of Anxiety Disorders, 16: 455–474.

Pohl R, Yeragani VK, Balon R, et al. 1992. Smoking in patients with panic disorder. Psychiatry Research, 43: 253–262.

Pohl RB, Feltner DE, Fieve RR, et al. 2005. Efficacy of pregabalin in the treatment of generalized anxiety disorder: Double-blind, placebo-controlled comparison of BID versus TID dosing. Journal of Clinical Psychopharmacology, 25: 151–158.

Pohl RB, Wolkow RM, Clary CM. 1998. Sertraline in the treatment of panic disorder: A double-blind multicenter trial. American Journal of Psychiatry, 155: 1189–1195.

Pollack M, Kinrys G, Krystal A, et al. 2008a. Eszopiclone coadministered with escitalopram in patients with insomnia and comorbid generalized anxiety disorder. Archives of General Psychiatry, 65: 551–562.

Pollack MH, Kornstein SG, Spann ME, et al. 2008b. Early improvement during duloxetine treatment of generalized anxiety disorder predicts response and remission at endpoint. Journal of Psychiatric Research, 42: 1176–1184.

Pollack MH, Lepola U, Koponen H, et al. 2007. A double-blind study of the efficacy of venlafaxine extended-release, paroxetine, and placebo in the treatment of panic disorder. Depression and Anxiety, 24: 1–14.

Pollack MH, Otto MW, Tesar GE, et al. 1993. Long-term outcome after acute treatment with alprazolam or clonazepam for panic disorder. Journal of Clinical Psychopharmacology, 13: 257–263.

Pollack MH, Otto MW, Worthington JJ, et al. 1998. Sertraline in the treatment of panic disorder: A flexible-dose multicenter trial. Archives of General Psychiatry, 55: 1010–1016.

Pollack MH, Simon NM, Worthington JJ, et al. 2003. Combined paroxetine and clonazepam treatment strategies compared to paroxetine monotherapy for panic disorder. Journal of Psychopharmacology, 17: 276–282.

Pollack MH, Simon NM, Zalta AK, et al. 2006. Olanzapine augmentation of fluoxetine for refractory generalized anxiety disorder: A placebo-controlled study. Biological Psychiatry, 59: 211–215.

Pollack MH, Tiller J, Xie F, et al. 2008c. Tiagabine in adult patients with generalized anxiety disorder: Results from 3 randomized, double-blind, placebo-controlled, parallel-group studies. Journal of Clinical Psychopharmacology, 28: 308–316.

Pollack MH, Worthington JJ, Manfro GG, et al. 1997. Abecarnil for the treatment of generalized anxiety disorder: A placebo-controlled comparison of two dosage ranges of abecarnil and buspirone. Journal of Clinical Psychiatry, 58 (Suppl. 11): 19–23.

Pollack MH, Zaninelli R, Goddard A, et al. 2001. Paroxetine in the treatment of generalized anxiety disorder: Results of a placebo-controlled, flexible-dosage trial. Journal of Clinical Psychiatry, 62: 350–357.

Post RM, Weiss SR, Smith M, et al. 1997. Kindling versus quenching: Implications for the evolution and treatment of posttraumatic stress disorder. Annals of the New York Academy of Sciences, 821: 285–295.

Power KG, Simpson RJ, Swanson V, et al. 1990. A controlled comparison of cognitive-behavior therapy, diazepam, and placebo, alone and in combination, for the treatment of generalized anxiety disorder. Journal of Anxiety Disorders, 4: 267–292.

Prigerson HG, Jacobs SC. 2001. Traumatic grief as a distinct disorder: A rationale, consensus criteria, and a preliminary empirical test. In Stroebe MS, Hansson RO, Stroebe W, Schut H, editors: Handbook of Bereavement Research: Consequences, Coping, and Care. Washington, DC: American Psychological Association, pp. 613–645.

Prochaska JO. 1991. Prescribing to the stage and level of phobic patients. Psychotherapy, 28: 463–468.

Purdon C, Clark DA. 1994. Perceived control and appraisal of obsessional intrusive thoughts: A replication and extension. Behavioural and Cognitive Psychotherapy, 22: 269–285.

Quitkin FM, Harrison W, Stewart JW, et al. 1991. Response to phenelzine and imipramine in placebo nonresponders with atypical depression: A new application of the crossover design. Archives of General Psychiatry, 48: 319–323.

Rabinowitz I, Baruch Y, Barak Y. 2008. High-dose escitalopram for the treatment of obsessive-compulsive disorder. International Clinical Psychopharmacology, 23: 49–53.

Rachman S. 1991. Neo-conditioning and the classical theory of fear acquisition. Clinical Psychology Review, 11: 155–173.

Rachman S. 2002. A cognitive theory of compulsive checking. Behaviour Research and Therapy, 40: 625–639.

Rachman SJ. 1997. A cognitive theory of obsessions. Behaviour Research and Therapy, 35: 793–802.

Rachman SJ. 1998. A cognitive theory of obsessions: Elaborations. Behaviour Research and Therapy, 36: 385–401.

Rachman SJ, Hodgson RJ. 1980. Obsessions and Compulsions. Englewood Cliffs, NJ: Prentice-Hall.

Rachman S, Lopatka C, Levitt K. 1988. Experimental analyses of panic: II. Panic patients. Behaviour Research and Therapy, 26: 33–40.

Radomsky AS, Rachman S. 1999. Memory bias in obsessive-compulsive disorder (OCD). Behaviour Research and Therapy, 37: 605–618.

Radomsky AS, Rachman S, Teachman BA, et al. 1998. Why do episodes of panic stop? Journal of Anxiety Disorders, 12: 263–270.

Raguram R, Bhide AY. 1985. Patterns of phobic neurosis: A retrospective study. British Journal of Psychiatry, 147: 557–560.

Rajkumar RP, Reddy YCJ, Kandavel T. 2008. Clinical profile of "schizo-obsessive" disorder: A comparative study. Comprehensive Psychiatry, 49: 262–268.

Ralevski E, Sanislow CA, Grilo CM, et al. 2005. Avoidant personality disorder and social phobia: Distinct enough to be separate disorders? Acta Psychiatrica Scandinavica, 112: 208–214.

Ramesh C, Yeragani VK, Balon R, et al. 1991. A comparative study of immune status in panic disorder patients and controls. Acta Psychiatrica Scandinavica, 84: 396–397.

Randall CL, Johnson MR, Thevos AK, et al. 2001. Paroxetine for social anxiety and alcohol use in dual-diagnosed patients. Depression and Anxiety, 14: 255–262.

Rapee RM. 1985. Distinctions between panic disorder and generalised anxiety disorder: Clinical presentations. Australian and New Zealand Journal of Psychiatry, 19: 227–232.

Rapee RM. 1991. Generalized anxiety disorder: A review of clinical features and theoretical concepts. Clinical Psychology Review, 11: 419–440.

Rapee RM. 1997. Potential role of childrearing practices in the development of anxiety and depression. Clinical Psychology Review, 17: 47–67.

Rapee RM, Craske MG, Barlow DH. 1990a. Subject-described features of panic attacks using self-monitoring. Journal of Anxiety Disorders, 4: 171–181.

Rapee RM, Heimberg RG. 1997. A cognitive-behavioral model of anxiety in social phobia. Behaviour Research and Therapy, 35: 741–756.

Rapee RM, Lim L. 1992. Discrepancy between self and observer ratings of performance in social phobics. Journal of Abnormal Psychology, 101: 727–731.

Rapee RM, Litwin EM, Barlow DH. 1990b. Impact of life events on subjects with panic disorder and on comparison subjects. American Journal of Psychiatry, 147: 640–644.

Rapee RM, Murrell E. 1988. Predictors of agoraphobic avoidance. Journal of Anxiety Disorders, 2: 203–217.

Raskin M, Peeke HVS, Dickman W, et al. 1982. Panic and generalized anxiety disorders: Developmental antecedents and precipitants. Archives of General Psychiatry, 39: 687–689.

Raskind MA, Peskind ER, Kanter ED, et al. 2003. Reduction of nightmares and other PTSD symptoms in combat veterans by prazosin: A placebo-controlled study. American Journal of Psychiatry, 160: 371–373.

Rasmussen SA. 1994. Obsessive compulsive spectrum disorders. Journal of Clinical Psychiatry, 55: 89–91.

Rasmussen SA, Eisen JL. 1988. Clinical and epidemiologic findings of significance to neuropharmacologic trials in OCD. Psychopharmacology Bulletin, 24: 466–470.

Rasmussen SA, Eisen JL. 1990. Epidemiology of obsessive-compulsive disorder. Journal of Clinical Psychiatry, 51 (Suppl. 2): 10–13.

Rasmussen SA, Eisen JL. 1991. Phenomenology of obsessive-compulsive disorder: Clinical subtypes, heterogeneity and coexistence. In Zohar J, Insel T, Rasmussen S, editors: Psychobiology of Obsessive- Compulsive Disorder. New York: Springer-Verlag, pp. 743–758.

Rasmussen SA, Eisen JL. 1992. The epidemiology and clinical features of obsessive-compulsive disorder. Psychiatric Clinics of North America, 15: 743–758.

Rasmussen S, Hackett E, DuBoff E, et al. 1997. A 2-year study of sertraline in the treatment of obsessive-compulsive disorder. International Clinical Psychopharmacology, 12: 309–316.

Rasmussen SA, Tsuang MT. 1986. DSM-III obsessive-compulsive disorder: Clinical characteristics and family history. American Journal of Psychiatry, 143: 317–322.

Rassin E, Merckelbach H, Muris P. 2000. Paradoxical and less paradoxical effects of thought suppression: A critical review. Clinical Psychology Review, 20: 973–995.

Rauch SL, Jenike MA 1993. Neurobiological models of obsessive-compulsive disorder. Psychosomatics, 34: 20–32.

Rauch SL, Jenike MA, Alpert NM, et al. 1994. Regional cerebral blood flow measured during symptom provocation in obsessive-compulsive disorder using oxygen 15-labeled carbon dioxide and positron emission tomography. Archives of General Psychiatry, 51: 62–70.

Rauch SL, van der Kolk BA, Fisler RE, et al. 1996. A symptom provocation study of posttraumatic stress disorder using positron emission tomography and script-driven imagery. Archives of General Psychiatry, 53: 380–387.

Ravizza L, Barzega G, Bellino S, et al. 1995. Predictors of drug treatment response in obsessive-compulsive disorder. Journal of Clinical Psychiatry, 56: 368–373.

Redmond DE. 1979. New and old evidence for the involvement of a brain norepinephrine system in anxiety. In Fann WE, Karacan I, Pokorny AD, et al., editors: Phenomenology and Treatment of Anxiety. New York: Spectrum Press, pp. 153–203.

Regier DA, Boyd JH, Burke JD, et al. 1988. One-month prevalence of mental disorders in the United States based on five Epidemiologic Catchment Area sites. Archives of General Psychiatry, 45: 977–986.

Regier DA, Narrow WE, Rae DS. 1990. The epidemiology of anxiety disorders: The Epidemiologic Catchment Area (ECA) experience. Journal of Psychiatric Research, 24: 3–14.

Regier DA, Rae DS, Narrow WE, et al. 1998. Prevalence of anxiety disorders and their comorbidity with mood and addictive disorders. British Journal of Psychiatry, 173 (Suppl. 34): 24–28.

Reich DB, Winternitz S, Hennen J, et al. 2004. A preliminary study of risperidone in the treatment pf posttraumatic stress disorder related to childhood abuse in women. Journal of Clinical Psychiatry, 65: 1601–1606.

Reich J. 2000. The relationship of social phobia to avoidant personality disorder: A proposal to reclassify avoidant personality disorder based on clinical empirical findings. European Psychiatry, 15: 151–159.

Reich J, Goldenberg I, Vasile R, et al. 1994. A prospective follow-along study of the course of social phobia. Psychiatry Research, 54: 249–258.

Reich J, Noyes R, Yates W. 1988. Anxiety symptoms distinguishing social phobia from panic and generalized anxiety disorders. Journal of Nervous and Mental Disease, 176: 510–513.

Reich J, Troughton E. 1988. Frequency of DSM-III personality disorders in patients with panic disorder: Comparison with psychiatric and normal control subjects. Psychiatry Research, 26: 89–100.

Reich J, Yates W. 1988. Family history of psychiatric disorders in social phobia. Comprehensive Psychiatry, 29: 72–75.

Reichborn-Kjennerud T, Czajkowski N, Torgersen S, et al. 2007. The relationship between avoidant personality disorder and social phobia: A population-based twin study. American Journal of Psychiatry, 164: 1722–1728.

Reiss S. 1991. Expectancy model of fear, anxiety, and panic. Clinical Psychology Review, 11: 141–153.

Reiss S, McNally RJ. 1985. Expectancy model of fear. In Reiss S, Bootzin RR, editors: Theoretical Issues in Behavioral Therapy. San Diego: Academic Press, pp. 107–121.

Reiss S, Peterson RA, Gursky DM. et al. 1986. Anxiety sensitivity, anxiety frequency and the prediction of fearfulness. Behaviour Research and Therapy, 24: 1–8.

Resick PA, Nishith P, Weaver TL, et al. 2002. A comparison of cognitive-processing therapy with prolonged exposure and a waiting condition for the treatment of chronic posttraumatic stress disorder in female rape victims. Journal of Consulting and Clinical Psychology, 70: 867–879.

Resnick PJ. 2003. Guidelines for evaluation of malingering in PTSD. In Simon RI, editor: Posttraumatic Stress Disorder in Litigation: Guidelines for Forensic Assessment, 2nd Edition. Washington, DC: American Psychiatric Press, pp. 187–205.

Ressler KJ, Rothbaum BO, Tannenbaum L, et al. 2004. Cognitive enhancers as adjuncts to psychotherapy: Use of D-cycloserine in phobic individuals to facilitate extinction of fear. Archives of General Psychiatry, 61: 1136–1144.

Rickels K, Downing R, Schweizer E, et al. 1993. Antidepressants for the treatment of generalized anxiety disorder: A placebo-controlled comparison of imipramine, trazodone, and diazepam. Archives of General Psychiatry, 50: 884–895.

Rickels K, Mangano R, Khan A. 2004. A double-blind, placebo-controlled study of a flexible dose of venlafaxine ER in adult outpatients with generalized social anxiety disorder. Journal of Clinical Psychopharmacology, 24: 488–496.

Rickels K, Pollack MH, Feltner DE, et al. 2005. Pregabalin for treatment of generalized anxiety disorder: A 4-week, multicenter, double-blind, placebo-controlled trial of pregabalin and alprazolam. Archives of General Psychiatry, 62: 1022–1030.

Rickels K, Pollack MH, Sheehan DV, et al. 2000. Efficacy of extended-release venlafaxine in nondepressed outpatients with generalized anxiety disorder. American Journal of Psychiatry, 157: 968–974.

Rickels K, Rynn MA. 2001. What is generalized anxiety disorder? Journal of Clinical Psychiatry, 62 (Suppl. 11): 4–12.

Rickels K, Schweizer E, DeMartinis N, et al. 1997. Gepirone and diazepam in generalized anxiety disorder: A placebo-controlled trial. Journal of Clinical Psychopharmacology, 17: 272–277.

Rickels K, Wiseman K, Norstad N, et al. 1982. Buspirone and diazepam in anxiety: A controlled study. Journal of Clinical Psychiatry, 43: 81–86.

Rickels K, Zaninelli R, McCafferty J, et al. 2003. Paroxetine treatment of generalized anxiety disorder: A double-blind, placebo-controlled study. American Journal of Psychiatry, 160: 749–756.

Riddle MA, Scahill L, King R, et al. 1990. Obsessive compulsive disorder in children and adolescents. Journal of the American Academy of Child and Adolescent Psychiatry, 29: 766–772.

Risse SC, Whitters A, Burke J, et al. 1990. Severe withdrawal symptoms after discontinuation of alprazolam in eight patients with combat-induced posttraumatic stress disorder. Journal of Clinical Psychiatry, 51: 206–209.

Robins LN, Regier DA. 1991. Psychiatric Disorders in America. New York: Macmillan.

Rocca P, Fonzo V, Scotta M, et al. 1997. Paroxetine efficacy in the treatment of generalized anxiety disorder. Acta Psychiatrica Scandinavica, 95: 444–450.

Rogers MP, Warshaw MG, Goisman RM, et al. 1999. Comparing primary and secondary generalized anxiety disorder in a long-term naturalistic study of anxiety disorders. Depression and Anxiety, 10: 1–7.

Romano S, Goodman W, Tamura R, et al. 2001. Long-term treatment of obsessive-compulsive disorder after an acute response: A comparison of fluoxetine versus placebo. Journal of Clinical Psychopharmacology, 21: 46–52.

Rosa-Alcázar AI, Sánchez-Meca J, Gómez-Conesa A, et al. 2008. Psychological treatment of obsessive-compulsive disorder: A meta-analysis. Clinical Psychology Review, 28: 1310–1325.

Rosario-Campos MC, Leckman JF, Mercadante MT, et al. 2001. Adults with early-onset obsessive-compulsive disorder. American Journal of Psychiatry, 158: 1899–1903.

Rose S, Bisson J. 1998. Brief early psychological interventions following trauma: A systematic review of the literature. Journal of Traumatic Stress, 11: 697–710.

Rose S, Bisson J, Wessely S. 2003. A systematic review of single-session psychological interventions ("debriefing") following trauma. Psychotherapy and Psychosomatics, 72: 176–184.

Rosen GM. 2004. Litigation and reported rates of posttraumatic stress disorder. Personality and Individual Differences, 36: 1291–1294.

Rosen GM, Lilienfeld SO. 2008. Posttraumatic stress disorder: An empirical evaluation of core assumptions. Clinical Psychology Review, 28: 837–868.

Rosen GM, Spitzer RL, McHugh PR. 2008. Problems with the post-traumatic stress disorder diagnosis and its future in DSM-V. British Journal of Psychiatry, 192: 3–4.

Rosen GM, Taylor S. 2007. Pseudo-PTSD. Journal of Anxiety Disorders, 21: 201–210.

Rosenbaum JF, Biederman J, Gersten M, et al. 1988. Behavioral inhibition in children of parents with panic disorder and agoraphobia: A controlled study. Archives of General Psychiatry, 45: 463–470.

Rosenbaum JF, Biederman J, Hirshfeld DR, et al. 1991. Further evidence of an association between behavioral inhibition and anxiety disorders: Results from a family study of children from a non-clinical sample. Journal of Psychiatric Research, 25: 49–65.

Rosenbaum JF, Moroz G, Bowden CL. 1997. Clonazepam in the treatment of panic disorder with or without agoraphobia: A dose-response study of efficacy, safety, and discontinuance. Journal of Clinical Psychopharmacology, 17: 390–400.

Rosenberg DR, Keshavan MS, O'Hearn KM, et al. 1997. Frontostriatal measurement in treatment-naive children with obsessive-compulsive disorder. Archives of General Psychiatry, 54: 824–830.

Rosenberg DR, MacMaster FP, Keshavan MS, et al. 2000. Decrease in caudate gluta-matergic concentrations in pediatric obsessive-compulsive disorder patients taking paroxetine. Journal of the American Academy of Child and Adolescent Psychiatry, 39: 1096–1103.

Roth D, Antony MM, Swinson RP. 2001. Interpretations for anxiety symptoms in social phobia. Behaviour Research and Therapy, 39: 129–138.

Rothbaum BO, Hodges L, Smith S, et al. 2000. A controlled study of virtual reality exposure therapy for the fear of flying. Journal of Consulting and Clinical Psychology, 68: 1020–1026.

Rothbaum BO, Killeen TK, Davidson JR, et al. 2008. Placebo-controlled trial of risperidone augmentation for selective serotonin reuptake inhibitor-resistant civilian posttraumatic stress disorder. Journal of Clinical Psychiatry, e1–e6.

Roy MA, Neale MC, Pedersen NL, et al. 1995. A twin study of generalized anxiety disorder and major depression. Psychological Medicine, 25: 1037–1049.

Roy-Byrne PP, Cowley DS, Greenblatt DJ, et al. 1990. Reduced benzodiazepine sensitivity in panic disorder. Archives of General Psychiatry, 47: 534–538.

Roy-Byrne PP, Craske MG, Stein MB, et al. 2005. A randomized effectiveness trial of cognitive-behavioral therapy and medication for primary care panic disorder. Archives of General Psychiatry, 62: 290–298.

Roy-Byrne PP, Geraci M, Uhde TW. 1986. Life events and the onset of panic disorder. American Journal of Psychiatry, 143: 1424–1427.

Rubio G, López-Ibor JJ. 2007. Generalized anxiety disorder: A 40-year follow-up study. Acta Psychiatrica Scandinavica, 115: 372–379.

Rück C, Karlsson A, Steele JD, et al. 2008. Capsulotomy for obsessive-compulsive disorder: Long-term follow-up of 25 patients. Archives of General Psychiatry, 65: 914–922.

Rufer M, Grothusen A, Mass R, et al. 2005. Temporal stability of symptom dimen-sions in adult patients with obsessive-compulsive disorder. Journal of Affective Disorders, 88: 99–102.

Ruscio AM. 2002. Delimiting the boundaries of generalized anxiety disorder: Differentiating high worriers with and without GAD. Journal of Anxiety Disorders, 16: 377–400.

Ruscio AM, Borkovec TD. 2004. Experience and appraisal of worry among high worriers with and without generalized anxiety disorder. Behaviour Research and Therapy, 42: 1469–1482.

Ruscio AM, Brown TA, Chiu WT, et al. 2008. Social fears and social phobia in the USA: Results from the National Comorbidity Survey Replication. Psychological Medicine, 38: 15–28.

Ruscio AM, Lane M, Roy-Byrne P, et al. 2005. Should excessive worry be required for a diagnosis of generalized anxiety disorder? Results from the US National Comorbidity Survey Replication. Psychological Medicine, 35: 1761–1772.

Ruscio AM, Weathers FW, King LA, et al. 2002. Male war-zone veterans' perceived relationships with their children: The importance of emotional numbing. Journal of Traumatic Stress, 15: 351–357.

Russell JL, Kushner MG, Beitman BD, et al. 1991. Nonfearful panic disorder in neurology patients validated by lactate challenge. American Journal of Psychiatry, 148: 361–364.

Rynn M, Khalid-Khan S, Garcia-Espana JF, et al. 2006. Early response and 8- week treatment outcome in GAD. Depression and Anxiety, 23: 461– 465.

Rynn M, Russell J, Erickson J, et al. 2008. Efficacy and safety of duloxetine in the treatment of generalized anxiety disorder: A flexible-dose, progressive-titration, placebo-controlled trial. Depression and Anxiety, 25: 182–189.

Sachdev P, Hay P. 1995. Does neurosurgery for obsessive-compulsive disorder produce personality change? Journal of Nervous and Mental Disease, 183: 408–413.

Sachdev PS, McBride R, Loo CK, et al. 2001. Right versus left prefrontal transcranial magnetic stimulation for obsessive-compulsive disorder: A preliminary investigation. Journal of Clinical Psychiatry, 62: 981–984.

Sack M, Lahmann C, Jaeger B, et al. 2007. Trauma prevalence and somatoform symptoms: Are there specific somatoform symptoms related to traumatic experiences? Journal of Nervous and Mental Disease, 195: 928–933.

Sack WH, McSharry S, Clarke GN, et al. 1994. The Khmer Adolescent Project: I. Epidemiologic findings in two generations of Cambodian refugees. Journal of Nervous and Mental Disease, 182: 387–395.

Salaberria K, Echeburua E. 1998. Long-term outcome of cognitive therapy's contribution to self-exposure in vivo to the treatment of generalized social phobia. Behavior Modification, 22: 262–284.

Salkovskis PM. 1985. Obsessional-compulsive problems: A cognitive-behavioural analysis. Behaviour Research and Therapy, 23: 571–583.

Salkovskis PM. 1989. Cognitive-behavioural factors and the persistence of intrusive thoughts in obsessional problems. Behaviour Research and Therapy, 27: 677–682.

Salkovskis PM. 1996. Cognitive-behavioral approaches to the understanding of obsessional problems. In Rapee RM, editor: Current Controversies in the Anxiety Disorders. New York: Guilford Press, pp. 103–133.

Salkovskis PM. 1999. Understanding and treating obsessive-compulsive disorder. Behaviour Research and Therapy, 37 (Suppl. 1): S29–S52.

Salkovskis PM, Clark DM. 1993. Panic disorder and hypochondriasis. Advances in Behaviour Research and Therapy, 15: 23–48.

Salkovskis P, Shafran R, Rachman S, et al. 1999. Multiple pathways to inflated responsibility beliefs in obsessional problems: Possible origins and implications for therapy and research. Behaviour Research and Therapy, 37: 1055–1072.

Salvador-Carulla L, Segui J, Fernandez-Cano P, et al. 1995. Costs and offset effect in panic disorders. British Journal of Psychiatry, 166 (Suppl. 27): 23–28.

Salzman C, Miyawaki EK, le Bars P, et al. 1993. Neurobiologic basis of anxiety and its treatment. Harvard Review of Psychiatry, 1: 197–206.

Salzman L. 1968. The Obsessive Personality: Origins, Dynamics, and Therapy. New York: Science House.

Samuels JF, Bienvenu OJ, Pinto A, et al. 2007. Hoarding in obsessive-compulsive disorder: Results from the OCD Collaborative Genetics Study. Behaviour Research and Therapy, 45: 673–686.

Sanavio E. 1988. Obsessions and compulsions: The Padua Inventory. Behaviour Research and Therapy, 26: 169–177.

Sanderson W, Rapee R, Barlow D. 1989. The influence of an illusion of control on panic attacks induced via inhalation of 5.5% carbon dioxide-enriched air. Archives of General Psychiatry, 46: 157–162.

Sanderson WC, DiNardo PA, Rapee RM, et al. 1990. Syndrome comorbidity in patients diagnosed with a DSM-III-R anxiety disorder. Journal of Abnormal Psychology, 99: 308–312.

Sapolsky RM. 1995. Why stress is bad for your brain. Science, 273: 749–750.

Sareen J, Cox BJ, Afifi TO, et al. 2005. Anxiety disorders and risk for suicidal ideation and suicide attempts: A population-based longitudinal study of adults. Archives of General Psychiatry, 62: 1249–1257.

Scheibe G, Albus M. 1994. Prospective follow-up study lasting 2 years in patients with panic disorder with and without depressive disorders. European Archives of Psychiatry and Clinical Neuroscience, 244: 39–44.

Scher CD, Stein MB. 2003. Developmental antecedents of anxiety sensitivity. Journal of Anxiety Disorders, 17: 253–269.

Schlenker B, Leary M. 1982. Social anxiety and self-presentation: A conceptualization and model. Psychological Bulletin, 92: 641–669.

Schmidt NB, Lerew DR, Jackson RJ. 1997. The role of anxiety sensitivity in the pathogenesis of panic: Prospective evaluation of spontaneous panic attacks during acute stress. Journal of Abnormal Psychology, 106: 355–364.

Schmidt NB, Lerew DR, Jackson RJ. 1999. Prospective evaluation of anxiety sensitivity in the pathogenesis of panic: Replication and extension. Journal of Abnormal Psychology, 108: 532–537.

Schneier F, Liebowitz MR, Abi-Dargham A, et al. 2000. Low dopamine D2 binding potential in social phobia. American Journal of Psychiatry, 157: 457–459.

Schneier FR, Goetz D, Campeas R, et al. 1998. Placebo-controlled trial of moclobemide in social phobia. British Journal of Psychiatry, 172: 70–77.

Schneier FR, Johnson J, Hornig CD, et al. 1992. Social phobia: Comorbidity and morbidity in an epidemiological sample. Archives of General Psychiatry, 49: 282–288.

Schneier FR, Martin LY, Liebowitz MR, et al. 1989. Alcohol abuse in social phobia. Journal of Anxiety Disorders, 3: 15–23.

Schneier FR, Spitzer RL, Gibbon M, et al. 1991. The relationship of social phobia subtypes and avoidant personality disorder. Comprehensive Psychiatry, 32: 496–502.

Schnurr PP, Friedman MJ, Foy DW, et al. 2003. Randomized trial of trauma-focused group therapy for posttraumatic stress disorder: Results from a Department of Veterans Affairs Cooperative Study. Archives of General Psychiatry, 60: 481–489.

Schnyder U, Moergeli H, Klaghofer R, et al. 2001. Incidence and prediction of posttraumatic stress disorder symptoms in severely injured accident victims. American Journal of Psychiatry, 158: 594–599.

Scholing A, Emmelkamp PMG. 1996. Treatment of generalized social phobia: Results at long-term follow-up. Behaviour Research and Therapy, 34: 447–452.

Schwab-Stone M, Ayers T, Kasprow W, et al. 1995. No safe haven: A study of violence exposure in an urban community. Journal of the American Academy of Child and Adolescent Psychiatry, 34: 1343–1352.

Schwartz JM, Stoessel PW, Baxter LR, et al. 1996. Systematic changes in cerebral glucose metabolic rate after successful behavior modification treatment of obsessive-compulsive disorder. Archives of General Psychiatry, 53: 109–113.

Schweizer E, Rickels K, Lucki I. 1986. Resistance to the anti-anxiety effect of buspirone in patients with a history of benzodiazepine use. New England Journal of Medicine, 314: 719–720.

Schweizer E, Rickels K, Weiss S, et al. 1993. Maintenance drug treatment of panic disorder: I. Results of a prospective, placebo-controlled comparison of alprazolam and imipramine. Archives of General Psychiatry, 50: 51–60.

Scott MJ, Stradling SG. 1994. Post-traumatic stress disorder without the trauma. British Journal of Clinical Psychology, 33: 71–74.

Scrignar CB. 1984. Post-Traumatic Stress Disorder: Diagnosis, Treatment, and Legal Issues. New York: Praeger.

Seedat S, Stein DJ, Emsley RA. 2000. Open trial of citalopram in adults with post-traumatic stress disorder. International Journal of Neuropsychopharmacology, 3: 135–140.

Seedat S, Stein MB. 2004. Double-blind, placebo-controlled assessment of combined clonazepam with paroxetine compared with paroxetine monotherapy for generalized social anxiety disorder. Journal of Clinical Psychiatry, 65: 244–248.

Segerstrom SC, Tsao JCI, Alden LE, et al. 2000. Worry and rumination: Repetitive thought as a concomitant and predictor of negative mood. Cognitive Therapy and Research, 24: 671–688.

Seidler GH, Wagner FE. 2006. Comparing the efficacy of EMDR and trauma- focused cognitive-behavioral therapy in the treatment of PTSD: A meta-analytic study. Psychological Medicine, 36: 1515–1522.

Seligman MEP. 1971. Phobias and preparedness. Behavior Therapy, 2: 307–320.

Sepede G, De Berardis D, Gambi F et al. 2006. Olanzapine augmentation in treatment-resistant panic disorder: A 12-week, fixed-dose, open-label trial. Journal of Clinical Psychopharmacology, 26: 45–49.

Sevy S, Papadimitriou G, Surmont W, et al. 1989. Noradrenergic function in generalized anxiety disorder, major depressive disorder, and healthy subjects. Biological Psychiatry, 25: 141–152.

Shafran R, Thordarson DS, Rachman S. 1996. Thought-action fusion in obsessive compulsive disorder. Journal of Anxiety Disorders, 10: 379–391.

Shalev A, Rogel-Fuchs Y. 1992. Auditory startle reflex in post-traumatic stress disorder patients treated with clonazepam. Israel Journal of Psychiatry and Related Sciences, 29: 1–6.

Shalev AY, Bleich A, Ursano RJ. 1990. Posttraumatic stress disorder: Somatic comorbidity and effort tolerance. Psychosomatics, 31: 197–203.

Shalev AY, Freedman S, Brandes D, et al. 1997. Predicting PTSD in civilian trauma survivors: Prospective evaluation of self report and clinician administered instruments. British Journal of Psychiatry, 170: 558–564.

Shalev AY, Freedman S, Peri T, et al. 1998a. Prospective study of posttraumatic stress disorder and depression following trauma. American Journal of Psychiatry, 155: 630–637.

Shalev AY, Peri T, Canetti L, et al. 1996. Predictors of PTSD in injured trauma survivors: A prospective study. American Journal of Psychiatry, 153: 219–225.

Shalev AY, Sahar T, Freedman S, et al. 1998b. A prospective study of heart rate response following trauma and the subsequent development of posttraumatic stress disorder. Archives of General Psychiatry, 55: 553–559.

Shapiro AK, Shapiro E. 1992. Evaluation of the reported association of obsessive-compulsive symptoms or disorder with Tourette's disorder. Comprehensive Psychiatry, 33: 152–165.

Shapiro D. 1965. Neurotic Styles. New York: Basic Books.

Shapiro F. 1995. Eye Movement Desensitization and Reprocessing: Basic Principles, Protocols, and Procedures. New York: Guilford Press.

Shavitt RG, Gentil V, Mandetta R. 1992. The association of panic/agoraphobia and asthma: Contributing factors and clinical implications. General Hospital Psychiatry, 14: 420–423.

Shear K, Belnap BH, Mazumdar S, et al. 2006. Generalized Anxiety Disorder Severity Scale (GADSS): A preliminary validation study. Depression and Anxiety, 23: 77–82.

Shear MK, Brown TA, Barlow DH, et al. 1997. Multicenter Collaborative Panic Disorder Severity Scale. American Journal of Psychiatry, 154: 1571–1575.

Shear MK, Cooper AM, Klerman GL, et al. 1993. A psychodynamic model of panic disorder. American Journal of Psychiatry, 150: 859–866.

Sheehan DV, Ballenger J, Jacobson G. 1980. Treatment of endogenous anxiety with phobic, hysterical and hypochondriacal symptoms. Archives of General Psychiatry, 37: 51–59.

Sheehan D, Janavs J, Baker R, et al. 2000. The Worry-Anxiety-Tension Scale. Adapted from the M.I.N.I. International Neuropsychiatric Interview. Tampa FL: University of South Florida.

Sheeran T, Zimmerman M. 2002. Social phobia: Still a neglected anxiety disorder? Journal of Nervous and Mental Disease, 190: 786–788.

Shetti CN, Reddy YCJ, Kandavel T, et al. 2005. Clinical predictors of drug nonresponse in obsessive-compulsive disorder. Journal of Clinical Psychiatry, 66: 1517–1523.

Shin LM, Kosslyn SM, McNally RJ, et al. 1997. Visual imagery and perception in posttraumatic stress disorder: A positron emission tomographic investigation. Archives of General Psychiatry, 54: 233–241.

Shin LM, McNally RJ, Kosslyn SM, et al. 1999. Regional cerebral blood flow during script-driven imagery in childhood sexual abuse-related PTSD: A PET investigation. American Journal of Psychiatry, 156: 575–584.

Shore JH, Tatum E, Vollmer WM. 1986. Psychiatric reactions to disaster: The Mt. St. Helen's experience. American Journal of Psychiatry, 143: 590–595.

Silove D, Manicavasagar V, O'Connell D, et al. 1993. Reported early separation anxiety symptoms in patients with panic and generalized anxiety disorders. Australian and New Zealand Journal of Psychiatry, 27: 489–494.

Silove D, Manicavasagar V, O'Connell D, et al. 1995. Genetic factors in early separation anxiety: Implications for the genesis of adult anxiety disorders. Acta Psychiatrica Scandinavica, 92: 17–24.

Silove D, Parker G, Hadzi-Pavlovic D, et al. 1991. Parental representations of patients with panic disorder and generalized anxiety disorder. British Journal of Psychiatry, 159: 835–841.

Simon NM, Safren SA, Otto MW, et al. 2002. Longitudinal outcome with pharmacotherapy in a naturalistic study of panic disorder. Journal of Affective Disorders, 69: 201–208.

Simpson HB, Foa EB, Liebowitz MR, et al. 2008. A randomized, controlled trial of cognitive-behavioral therapy for augmenting pharmacotherapy in obsessive-compulsive disorder. American Journal of Psychiatry, 165: 621–630.

Simpson HB, Gorfinkle KS, Liebowitz MR. 1999. Cognitive-behavioral therapy as an adjunct to serotonin reuptake inhibitors in obsessive-compulsive disorder: An open trial. Journal of Clinical Psychiatry, 60: 584–590.

Skapinakis P, Papatheodorou T, Mavreas V. 2007. Antipsychotic augmentation of serotonergic antidepressants in treatment-resistant obsessive-compulsive disorder: A meta-analysis of the randomized controlled trials. European Neuropsychopharmacology, 17: 79–93.

Skoog G, Skoog I. 1999. A 40-year follow-up of patients with obsessive-compulsive disorder. Archives of General Psychiatry, 56: 121–127.

Skre I, Ontad S, Torgersen S, et al. 1993. A twin study of DSM-III-R anxiety disorders. Acta Psychiatrica Scandinavica, 88: 85–92.

Slade T, Watson D. 2006. The structure of common DSM-IV and ICD-10 mental disorders in the Australian general population. Psychological Medicine, 36: 1593–1600.

Smail P, Stockwell T, Canter S, et al. 1984. Alcohol dependence and phobic anxiety states. British Journal of Psychiatry, 144: 53–57.

Smith K, Bryant RA. 2000. The generality of cognitive bias in acute stress disorder. Behaviour Research and Therapy, 38: 709–715.

Smits JAJ, Telch MJ, Randall PK. 2002. An examination of the decline in fear and disgust during exposure-based treatment. Behaviour Research and Therapy, 40: 1243–1253.

Smoller JW, Pollack MH, Wassertheil-Smoller S, et al. 2007. Panic attacks and risk of incident cardiovascular events among postmenopausal women in the Women's Health Initiative Observational Study. Archives of General Psychiatry, 64: 1153–1160.

Solomon Z, Benbenishty R, Mikulincer M. 1991. The contribution of wartime, pre-war, and post-war factors to self-efficacy: A longitudinal study of combat stress reaction. Journal of Traumatic Stress, 4: 345–361.

Solomon Z, Kotler M, Shalev A, et al. 1989a. Delayed post-traumatic stress disorder. Psychiatry, 52: 428–436.

Solomon Z, Mikulincer M, Benbenishty R. 1989b. Locus of control and combat-related post-traumatic stress disorder: The intervening role of battle intensity, threat appraisal, and coping. British Journal of Clinical Psychology, 28: 131–144.

Somers JM, Goldner EM, Waraich P, et al. 2006. Prevalence and incidence studies of anxiety disorders: A systematic review of the literature. Canadian Journal of Psychiatry, 51: 100–113.

Southwick SM, Krystal JH, Bremner JD, et al. 1997. Noradrenergic and serotonergic function in posttraumatic stress disorder. Archives of General Psychiatry, 54: 749–758.

Southwick SM, Krystal JH, Morgan CA, et al. 1993. Abnormal noradrenergic function in posttraumatic stress disorder. Archives of General Psychiatry, 50: 266–274.

Spiegel DA, Bruce TJ. 1997. Benzodiazepines and exposure-based cognitive behavior therapies for panic disorder: Conclusions from combined treatment trials. American Journal of Psychiatry, 154: 773–781.

Spiegel DA, Bruce TJ, Gregg SF, et al. 1994. Does cognitive behavior therapy assist slow-taper alprazolam discontinuation in panic disorder? American Journal of Psychiatry, 151: 876–881.

Spitzer RL, First MB, Wakefield JC. 2007. Saving PTSD from itself in DSM-V. Journal of Anxiety Disorders, 21: 233–241.

Staab JP, Grieger TA, Fullerton CS, et al. 1996. Acute stress disorder, subsequent posttraumatic stress disorder and depression after a series of typhoons. Anxiety, 2: 219–225.

Stahl SM, Gergel I, Li D. 2003. Escitalopram in the treatment of panic disorder: A randomized, double-blind, placebo-controlled trial. Journal of Clinical Psychiatry, 64: 1322–1327.

Stangier U, Heidenreich T, Peitz M, et al. 2003. Cognitive therapy for social phobia: Individual versus group treatment. Behaviour Research and Therapy, 41: 991–1007.

Starcevic V. 1992. Comorbidity models of panic disorder/agoraphobia and personality disturbance. Journal of Personality Disorders, 6: 213–225.

Starcevic V. 1995. Pathological worry in major depression: A preliminary report. Behaviour Research and Therapy, 33: 55–56.

Starcevic V. 1998. Treatment goals for panic disorder. Journal of Clinical Psychopharmacology, 18 (Suppl. 2): 19S–26S.

Starcevic V. 2007. The conceptual validity of panic disorder and agoraphobia. In: Castle D, Hood S, Kyrios M, editors: Anxiety Disorders: Current

Controversies, Future Directions. Melbourne: Australian Postgraduate Medicine, pp. 1–10.

Starcevic V. 2008. Anxiety disorders no more? Australasian Psychiatry, 16: 317–321.

Starcevic V, Berle D, Milicevic D, et al. 2007. Pathological worry, anxiety disorders and the impact of co-occurrence with depressive and other anxiety disorders. Journal of Anxiety Disorders, 21: 1016–1027.

Starcevic V, Bogojevic G. 1997. Comorbidity of panic disorder with agoraphobia and specific phobia: Relationship with the subtypes of specific phobia. Comprehensive Psychiatry, 38: 315–320.

Starcevic V, Bogojevic G. 1999. The concept of generalized anxiety disorder: Between the too narrow and too wide diagnostic criteria. Psychopathology, 32: 5–11.

Starcevic V, Brakoulias V. 2008. Symptom subtypes of obsessive-compulsive disorder: Are they relevant for treatment? Australian and New Zealand Journal of Psychiatry, 42: 651–661.

Starcevic V, Eric Lj, Kelin K, et al. 1994b. The structure of discrete social phobias. European Journal of Psychiatry, 8: 140–148.

Starcevic V, Fallon S, Uhlenhuth EH. 1994a. The frequency and severity of generalized anxiety disorder symptoms: Toward a less cumbersome conceptualization. Journal of Nervous and Mental Disease, 182: 80–84.

Starcevic V, Kellner R, Uhlenhuth EH, et al. 1992a. Panic disorder and hypochondriacal fears and beliefs. Journal of Affective Disorders, 24: 73–85.

Starcevic V, Kellner R, Uhlenhuth EH, et al. 1993a. The phenomenology of panic attacks in panic disorder with and without agoraphobia. Comprehensive Psychiatry, 34: 36–41.

Starcevic V, Kolar D, Latas M, et al. 2002. Panic disorder patients at the time of air strikes. Depression and Anxiety, 16: 152–156.

Starcevic V, Linden M, Uhlenhuth EH, et al. 2004. Treatment of panic disorder with agoraphobia in an anxiety disorders clinic: Factors influencing psychiatrists' treatment choices. Psychiatry Research, 125: 41–52.

Starcevic V, Uhlenhuth EH, Kellner R, et al. 1992b. Patterns of comorbidity in panic disorder and agoraphobia. Psychiatry Research, 42: 171–183.

Starcevic V, Uhlenhuth EH, Kellner R, et al. 1993b. Comorbidity in panic disorder: II. Chronology of appearance and pathogenic comorbidity. Psychiatry Research, 46: 285–293.

Stein DJ. 2007. The Cape Town Consensus Statement on obsessive-compulsive disorder. International Journal of Psychiatry in Clinical Practice, 11 (Suppl. 2): 11–15.

Stein DJ, Andersen EW, Overo KF. 2007a. Response of symptom dimensions in obsessive-compulsive disorder to treatment with citalopram or placebo. Revista Brasileira de Psiquiatria, 29: 303–307.

Stein DJ, Andersen EW, Tonnoir B, et al. 2007b. Escitalopram in obsessive-compulsive disorder: A randomized, placebo-controlled, paroxetine-referenced, fixed-dose, 24-week study. Current Medical Research and Opinion, 23: 701–711.

Stein DJ, Baldwin DS, Baldinetti F, et al. 2008. Efficacy of pregabalin in depressive symptoms associated with generalized anxiety disorder: A pooled analysis of 6 studies. European Neuropsychopharmacology, 18: 422–430.

Stein DJ, Cameron A, Amrein R, et al. 2002a. Moclobemide is effective and well tolerated in the long-term pharmacotherapy of social anxiety disorder with or without comorbid anxiety disorder. International Clinical Psychopharmacology, 17: 161–170.

Stein DJ, Seedat S, Potocnik F. 1999. Hoarding: A review. Israel Journal of Psychiatry and Related Sciences, 36: 35–46.

Stein DJ, Spadaccini E, Hollander E. 1995. Meta-analysis of pharmacotherapy trials for obsessive-compulsive disorder. International Clinical Psychopharmacology, 10: 11–18.

Stein DJ, Stein MB, Pitts CD, et al. 2002b. Predictors of response to pharmacotherapy in social anxiety disorder: An analysis of 3 placebo-controlled paroxetine trials. Journal of Clinical Psychiatry, 63: 152–155.

Stein DJ, van der Kolk BA, Austin C, et al. 2006. Efficacy of sertraline in posttraumatic stress disorder secondary to interpersonal trauma or childhood abuse. Annals of Clinical Psychiatry, 18: 243–249.

Stein DJ, Versiani M, Hair T, et al. 2002c. Efficacy of paroxetine for relapse prevention in social anxiety disorder: A 24-week study. Archives of General Psychiatry, 59: 1111–1118.

Stein MB, Chartier MJ, Hazen AL, et al. 1998a. A direct-interview family study of generalized social phobia. American Journal of Psychiatry, 155: 90–97.

Stein MB, Forde DR, Anderson G, et al. 1997a. Obsessive-compulsive disorder in the community: An epidemiological study with clinical reappraisal. American Journal of Psychiatry, 154: 1120–1126.

Stein MB, Fuetsch M, Müller N, et al. 2001. Social anxiety disorder and the risk of depression: A prospective community study of adolescents and young adults. Archives of General Psychiatry, 58: 251–256.

Stein MB, Fyer AJ, Davidson JRT, et al. 1999b. Fluvoxamine treatment of social phobia (social anxiety disorder): A double-blind, placebo-controlled study. American Journal of Psychiatry, 156: 756–760.

Stein MB, Goldin PR, Sareen J, et al. 2002a. Increased amygdala activation to angry and contemptuous faces in generalized social phobia. Archives of General Psychiatry, 59: 1027–1034.

Stein MB, Heuser IJ, Juncos JL, et al. 1990a. Anxiety disorders in patients with Parkinson's disease. American Journal of Psychiatry, 147: 217–220.

Stein MB, Jang KJ, Livesley WJ. 1999a. Heritability of anxiety sensitivity: A twin study. American Journal of Psychiatry, 156: 246–251.

Stein MB, Kean YM. 2000. Disability and quality of life in social phobia: Epidemiologic findings. American Journal of Psychiatry, 157: 1606–1613.

Stein MB, Kline NA, Matloff JL. 2002b. Adjunctive olanzapine for SSRI-resistant combat-related PTSD: A double-blind, placebo-controlled study. American Journal of Psychiatry, 159: 1777–1779.

Stein MB, Liebowitz MR, Lydiard RB, et al. 1998b. Paroxetine treatment of generalized social phobia (social anxiety disorder): A randomized controlled trial. Journal of the American Medical Association, 280: 708–713.

Stein MB, Pollack MH, Bystritsky A, et al. 2005. Efficacy of low and higher dose extended-release venlafaxine in generalized social anxiety disorder: A 6-month randomized controlled trial. Psychopharmacology, 177: 280–288.

Stein MB, Tancer ME, Gelernter CS, et al. 1990b. Major depression in patients with social phobia. American Journal of Psychiatry, 147: 637–639.

Stein MB, Torgrud LJ, Walker JR. 2000. Social phobia symptoms, subtypes, and severity: Findings from a community survey. Archives of General Psychiatry, 57: 1046–1052.

Stein MB, Walker JR, Forde DR. 1994. Setting diagnostic thresholds for social phobia: Considerations from a community survey of social anxiety. American Journal of Psychiatry, 151: 408–412.

Stein MB, Walker JR, Hazen AL, et al. 1997b. Full and partial posttraumatic stress disorder: Findings from a community survey. American Journal of Psychiatry, 154: 1114–1119.

Steketee G, Eisen J, Dyck I, et al. 1999. Predictors of course in obsessive-compulsive disorder. Psychiatry Research, 89: 229–238.

Steketee G, Frost RO. 2006. Compulsive Hoarding and Acquiring: Therapist Guide. Oxford: Oxford University Press.

Stemberger RT, Turner SM, Beidel DC, et al. 1995. Social phobia: An analysis of possible developmental factors. Journal of Abnormal Psychology, 104: 526–531.

Stinson FS, Dawson DA, Chou SP, et al. 2007. The epidemiology of DSM-IV specific phobia in the USA: Results from the National Epidemiologic Survey on Alcohol and Related Conditions. Psychological Medicine, 37:1047–1059.

Stocchi F, Nordera G, Jokinen RH, et al. 2003. Efficacy and tolerability of paroxetine for the long-term treatment of generalized anxiety disorder. Journal of Clinical Psychiatry, 64: 250–258.

Stopa L, Clark DM. 1993. Cognitive processes in social phobia. Behaviour Research and Therapy, 31: 255–267.

Stopa L, Clark DM. 2000. Social phobia and interpretation of social events. Behaviour Research and Therapy, 38: 273–283.

Storch EA, Abramowitz J, Goodman WK. 2008. Where does obsessive-compulsive disorder belong in DSM-V? Depression and Anxiety, 25: 336–347.

Storch EA, Merlo LJ, Bengtson M, et al. 2007. D-cycloserine does not enhance exposure-response prevention therapy in obsessive-compulsive disorder. International Clinical Psychopharmacology, 22: 230–237.

Straube T, Mentzel HJ, Miltner WH. 2005. Common and distinct brain activation to threat and safety signals in social phobia. Neuropsychobiology, 52: 163–168.

Straube T, Mentzel HJ, Miltner WH. 2006. Neural mechanisms of automatic and direct processing of phobogenic stimuli in specific phobia. Biological Psychiatry, 59: 162–170.

Stravynski A, Lamontagne Y, Lavellee Y-J. 1986. Clinical phobias and avoidant personality disorder among alcoholics admitted to an alcoholism rehabilitation setting. Canadian Journal of Psychiatry, 31: 714–719.

Stravynski A, Marks I, Yule W. 1982. Social skills problems in neurotic outpatients: Social skills training with and without cognitive modification. Archives of General Psychiatry, 39: 1378–1385.

Struzik L, Vermani M, Duffin J, et al. 2004. Anxiety sensitivity as a predictor of panic attacks. Psychiatry Research, 129: 273–278.

Summerfeldt LJ. 2004. Understanding and treating incompleteness in obsessive-compulsive disorder. Journal of Clinical Psychology, 60: 1155–1168.

Summerfield D. 2004. Cross-cultural perspectives on the medicalization of human suffering. In Rosen GM, editor: Posttraumatic Stress Disorder: Issues and Controversies. New York: Wiley, pp. 233–244.

Suzuki K, Takei N, Kawai M, et al. 2003. Is taijin kyofusho a culture-bound syndrome? American Journal of Psychiatry, 160: 1358.

Swedo SE. 1994. Sydenham's chorea: A model for autoimmune neuropsychiatric disorders. Journal of the American Medical Association, 272: 1788–1791.

Swedo SE, Leonard HL, Garvey M, et al. 1998. Pediatric Autoimmune Neuropsychiatric Disorders Associated with Streptococcus Infection (PANDAS): Clinical description of the first 50 cases. American Journal of Psychiatry, 155: 264–271.

Swedo SE, Leonard HL, Kiessling LS. 1994. Speculations on antineuronal antibody-mediated neuropsychiatric disorders of childhood. Pediatrics, 93: 323–326.

Swedo SE, Rapoport JL, Leonard H, et al. 1989a. Obsessive compulsive disorder in children and adolescents: Clinical phenomenology of 70 consecutive cases. Archives of General Psychiatry, 46: 335–341.

Swedo SE, Schapiro MB, Grady CL, et al. 1989b. Cerebral glucose metabolism in childhood-onset obsessive-compulsive disorder. Archives of General Psychiatry, 46: 518–523.

Swoboda H, Amering M, Windhaber J, et al. 2003. The long-term course of panic disorder – An 11 year follow-up. Journal of Anxiety Disorders, 17: 223–232.

Szegedi A, Wetzel H, Leal M, et al. 1996. Combination treatment with clomipramine and fluvoxamine: Drug monitoring, safety, and tolerability data. Journal of Clinical Psychiatry, 57: 257–264.

Szeszko PR, Robinson D, Alvir JMJ, et al. 1999. Orbital frontal and amygdala volume reductions in obsessive-compulsive disorder. Archives of General Psychiatry, 56: 913–919.

Tarrier N, Pilgrim H, Sommerfield C, et al. 1999. A randomized trial of cognitive therapy and imaginal exposure in the treatment of chronic posttraumatic stress disorder. Journal of Consulting and Clinical Psychology, 67: 13–18.

Taylor F, Cahill L. 2002. Propranolol for reemergent posttraumatic stress disorder following an event of retraumatization: A case study. Journal of Traumatic Stress, 15: 433–437.

Taylor S. 1996. Meta-analysis of cognitive-behavioral treatment for social phobia. Journal of Behavior Therapy and Experimental Psychiatry, 27: 1–9.

Taylor S, Koch WJ, McNally RJ. 1992. How does anxiety sensitivity vary across the anxiety disorders? Journal of Anxiety Disorders, 6: 249–259.

Taylor S, Koch WJ, Woody S, et al. 1996. Anxiety sensitivity and depression: How are they related? Journal of Abnormal Psychology, 105: 474–479.

Taylor S, Thordarson DS, Maxfield L, et al. 2003. Comparative efficacy, speed, and adverse effects of three PTSD treatments: Exposure therapy, EMDR, and relaxation training. Journal of Consulting and Clinical Psychology, 71: 330–338.

Telch MJ, Agras WS, Taylor CB, et al. 1985. Combined pharmacological and behavioral treatment for agoraphobia. Behaviour Research and Therapy, 23: 325–335.

Telch MJ, Brouillard M, Telch CF, et al. 1989a. Role of cognitive appraisal in panic-related avoidance. Behaviour Research and Therapy, 27: 373–383.

Telch MJ, Lucas JA, Nelson P. 1989b. Nonclinical panic in college students: An investigation of prevalence and symptomatology. Journal of Abnormal Psychology, 98: 300–306.

Telch MJ, Lucas JA, Schmidt NB, et al. 1993. Group cognitive-behavioral treatment of panic disorder. Behaviour Research and Therapy, 31: 279–287.

Tesar GE, Rosenbaum JF, Pollack MH, et al. 1991. Double-blind, placebo-controlled comparison of clonazepam and alprazolam for panic disorder. Journal of Clinical Psychiatry, 52: 69–76.

Thayer JF, Friedman BH, Borkovec TD. 1996. Autonomic characteristics of generalized anxiety disorder and worry. Biological Psychiatry, 39: 255–266.

Thomas SE, Thevos AK, Randall CL. 1999. Alcoholics with and without social phobia: A comparison of substance use and psychiatric variables. Journal of Studies on Alcohol, 60: 472–479.

Thompson AH, Bland RC, Orn HT. 1989. Relationship and chronology of depression, agoraphobia, and panic disorder in the general population. Journal of Nervous and Mental Disease, 177: 456–463.

Thordarson DS, Radomsky AS, Rachman S, et al. 2004. The Vancouver Obsessional Compulsive Inventory (VOCI). Behaviour Research and Therapy, 42: 1289–1314.

Thoren P, Asberg M, Cronholm B, et al. 1980. Clomipramine treatment of obsessive-compulsive disorder: I. A controlled clinical trial. Archives of General Psychiatry, 37: 1281–1285.

Thorpe SJ, Salkovskis PM. 1995. Phobic beliefs: Do cognitive factors play a role in specific phobias? Behaviour Research and Therapy, 33: 805–816.

Thyer B, Himle J. 1985. Temporal relationship between panic attack onset and phobic avoidance in agoraphobia. Behaviour Research and Therapy, 23: 607–608.

Tiihonen J, Kuikka J, Rasanen P, et al. 1997. Cerebral benzodiazepine receptor binding and distribution in generalized anxiety disorder: A fractional analysis. Molecular Psychiatry, 2: 463–471.

Tiller JW, Biddle N, Maguire KP, et al. 1988. The dexamethasone suppression test and plasma dexamethasone in generalized anxiety disorder. Biological Psychiatry, 23: 261–270.

Tollefson GD, Rampey AH, Potvin JH, et al. 1994. A multicenter investigation of fixed-dose fluoxetine in the treatment of obsessive-compulsive disorder. Archives of General Psychiatry, 51: 559–567.

Tolin DF, Abramowitz JS, Brigidi BD, et al. 2003. Intolerance of uncertainty in obsessive-compulsive disorder. Journal of Anxiety Disorders, 17: 233–242.

Tolin DF, Lohr JM, Sawchuk CN, et al. 1997. Disgust and disgust sensitivity in blood-injection-injury and spider phobia. Behaviour Research and Therapy, 35: 949–953.

Toni C, Perugi G, Frare F, et al. 2000. A prospective naturalistic study of 326 panic-agoraphobic patients treated with antidepressants. Pharmacopsychiatry, 33: 121–131.

Torgersen S. 1983. Genetic factors in anxiety disorders. Archives of General Psychiatry, 40: 1085–1089.

Trower P, Yardley K, Bryant B, et al. 1978. The treatment of social failure: A comparison of anxiety-reduction and skills-acquisition procedures on two social problems. Behavior Modification, 2: 41–60.

True WR, Rice J, Eisen SA, et al. 1993. A twin study of genetic and environmental contributions to liability for posttraumatic stress symptoms. Archives of General Psychiatry, 50: 257–264.

Trull TJ, Nietzel MT, Main A. 1988. The use of meta-analysis to assess the clinical significance of behavior therapy for agoraphobia. Behavior Therapy, 19: 527–538.

Tsao S, McKay D. 2004. Behavioral avoidance tests and disgust in contamination fear: Distinctions from trait anxiety. Behaviour Research and Therapy, 42: 207–216.

Tsuang M, Domschke K, Jerkey BA, et al. 2004. Agoraphobic behavior and panic attack: A study of male twins. Journal of Anxiety Disorders, 18: 799–807.

Tucker P, Potter-Kimball R, Wyatt D, et al. 2003. Can physiologic assessment and side effects tease out differences in PTSD trials? A double-blind comparison of citalopram, sertraline, and placebo. Psychopharmacology Bulletin, 37: 135–149.

Tucker P, Zaninelli R, Yehuda R, et al. 2001. Paroxetine in the treatment of chronic posttraumatic stress disorder: Results of a placebo-controlled, flexible-dosage trial. Journal of Clinical Psychiatry, 62: 860–868.

Tundo A, Salvati L, Busto G, et al. 2007. Addition of cognitive-behavioral therapy for nonresponders to medication for obsessive-compulsive disorder: A naturalistic study. Journal of Clinical Psychiatry, 68: 1552–1556.

Turner SM, Beidel DC, Borden JW, et al. 1991. Social phobia: Axis I and II correlates. Journal of Abnormal Psychology, 100: 102–106.

Turner SM, Beidel DC, Cooley-Quille MR. 1995. Two-year follow-up of social phobics treated with social effectiveness therapy. Behaviour Research and Therapy, 33: 553–555.

Turner SM, Beidel DC, Dancu CV, et al. 1989. An empirically derived inventory to measure social fears and anxiety: The Social phobia and Anxiety Inventory. Psychological Assessment, 1: 35–40.

Turner SM, Beidel DC, Jacob RG. 1994. Social phobia: A comparison of behavior therapy and atenolol. Journal of Consulting and Clinical Psychology, 62: 350–358.

Turner SM, Beidel DC, Townsley RM. 1990. Social phobia: Relationship to shyness. Behaviour Research and Therapy, 28: 497–505.

Turner SM, Beidel DC, Townsley RM. 1992. Social phobia: A comparison of specific and generalized subtypes and avoidant personality disorder. Journal of Abnormal Psychology, 101: 326–331.

Tyrer P. 1984. Classification of anxiety. British Journal of Psychiatry, 144: 78–83.

Tyrer P. 1985. Neurosis divisible? Lancet, I: 685–688.

Tyrer P. 1999. Anxiety: A Multidisciplinary Review. Singapore: World Scientific Publishing Company.

Tyrer P. 2001. The case for cothymia: Mixed anxiety and depression as a single diagnosis. British Journal of Psychiatry, 179: 191–193.

Tyrer P, Seivewright N, Ferguson B, et al. 1992. The general neurotic syndrome: A coaxial diagnosis of anxiety, depression and personality disorder. Acta Psychiatrica Scandinavica, 85: 201–206.

Tyrer P, Seivewright H, Johnson T. 2004. The Nottingham Study of Neurotic Disorder: Predictors of 12-year outcome of dysthymic, panic and generalized anxiety disorder. Psychological Medicine, 34: 1385–1394.

Uchida RR, Del-Ben CM, Busatto GF, et al. 2008. Regional gray matter abnormalities in panic disorder: A voxel-based morphometry study. Psychiatry Research, 163: 21–29.

Uhde T, Boulenger J, Geraci H, et al. 1985. Longitudinal course of panic disorder. Progress in Neuropsychopharmacology and Biological Psychiatry, 9: 39–51.

Uhlenhuth EH, Balter MB, Ban TA, et al. 1999. International Study of Expert Judgment on Therapeutic Use of Benzodiazepines and Other Psychotherapeutic Medications: VI. Trends in recommendations for the pharmacotherapy of anxiety disorders, 1992–1997. Depression and Anxiety, 9: 107–116.

Uhlenhuth EH, Balter MB, Mellinger GD, et al. 1983. Symptom checklist syndromes in the general population: Correlations with psychotherapeutic drug use. Archives of General Psychiatry, 40: 1167–1173.

Uhlenhuth EH, DeWit H, Balter MB, et al. 1988. Risks and benefits of long-term benzodiazepine use. Journal of Clinical Psychopharmacology, 8: 161–167.

Uhlenhuth EH, Leon AC, Matuzas W. 2006. Psychopathology of panic attacks in panic disorder. Journal of Affective Disorders, 92: 55–62.

Uhlenhuth EH, Matuzas W, Warner TD, et al. 2000. Do antidepressants selectively suppress spontaneous (unexpected) panic attacks? A replication. Journal of Clinical Psychopharmacology, 20: 622–627.

Uhlenhuth EH, Warner TD, Matuzas W. 2002. Interactive model of therapeutic response in panic disorder: Moclobemide, a case in point. Journal of Clinical Psychopharmacology, 22: 275–284.

Ullman SE, Filipas HH. 2001. Predictors of PTSD symptom severity and social reactions in sexual assault victims. Journal of Traumatic Stress, 14: 369–389.

Ursano RJ, Fullerton CS, Epstein RS, et al. 1999a. Peritraumatic dissociation and posttraumatic stress disorder following motor vehicle accidents. American Journal of Psychiatry, 156: 1808–1810.

Ursano RJ, Fullerton CS, Epstein RS, et al. 1999b. Acute and chronic posttraumatic stress disorder in motor vehicle accident victims. American Journal of Psychiatry, 156: 589–595.

Ustun TB, Sartorius N. 1995. Mental Illness in General Health Care: An International Study. Chichester: Wiley.

Vaiva G, Ducrocq F, Jezequel K, et al. 2003. Immediate treatment with propranolol decreases posttraumatic stress disorder two months after trauma. Biological Psychiatry, 54: 947–949.

Vallejo J, Olivares J, Marcos T, et al. 1992. Clomipramine versus phenelzine in obsessive-compulsive disorder: A controlled clinical trial. British Journal of Psychiatry, 161: 665–670.

Van Ameringen M, Mancini C, Styan G, et al. 1991. Relationship of social phobia with other psychiatric illness. Journal of Affective Disorders, 21: 93–99.

Van Ameringen M, Mancini C, Wilson C. 1996. Buspirone augmentation of selective serotonin reuptake inhibitors (SSRIs) in social phobia. Journal of Affective Disorders, 39: 115–121.

Van Ameringen MA, Lane RM, Walker JR, et al. 2001. Sertraline treatment of generalized social phobia: A 20-week, double-blind, placebo-controlled study. American Journal of Psychiatry, 158: 275–281.

van Apeldoorn FJ, van Hout WJPJ, Mersch PPA, et al. 2008. Is a combined therapy more effective than either CBT or SSRI alone? Results of a multicenter trial on panic disorder with or without agoraphobia. Acta Psychiatrica Scandinavica, 117: 260–270.

van Balkom AJLM, Bakker A, Spinhoven P, et al. 1997. A meta-analysis of the treatment of panic disorder with or without agoraphobia: A comparison of psychopharmacological, cognitive-behavioral, and combination treatments. Journal of Nervous and Mental Disease, 185: 510–516.

van Balkom AJ, de Haan E, van Oppen P, et al. 1998. Cognitive and behavioral therapies alone versus in combination with fluvoxamine in the treatment of obsessive-compulsive disorder. Journal of Nervous and Mental Disease, 186: 492–499.

van den Hout M, Arntz A, Hoekstra R. 1994. Exposure reduced agoraphobia but not panic and cognitive therapy reduced panic but not agoraphobia. Behaviour Research and Therapy, 32: 447–451.

van den Hout M, Kindt M. 2003a. Repeated checking causes memory distrust. Behaviour Research and Therapy, 41: 301–316.

van den Hout M, Kindt M. 2003b. Phenomenological validity of an OCD-memory model and the remember/know distinction. Behaviour Research and Therapy, 41: 369–378.

van der Kolk BA, Dreyfuss D, Michaels B, et al. 1994. Fluoxetine treatment in posttraumatic stress disorder. Journal of Clinical Psychiatry, 55: 517–522.

van der Kolk BA, McFarlane AC, Weiseath L, editors. 1996. Traumatic Stress: The Effects of Overwhelming Experience on Mind, Body, and Society. New York: Guilford Press.

van der Kolk BA, Spinazzola J, Blaustein ME, et al. 2007. A randomized clinical trial of eye movement desensitization and reprocessing (EMDR), fluoxetine, and pill placebo in the treatment of posttraumatic stress disorder: Treatment effects and long-term maintenance. Journal of Clinical Psychiatry, 68: 37–46.

Vandervoort D, Rokach A. 2004. Abusive relationships: Is a new category for traumatization needed? Current Psychology: Developmental, Learning, Personality, Social, 23: 68–76.

van Dyck R, van Balkom AJLM. 1997. Combination therapy for anxiety disorders. In den Boer JA, editor: Clinical Management of Anxiety. New York: Marcel Dekker, pp. 109–136.

Van Emmerick AAP, Kamphuis JH, Hulsbosch AM, et al. 2002. Single session debriefing after psychological trauma: A meta-analysis. Lancet, 360: 766–771.

van Oppen P, De Haan E, Van Balkom AJLM, et al. 1995. Cognitive therapy and exposure in vivo in the treatment of obsessive compulsive disorder. Behaviour Research and Therapy, 33: 379–390.

van Velzen CJM, Emmelkamp PMJ, Scholing A. 2000. Generalized social phobia versus avoidant personality disorder: Differences in psychopathology, personality traits, and social and occupational functioning. Journal of Anxiety Disorders, 14: 395–411.

van Vliet IM, den Boer JA, Westenberg HGM. 1994. Psychopharmacological treatment of social phobia: A double-blind placebo controlled study with fluvoxamine. Psychopharmacology, 115: 128–134.

Verburg K, Griez E, Meijer J, et al. 1995. Discrimination between panic disorder and generalized anxiety disorder by 35% carbon dioxide challenge. American Journal of Psychiatry, 152: 1081–1083.

Vermetten E, Vythilingam M, Southwick SM, et al. 2003. Long-term treatment with paroxetine increases verbal declarative memory and hippocampal volume in posttraumatic stress disorder. Biological Psychiatry, 54: 693–702.

Versiani M, Cassano G, Perugi G, et al. 2002. Reboxetine, a selective norepinephrine reuptake inhibitor, is an effective and well-tolerated treatment for panic disorder. Journal of Clinical Psychiatry, 63: 31–37.

Versiani M, Mundim FD, Nardi AE, et al. 1988. Tranylcypromine in social phobia. Journal of Clinical Psychopharmacology, 8: 279–283.

Versiani M, Nardi AE, Mundim FD, et al. 1992. Pharmacotherapy of social phobia: A controlled study with moclobemide and phenelzine. British Journal of Psychiatry, 161: 353–360.

Vickers K, McNally RJ. 2004. Panic disorder and suicide attempt in the National Comorbidity Survey. Journal of Abnormal Psychology, 113: 582–591.

Villeponteaux VA, Lydiard RB, Laraia MT, et al. 1992. The effects of pregnancy on preexisting panic disorder. Journal of Clinical Psychiatry, 53: 201–203.

Vogel PA, Stiles TC, Götesman KG. 2004. Adding cognitive therapy elements to exposure therapy for obsessive-compulsive disorder: A controlled study. Behavioural and Cognitive Psychotherapy, 32: 275–290.

Vollebergh WAM, Iedema J, Bijl RV, et al. 2001. The structure and stability of common mental disorders: The NEMESIS study. Archives of General Psychiatry, 58: 597–603.

Von Korff M, Eaton WW, Keyl P. 1985. The epidemiology of panic attacks and panic disorder: Results of three community surveys. American Journal of Epidemiology, 122: 970–981.

Vrana SR, Cuthbert BN, Lang PJ. 1986. Fear imagery and text processing. Psychophysiology, 23: 247–253.

Vythilingam M, Anderson ER, Goddard A, et al. 2000. Temporal lobe volume in panic disorder – A quantitative magnetic resonance imaging study. Psychiatry Research, 99: 75–82.

Vythilingum B, Stein DJ, Soifer S. 2002. Is "shy bladder syndrome" a subtype of social phobia? A survey of people with paruresis. Depression and Anxiety, 16: 84–87.

Wacker HR, Mullejans R, Klein KH, et al. 1992. Identification of cases of anxiety disorders and affective disorders in the community according to ICD-10 and DSM-III-R by using the Composite International Diagnostic Interview (CIDI). International Journal of Methods of Psychiatric Research, 2: 91–100.

Waddington A, Ampelas JF, Mauriac F, et al. 2003. Post-traumatic stress disorder (PTSD): The syndrome with multiple faces. Encephale, 29: 20–27.

Wade AG, Lepola U, Koponen HJ, et al. 1997. The effects of citalopram in panic disorder. British Journal of Psychiatry, 170: 549–553.

Wakefield JC, Horwitz AV, Schmitz MF. 2005. Are we overpathologizing the socially anxious? Social phobia from a harmful dysfunction perspective. Canadian Journal of Psychiatry, 50: 317–319.

Walker EA, Roy-Byrne PP, Katon W, et al. 1990. Psychiatric illness and irritable bowel syndrome: A comparison with inflammatory bowel disease. American Journal of Psychiatry, 147: 1656–1661.

Walker JR, Van Ameringen MA, Swinson R, et al. 2000. Prevention of relapse in generalized social phobia: Results of a 24-week study in responders to 20 weeks of sertraline treatment. Journal of Clinical Psychopharmacology, 20: 636–644.

Wallace ST, Alden LE. 1997. Social phobia and positive social events: The price of success. Journal of Abnormal Psychology, 106: 416–424.

Warda G, Bryant RA. 1998a. Cognitive bias in acute stress disorder. Behaviour Research and Therapy, 36: 1177–1183.

Warda G, Bryant RA. 1998b. Thought control strategies in acute stress Disorder. Behaviour Research and Therapy, 36: 1171–1175.

Wardle J. 1990. Behaviour therapy and benzodiazepines: Allies or antagonists? British Journal of Psychiatry, 156: 163–168.

Wardle J, Hayward P, Higgitt A, et al. 1994. Effects of concurrent diazepam treatment on the outcome of exposure therapy in agoraphobia. Behaviour Research and Therapy, 32: 203–215.

Warshaw MG, Dolan RT, Keller MB. 2000. Suicidal behavior in patients with current or past panic disorder: Five years of prospective data from the Harvard/Brown Anxiety Research Program. American Journal of Psychiatry, 157: 1876–1878.

Warshaw MG, Fierman E, Pratt L, et al. 1993. Quality of life and dissociation in anxiety disorder patients with histories of trauma or PTSD. American Journal of Psychiatry, 150: 1512–1516.

Watanabe N, Churchill R, Furukawa TA. 2007. Combination of psychotherapy and benzodiazepines versus either therapy alone for panic disorder: A systematic review. BMC Psychiatry, 7: 18.

Watkins E, Moulds M, Mackintosh B. 2005. Comparisons between rumination and worry in a non-clinical population. Behaviour Research and Therapy, 43: 1577–1585.

Watson D. 2005. Rethinking the mood and anxiety disorders: A quantitative hierarchical model for DSM-V. Journal of Abnormal Psychology, 114: 522–536.

Watson D, Gamez W, Simms LJ. 2005. Basic dimensions of temperament and their relation to anxiety and depression: A symptom-based perspective. Journal of Research in Personality, 39: 46–66.

Watson JB, Rayner R. 1920. Conditioned emotional reactions. Journal of Experimental Psychology, 3: 1–14.

Watt MC, Stewart SH. 2000. Anxiety sensitivity mediates the relationships between childhood learning experiences and elevated hypochondriacal concerns in young adulthood. Journal of Psychosomatic Research, 49: 107–118.

Watt MC, Stewart SH, Cox BJ. 1998. A retrospective study of the learning history origins of anxiety sensitivity. Behaviour Research and Therapy, 36: 505–525.

Weiller E, Bisserbe JC, Boyer P, et al. 1996. Social phobia in general health care: An unrecognised undertreated disabling disorder. British Journal of Psychiatry, 168: 169–174.

Weiss DS, Marmar CR. 1996. The Impact of Event Scale – Revised. In Wilson JP, Keane TM, editors: Assessing Psychological Trauma and PTSD. New York: Guilford Press, pp. 399–411.

Weissman MM. 1993. Family genetic studies of panic disorder. Journal of Psychiatric Research, 27 (Suppl. 1): 69–78.

Weissman MM, Bland RC, Canino GJ, et al. 1994. The cross national epidemiology of obsessive compulsive disorder. Journal of Clinical Psychiatry, 55 (Suppl. 3): 5–10.

Weissman MM, Klerman GL, Markowitz JS, et al. 1989. Suicidal ideation and suicide attempts in panic disorder. New England Journal of Medicine, 321: 1209–1214.

Weissman MM, Markowitz JS, Ouellette R, et al. 1990. Panic disorder and cardiovascular/cerebrovascular problems: Results from a community survey. American Journal of Psychiatry, 147: 1504–1508.

Wells A. 1994. Attention and the control of worry. In Davey GCL, Tallis F, editors: Worrying: Perspectives on Theory, Assessment and Treatment. New York: Wiley, pp. 91–114.

Wells A. 1995. Meta-cognition and worry: A cognitive model of generalized anxiety disorder. Behavioural and Cognitive Psychotherapy, 23: 301–320.

Wells A. 1997. Cognitive Therapy of Anxiety Disorders: A Practice Manual and Conceptual Guide. Chichester, UK: Wiley.

Wells A, Papageorgiou C. 1999. The observer perspective: Biased imagery in social phobia, agoraphobia, and blood/injury phobia. Behaviour Research and Therapy, 37: 653–658.

Wells A, Papageorgiou C. 2001. Social phobic interoception: Effects of bodily information on anxiety, beliefs and self-processing. Behaviour Research and Therapy, 39: 1–11.

Wessely S. 2003. In debate: Psychological debriefing is a waste of time. For. British Journal of Psychiatry, 183: 12–13.

Westenberg HG, Stein DJ, Yang H, et al. 2004. A double-blind placebo-controlled study of controlled release fluvoxamine for the treatment of generalized social anxiety disorder. Journal of Clinical Psychopharmacology, 24: 49–55.

Westra HA, Stewart SH, Conrad BE. 2002. Naturalistic manner of benzodiazepine use and cognitive behavioral therapy outcome in panic disorder with agoraphobia. Journal of Anxiety Disorders, 16: 233–246.

White KS, Raffa SD, Jakle KR, et al. 2008. Morbidity of DSM-IV axis I disorders in patients with noncardiac chest pain: Psychiatric morbidity linked with increased pain and health care utilization. Journal of Consulting and Clinical Psychology, 76: 422–430.

White WB, Baker CH. 1986. Episodic hypertension secondary to panic disorder. Archives of Internal Medicine, 146: 1129–1130.

Whittal ML, Robichaud M, Thordarson DS, et al. 2008. Group and individual treatment of obsessive-compulsive disorder using cognitive therapy and exposure plus response prevention: A 2-year follow-up of two randomized trials. Journal of Consulting and Clinical Psychology, 76: 1003–1014.

Whittal ML, Thordarson DS, McLean PD. 2005. Treatment of obsessive- compulsive disorder: Cognitive behavior therapy vs exposure and response prevention. Behaviour Research and Therapy, 43: 1559–1576.

Wiborg IM, Dahl AA. 1996. Does brief dynamic psychotherapy reduce the relapse rate of panic disorder? Archives of General Psychiatry, 53: 689–694.

Wilhelm S, Buhlmann U, Tolin DF, et al. 2008. Augmentation of behaviour therapy with D-cycloserine for obsessive-compulsive disorder. American Journal of Psychiatry, 165: 335–341.

Windle M, Windle RC, Scheidt DM, et al. 1995. Physical and sexual abuse and associated mental disorders among alcoholic inpatients. American Journal of Psychiatry, 152: 1322–1328.

Winfield I, George LK, Swartz M, et al. 1990. Sexual assault and psychiatric disorders among a community sample of women. American Journal of Psychiatry, 147: 335–341.

Winsberg ME, Cassic KS, Koran LM. 1999. Hoarding in obsessive-compulsive disorder: A report of 20 cases. Journal of Clinical Psychiatry, 60: 591– 597.

Wittchen H-U. 2004. Generalized anxiety disorder: Prevalence, burden, and cost to society. Depression and Anxiety, 16: 162–171.

Wittchen H-U, Beesdo K, Bittner A, et al. 2003. Depressive episodes – evidence for a causal role of primary anxiety disorders? European Psychiatry, 18: 384–393.

Wittchen H-U, Carter RM, Pfister H, et al. 2000a. Disabilities and quality of life in pure and comorbid generalized anxiety disorder and major depression in a national survey. International Clinical Psychopharmacology, 15: 319–328.

Wittchen H-U, Fuetsch M, Sonntag H, et al. 2000b. Disability and quality of life in pure and comorbid social phobia: Findings from a controlled study. European Psychiatry, 15: 46–58.

Wittchen H-U, Jacobi F. 2005. Size and burden of mental disorders in Europe – a critical review and appraisal of 27 studies. European Neuropsychopharmacology, 15: 357–376.

Wittchen H-U, Kessler RC, Beeselo K, et al. 2002. Generalized anxiety and depression in primary care: Prevalence, recognition and management. Journal of Clinical Psychiatry, 63: 24–34.

Wittchen H-U, Nocon A, Beesdo K, et al. 2008. Agoraphobia and panic: Prospective-longitudinal relations suggest a rethinking of diagnostic concepts. Psychotherapy and Psychosomatics, 77: 147–157.

Wittchen H-U, Reed V, Kessler RC. 1998. The relationship of agoraphobia and panic in a community sample of adolescents and young adults. Archives of General Psychiatry, 55: 1017–1024.

Wittchen H-U, Stein MB, Kessler RC. 1999. Social fears and social phobia in a community sample of adolescents and young adults: Prevalence, risk factors and co-morbidity. Psychological Medicine, 29: 309–323.

Wittchen H-U, Zhao S, Kessler RC, et al. 1994. DSM-III-R generalized anxiety disorder in the National Comorbidity Survey. Archives of General Psychiatry, 51: 355–364.

Wlazlo Z, Schroeder-Hartwig K, Hand I, et al. 1990. Exposure in vivo vs. social skills training for social phobia: Long-term outcome and differential effects. Behaviour Research and Therapy, 28: 181–193.

Wolitzky-Taylor KB, Horowitz JD, Powers MB, et al. 2008. Psychological approaches in the treatment of specific phobias: A meta-analysis. Clinical Psychology Review, 28: 1021–1037.

Wolpe J. 1958. Psychotherapy by Reciprocal Inhibition. Stanford, CA: Stanford University Press.

Wolpe J, Lang PJA. 1964. A Fear Survey Schedule for use in behavior therapy. Behaviour Research and Therapy, 2: 27–30.

Wolpe J, Lazarus AA. 1966. Behavior Therapy Techniques. New York: Pergamon Press.

Wolpe J, Rowan VC. 1988. Panic disorder: A product of classical conditioning. Behaviour Research and Therapy, 26: 441–450.

Woodman CL, Noyes R, Black DW, et al. 1999. A 5-year follow-up study of generalized anxiety disorder and panic disorder. Journal of Nervous and Mental Disease, 187: 3–9.

Woody SR. 1996. Effects of focus of attention on social phobics' anxiety and social performance. Journal of Abnormal Psychology, 105: 61–69.

World Health Organization. 1992. The ICD-10 (International Classification of Diseases) Classification of Mental and Behavioural Disorders: Clinical Descriptions and Diagnostic Guidelines. Geneva: World Health Organization.

Worthington JJ, Pollack MH, Otto MW, et al. 1998. Long-term experience with clonazepam in patients with a primary diagnosis of panic disorder. Psychopharmacology Bulletin, 34: 199–205.

Wu JC, Buchsbaum MS, Hershey TG, et al. 1991. PET in generalized anxiety disorder. Biological Psychiatry, 29: 1181–1199.

Yaryura-Tobias JA, Neziroglu FA. 1996. Venlafaxine in obsessive-compulsive disorder. Archives of General Psychiatry, 53: 653–654.

Yehuda R, McFarlane AC, Shalev AY. 1998a. Predicting the development of post-traumatic stress disorder from the acute response to a traumatic event. Biological Psychiatry, 44: 1305–1313.

Yehuda R, Schmeidler J, Wainberg M, et al. 1998b. Vulnerability to posttraumatic stress disorder in adult offspring of Holocaust survivors. American Journal of Psychiatry, 155: 1163–1171.

Yehuda R, Siever LJ, Teicher MH, et al. 1998c. Plasma norepinephrine and 3-methoxy-4-hydroxyphenylglycol concentrations and severity of depression in combat posttraumatic stress disorder and major depressive disorder. Biological Psychiatry, 44: 56–63.

Yehuda R, Southwick SM, Nussbaum G, et al. 1990. Low urinary cortisol excretion in PTSD. Journal of Nervous and Mental Disease, 178: 366–369.

Yellowlees PM, Alpers JH, Bowden JJ, et al. 1987. Psychiatric morbidity in patients with chronic airflow obstruction. Medical Journal of Australia, 146: 305–307.

Yerkes RM, Dodson JD. 1908. The relation of strength of stimulus to rapidity of habit-formation. Journal of Comparative Neurology and Psychology, 18: 459–482.

Yonkers KA, Dyck IR, Warshaw M, et al. 2000. Factors predicting the course of generalized anxiety disorder. British Journal of Psychiatry, 176: 544–549.

Yonkers KA, Zlotnick C, Allsworth J, et al. 1998. Is the course of panic disorder the same in women and men? American Journal of Psychiatry, 155: 596–602.

Young EA, Breslau N. 2004. Cortisol and catecholamines in posttraumatic stress disorder: An epidemiologic community study. Archives of General Psychiatry, 61: 394–401.

Zaidi LY, Foy DW. 1994. Childhood abuse and combat-related PTSD. Journal of Traumatic Stress, 7: 33–42.

Zandbergen J, Bright M, Pols H, et al. 1991. Higher lifetime prevalence of respiratory diseases in panic disorder. American Journal of Psychiatry, 148: 1583–1585.

Zebb BJ, Beck JG. 1998. Worry versus anxiety: Is there really a difference? Behavior Modification, 22: 45–61.

Zinbarg RE, Barlow DH, Brown TA. 1997. Hierarchical structure and general factor saturation of the Anxiety Sensitivity Index: Evidence and implications. Psychological Assessment, 9: 277–284.

Zisook S, Braff DL, Click MA. 1985. Monoamine oxidase inhibitors in the treatment of atypical depression. Journal of Clinical Psychopharmacology, 5: 131–137.

Zitrin CM, Klein DF, Woerner MG. 1980. Treatment of agoraphobia with group exposure in vivo and imipramine. Archives of General Psychiatry, 37: 63–72.

Zitrin CM, Ross DC. 1988. Early separation anxiety and adult agoraphobia. Journal of Nervous and Mental Disease, 176: 621–625.

Zlotnick C, Shea MT, Rosen KH, et al. 1997. An affect-management group for women with posttraumatic stress disorder and histories of childhood sexual abuse. Journal of Traumatic Stress, 10: 425–436.

Zlotnick C, Warshaw M, Shea MT, et al. 1999. Chronicity in posttraumatic stress disorder (PTSD) and predictors of course of comorbid PTSD in patients with anxiety disorders. Journal of Traumatic Stress, 12: 89–100.

Zoellner LA, Foa EB, Bartholomew DB. 1999. Interpersonal friction and PTSD in female victims of sexual and nonsexual assault. Journal of Traumatic Stress, 12: 689–700.

Zohar J. 1997. Is there room for a new diagnostic subtype: The schizo-obsessive subtype? CNS Spectrums, 2: 49–50.

Zohar J, Amital D, Miodownik C, et al. 2002. Double-blind placebo-controlled pilot study of sertraline in military veterans with posttraumatic stress disorder. Journal of Clinical Psychopharmacology, 22: 190–195.

Zohar J, Hollander E, Stein DJ, et al. 2007. Consensus statement. CNS Spectrums, 12 (Suppl. 3): 59–63.

Zohar J, Judge R. 1996. Paroxetine versus clomipramine in the treatment of obsessive-compulsive disorder. OCD Paroxetine Study Investigators. British Journal of Psychiatry, 169: 468–474.

Index

Note: Page numbers followed by the notations *f* and *t* refer to pages containing figures and tables respectively.